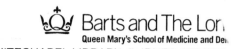
Epilepsy
# Treatment

## Forms, Causes and Therapy
## in Children and Adults

# HANDBOOK OF
# Epilepsy Treatment

## Forms, Causes and Therapy in Children and Adults

## Simon D Shorvon

MA MB BChir MD FRCP
Professor in Clinical Neurology and Clinical Subdean, Instit
University College London
Consultant Neurologist, National Hospital for Neurolo
Queen Square
London WC1N 3BG
Past Vice President, International League Against epsy
Neurology
Neurosurgery

## 2nd edition

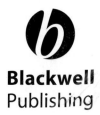

**Blackwell**
Publishing

© 2005 by Blackwell Publishing Ltd

Blackwell Publishing, Inc., 350 Main Street, Malden, Massachusetts 02148-5020, USA
Blackwell Publishing Ltd, 9600 Garsington Road, Oxford OX4 2DQ, UK
Blackwell Publishing Asia Pty Ltd, 550 Swanston Street, Carlton, Victoria 3053, Australia

The right of the Author to be identified as the Author of this Work has been asserted
in accordance with the Copyright, Designs and Patents Act 1988.

First published 2000
Reprinted 2000
American version 2000
Second edition 2005

Library of Congress Cataloging-in-Publication Data
Shorvon, S. D. (Simon D.)
   Handbook of epilepsy treatment / Simon D. Shorvon. — 2nd ed.
      p. ; cm.
      udes index.
      ISB3: 978-1-4051-3134-6
         1. 1-4051-3134-9
      manuapsy—Handbooks, manuals, etc.   2. Anticonvulsants—Handbooks,
      [DNLM:    I. Title.
   RC372.S528 Epilepsy—therapy.   WL 385 S559h 2005]
   616.8′5306—dc2

                                                            2004028334

   ISBN-13: 978-1-4051-
   ISBN-10: 1-4051-3134-9-6

A catalogue record for this is available from the British Library

Set in 10/12pt Minion by Grap aft Limited, Hong Kong
Printed and bound in India by R ka Press Pvt., Ltd

Development Editor: Rebecca Huxl
Commissioning Editor: Stuart Taylor
Production Controller: Kate Charman

For further information on Blackwell Publing, visit our website:
http://www.blackwellpublishing.com

The publisher's policy is to use permanent paper from mills that operate a sustainable
forestry policy, and which has been manufactured from pulp processed using acid-free
and elementary chlorine-free practices. Furthermo the publisher ensures that the text
paper and cover board used have met acceptable environmental accreditation standards.

The drawing on the cover is by Jonathan Cusick. The idea of *pills filling the head* is
intended as an ironic reflection on inappropriate prescribing practice. This book
endeavours to show that there is indeed far more to the treatment of epilepsy than the
simple prescription of drugs.

# Contents

# Preface

This monograph is part of *Blackwell Publishing*'s series of 'Handbooks' which are produced to accompany their multi-authored textbooks. This handbook (a *handbuch* in the German sense) is, like the accompanying textbook, now in its second edition. The first edition was published 5 years ago, was generously received and, I hope, fulfilled at least in part its purpose of informing and improving epilepsy therapy. However, in epilepsy as in all of medicine, treatment has moved on, knowledge has increased and fashions have changed. The writing of a second edition is an opportunity to reflect these changes, and also to correct the previous edition's all too obvious deficiencies.

This resulting book now contains pretty much everything I know about epilepsy therapy. It is a worrying thought that all one's professional knowledge can be compressed into a couple of megabytes, but this is the sad reality. Worrying also is the bias that single-authorship inevitably carries. My defence is that the book is embedded in the experience gained from my own clinical practice (now over 25 years of specialization in epilepsy) and is heavily influenced by this. This is a disadvantage of single-authorship generally, but one that needs to be weighed against the advantages of coherence and lack of omission, repetition or inconsistency. Avoiding these in the writing of this book has been a constant preoccupation. Whether a balance has been achieved is for the reader to decide.

The aim has been to summarize the many and various treatments of epilepsy in a clear yet comprehensive, and concise yet balanced and practical manner. Surgical as well as medical therapy is included, as is the treatment of epilepsy in adults and children. Rare as well as common clinical problems are covered, and rarely- as well as commonly-used therapies. It is intended to be a hands-on text which will guide clinical practice and rational therapy, and to be a source of ready reference; a catalogue of epilepsy therapy. There is an emphasis on factual information, which I have tried to give in a parsimonious and easily-digested form, but one that still gives the reader a clear idea of the scientific basis of current practice. This scientific perspective is important and, where possible, the text has endeavoured to be science- and evidence-based. In some areas of therapy an evidence base, however, is lacking (perhaps especially in the area of epilepsy surgery), and data informing longer-term outcome, risk and benefit in particular are missing. In these areas the book inevitably reflects the author's own prejudices and anecdotal experience. The book also is embedded in the style of epilepsy practice at the National Hospital for Neurology and Neurosurgery, Queen Square, London, where I have practised since 1979, and in the work of the International League Against Epilepsy, on whose executive committee I have worked for 12 years; these provide a distinctive perspective which I hope adds coherence and interest.

Since the publication of the first edition, three developments in epilepsy therapy deserve special mention, as these have influenced the writing approach. The first is the impact of molecular genetics, which has swept like a tidal wave over medicine, leaving few areas dry—and epilepsy is no exception. The molecular advances have enormously clarified the aetiology and clinical forms of many forms of congenital and idiopathic epilepsy, and informed many aspects of treatment. Much more remains to be discovered and the elusive goal of tailoring therapy to individuals on the basis of their molecular profile has yet to be achieved—a prize perhaps for a third edition? The second important change increasingly making its mark on epilepsy therapy is the proliferation of clinical guidelines and of evidence-based methodologies (notably the controlled clinical trial). This is a bureaucracy that has generally been a power for good, and the improvements in minimum standards of therapy all over the world are self-evident. There are, however, clear downsides to this tendency. The stifling of innovation and the bureaucratization of decisions by committee-driven consensus are also all too obvious, and scientific progress can only be made by dissenting voices. In this book, alternative views are reflected where appropriate; it remains important that committees and quangos do not impose bland uniformity. The third change worthy of comment is the recognition of the importance of patient involvement in medical decisions. Too often in the past the patients' own views have been ignored and medical advice has been given without discussion or without option-appraisal. In this edition, the importance of two-way communication and of patient choice is emphasized.

As in the sister textbook, therefore, a dual approach is attempted, mixing scientifically-based evidential medicine with a patient-focused orientation—a powerful combination if successfully achieved.

In writing this book, a number of editorial decisions were made which should be noted here. Emphasis has been put on tables, so that some of the factual information can be easily referred to; and to this end, also, a *pharmacopoeia* section has been added. Tabulating data (particularly pharmacological and pharmacokinetic data) where conflicting information exists can be contentious, and the tables include what the author considers to be the most reliable data. It is important to recognize also that data do vary, and in some places the data in the tables and *pharmacopoeia* are not universally applicable. In the interests of readability and clarity, citations to the literature in the text have been omitted. In the age of PubMed© and Medline© literature is now easily tracked, and citations can be found in the relevant chapters of the associated textbook. In place of this, a 'further reading section', listing key articles, books and review articles, with an emphasis on recent publications, has been included; this seemed to the author to be of more general utility. Finally, the sections on the clinical forms and causes of epilepsy have been expanded, as these underpin rational therapy.

This book, like its predecessor, is conceptually, and in many places actually, a condensation of the multi-authored textbook of epilepsy therapy *The Treatment of Epilepsy*, edited by Shorvon SD, Perucca E, Fish DR, Dodson WE (Blackwell 2004). The information in this book has been the basis of much of what is written here and the borrowing has often been heavy and the influence great. I would like to acknowledge here my debt of gratitude to my co-editors of this textbook, Professor Emilio Perucca, Professor David Fish and Professor Ed Dodson. Without their work this book could not have been attempted or even contemplated. I would also like to acknowledge and to thank the contributors to the multi-authored book, which remains a landmark in the bibliography of epilepsy therapy. I would also like to thank Jonathan Cusick, an exceptional graphic artist and friend, for his illustration on the cover. The idea of *pills filling the head* is an ironic commentary on the tendency, misguided but widespread, to treat epilepsy by handing out increasing quantities of medication. If there is one message to be taken from this book, it is that therapy should be multifaceted and attend broadly to all aspects of a patient's predicament. Treatment is far more than simply pouring pharmaceuticals on a troubled brain. I offer my grateful thanks also to the Blackwell publication team, for their forbearance in dealing with an obsessional neurologist and their advice, humour, and friendship—and in particular to Rebecca Huxley, Kate Brothwell and Stuart Taylor. Modern practice and research are sometimes mired in Machiavellian politics and professional jealousy, which work wholly against the interests of patients we serve. I have had recent experience of this, and this book is therefore dedicated to these patients, to Christina Milne, who is a true champion of truth and moral standards in medicine, and to Lynne and Matthew, for whom the writing of this book has meant lost time and the smoke of much midnight oil.

Finally, a health warning: whilst every effort has been made in the preparation of this book to ensure that the details given are correct, it is possible that errors have been overlooked (for instance in pharmaceutical or pharmacokinetic data). The reader is advised to refer to published information from the pharmaceutical companies and other reference works to check accuracy.

Simon Shorvon
London 2005

# Acknowledgements

In the preparation of the text of this book, I am heavily indebted to the contributors to the textbook *The Treatment of Epilepsy*. The *Handbook of Epilepsy Treatment* is modelled on this sister book, and the text and tables are in places borrowed and transposed from this book. I thank Blackwell Publishing Ltd for permission for this, and also offer my thanks and acknowledgement to the following individuals who were the contributors to the *Treatment of Epilepsy*:

Michael J Aminoff, Santiago Arroyo, Giuliano Avanzini, Viktor Bartanusz, Ettore Beghi, Antonio Belli, Elinor Ben-Menachem, Victor Biton, Eilis A Boudreau, Eylert Brodtkorb, Thomas R Browne, Katharina Buchheim, Gregory Cascino, David Chadwick, Catherine Chiron, Hannah R Cock, Aaron A Cohen-Gadol, Mark Cook, J Helen Cross, Mogens A Dalby, Ronan Dardis, Luciano De Paola, Jelena Djordjevic, W Edwin Dodson, Michael S Duchowny, Mervyn J Eadie, Christian E Elger, Edward Faught, Katrina S Firlik, David R Fish, Andrew Fisher, Lars Forsgren, Silvana Franceschetti, Jacqueline A French, Buichi Fujitani, John R Gates, Tracey A Glauser, L John Greenfield Jr, Yvonne M Hart, Ruediger Hopfengärtner, Cornelia Hummel, Marilyn Jones-Gotman, Reetta Kälviäinen, Neil David Kitchen, Mathias J Koepp, Eric H Kossoff, Gunter Krämer, Ennapadam S Krishnamoorthy, Alan R Kugler, Yvonne Langan, John A Lawson, Ilo E Leppik, Nita Limdi, Fumisuke Matsuo, François Mauguière, Andrew W McEvoy, Hartmut Meierkord, Isabelle Merlet, Roberto Michelucci, Andrew N Miles, Lina Nashef, Miri Y Neufeld, Dang K Nguyen, Karen E Nilsen, George A Ojemann, Jeffrey G Ojemann, Hian-Tat Ong, Jack M Parent, Tae Sung Park, Philip N Patsalos, Emilio Perucca, Charles E Polkey, Flavia Pryor, Kurupath Radhakrishnan, R Eugene Ramsay, Howard C Rosenberg, Ahmed Sadek, Bernard Sadzot, Afraim Salek-Haddadi, Josemir Sander, Sasumo Sato, Steven C Schachter, Maria Gabriella Scordo, Masakazu Seino, Richard Selway, Jon A Sen, Matti Sillanpää, Sanjay M Sisodiya, Martin Smith, Elson Lee So, Dennis D Spencer, Susan S Spencer, Edoardo Spina, Herman Stefan, Raymond C Tallis, Carlo Alberto Tassinari, Torbjörn Tomson, Bijal M Trivedi, Win can Paesschen, Jean-Guy Villemure, Eileen PG Vining, Joachim von Oertzen, Matthew C Walker, Nicholas M Wetjen, Steve H White, Thomas E Whitmarsh, Federico Zara.

I also am grateful for permission to reproduce the illustrations, text and tables from the following sources.

## Section 1

Figures 1.1 and 1.2 redrawn from Forsgren L 2004. Epidemiology and prognosis of epilepsy and its treatment. In: Shorvon SD *et al.* (eds) *The Treatment of Epilepsy* (2nd edn). Blackwell Publishing, Oxford: 21–42. Figure 1.1 was based on data from: Jensen P 1986. *Acta Neurol Scand*, **74**: 150–155; Olafsson E *et al.* 1996 *Epilepsia* **37**: 951–955; Fosgren L *et al.* 1996. *Epilepsia*, **37**: 224–229; Hauser WA *et al.* 1993 *Epilepsia*, **34**: 453–468; Sidenvall R *et al.* 1993. *Acta Paediatr*, **82**: 62–65.

Table 1.3 from the Commission for the Classification and Terminology of the International Leagues Against Epilepsy. 1981. *Epilepsia*, **22**: 489–501.

Tables 1.4, 1.5, 1.11, 1.13 and 1.16 (and also borrowings of text) derived from Duncan JS, Fish DR and Shorvon SD 1995. *Clinical Epilepsy*. Churchill Livingstone, Edinburgh.

Table 1.7 from the Commission for the Classification and Terminology of the International Leagues Against Epilepsy. 1989. *Epilepsia*, **30**: 389–99.

Table 1.8 derived from Loiseau P *et al.* 1990. *Epilepsia*, **31**: 391–6.

Table 1.27 derived from Roach E *et al.* 1998. *J Child Neurol*, **13**: 624–8.

Table 1.29 derived from Gutmann E *et al.* 1997. *JAMA*, **278**: 51–7.

Table 1.31 derived from Kennedy P 2004. *J Neurol Neurosurg Psychiat*, **75** (suppl. 1): 110–155.

## Section 2

Figure 2.1 from Richens A *et al.* 1985. In: Williams DC and Marks V (eds) *Biochemistry in Clinical Practice*. Elsevier, Amsterdam.

Figure 2.2 from Shorvon SD 2004. The choice of drugs and approach to drug treatments in partial epilepsy. In:

Shorvon SD *et al.* (eds) *The Treatment of Epilepsy* (2nd edn) Blackwell Publishing, Oxford: 317–33. Derived from Marson AG *et al.* 1997. *Epilepsia*, **38**: 859–80.

Figure 2.3 adapted from Shorvon SD. The choice of drugs and approach to drug treatments in partial epilepsy. In: Shorvon SD *et al.* (eds) 2004. *The Treatment of Epilepsy* (2nd edn) Blackwell Publishing, Oxford: 317–33. Derived from Marson AG *et al.* 1997 *Epilepsia*, **38**: 859–80; Chadwick DW *et al.* 1996. *Epilepsia*, **37** (Suppl. 6): S17–22.

Figures 2.4 and 2.5 from Hart Y *et al.* 1991. *Lancet*, **337**: 1175–80.

Figure 2.6 from MRC Antiepileptic Drug Withdrawal Study Group. 1991. *Lancet*, **332**: 1175–80.

Figure 2.7 from Wallace H *et al.* 1998. *Lancet*, **352**: 1970–3.

Table 2.9 derived from *Newer Drugs for Epilepsy in Adults.* NICE Technology Appraisal 76, March 2004.

Table 2.11 derived from Perucca E *et al.* 2000. *Epilepsy Res*, **41**: 107–39.

Table 2.12 derived from McCorry D *et al.* 2004. *Lancet Neurology*, **3**: 729–735.

Table 2.19 derived from Moran D *et al.* 2004. *Seizure*, **13**: 425–73.

Table 2.23 from Chadwick D 2004. Management of epilepsy in remission. In: Shorvon SD *et al.* (eds) *The Treatment of Epilepsy* (2nd edn) Blackwell Publishing, Oxford: 174–9.

**Section 3**

Figure 3.1 from Kutt H 1995. In: Levy R *et al.* (eds) *Antiepileptic Drugs* (4th edn) Raven Press, New York.

Figure 3.2 adapted from Mattson RH 1998. In: Engel J and Pedley TA (eds) *Epilepsy: A Comprehensive Textbook*, Vol 2. Lippencott-Raven, New York: 1497.

Figure 3.3 from Rupp R *et al.* 1979. *Br J Clin Pharmacol*, **7** (Suppl. 1): 219–34.

Figure 3.4 from Kasteleijn-Nolst Trenité DGA *et al.* 1996. *Epilepsy Res*, **25**: 227.

Figure 3.5 from Faught E 2004. Oxcarbazepine. In: Shorvon SD *et al.* (eds) *The Treatment of Epilepsy* (2nd edn) Blackwell Publishing, Oxford: 451–60.

Figure 3.6 from Wilenski AJ *et al.* 1982. *Eur J Clin Pharmacol*, **23**: 87–92.

Figure 3.7 from Michelucci R and Tassinari CA 2004. Phenobarbital, primidone and other barbituates. In: Shorvon SD *et al.* (eds) *The Treatment of Epilepsy* (2nd edn) Blackwell Publishing, Oxford: 461–74.

Figure 3.8 from Eadie MJ 2004. Phenytoin. In: Shorvon SD *et al.* (eds) *The Treatment of Epilepsy* (2nd edn) Blackwell Publishing, Oxford: 475–88.

Figure 3.9 from Richens A and Dunlop A 1975. *N Engl J Med*, **2**: 347–8.

Figure 3.10 Derived from Imai J *et al.* 2000. Pharmacogenetics. **10**: 85–9.

Figure 3.11 with grateful thanks to Mr James Acheson.

Figure 3.12 from Greenfield LJ and Rosenberg HC 2004. Short-acting and other benzodiazepines. In: Shorvon SD *et al.* (eds) *The Treatment of Epilepsy* (2nd edn) Blackwell Publishing, Oxford: 374–90.

Table 3.4 data from Mattson RH *et al.* 1992. *N Engl J Med*, **327**: 765–71.

Table 3.5 from Dalby MA Clobazam. In: Shorvon SD *et al.* (eds) 2004. *The Treatment of Epilepsy* (2nd edn) Blackwell Publishing, Oxford: 358–364. Based on articles by Shorvon S, 1995, in Levy *et al.* (eds), *Antiepileptic Drugs*, New York: Raven Press, 763–768; and D Koeppen 1985, in I Hindmarch *et al.* (eds), *Clobazam, Human Psychopharmacology and Clinical Applications*, London: Royal Society of Medicine, 1207–15.

Table 3.6 from Glauser TA 2004. Ethosuximide. In: Shorvon SD *et al.* (eds) *The Treatment of Epilepsy* (2nd edn) Blackwell Publishing, Oxford: 391–402. Derived from Browne T 1983. Ethosuximide (zarontin) and other succinimides. In: Browne T and Feldman R (eds) *Epilepsy, Diagnosis and Management*. Boston: Little, Brown: 215–24.

Table 3.7 derived from Chadwick D 1994. *Lancet*, **343**: 89–91.

Table 3.8 from Matsuo F 2004. Lamotrigine. In: Shorvon SD *et al.* (eds) *The Treatment of Epilepsy* (2nd edn) Blackwell Publishing, Oxford: 425–42. Derived from Brodie MJ, Richens A and Yuen AWC 1995. *Lancet*, **345**: 476–9; Reunanen OM, Dam M and Yuen AWC 1996. *Epilepsy Res*, **23**: 149–55; Steiner TJ, Dellaportas CI, Findley LJ *et al.* 1999. *Epilepsia*, **40**: 601–7.

Table 3.9 derived from Schachter S 1995 *J Epilepsy*, **8**: 201–210.

Table 3.10 from Matsuo F 2004. Lamotrigine. In: Shorvon SD *et al.* (eds) *The Treatment of Epilepsy* (2nd edn) Blackwell Publishing, Oxford: 425–42. Derived from Messenheimer JA, Giorgi L and Risner ME 2000. The tolerability of lamotrigine in children. *Drug Saf*, **22**: 303–12.

Table 3.11 and 3.12 from Matsuo F 2004. Lamotrigine. In: Shorvon SD *et al.* (eds) *The Treatment of Epilepsy* (2nd edn) Black-well Publishing, Oxford: 425–42.

Table 3.13 Data from UCB Pharma internal database.

Table 3.14 Derived from Sadek A and French JA 2004. Levetiracetam. In: Shorvon SD *et al.* (eds) *The Treatment of Epilepsy* (2nd edn) Blackwell Publishing, Oxford: 443–50.

Table 3.15 derived from Sadek A and French JA 2001 *Epilepsia* **42** (Suppl. 4): 40–43.

Table 3.16 from Faught E 2004. Oxcarbazepine. In: Shorvon SD *et al.* (eds) *The Treatment of Epilepsy* (2nd edn) Black-well Publishing, Oxford: 451–60. Derived from Barcs G, Walker EB and Elger CE *et al.* 2000. *Epilepsia*, **41**: 1597–607; Glauser TA, Nigro M, Sachdeo R *et al.* 2000. *Neurology*, **54**: 2237–44.

Tables 3.19 and 3.20 from Brodie M 2004. *Epilepsia*, **45** (Suppl. 6): 19–27.

Table 3.21 Derived from Leppik *et al.* 1999. *Epilepsy Res*, **33**: 235–46.

Table 3.22 from Shorvon SD 1996. *Epilepsia*, **37**: S18–22.

Table 3.23 from Cross JH 2004. Topiramate. In: Shorvon SD *et al.* (eds) *The Treatment of Epilepsy* (2nd edn) Blackwell Publishing, Oxford: 515–27.

Table 3.24 from Ben-Menarchem E 1997. *Exp Clin Invest Drugs*, **6**: 1088–9.

Table 3.26 from Ben-Menachem E and French J 1998. In: Engel J and Pedley TA (eds) *Epilepsy: A Comprehensive Textbook*, Vol 2. Lippencott-Raven, New York: 1613.

Tables 3.27 and 3.28 from Seino M and Fujitani B Zonisamide. In: Shorvon SD *et al.* (eds) *The Treatment of Epilepsy* (2nd edn) Blackwell Publishing, Oxford: 548–59.

## Section 4

Figure 4.1 from Kapur J and MacDonald RL 1997. *J Neuroscience*, **17**: 7532–40.

Figure 4.2 from Lothman EW 1990. *Neurology*, **40** (Suppl. 2): 13–23.

Tables 4.1, 4.2, 4.3 and 4.4 Derived from Shorvon S 1994. *Status Epilepticus: Its Clinical Features and Treatment in Children and Adults*. Cambridge University Press, Cambridge.

Tables 4.5 and 4.6 Derived from Walker MC and Shorvon SD 2004. Emergency treatment of seizures and status epilepticus. In: Shorvon SD *et al.* (eds) *The Treatment of Epilepsy* (2nd edn) Blackwell Publishing, Oxford: 227–43.

## Section 5

Figure 5.1 derived from Scaravilli F 1980. Structure, Function and Connection. In: Scaravilli F (ed) *Neuropathology in Epilepsy*. Scientific Publishing Company plc: 20.

Figures 5.2 and 5.3 from Cook MC and Sisodiya S 1996. Magnetic resonance imaging evaluation for epilepsy surgery. In: Shorvon SD *et al. The Treatment of Epilepsy* (1st edn) Blackwell Science, Oxford: 589–604.

Figures 5.4, 5.5, 5.13–5.16 and 5.18–5.21 from Fish D 1996. The role of scalp electoencephalography evaluation for epilepsy surgery. In: Shorvon SD *et al. The Treatment of Epilepsy* (1st edn) Blackwell Science, Oxford: 542–561.

Figure 5.6 from Spencer SS and Lamoureux D 1996. Invasive electoencephalography evaluation for epilepsy surgery. In: Shorvon SD *et al. The Treatment of Epilepsy* (1st edn) Blackwell Science, Oxford.

Figure 5.7 from Raymond AA *et al.* 1994. *Neurology*, **44**: 1841–5.

Figure 5.8 from Olivier A. 1996. Surgery of mesial temporal epilepsy. In: Shorvon SD *et al. The Treatment of Epilepsy* (1st edn) Blackwell Science, Oxford: 689–698.

Figure 5.9 from Kitchen ND and Thomas DGT 1996. Stereotactic neurosurgery for epilepsy. In: Shorvon SD *et al. The Treatment of Epilepsy* (1st edn) Blackwell Science, Oxford: 759–771.

Figures 5.10 and 5.11 from Kitchen ND *et al.* 2004. Resective surgery of vascular and infective lesions for epilepsy. In: Shorvon SD *et al.* (eds) *The Treatment of Epilepsy* (2nd edn) Blackwell Publishing, Oxford: 742–62.

Figure 5.12 from Schweitzer JS and Spencer DD 1996. Surgery of congenital, traumatic and infectious lesions and those of uncertain aetiology. In: Shorvon SD *et al. The Treatment of Epilepsy* (1st edn) Blackwell Science, Oxford: 669–688.

Figure 5.17 derived from Nguyen DK and Spencer SS 2004. Invasive EEG in presurgical evaluation of epilepsy. In: Shorvon SD *et al. The Treatment of Epilepsy* (2nd edn) Blackwell Science, Oxford: 609–34.

Figure 5.22 from Gates JR and De Paola L 2004. Corpus callosum section for epilepsy. In: Shorvon SD *et al. The Treatment of Epilepsy* (2nd edn) Blackwell Science, Oxford: 798–811.

Figure 5.23 from Selway R and Dardis R 2004. Multiple subpial transection for epilepsy. In: Shorvon SD *et al. The Treatment of Epilepsy* (2nd edn) Blackwell Science, Oxford: 812–23.

Figure 5.24 from Schachter S 2004. Vagal nerve stimulation. In: Shorvon SD *et al. The Treatment of Epilepsy* (2nd edn) Blackwell Science, Oxford: 873–83.

Table 5.3 from Shorvon SD 2004. Introduction to epilepsy surgery and its presurgical assessment. In: Shorvon SD *et al.* (eds) *Treatment of Epilepsy* (2nd edn) Blackwell Publishing, Oxford: 579–98.

Tables 5.7, 5.8 and 5.9 Derived from Schachter SC 2004. Vagus nerve stimulation. In: Shorvon SD *et al.* (eds) *The Treatment of Epilepsy* (2nd edn) Blackwell Publishing, Oxford: 873–83.

# 1 The clinical forms and causes of epilepsy

## EPILEPSY

Epilepsy is—rather like headache—a *symptom* of neurological dysfunction. It has many forms and underlying causes, and biological and non-biological facets which extend well beyond the simple occurrence of seizures. Treatment approaches vary considerably in the different types of epilepsy and in this section of the book, the various clinical forms and causes of epilepsy are described. The forms of epilepsy can be classified in three main ways: by seizure type, syndrome or—in the cases of partial (focal) seizures—by the anatomical site of seizure onset. Each classification is described here. The causes can be subdivided into genetic and developmental, and acquired categories. There is often some overlap, but these general divisions are useful in clinical practice.

## Definitions

### Epileptic seizure (epileptic fit)

An epileptic seizure is defined as *the transient clinical manifestations that result from an episode of epileptic neuronal activity*. The epileptic neuronal activity is a specific dysfunction, characterized by abnormal synchronization, excessive excitation and/or inadequate inhibition, and can affect small or large neuronal populations (aggregates). The clinical manifestations are sudden, transient and usually brief. They include motor, psychic, autonomic and sensory phenomena, with or without alteration in consciousness or awareness. The symptoms depend on the part of the brain involved in the epileptic neuronal discharge, and the intensity of the discharge. The signs of a seizure vary from the only-too-evident wild manifestations of a generalized convulsion, to other seizures where subtle changes are apparent only to the patient. Some neuronal epileptic discharges, detectable by electroencephalography (EEG), are not accompanied by any evident symptoms or signs and this complicates definition. For most purposes these 'subclinical' or 'interictal' changes are not considered to be epileptic seizures, although the physiological changes can be identical to overt attacks, and the difference is largely one of degree. Furthermore, subtle impairment of psychomotor performance can be demonstrated due to interictal spiking, for instance, of which the patient may be unaware.

### Epilepsy

Epilepsy is a *disorder of brain characterized by an ongoing liability to recurrent epileptic seizures*. This definition is unsatisfactory for various reasons. First, it is difficult clearly to define, in many cases, to what extent recurrent attacks are likely—a definition based on crystal-ball gazing is inherently unsatisfactory. In the clinical setting, for pragmatic reasons, a 'liability to further attacks' is often said to be present when two or more spontaneous attacks have occurred, on the basis that this means that more are likely. However, this arbitrary definition is inadequate, for instance, in patients after a single attack who have a clear liability to further seizures, for patients who have had more than one provoked attack (see below) or for those whose epilepsy has remitted and whose liability for further attacks has lapsed. Furthermore, in physiological terms, the distinction between single and recurrent attacks is often meaningless. A second problem is that 'epilepsy' occurs with a wide variety of cerebral pathologies; like 'anaemia' or 'headache' in this sense it is a symptom masquerading as a disease. The standard definition is also inadequate in epileptic states in which physiological changes occur without obvious seizures. In these so-called epileptic encephalopathies, alterations in cognition and other cortical functions are major features unrelated to overt seizures (examples include the Landau–Kleffner syndrome or the childhood epileptic encephalopathies). Patients with subclinical discharges also sometimes have progressive cerebral dysfunction which could be characterized as epileptic in origin (for instance in examples of non-convulsive status). There are also certain non-epileptic conditions where differentiation from epilepsy is problematic. These are sometimes called borderline conditions, and include certain psychiatric conditions, some cases of migraine and some forms of movement disorder. Finally, the fact of 'being epileptic' involves far more than the risk of recurrent seizures, but incorporates prejudice and stigmatization, psychosocial and developmental issues which may, indeed, be more problematic than the seizures themselves. A comprehensive definition should ideally incorporate broader psychosocial, developmental and cognitive aspects.

## Status epilepticus

This is defined as a condition in which epileptic seizures continue, or are repeated without recovery, for a period of 30 minutes or more. This is the maximal expression of epilepsy, and often requires emergency therapy (see pp. 212–25). There are physiological and neurochemical changes that distinguish status epilepticus from ordinary epileptic seizures. Recent debate has revolved around the minimum duration of seizures necessary to define this condition, with suggestions ranging from 10 to 60 minutes; the usual 30 minutes is to some extent a compromise. As with the definitions of epilepsy and of epileptic seizures, there is a range of boundary conditions that do not fall easily into the simple clinical definitions.

## Epileptic seizures not considered to warrant a diagnosis of epilepsy

There are two categories of epileptic seizures—provoked seizures (acute symptomatic seizures) and childhood febrile seizures—that usually are not considered to warrant the diagnosis of epilepsy, on the basis that they do not indicate a continuing liability for recurrence. This is again rather arbitrary as recurrence is not uncommon in either category.

### Provoked seizures

Provoked seizures (acute symptomatic seizures) are defined as seizures that have an obvious and immediate preceding cause (for instance an acute systemic or metabolic disturbance or exposure to toxins or drugs), or which are the direct result of recent acute cerebral damage (for instance stroke, trauma, infection). Seizures following acute metabolic disturbance or toxin/drug exposure often do not recur when the cause is removed, and the term has utility in this context. The use of the term to include seizures after acute cerebral damage, however, is rather unsatisfactory as the damage is not reversible and the propensity for seizure recurrence is higher (see p. 57).

### Febrile seizures

A febrile seizure is an epileptic attack occurring in children under the age of 5 years (usually between 2 and 5 years) in the setting of a rise in body temperature. For most purposes, such seizures are not included within the rubric of 'epilepsy', as they are very common (2–5% of children in the West have at least one febrile seizure, and 9% in Japan), presumably have a specific physiological basis which is distinct from epilepsy, and have clinical implications that are very different from those of epilepsy. Febrile seizures are discussed further on pp. 21–22.

## Epileptic encephalopathy

An epileptic encephalopathy is a term used to describe a clinical state in which epilepsy is a prominent feature, and in which changes in cognition or other cerebral functions are, at least in part, likely to be due to ongoing epileptic processes in the brain. The epileptic encephalopathies are more common in children than in adults.

## Idiopathic, symptomatic and cryptogenic epilepsy

Epilepsy can have many causes. Where the cause is clearly identified, the epilepsy is categorized as 'symptomatic' (i.e. of known cause). Where no cause is known, the epilepsy is known as 'cryptogenic' (i.e. hidden cause). Where the epilepsy is part of the genetic syndrome of 'idiopathic generalized epilepsy' it is known as idiopathic. However, all is not as straightforward as this implies. In many cases—indeed perhaps in all cases—the epilepsy is multifactorial, reflecting the interaction of genetic and environmental factors (see p. 26). The attribution to a particular causal category can thereby be rather subjective and difficult to apply strictly. In clinical practice, for pragmatic reasons, the categorization is usually applied based on the presumed predominant aetiology.

## Active epilepsy and epilepsy in remission

A person is said to have active epilepsy when at least one epileptic seizure has occurred in the preceding period (usually 2–5 years). Conversely, epilepsy is said to be in remission when no seizures have occurred in this preceding period. The period of time used in these definitions varies in different studies, and furthermore some definitions of remission require the patient not only to be seizure-free but also off medication. An interesting question, and one of great importance to those with epilepsy, is after what period of remission can the person claim no longer to have the condition? Logically, the condition has remitted as soon as the last seizure has occurred, but this cannot be known except retrospectively. In practice, it is reasonable to consider epilepsy to have ceased in someone off therapy if 2–5 years have passed since the last attack.

## Acute symptomatic, remote symptomatic and congenital epilepsy

A categorization of epilepsy, for epidemiological studies, divides epilepsy into four types: acute symptomatic epilepsy, where there is an acute cause; remote symptomatic, where there is a cause that has been present for at least 3 months; congenital, where the cause existed at birth; and idiopathic, where the cause is not known. In view of the considerable grey area between acute and remote symptomatic epilepsies, the multifactorial nature of epilepsy and the subjectivity in idiopathic epilepsy, this classification has little value and should not now be used.

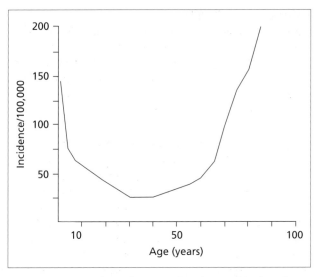

**Figure 1.1** Age-specific incidence rates based on combined results from studies in USA, Iceland and Sweden.

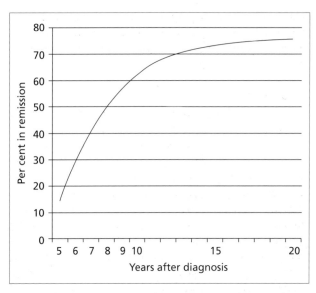

**Figure 1.2** Proportion of patients in 5-year remission by years after diagnosis of epilepsy (figures based on four population-based studies).

## Frequency and population features of epilepsy

Epilepsy is a common condition. Its incidence is in the region of 80 cases per 100,000 persons per year, with different studies showing rates varying between 50 and 120 per 100,000 per year. Its point prevalence is about 4–10 cases per 1000 persons. The prevalence is higher in underdeveloped countries, perhaps due to poorer perinatal care and standards of nutrition and public hygiene, and the greater risk of brain injury, cerebral infection or other symptomatic cerebral conditions. The frequency of epilepsy is also slightly higher in lower socio-economic classes. However, more striking than any differences in frequency, is the fact that epilepsy occurs in all parts of the world and can affect all strata in a population. Males may be slightly more likely to develop epilepsy than females, and there are no differences in rate in large ethnic populations. The incidence of seizures is age-dependent, with the highest rates in the first year of life and a second peak in late life (Figure 1.1). About 40% of patients develop epilepsy below the age of 16 years and about 20% over the age of 65 years. In recent times, the rate in children has been falling, possibly owing to better public health and living standards and better perinatal care. Conversely, the rate in the elderly is rising largely due to cerebrovascular disease.

An isolated (first and only) seizure occurs in about 20 persons per 100,000 each year. The cumulative incidence of epilepsy—the risk of an individual developing epilepsy in his/her lifetime—is between 3 and 5%. The fact that prevalence is much lower than cumulative incidence demonstrates that in many cases epilepsy remits. In fact the prognosis is generally good, and within 5 years of the onset of seizures, 50–60% of patients will have entered long remission (Figure 1.2). However, in about 20% of cases, epilepsy, once developed, never remits. Fertility rates are reduced by about 30% in women with epilepsy (see pp. 101–2). Standardized mortality rates are also 2–3 times higher in patients with epilepsy than in others in the population. The excess mortality is due largely to the underlying cause of the epilepsy. However, some deaths are directly related to seizures and there are higher rates of accidents, sudden unexpected deaths and suicides amongst patients with epilepsy when compared with the general population. The rates of death are highest in the first few years after diagnosis, reflecting the underlying cerebral disease (tumour, stroke, etc.). In chronic epilepsy, the more severe the epilepsy, the higher the mortality rate, an excess due largely to sudden unexpected death in epilepsy (SUDEP), and rates of SUDEP range from about one death per 2500 persons per year in mild epilepsy to one death per 250 patients per year amongst those with severe and intractable epilepsy. Life expectancy estimates at a population level have been recently calculated, showing a reduction of expectancy in idiopathic/cryptogenic epilepsy of up to 2 years and in symptomatic epilepsy of up to 10 years.

Table 1.1 shows an approximate breakdown of epilepsy in a typical Western population of 1,000,000 persons. This gives some indication of the burden of epilepsy. In populations of patients on therapy for epilepsy, about two-thirds had 'mild epilepsy' (i.e. seizures less than once a month) which required only minor medical input, and 50% had no seizures in the prior 12 months. However, about 5–10% had seizures at a greater than weekly frequency, required intensive medical resources for their epilepsy and incurred significant medical costs.

As mentioned above, almost every brain disorder can cause epileptic seizures and aetiology differs greatly in

**Table 1.1** The characteristics of epilepsy in a population of 1,000,000 persons (approximate estimates).

| | |
|---|---|
| *Incident cases* (new cases each year) | |
| Febrile seizures (annual incidence rate 50/100,000) | 500 |
| Single seizures (annual incidence rate 20/100,000) | 200 |
| Epilepsy (annual incidence rate 50/100,000) | 500 |
| | |
| *Prevalent cases* (cases with established epilepsy) | |
| Active epilepsy (prevalence rate 5/1000) | 5000 |
| Epilepsy in remission | 15,000 |
| | |
| *Severity of cases* (in patients taking antepileptic drugs; seizures in previous year) | |
| More than one seizure per week | 10% |
| Between one seizure per week and one per year | 40% |
| No seizures | 50% |
| | |
| *Type of seizure* | |
| Partial seizures alone | 15% |
| Partial and secondarily generalized | 60% |
| Generalized tonic–clonic | 20% |
| Other generalized seizures | 5% |
| | |
| *Medical care required* (in prevalent cases) | |
| Occasional medical attention | 65% |
| Regular medical attention | 30% |
| Residential or institutional care | 5% |

**Table 1.2** The range of causes of epilepsy in a typical Western population (approximate figures based on a range of published studies of prevalence; the figures exclude childhood febrile convulsions).

| | Approximate frequency (%) |
|---|---|
| Idiopathic† | 10–30 |
| Vascular†† | 10–20 |
| Congenital malformations†††* | 2–10 |
| Degenerative disorders | 2–10 |
| Hippocampal sclerosis* | 2–10 |
| Neoplasm | 2–10 |
| Trauma | 2–5 |
| Epilepsy syndromes of childhood†††† | 2–5 |
| Infection | 2–5 |
| Genetic – single gene disorder* | 1–2 |
| Unknown (cryptogenic epilepsy)* | 25–40 |

*, Figures adjusted to account for the increased identification of hippocampal sclerosis/genetic disorders/congenital malformations possible with modern neuro-imaging and genetics, which were not available to most of the population-based studies); †, idiopathic generalized epilepsies and benign partial epilepsies; ††, ischaemic (approximately 80%) and haemorrhagic (approximately 20%); †††, including cortical dysplasias and other congenital cerebral malformations; ††††, epilepsy syndromes not included in other categories (e.g. cryptogenic Lennox–Gastaut syndrome, cryptogenic West syndrome, etc.).

different populations, geographic locations, and in different age groups. The aetiologies of epilepsy are described on pp. 26–54. The main aetiological categories of epilepsy in a typical Western population are given in Table 1.2.

About one-third to half of children and about one-fifth of adults with epilepsy have additional learning disability; similarly, epilepsy occurs in about 20% of those with learning disability (7–18% of those with intelligence quotients [IQs] rated between 50 and 70, and 35–44% in those with IQ ratings below 50), equating to a prevalence rate of 1.2 per 1000. Of adults with newly diagnosed epilepsy, 18% show additional dementia, 6% motor disabilities (usually hemiplegia due to stroke) and 6% severe psychiatric disorders. About one in 15 persons with epilepsy is dependent on others for daily living because of epilepsy and the associated handicaps. In terms of direct medical care costs, epilepsy accounts for about 0.25% of general practitioner costs, 0.63% of hospital costs and 0.95% of pharmaceutical costs in the UK National Health Service. Epilepsy results in social exclusion and isolation, and causes problems in education, employment, personal development, personal relationships and family life, and dependency. These secondary handicaps are to a large extent culturally determined. Taking a broad brush, the World Health Organization (WHO) has estimated that epilepsy causes 6.4 million disability-adjusted life years (DALYs) and 1.32 million years of life lost (YLL) world-

wide, second amongst neurological diseases only to stroke and dementia in its impact. Stigmatization of patients with epilepsy is common, and social attitude change would alleviate many of the problems encountered by patients with epilepsy; this is as important as any medical therapy.

## ILAE CLASSIFICATION OF SEIZURE TYPE

Epilepsy is a variable condition, and it is therefore appropriate to devise a system of classification. The International League Against Epilepsy (ILAE) has been engaged on this task for over 40 years, proposing and then revising various systems. The classification most widely accepted is a classification of seizure type (i.e. of the phenomenology of seizures rather than of epilepsies). Such a classification could be based on various criteria, for instance the cerebral region in which the seizure arises (the anatomical site), the cause of the seizures, the age or neuropsychiatric status of the patient, or the response to treatment. In fact, the commonly used classification, the 1981 ILAE classification, uses only two criteria: the clinical form and the EEG abnormality. This is therefore an entirely descriptive classification, with few pretensions.

The 1981 ILAE classification divides seizures into generalized and partial categories (Table 1.3). Generalized seizures are those that arise from large areas of cortex in

**Table 1.3** The 1981 International League Against Epilepsy (ILAE) Classification of Seizure Type.

*I Partial (focal, local) seizures*
A  Simple partial seizures
   1  With motor signs
   2  With somatosensory or special sensory symptoms
   3  With autonomic symptoms or signs
   4  With psychic symptoms

B  Complex partial seizures
   1  Simple partial onset followed by impairment of consciousness
   2  With impairment of consciousness at onset

C  Partial seizures evolving to secondarily generalized seizures (tonic–clonic, tonic, or clonic)
   1  Simple partial seizures evolving to generalized seizures
   2  Complex partial seizures evolving to generalized seizures
   3  Simple partial seizures evolving to complex partial seizures evolving to generalized seizures

*II Generalized seizures (convulsive and non-convulsive)*
A  Absence seizures
   1  Absence seizures
   2  Atypical absence seizures
B  Myoclonic seizures
C  Clonic seizures
D  Tonic seizures
E  Tonic–clonic seizures
F  Atonic seizures (astatic seizures)

*III Unclassified epileptic seizures*

both hemispheres, and in which consciousness is always lost. Generalized seizures are subdivided into seven categories. Partial seizures are those that arise in specific, often small, loci of cortex in one hemisphere. They are divided into simple partial seizures which occur without alteration of consciousness and complex partial seizures in which consciousness is impaired or lost. A secondarily generalized seizure is a seizure with a partial onset (the aura) which spreads to become a generalized attack. Simple partial seizures may spread to become complex partial seizures and either can spread to become secondarily generalized. Although this is a classification based entirely on clinical and EEG phenomenology, it should be realized that some of the generalized seizure types occur only in specific types of epilepsy, and this is discussed further below. Partial seizures invariably imply focal brain pathology, although this may not necessarily be demonstrated by conventional clinical investigation. About two-thirds of newly diagnosed epilepsies are partial and/or secondarily generalized.

The limitations of a classification based only on clinical and EEG appearance should not be underestimated, and the current classification is inadequate for many clinical and research purposes. The more recent ILAE *Classification of the Epilepsies and Epileptic Syndromes* was devised to be more comprehensive, and this is discussed further below (pp. 11–13). There have been other criticisms of the ILAE classification. The subdivision of partial seizures on the basis of consciousness is criticized because of the difficulty of deciding in many cases whether or not consciousness is altered. Many seizures do not fit well into any of the categories, and treatment can also modify the clinical form. With advances in imaging and neurophysiology, it has become clear that some generalized seizures do in fact have underlying focal brain disorders. Some partial seizures are underpinned by a large neuronal network akin to that of some generalized epilepsies. From the perspective of this book, devoted to therapy, a damning criticism of the classification is that as a general rule it generally does not help in choosing treatment or defining prognosis. There are obvious exceptions (the use of valproate or ethosuximide in generalized absence attacks, for instance) but the lack of treatment specificity for individual categories is striking.

The ILAE classifications of seizure type and of the epilepsies and epileptic syndromes are currently undergoing revision and are increasingly challenged by alternative systems. However, the main value of the *International Classification of Seizure Type* lies is its widespread clinical acceptance and, in spite of all its problems, this classification has become adopted universally in clinical practice.

## Partial seizures
### Simple partial seizures
Simple partial seizures are defined as partial seizures in which consciousness is not impaired. They are due to focal cerebral disease. Any cortical region may be affected, the most common sites being the frontal and temporal lobes. The symptoms are useful in predicting the anatomical localization of the seizures. The form of the seizures usually has no pathological specificity, and can occur at any age. Most simple partial seizures last only a few seconds. Their clinical form depends on the anatomical location within the cerebral cortex of the seizure discharge.

*Motor manifestations*
The most common manifestations are jerking (clonus), spasm or posturing. These occur in epilepsies arising in frontal or central regions, although they can also occur with spread of the epileptic discharges from other regions. The clonic jerks can spread from one part of the body to another (the so-called Jacksonian march) as the focal discharges spread along the motor cortices of the brain. Speech arrest occurs if the simple partial seizure involves the efferent speech areas, and anarthria, dysarthria or choking sensations can occur in seizures involving areas of the brain involved with muscles of articulation.

Turning (known usually as 'version') of the head or eyes, or less commonly rotation of the whole body, can occur in epilepsy arising in many cortical areas. It is of little localizing value unless it is the first symptom in a seizure and in full consciousness in which case the epilepsy arises usually from the contralateral anterior frontal lobe.

Todd paralysis is a term used to refer to a reversible unilateral weakness that occurs after a partial seizure which involves the motor cortex. It can last minutes or hours, but is never prolonged beyond 24 hours (prolonged paralysis indicates that cortical damage has occurred, unrelated to epilepsy *per se*). The occurrence of a Todd paralysis has reliable localizing value, indicating that the epilepsy arises in the contralateral motor cortex.

### Somatosensory or special sensory manifestations (simple hallucinations)

These take the form of tingling or numbness, or less commonly as an electrical shock-like feeling, burning, pain or a feeling of heat. The epileptic focus is usually in the central or parietal region, although similar symptoms occur with spread from epileptic foci in other locations. Simple visual phenomena such as flashing lights and colours occur if the calcarine cortex is affected. A rising epigastric sensation is the most common manifestation of a simple partial seizure arising in the mesial temporal lobe.

### Autonomic manifestations

Autonomic symptoms such as changes in skin colour, blood pressure, heart rate, pupil size and piloerection can be isolated phenomena in simple partial seizures, but more commonly are a component of generalized or complex partial seizures of frontal or temporal origin.

### Psychic manifestations

Psychic 'auras' can take various forms, and are more common in complex partial than in simple partial seizures. They can occur in epilepsy arising from a temporal, frontal or parietal focus. There are six principal categories:

*Dysphasic symptoms* are prominent if cortical speech areas (frontal or temporoparietal) are affected. Speech usually ceases or is severely reduced, and postictal dysphasia is a very reliable sign localizing the seizure discharge to the dominant hemisphere. Repetitive vocalization with formed words may occur in a complex partial seizure of origin in the non-dominant temporal lobe. Palilalia can occur in epilepsy arising in the dominant hemisphere. Dysphasia should be distinguished where possible from anarthria (speech arrest), which suggests a fronto-central origin.

*Dysmnestic symptoms* (disturbance of memory) may take the form of flashbacks, *déjà vu*, *jamais vu* or panoramic experiences (recollections of previous experiences, former life or childhood), and are most common in mesial temporal lobe seizures. However, similar symptoms also occur in inferior frontal or lateral temporal lobe seizures.

*Cognitive symptoms* include dreamy states and sensations of unreality or depersonalization, and occur primarily in temporal lobe seizures.

*Affective symptoms* include fear (the most common symptom), depression, anger and irritability. Elation, erotic thoughts, serenity or exhilaration may occur. Affective symptomatology is most commonly seen with mesial temporal lobe foci. Laughter (without mirth) is a feature of the automatism of seizures (known as gelastic seizures) which arise in frontal areas, and are a consistent feature of the epilepsy associated with hypothalamic hamartomas.

*Illusions* of size (macropsia, micropsia), shape, weight, distance or sound are usually features of temporal or parieto-occipital epileptic foci.

*Structured hallucinations* of visual, auditory, gustatory or olfactory forms, which can be crude or elaborate, are usually due to epileptic discharges in the temporal or parieto-occipital association areas. Hallucinations of taste, usually an unpleasant taste, are a frequent symptom of temporal lobe epilepsy. Visual hallucinations can vary greatly in sophistication from simple colours or flashing lights in epilepsy arising in the calcarine cortex to complex visual perceptual hallucinations in posterior temporal association areas. Auditory hallucinations also vary in complexity, and most commonly occur in seizures arising in Herschel's gyrus. Vertigo is a common perceptual change in temporal lobe epilepsy, and unlike vertigo of vestibular origin, epileptic vertigo is rarely associated with nausea and is usually not severe or incapacitating.

The scalp EEG, both interictally and also during a simple partial seizure, is often normal, because the epileptic disturbance is too small or too deep to be detected by the scalp electrodes. If an interictal abnormality is present, it will take the form of spikes, sharp waves, focal slow activity or suppression of normal rhythms. Before the seizure, the interictal EEG may show a sudden reduction in the frequency of interictal spike or sharp waves. Ictal abnormalities can take the form of rhythmic theta activity, focal spike-wave activity or runs of fast activity (13–30 Hz).

## Complex partial seizures

Complex partial seizures arise from the temporal lobe in about 60% of cases, the frontal lobe in about 30%, and from other cortical areas in about 10% of cases. The clinical features reflect the site of onset of the seizures, and the clinical features characteristic of specific sites of onset are described on pp. 13–15. Complex partial seizures vary considerably in duration. In one series of temporal lobe epilepsy, the ictal phase lasted 3 and 343 seconds (mean, 54 seconds), the postictal phase 3–767 seconds, and the total seizure duration 5–998 seconds (mean, 128 seconds), although longer seizures (occasionally lasting hours) are sometimes encountered.

Complex partial seizures of temporal or frontal lobe origin can have three components.

### Aura

These are equivalent to simple partial seizures, and can take any of the forms described above. The aura is usually short-lived, lasting a few seconds or so, although in rare cases a prolonged aura persists for minutes, hours or even days. Many patients experience isolated auras as well as full-blown complex partial seizures.

### Altered consciousness

This follows the aura or evolves simultaneously. The altered consciousness takes the form of an absence and motor arrest, during which the patient is motionless and inaccessible and appears vacant or glazed (the so-called 'motionless stare'). Sometimes there are no outward signs at all, and at other times there may be associated spasm, posturing or mild tonic jerking.

### Automatisms

Automatisms are defined as involuntary motor actions that occur during or in the aftermath of epileptic seizures, in a state of impaired awareness. The patient is totally amnesic for the events of the automatism. Sometimes the actions have purposeful elements, are affected by the environment and can involve quite complex activity. Automatisms should be distinguished from postictal confusion. Automatisms are most common in temporal and frontal lobe seizures. They are usually divided into:

*Oro-alimentary*: orofacial movements such as chewing, lip smacking, swallowing or drooling. These are most common in partial seizures of mesial temporal origin.

*Mimicry*: including displays of laughter or fear, anger or excitement.

*Gestural*: fiddling movements with the hands, tapping, patting, or rubbing, ordering and tidying movements. Complex actions such as undressing are quite common, as are genitally-directed actions.

*Ambulatory automatisms*: walking, circling, running.

*Verbal automatisms*: meaningless sounds, humming, whistling, grunting, words which may be repeated, formed sentences.

*Responsive automatisms*: quasi-purposeful behaviour, seemingly responsive to environmental stimuli.

*Violent behaviour* can occur in an automatism, and is best considered as a response in an acutely confused person. It is especially likely if the patient is restrained. The violent actions of the epileptic automatism are never premeditated, never remembered, never highly co-ordinated or skilful, and seldom goal-directed; these are useful diagnostic features in a forensic context.

In about 10–30% of seizures, the scalp EEG is unchanged and in the rest, runs of fast activity, localized spike-wave complexes, spikes or sharp waves or slow activity may occur, or the EEG may simply show flattening (desynchronization). The patterns can be focal (indicating the site or origin of the seizure), lateralized, bilateral or diffuse.

### Partial seizures evolving to secondarily generalized seizures

Partial seizures (simple, complex or simple evolving to complex) may spread to become generalized. The partial seizure is often experienced as an aura in the seconds before the generalized seizure. The generalized seizure is usually tonic–clonic, tonic or atonic.

## Generalized seizures

Consciousness is almost invariably impaired from the onset of the attack (owing to the extensive cortical and subcortical involvement), motor changes are bilateral and more or less symmetric, and the EEG patterns are bilateral and grossly synchronous and symmetrical over both hemispheres.

### Typical absence seizures (petit mal seizures)

The seizure comprises an abrupt loss of consciousness (the absence) and cessation of all motor activity. Tone is usually preserved, and there is no fall. The patient is not in contact with the environment, is inaccessible, and often appears glazed or vacant. The attack ends as abruptly as it started, and previous activity is resumed as if nothing had happened. There is no confusion, but the patient is often unaware that an attack has occurred. Most absence seizures (> 80%) last less than 10 seconds. Other clinical phenomena including blinking, slight clonic movements of the trunk or limbs, alterations in tone and/or brief automatisms can occur particularly in longer attacks. The attacks can be repeated, sometimes hundreds of times a day, often cluster and are often worse when the patient is awakening or drifting off to sleep.

Absences may be precipitated by fatigue, drowsiness, relaxation, photic stimulation or hyperventilation. Typical absence seizures develop in childhood or adolescence and are encountered almost exclusively in the syndrome of idiopathic generalized epilepsy (see pp. 17–19). Variations from this typical form include the myoclonic absence, absence with perioral myoclonia or with eyelid myoclonia. Whether or not these are distinct entities is controversial (see pp. 17–18).

The EEG during a typical absence has a very striking pattern. A regular, symmetric and synchronous 3 Hz spike-wave paroxysm is the classic form, although in longer attacks and in older patients the paroxysms may not be entirely regular and frequencies vary between 2 and 4 Hz. The interictal EEG has normal background activity and there may be intermittent short-lived bursts of spike-wave. These spike-wave paroxysms can frequently be induced by hyperventilation and less commonly by photic stimulation.

The features useful in differentiating a complex partial seizure and a typical absence are shown in Table 1.4.

### Atypical absence seizures

Atypical absence seizures, like typical absence seizures, take the form of loss of awareness (absence) and hypo-motor behaviour. They differ from typical absences in clinical form, EEG, aetiology and clinical context (Table 1.5). Their duration is longer, loss of awareness is often incomplete

| | Typical absence seizure | Complex partial seizure |
|---|---|---|
| Age of onset | Childhood or early adult | Any age |
| Aetiology/syndrome | Idiopathic generalized epilepsy | Any focal aetiology (or cryptogenic epilepsy) |
| Underlying focal anatomical lesion | None | Limbic structures, neocortex |
| Duration of attack | Short (usually < 10 s) | Longer, usually several minutes |
| Other clinical features | Slight (blinking, nodding or mild loss of tone) | Can be prominent, including aura, automatism |
| Postictal | None | Confusion, headache, emotional disturbance are common |
| Frequency | May be very numerous (hundreds a day) and cluster | Usually less frequent |
| Ictal and interictal EEG | 3 Hz spike-wave | Variable focal disturbance |
| Photosensitivity | 10–30% | None |
| Effect of hyperventilation on EEG | Often marked increase | None, modest increase |

**Table 1.4** Clinical features that help differentiate typical absence seizures from complex partial seizures.

and much less marked, and associated tone changes are more severe than in typical absence seizures. The onset and cessation of the attacks are not so abrupt. Amnesia may not be complete and the subject may be partially responsive. The patient appears relatively inaccessible, may be ambulant although often stumbling or clumsy and needing guidance or support, and there can be atonic, clonic or tonic phenomena, autonomic disturbance and automatism. The attacks can wax and wane and may be of long duration.

The ictal EEG shows usually diffuse but often asymmetric and irregular spike-wave bursts at 2–2.5 Hz, and sometimes fast activity or bursts of spikes and sharp waves. The background interictal EEG is usually abnormal, with continuous slowing, spikes or irregular spike-wave activity, and the ictal and interictal EEGs may be similar. The seizures are often not induced by hyperventilation or photic stimulation.

Atypical absences occur in the symptomatic epilepsies, are usually associated with learning disability, other neurologic abnormalities or multiple seizure types. They form part of the Lennox–Gastaut syndrome and they may occur at any age.

## Myoclonic seizures

A myoclonic seizure is a brief contraction of a muscle, muscle group or several muscle groups due to a cortical discharge. It can be single or repetitive, varying in severity from an almost imperceptible twitch to a severe jerking, resulting, for instance, in a sudden fall or the propulsion of hand-held objects (the 'flying saucer' syndrome). Recovery is immediate, and the patient often maintains that consciousness was not lost. During a myoclonic jerk, the electromyogram shows biphasic or polyphasic potentials

| | Typical absence seizure | Atypical absence seizure |
|---|---|---|
| Context | No other neurological signs or symptoms | Usually in context of learning difficulty, and other neurological abnormalities |
| Aetiology | Idiopathic generalized epilepsy | Lennox–Gastaut syndrome and other secondarily generalized and cryptogenic generalized epilepsies |
| Consciousness | Totally lost | Often only partially impaired |
| Focal signs in seizures | Nil | May be present |
| Onset/offset of seizures | Abrupt | Often gradual |
| Co-existing seizure types | Sometimes tonic–clonic and myoclonic | Mixed seizure disorder common, all seizure types |

**Table 1.5** Clinical features that help differentiate typical and atypical absence seizures.

of 20–120 ms in duration followed by tonic contraction or hypotonia. Myoclonus can be induced by action, noise, startle, photic stimulation or percussion.

Myoclonic seizures occur in very different types of epilepsy. They are one of the three seizure types in the syndrome of idiopathic generalized epilepsy (the other two being absence and tonic–clonic seizures) and in this syndrome the myoclonus usually has a strong diurnal pattern, occurring mainly in the first few hours after waking or when dropping off to sleep. Myoclonic seizures also occur in the epileptic encephalopathies (e.g. Lennox–Gastaut syndrome) and in epilepsy associated with other forms of childhood myoclonic encephalopathy. Focal myoclonus is a feature of focal occipital lobe epilepsy and epilepsy arising in the central areas (and if continuous is named *epilepsia partialis continua*). Generalized myoclonus can also occur in symptomatic epilepsies due to cerebral anoxia, cerebral infections, hereditary or acquired metabolic disease, drugs, toxins or poisoning. Myoclonus is also the major seizure type in the progressive myoclonic epilepsies. Epileptic myoclonus needs to be differentiated from non-epileptic myoclonus of spinal and subcortical origin.

The ictal EEG usually shows a generalized spike, spike-wave, or polyspike-wave discharge, which is often asymmetric or irregular and frequently has a frontal predominance. The cortical origin of some myoclonic jerks, however, can be detected only on back averaging of the EEG. The inter-ictal EEG varies with the cause, being usually normal in idiopathic generalized epilepsy, and abnormal in other types of myoclonic epilepsy showing generalized changes.

### Clonic seizures

Clonic seizures consist of clonic jerking which is often asymmetric and irregular. Clonic seizures are most frequent in neonates, infants or young children, and are always symptomatic. The EEG may show fast activity (10 Hz), fast activity mixed with larger amplitude slow waves, or more rarely polyspike-wave or spike-wave discharges. These should not be confused with bilateral clonic jerking (with or without loss of consciousness, even if involving all four limbs), which is a form of partial seizure arising in the frontal lobe.

### Tonic seizures

Tonic seizures take the form of a tonic muscle contraction with altered consciousness without a clonic phase. The tonic contraction causes extension of the neck; contraction of the facial muscles, with the eyes opening widely; upturning of the eyeballs; contraction of the muscles of respiration; and spasm of the proximal upper limb muscles causing the abduction and elevation of the semiflexed arms and the shoulders. If the tonic contractions spread distally, the arms rise up and are held as if defending the head against a blow and the lower limbs become forcibly extended or contracted in triple flexion. There may be a cry

followed by apnoea. The spasm may fluctuate during the seizure, causing head nodding or slight alterations in the posture of the extended limbs, and autonomic changes can be marked. Tonic seizures last less than 60 seconds.

The ictal EEG may show flattening (desynchronization), fast activity (15–25 Hz) with increasing amplitude (to about 100 µV) as the attack progresses, or a rhythmic 10 Hz discharge similar to that seen in the tonic phase of the tonic–clonic seizure. On a scalp recording, however, the ictal EEG changes are often obscured by artefact from muscle activity and movement. The interictal EEG is seldom normal, usually showing generalized changes.

Tonic seizures occur at all ages in the setting of diffuse cerebral damage and learning disability, and are invariably associated with other seizure types. Tonic seizures are the characteristic and defining seizure type in the Lennox–Gastaut syndrome, and this is their usual clinical setting. They should be differentiated from partial motor seizures, which can also show predominantly tonic features, and from partially treated tonic–clonic seizures.

### Tonic–clonic seizures (grand mal seizures)

This is the classic form of epileptic attack, the 'convulsion' or 'fit' that typifies epilepsy in the public imagination. It has a number of well-defined stages. It is sometimes preceded by a prodromal period during which an attack is anticipated, often by an ill-defined vague feeling or sometimes more specifically, for instance, by the occurrence of increasing myoclonic jerking. If an aura then occurs (in fact a simple or complex partial seizure) in the seconds before the full-blown attack, this indicates that the tonic–clonic seizure is secondarily generalized. The seizure is initiated by loss of consciousness, and sometimes the epileptic cry. The patient will fall if standing, there is a brief period of tonic flexion, and then a longer phase of rigidity and axial extension, with the eyes rolled up, the jaw clamped shut, the limbs stiff, adducted and extended, and the fists either clenched or held in the *main d'accoucheur* position. Respiration ceases and cyanosis is common. This tonic stage lasts on average 10–30 seconds and is followed by the clonic phase, during which convulsive movements usually of all four limbs, jaw and facial muscles occur; breathing can be stertorous; and saliva (sometimes blood-stained owing to tongue biting) may froth from the mouth. The convulsive movements decrease in frequency (eventually to about four clonic jerks per second), and increase in amplitude as the attack progresses.

Autonomic features such as flushing, changes in blood pressure, changes in pulse rate and increased salivation are common. The clonic phase lasts between 30 and 60 seconds and is followed by a further brief tonic contraction of all muscles, sometimes with incontinence. The final phase lasts between 2 and 30 minutes and is characterized by flaccidity of the muscles. Consciousness is slowly regained.

The plantar responses are usually extensor at this time and the tendon jerks are diminished. Confusion is invariable in the postictal phase. The patient often has a severe headache, feels dazed and extremely unwell, and often lapses into deep sleep. On awakening minutes or hours later, there may be no residual symptoms or, more commonly, persisting headache, dysthymia, lethargy, muscle aching and soreness (including stiffness of the jaw).

Tonic–clonic seizures can occur at any age and are encountered in many different types of epilepsy, including idiopathic generalized epilepsy, symptomatic generalized epilepsies, epileptic encephalopathies, in various epilepsy syndromes, in febrile convulsions, and in acute symptomatic seizures. They have no pathological specificity.

The interictal EEG has a variable appearance, depending on the cause of the tonic–clonic seizures. During the tonic phase, the ictal EEG may show generalized flattening (desynchronization). This is followed by low-voltage fast activity and then 10 Hz rhythms appear and increase in amplitude (recruiting rhythms). These are followed some seconds later by slow waves increasing in amplitude and decreasing in frequency from 3 to 1 Hz. During the clonic phase, the slow waves are interrupted by bursts of faster activity (at about 10 Hz) corresponding to the clonic jerks, and as the phase progresses, the slow waves widen and these bursts become less frequent. With scalp recordings, however, these EEG patterns will often be obscured by artefact from muscle and movement. As the jerks cease, the EEG becomes silent and then slow delta activity develops. This persists for a variable period and the EEG background rhythms then slowly increase in frequency. Minutes or hours usually elapse before the EEG activity returns to normal. In patients with idiopathic generalized epilepsy, the EEG in the pre-ictal period may show increasing abnormalities with spike-wave or spike paroxysms.

### Atonic seizures

The most severe form is the classic drop attack (astatic seizure) in which all postural tone is suddenly lost causing collapse to the ground like a rag doll. The tone change can be more restricted, resulting for instance in nodding of the head, a bowing movement or sagging at the knees. The seizures are short and are followed by immediate recovery. Longer (inhibitory) atonic attacks can develop in a stepwise fashion with progressively increasing nodding, sagging or folding.

The seizures occur at any age, and are always associated with diffuse cerebral damage, learning disability and are common in severe symptomatic epilepsies (especially in the Lennox–Gastaut syndrome and in myoclonic astatic epilepsy). The ictal EEG shows irregular spike-wave, polyspike-wave, slow wave, or low amplitude fast activity, or a mixture of these and may be obscured by movement artefact. The interictal EEG usually shows diffuse abnormalities.

### Unclassifiable seizures

Up to one-third of seizures in many clinical series are considered unclassifiable using the current ILAE classification scheme, taking forms that do not conform to the typical clinical and EEG patterns described above.

The clinical context of the different seizure types are summarized in Table 1.6. It is also important to recognize

**Table 1.6** The usual clinical contexts in which different seizure types occur.

| Seizure type | Clinical context |
|---|---|
| *Partial seizures* | |
| Simple, complex, secondarily generalized | Epilepsies due to any focal (or multifocal) cerebral pathology<br>Many forms of cryptogenic epilepsy |
| *Generalized seizures* | |
| Typical absence seizures | Idiopathic generalized epilepsy (IGE) |
| Atypical absence seizures | Lennox–Gastaut syndrome<br>Other severe cryptogenic or secondarily generalized epilepsies |
| Myoclonic seizures | Idiopathic generalized epilepsy (IGE)<br>Progressive myoclonus epilepsies<br>Myoclonic epilepsy syndromes of childhood<br>Focal occipital lobe epilepsies |
| Clonic, tonic, atonic | Lennox–Gastaut syndrome<br>Other epileptic encephalopathies<br>Focal frontal or parietal lobe epilepsy |
| Tonic–clonic seizures | Epilepsy in generalized or diffuse cerebral pathologies |

that treatment can markedly modify the form of an epileptic attack, and this can cause confusion. The seizures can be shortened, and the aura and the phasic nature of a prolonged seizure can be lost. Tonic–clonic seizures can, for example, be modified and appear more like tonic or atonic attacks.

## ILAE CLASSIFICATION OF THE EPILEPSIES AND EPILEPSY SYNDROMES

In an attempt to encompass a broader range of clinical features than is possible in a classification of seizure type, the ILAE published, in 1985, and revised in 1989, a *Classification of the Epilepsies and Epileptic Syndromes* (Table 1.7). An epileptic syndrome is defined as 'an epileptic disorder characterized by a cluster of signs and symptoms customarily occurring together'. The relationship between the epilepsy syndrome and the underlying disease is complex. While some syndromes represent a single disease, others can be the result of many diseases. A good example of the latter is the Lennox–Gastaut syndrome. Furthermore, the same

underlying disease can manifest as different epileptic syndromes; an example is tuberous sclerosis. The syndromes are often age-specific, and over time in individual patients one epileptic syndrome can evolve into another. Similarly, the same seizure type can occur in very different syndromes (for example, myoclonic seizures in the benign syndrome of juvenile myoclonic epilepsy and the refractory syndromes of the progressive myoclonic epilepsies). The advantages of the classification are its flexibility, the potential for change and expansion, and the acknowledgement of the complex interplay of factors underlying epilepsy.

There are, however, serious disadvantages. First, the classification is a complex system with very clumsy terminology, and for this reason alone is unlikely ever to gain widespread clinical usage, especially in non-specialist settings. A second problem is the maintenance of the distinction between focal and generalized epilepsies which in many types of epilepsy is difficult to justify and presumes an unrealistic knowledge of the underlying physiological processes. It is perhaps in recognition of this problem that the third category has been introduced, although it might have been better to avoid this distinction altogether.

**Table 1.7** International classification of epilepsies and epileptic syndromes.

1  Localization-related (focal, local, partial epilepsies and syndromes)
   **1.1** Idiopathic (with age-related onset)
     • Benign childhood epilepsy with centrotemporal spike
     • Childhood epilepsy with occipital paroxysms
     • Primary reading epilepsy
   **1.2** Symptomatic epilepsy
     • Chronic epilepsia partialis continua of childhood (Kojewnikow's syndrome)
     • Syndromes characterized by seizures with specific modes of precipitation
   **1.3** Cryptogenic
2  Generalized epilepsies and syndromes
   **2.1** Idiopathic (with age-related onset—listed in order of age)
     • Benign neonatal familial convulsions
     • Benign neonatal convulsions
     • Benign myoclonic epilepsy in infancy
     • Childhood absence epilepsy (pyknolepsy)
     • Juvenile myoclonic epilepsy (impulsive petit mal)
     • Epilepsy with grand mal (GTCS) seizures on awakening
     • Other generalized idiopathic epilepsies not defined above
     • Epilepsies with seizures precipitated by specific modes of activation
   **2.2** Cryptogenic or symptomatic (in order of age)
     • West syndrome (infantile spasms, Blitz–Nick–Salaam–Krämpfe)
     • Lennox–Gastaut syndrome
     • Epilepsy with myoclonic-astatic seizures
     • Epilepsy with myoclonic absences

   **2.3** Symptomatic
     **2.3.1** Non-specific aetiology
       • Early myoclonic encephalopathy
       • Early infantile epileptic encephalopathy with suppression-burst
       • Other symptomatic generalized epilepsies not defined above
     **2.3.2** Specific syndromes
       • Epileptic seizure may complicate many disease states Under this heading are diseases in which seizures are a presenting or predominant feature
3  Epilepsies and syndromes undetermined whether focal or generalized
   **3.1** With both generalized and focal seizures
     • Neonatal seizures
     • Severe myoclonic epilepsy in infancy
     • Epilepsy with continuous spike-waves during slow-wave sleep
     • Acquired epileptic aphasia (Landau–Kleffner)
     • Other undetermined epilepsies not defined above
   **3.2** Without unequivocal generalized or focal features. All cases with generalized tonic–clonic seizures in which clinical and EEG findings do not permit classification as clearly generalized or localization-related such as in many cases of sleep-grand mal (GTCS) are considered not to have unequivocal generalized or focal features
4  Special syndromes
   **4.1** Situation-related seizures (Gelegenheitsanfälle)
     • Febrile convulsions
     • Isolated seizures or isolated status epilepticus
     • Seizures occurring only when there is an acute metabolic or toxic event due to factors such as alcohol, drugs, eclampsia, non-ketotic hyperglycaemia

A third problem is that, in the attempt to be all-inclusive, this classification becomes unwieldy. Common syndromes are mixed in with those that are extremely rare and syndromes whose identity is contentious are also included. In normal clinical practice, the majority of epilepsy seen (66% in one series) will fall into categories 1.2, 2.3 and 4.1, each of which are poorly defined 'non-specific' categories—which undermines the purpose and value of the scheme. Another problem is the arbitrary nature of some categories (notably 3 and 4). This results in the grouping of epilepsies that have little else in common. Finally, it is the difficult to justify the full epithet 'syndrome' for some of the idiopathic conditions listed. Some prefer to see the idiopathic generalized epilepsies, for instance, as a 'neurobiological continuum' while others have split the conditions into at least 10 subdivisions. The incidence of different syndromes presenting in one geographical area is shown in Table 1.8.

The categorization is also of limited value from the perspective of therapy. Most of the categories can be treated by most of the available drug therapies (there are exceptions discussed under the relevant sections of this book) and this lack of specificity is disappointing.

## Localization-related epilepsies and syndromes

These epilepsies and syndromes are sometimes referred to as the partial or focal epilepsies.

### Idiopathic localization-related epilepsies and syndromes

Three conditions are included here, including benign childhood epilepsy with centro-temporal spikes (p. 20), which is said to account for up to 15% of childhood epilepsies, and two much less common syndromes, childhood epilepsy with occipital paroxysms (p. 20) and primary reading epilepsy (p. 57). Other genetic and idiopathic syndromes will no doubt be added as knowledge advances, such as the recently described syndrome of dominantly inherited nocturnal frontal lobe epilepsy.

### Symptomatic localization-related epilepsies and syndromes

This category includes the large number of epilepsies due to specific focal cerebral lesions (e.g. tumour, stroke) in which epilepsy is a variable feature. The epilepsies are divided into anatomical site and are described below. Chronic epilepsia partialis continua is also included, rather strangely, in this category.

### Cryptogenic localization-related epilepsies and syndromes

This category has been created to include symptomatic focal epilepsies in which the aetiology is unknown. With increasingly sophisticated neuroimaging techniques, the number of cases falling into this category has become much smaller than when the classification was first proposed.

## Generalized epilepsies and syndromes

These conditions, like the localization-related epilepsies, are divided into subcategories on the basis of presumed aetiology.

### Idiopathic generalized epilepsies and syndromes

The idiopathic generalized epilepsies (also called the primary generalized epilepsies) are genetic conditions in which epilepsy is the major clinical feature. Encompassed within this rubric are a variety of age-related syndromes, although to what extent the subdivisions are specific entities or simply a biological continuum is a matter of controversy. These common conditions are considered in more detail on pp. 17–19.

### Cryptogenic or symptomatic generalized epilepsies

This category includes the epileptic encephalopathies in which epilepsy is a major clinical feature of a diffuse encephalopathic condition. Included in this category are conditions described elsewhere in this book: West syndrome (pp. 22–3), Lennox–Gastaut syndrome (pp. 23–5), epilepsy with myoclonic astatic seizures (p. 12), and epilepsy with myoclonic absences. Also included are the rare myoclonic syndromes and epileptic encephalopathies of infancy. The relative nosological position of many of these

| International classification of epilepsies and epilepsy syndromes: category | Annual incidence per 100,000 population |
|---|---|
| 1.1  Idiopathic localization-related epilepsy | 1.68 |
| 1.2  Symptomatic localization-related epilepsy | 17.11 |
| 2.1  Idiopathic generalized epilepsies | 6.65 |
| 2.2  Symptomatic generalized epilepsies | 1.15 |
| 3  Epilepsies and syndromes undetermined whether focal or generalized | 2.92 |
| 4  Situation-related seizures | 37.33† |

†, Acute symptomatic epilepsy, 25.37; isolated unprovoked seizure, 11.70; television epilepsy, 0.26.

**Table 1.8** Annual incidence of different categories of epilepsy (from prospective study in south-west France).

conditions is often unclear, and there is considerable overlap between the core conditions. Also included here are the epilepsies due to malformations, inborn errors of metabolism, hereditary or congenital disorders.

## Epilepsies and syndromes undetermined as to whether they are focal or generalized

The existence of this category is an acknowledgement that the differentiation between focal and generalized epilepsy is not always easy to make. The category is divided into those syndromes with both focal and generalized seizures, and those without unequivocal generalized or focal features. Included in the first subdivision is a miscellany of 'syndromes', including neonatal seizures—which have a variety of forms which overlap with other categories—infantile myoclonic epilepsy, and electrical status epilepticus during slow wave sleep (ESES) and the Landau–Kleffner syndrome, which are epileptic encephalopathies of unknown pathophysiology. In the second subdivision are those epilepsies with tonic–clonic seizures in which clinical and EEG features do not allow categorization into focal or generalized groups.

## Special syndromes

This category includes the 'situational-related syndromes' (reflex epilepsy, pp. 56–7), febrile seizures (pp. 21–2), isolated seizures (including single seizures and isolated status epilepticus), and the acute symptomatic seizures precipitated by acute toxic or metabolic events (pp. 57–9).

## CLASSIFICATION OF PARTIAL SEIZURES BY ANATOMICAL SITE OF SEIZURE ONSET

From the point of view of epilepsy surgery it is clearly imperative to have a classification based on anatomical localization. Thus, various subclassifications of partial seizures have been devised based on the anatomical site of seizure onset. About 60% of complex partial seizures have their origin in the temporal lobe and about 40% are extratemporal and, although less well studied, a similar pattern probably also applies in the case of simple partial seizures. While the epilepsy arising in each region can have characteristic clinical features, in practice the distinction is often blurred, owing to the non-specific nature of many epileptic symptoms and the tendency for seizures arising in one cortical area to spread rapidly to another.

## Partial seizures arising in the temporal lobe

Sixty per cent of partial seizures arise in the temporal lobes, and these are an important target for surgical therapy. A number of subclassifications exist, the validity of which is open to question. The ambitious subcategorization, for instance, into opercular, temporal polar, basal or limbic

**Table 1.9** Complex partial seizures of mesial temporal lobe origin.

Tripartite seizure pattern (aura, absence, automatism; although only one feature may be present in any individual)

Partial awareness commonly preserved, especially in early stages, and slow evolution of seizure

Auras are common and include visceral, cephalic, gustatory, dysmnestic, affective, perceptual or autonomic auras

Dystonic posturing of the contralateral upper limb and ipsilateral automatisms common

In seizures arising in the dominant temporal lobe, speech arrest during the seizures and dysphasia postictally

Seizures typically last > 2 min, with a slow evolution and gradual onset/offset

Autonomic changes (e.g., pallor, redness and tachycardia) common

Automatisms usually take the form of oro-alimentary (lip smacking, chewing, swallowing), or gestural (e.g. fumbling, fidgeting, repetitive, motor actions, undressing, walking, sexually directed actions, walking, running) and are sometimes prolonged

Postictal confusion common

Seizures tend to cluster

Secondary generalization (to tonic–clonic seizure) infrequent

In patients with hippocampal sclerosis:
- Past history of febrile convulsions
- Onset in mid childhood or adolescence
- Initial response to therapy, lost after several years

types seems seldom to be valid or useful. The distinction into two categories—mesial temporal and lateral temporal—is more widely accepted, even though symptomatology overlaps owing to rapid spread from lateral to mesial cortex (and vice versa). This categorization has some utility in clinical practice (Table 1.9).

## Epilepsy arising in the mesial temporal lobe (limbic epilepsy)

The seizures take the form of simple or complex partial seizures. The simple partial seizures usually last for a matter of seconds only. The complex partial seizures typically evolve relatively gradually (compared with extratemporal seizures) over 1–2 minutes, have an indistinct onset with initially at least some retention of awareness, and last longer than most extratemporal complex partial seizures (2–10 minutes). The typical complex partial seizure of temporal lobe origin has three components.

### Aura

An aura can occur in isolation (in which case, the seizure is categorized as a 'simple partial seizure', or it can be the initial manifestation of a complex partial seizure. Typically, auras of mesial temporal origin are comprised of visceral, autonomic, cephalic, gustatory, dysmnestic or affective symptoms. The most common symptoms are a rising epigastric sensation (the most common), an abnormal sense of taste (almost invariably unpleasant) or smell, *déjà vu*, and a dreamy sensation. Fear is the most common affective symptom, although other complex emotional feelings occur. Common autonomic features in mesial temporal seizures include changes in skin colour (pallor or flushing), blood pressure, heart rate, pupil size and piloerection.

### Absence

Motor arrest or absence (the motionless stare) is prominent especially in the early stages of seizures arising in mesial temporal structures, and more so than in extratemporal lobe epilepsy. Speech usually ceases or is severely reduced if the seizure is in the dominant temporal lobe. In the nondominant lobe, speech may be retained throughout the seizure or meaningless repetitive vocalizations may occur. A 'dreamy' state is highly characteristic.

### Automatisms

The automatisms of mesio-basal temporal lobe epilepsy are typically less violent than in frontal lobe seizures, and are usually oro-alimentary (lip smacking, chewing, swallowing), or gestural (e.g. fumbling, fidgeting, repetitive motor actions, undressing, walking, sexually directed actions, walking, running) and sometimes prolonged.

Postictal confusion and headache are common after a temporal lobe complex partial seizure, and if dysphasia occurs this is a useful lateralizing sign indicating seizure originating in the dominant temporal lobe. Amnesia is the rule for the absence and the automatism. Secondary generalization is much less common than in extratemporal lobe epilepsy. Psychiatric or behavioural disturbances often accompany the epilepsy.

The most common pathology underlying this type of epilepsy is hippocampal sclerosis (Ammon's horn sclerosis, mesial temporal sclerosis). This is characteristically associated with a history of febrile convulsions and the subsequent development of complex partial seizures in late childhood or adolescence. Other aetiologies include dysembryoplastic neuroepithelioma and other benign tumours, arteriovenous malformations, glioma, neuronal migration defects, or gliotic damage as a result of encephalitis.

The EEG in mesial temporal lobe epilepsy often shows anterior or mid-temporal spikes. Superficial or deep sphenoidal electrodes can assist in their detection in some cases. Other changes include intermittent or persisting slow activity over the temporal lobes. The EEG signs can be unilateral or bilateral. Modern magnetic resonance imaging (MRI) will frequently reveal the abnormality underlying the epilepsy.

### Epilepsy arising in the lateral temporal neocortex

There is considerable overlap between the clinical and EEG features of mesial and lateral temporal lobe epilepsy, due presumably to rapid spread and dissemination of discharges between these two anatomical areas. However, differences

**Table 1.10** Complex partial seizures of lateral temporal lobe origin.

Features overlap with those of complex partial seizures of mesial temporal origin (Table 1.9) with the following differences in emphasis:
- Motor arrest and absence less prominent
- Aura more likely to take the form of complex perceptual changes, visual or auditory hallucinations
- Tonic posturing or jerking more common
- More frequent secondary generalization

in degree exist (Table 1.10). Simple auditory phenomena such as humming, buzzing, hissing and roaring may occur if the discharges occur in the superior temporal gyrus (Herschel gyrus); and olfactory sensations, which are usually unpleasant and difficult to define, with seizures in the sylvian region. More complex hallucinatory or illusionary states are produced with seizure discharges in association areas, for instance structured visual hallucinations, complex visual patterns, musical sounds and speech. Illusions of size (macropsia, micropsia), shape, weight, distance or sound can occur. A cephalic aura can also occur in focal temporal lobe seizures, although this is more typical of a frontal lobe focus. Affective, visceral or psychic auras are less common than in mesial temporal lobe epilepsy.

Lateral temporal lobe seizures typically have more motor activity, less prominent motor arrest and may more frequently secondarily generalize because of spread outside the temporal lobe. It is sometimes claimed that consciousness may be preserved for longer than in a typical mesial temporal seizure, but this distinction is seldom useful clinically. The automatisms can be unilateral and have more prominent motor manifestations than in mesial temporal lobe epilepsy. Postictal phenomena, amnesia for the attack and the psychiatric accompaniments are indistinguishable from those of the mesial temporal form.

There is usually a detectable underlying structural pathology, the most common being a glioma, angioma, cavernoma, hamartoma, dysembryoplastic neuroepithelial tumour, other benign tumour, neuronal migration defect and post-traumatic change. There is no association with a history of febrile convulsions. The age of onset of the epilepsy will depend on the aetiology.

The interictal EEG often shows spikes over the temporal region, maximal over the posterior or lateral temporal rather than inferomesial electrodes. MRI will reliably demonstrate the other structural lesions responsible for the epilepsy.

### Epilepsy arising in the frontal lobe

Seizures of frontal lobe origin can take the form of complex partial seizures, simple partial seizures, and secondarily generalized attacks. About 30% of complex partial seizures arise in the frontal lobe.

The clinical and EEG features of the complex partial seizures overlap with those of temporal lobe origin, not

**Table 1.11** Clinical features of complex partial seizures of frontal lobe origin which help differentiation from seizures of temporal lobe origin.

Frequent attacks with clustering

Brief stereotyped seizures (< 30 s)

Nocturnal attacks common

Sudden onset and cessation, with rapid evolution and awareness lost at onset

Absence of complex aura

Version of head or eyes common

Prominent motor activity (posturing, jerking and tonic spasm)

Prominent complex bilateral motor automatisms involving lower limbs (may be bizarre and misdiagnosed as pseudoseizures)

Absence of postictal confusion

Frequent secondary generalization

History of status epilepticus

least because of the rapid spread from seizure foci in the frontal lobe (especially the orbito-frontal cortex) and to the mesial temporal lobe. There are, however, several core features that are strongly suggestive of a frontal lobe origin (Table 1.11).

Typically, complex partial seizures of frontal lobe origin are frequent with a marked tendency to cluster. The attacks are brief, with a sudden onset and offset, without the gradual evolution of the temporal lobe seizure. Some types of frontal lobe seizure occur largely or exclusively during sleep, and in some patients the epilepsy comprises frequent short nocturnal attacks (sometimes known misleadingly as paroxysmal nocturnal dystonia). The tripartite pattern of aura/absence/automatism is seldom as well defined in frontal lobe as in mesial temporal lobe complex partial seizures. A brief non-specific 'cephalic aura' can occur, but not the rich range of auras of temporal lobe epilepsy. The absence (motor arrest) is usually short, and may be obscured by the prominent motor signs of the automatism. There are marked qualitative differences between frontal and temporal lobe automatisms, although these are often not specific enough to be reliably of diagnostic value. Frontal lobe automatisms are typically gestural, especially comprising bilateral leg movements (e.g. cycling, stepping, kicking) rather than oro-alimentary. The behaviour in the automatism is often highly excited, violent or bizarre and not infrequently leads to a misdiagnosis of non-epileptic attacks (pseudoseizures). In other frontal seizures, posturing or muscle spasms predominate. Urinary incontinence is frequent in frontal lobe complex partial seizures, as is vocalization. The automatisms are usually short, with minimal postictal confusion, and recovery is usually rapid. Frontal lobe partial seizures have a more marked tendency to evolve into secondarily generalized seizures than do those of temporal lobe origin, and the evolution is also more rapid. There is also commonly a history of status epilepticus, both of the tonic–clonic and non-convulsive types.

The manifestations of complex partial seizures from different frontal lobe regions may differ, but because of rapid spread of discharges, there is considerable overlap between types, and attempts to classify according to site of origin have been uniformly unsatisfactory. Various patterns of frontal lobe partial seizures occur, many with marked motor manifestations (clonic jerking or posturing) either bilateral or contralateral. Sometimes consciousness is retained in the presence of bilateral limb jerking, and these attacks are commonly misdiagnosed as non-epileptic attacks. Apparently generalized tonic–clonic seizures, without lateralizing features, are particularly characteristic of seizures arising in the cingulate or dorsolateral cortex, but can occur from other frontal lobe locations. Version of the head and eyes is common in many types of frontal lobe (and less frequently in temporal lobe epilepsy), and is sometimes the only seizure manifestation ('versive seizures'). When version occurs in full consciousness at the onset of a seizure, this is useful evidence of a focus in the contralateral frontal dorsolateral convexity, but in other situations the direction of version is of little lateralizing value. Occasionally, version is so marked that the patient actually circles round. Drop attacks are not uncommon in partial seizures arising especially medially or anteriorly. Autonomic features are common in frontal lobe epilepsy, and may occasionally be an isolated manifestation of an epileptic focus. Dysphasia in frontal seizures is often accompanied by versive or clonic movements. In epileptic discharges from the perisylvian areas, the aphasia is often preceded by numbness in the mouth and throat, or salivation, swallowing or laryngeal symptoms. Mesial frontal foci can result in absence seizures which can be almost indistinguishable from generalized absences.

Seizures arising in the dorsolateral convexity sometimes take the form of a sudden assumption of an abnormal posture (usually bilateral and asymmetrical) with or without loss of consciousness, lasting a second or two only and which cluster, with numerous attacks over a few minutes.

The scalp EEG in frontal lobe epilepsy is often rather disappointing. This is partly because the large area of frontal cortex is covered by relatively few scalp electrodes and also because much of the frontal cortex is hidden in sulci or on the medial or inferior surfaces of the frontal lobe which are distant from the dorsolaterally placed electrodes. Many frontal lobe seizures either fail to show a focus, or only demonstrate widespread and poorly localized foci. Apparently generalized irregular or bilateral and synchronous spike-wave or polyspike discharges with anterior predominance can occur. Sometimes, the interictal and ictal EEGs show non-specific generalized slow activity only.

### Epilepsy arising in the central (peri-rolandic) region

The primary manifestations are motor or sensory (Table 1.12). The motor features can take the form of jerking, dystonic spasm, posturing or occasionally paralysis,

**Table 1.12** Partial seizures of central origin.

Often no loss of consciousness (simple partial seizure)
Contralateral clonic jerking (which may or may not march)
Contralateral tonic spasm
Posturing, which is often bilateral, and version of head and eyes
Speech arrest and involvement of bulbar musculature (producing anarthria or choking, gurgling sounds)
Contralateral sensory symptoms
Short, frequently recurring attacks which cluster
Prolonged seizures with slow progression, and episodes of epilepsia partialis continua
Postictal Todd paralysis

often with clear consciousness (i.e. simple partial seizures). The jerking can affect any muscle group, usually unilaterally, the exact site depending on the part of the precentral gyrus involved in the seizure, and the jerks may 'march' (the Jacksonian march) from one part of the body to another as the discharge spreads over the motor cortex. The seizure discharge may remain limited to one small segment for long periods of time, and when it does spread it is typically very slow. The clonic jerks consist of brief tetanic contractions of all the muscles that co-operate in a single movement. The seizures spread through the cortex, producing clonic movements according to the sequence of cortical representation. A seizure that begins in the hand usually passes up the arm and down the leg and if it begins in the foot it passes up the leg and down the arm. A seizure beginning in the face is most likely to originate in the mouth because of the correspondingly large area of cortical representation. In seizures arising anywhere in the central region, head and eye version is common. Arrest of speech (anarthria) may occur if the motor area of the muscles of articulation is affected (phonatory seizure) and is usually associated with spasm or clonic movements of the jaw. After focal seizure activity, there may be localized paralysis in the affected limbs (Todd paralysis), which is usually short-lived.

If the seizure is initiated in or evolves to affect supplementary motor areas, posturing of the arms may develop, classically with adversive head and eye deviation, abduction and external rotation of the contralateral arm and flexion at the elbows. There may also be posturing of the legs, and speech arrest or stereotyped vocalizations. Consciousness is usually maintained unless secondary generalization occurs. The classical posture is named by Penfield the 'fencing posture' (resembling as it does the *en garde* position), but other postures also occur. The posturing is often bilateral and asymmetric. The fencing posture or fragments of it can also occur in seizures originating in various other frontal and temporal brain regions, presumably due to spread of the seizure discharge to the supplementary motor cortex. In contrast to Jacksonian seizures, supplementary motor

area seizures are often very brief, occur frequently and in clusters, sometimes hundreds each day, and are sometimes also precipitated by startle.

Somatosensory or special sensory manifestations (simple hallucinations) occur if the seizure discharge originates in, or spreads to, the post-central region. Typically, these take the form of tingling, numbness, an electrical shock-like feeling, a tickling or crawling feeling, burning, pain or a feeling of heat. These symptoms are usually accompanied by jerking, posturing or spasms as the epileptic discharges usually spread anteriorly. The sensory symptoms may remain localized or march in a Jacksonian manner. Ictal pain is occasionally a prominent symptom and can be severe and poorly localized.

Interictal and ictal scalp EEGs in focal epilepsy in central regions are often normal as the focus may be small and buried within the central gyri.

## Epilepsy arising in the parietal and occipital lobes

Focal seizures arise from foci in these locations less commonly than from frontal, central or temporal lobe regions. The typical manifestations of the seizures are subjective sensory and visual disturbances (Table 1.13). Additional features are common owing to spread to adjacent cortical regions.

Parietal lobe seizures typically comprise sensory manifestations. These may be tingling or a feeling of electricity which can be confined or march in a Jacksonian manner. Sensations of sinking, choking or nausea can occur. There may be accompanying loss of tone or a sensation of paralysis. Illusions of bodily distortion are characteristic, such as a feeling of swelling or shrinking, or lengthening or shortening particularly affecting the tongue, mouth or extremities. Ictal pain typically, but not exclusively, occurs in parietal seizures. Ictal apraxia, alexia and agnosia have been

**Table 1.13** Parietal and occipital lobe epilepsy.

Somatosensory symptoms (e.g. tingling, numbness or more complex sensations—may or may not march)
Sensation of inability to move
Sexual sensations
Illusions of change in body size/shape
Vertigo
Gustatory seizures
Elementary visual hallucinations (e.g. flashes, colours, shapes, patterns)
Complex visual hallucinations (e.g. objects, scenes, autoscopia, often moving)
Head turning (usually adversive, with sensation of following or looking at the visual hallucinations)
Visual–spatial distortions (e.g. of size [micropsia, macropsia], shape, position)
Loss or dulling of vision (amaurosis)
Eyelid fluttering, blinking, nystagmus

reported. Sexual feelings can occur sometimes with erection or ejaculation. Gustatory seizures have their origin in the suprasylvian region (adjacent to the mouth and throat primary sensory region). Ictal vertigo also originates in the suprasylvian region. Transient postictal sensory deficits or spatial disorientation occur.

Seizures from the occipital, parieto-occipital, and temporal-occipital cortex are usually characterized by visual symptoms. Elementary visual hallucinations (sensations of colours, shapes, flashes and patterns) are most common, which can be intermittent, stationary or appear to move across the visual field and to grow. More complex stereotyped hallucinations/illusions can take the form of scenes, animals, people (including self-images), or of topographical or spatial distortion, alterations of size and shape, perseveration or repetition of visual objects, or the break-up of visual objects or movement. Vision commonly blacks out in occipital lobe seizures, one of the few examples of negative epileptic symptomatology. The blindness typically is accompanied by the development of illusions of lights or colours. Forced head and eye turning are common, with the patient believing that the visual hallucination is being tracked voluntarily. Rapid blinking or eyelid flutter are frequent in some types of occipital seizures. Headache and nausea are common, and the attacks are not infrequently misdiagnosed as migraine. In the benign occipital epilepsies (pp. 20–1), the seizures can be very prolonged, but most focal seizures in adults last seconds or minutes only. Studies have shown that there are no clinical or EEG features that help differentiate epilepsy arising in the medial or lateral occipital cortex. Occasionally, occipital seizures denote mitochondrial disease, Lafora body disease, coeliac disease or metabolic disorders.

The EEG in occipital or parietal epilepsy can be normal or show appropriate focal discharges, although often the epileptic disturbance is poorly localized without correlation to the ictal symptoms. Occipital spike-wave is characteristic of some types of focal occipital seizures, which can be confused with primary generalized epilepsy.

## THE AGE-RELATED EPILEPSY SYNDROMES

There are a number of syndromes identified in the *ILAE Classification of the Epilepsies and Epilepsy Syndromes* that are common, age-related and which either have no specific identifiable cause or which can result from a variety of different identifiable conditions. The most important or most common are described here. It must be recognized that there is overlap between some of these syndromes and there is considerable disagreement about the exact nosology. It is assumed that the cryptogenic or idiopathic cases have a complex polygenic genetic basis, although environmental influences also play a part. Some of these syndromes are highly age-specific and assume characteristic clinical forms regardless of cause. These may be best conceptualized as generic age-related responses of disordered brain function or development.

### Neonatal seizures

The clinical and EEG features, the cause and the pathophysiology of seizures in the neonatal period differ from those in later life. Clinical signs are necessarily confined to motor features and are usually focal or multifocal, reflecting the immature synaptic connections in the neonatal brain. The EEG changes are variable and non-specific. Seizures can take the form of tonic attacks, clonic seizures, unilateral focal seizures, electrographic seizures without overt clinical changes and so-called subtle seizures. The seizures can have mild or atypical features such as grimacing, staring, eye movements, posturing or pedalling movements. Neonatal seizures occur in about 1% of all infants, with a higher frequency (up to 23%) in premature babies. While there is no doubt that most neonatal seizures are 'epileptic', some subtle and some tonic seizures are not associated with any EEG changes and may be subcortical in origin owing to abnormal brainstem release mechanisms. There are a large variety of potential causes, the most common being hypoxic-ischaemic encephalopathy, intracranial haemorrhage, neonatal infection and metabolic disorders (especially hypocalcaemia, hypomagnesaemia and hypoglycaemia). The development of neonatal seizures is an ominous sign, not only because they often indicate cerebral disease but also because the seizures themselves possibly damage the developing brain. The prognosis depends largely on the underlying cause. Overall, the immediate mortality rate is about 15%, 37% develop neurological deficits and only 48% develop normally. Prognosis is worse in premature infants, especially those with a gestational age under 31 weeks.

If the seizures are considered non-epileptic, antiepileptic drug treatment may not be indicated. Indeed, medication may worsen the phenomenon by decreasing the level of cortical inhibition over subcortical structures. Whether genuine (cortical) but slight (subtle) epileptic seizures require treatment is uncertain, especially in infants who are not paralysed for artificial ventilation. Not uncommonly, such seizure manifestations remit spontaneously after days or weeks and the usefulness of treatment in this situation is difficult to assess. Opinions vary about the need to treat infants with EEG evidence of seizure activity without overt clinical signs. There is also disagreement about the duration of therapy, although most would aim for as short a period as possible. Many neonatal seizures are self-limiting and over-long treatment carries its own risks.

### Idiopathic generalized epilepsy

The term idiopathic generalized epilepsy (IGE; also known as primary generalized epilepsy) is used to denote a very common and important group of conditions, with a probable genetic basis, and in which there is a characteristic clinical and electrographic pattern. It has been estimated that patients with IGE account for about 10–20% of all those with epilepsy. The identification of the genetic basis of IGE has proved elusive. This was the first 'pure' epilepsy in which an intensive genetic search was undertaken, on the basis that there may be a single underlying gene (albeit with markedly variable penetrance). None was found, and it is now believed that the syndromes of IGE have a polygenic basis, but disappointingly still no common susceptibility gene has been found. A contentious and unresolved issue, which itself may have confounded the search for genes, is the extent to which the 'syndrome' can or should be sub-categorized. Nowhere in the study of epilepsy is there more divergence of opinion between those who view this epilepsy type as a 'biological continuum' (possibly with a unitary genetic mechanism) and those who subdivide according to clinical pattern. It is not currently possible to know where nosological reality exists. Table 1.14 shows commonly proposed subdivisions, but even in this matter, different authorities subdivide to different extents. It is a dearly held expectation that, when the genetic basis is clarified, a more definitive subclassification will become apparent based on genotypic–phenotypic correlation.

Core clinical features shared to a greater or lesser extent by these syndromes (at least those with onset in later child-hood or early adult life) are shown in Table 1.15. The treat-ment of the idiopathic generalized epilepsies is described on p. 85.

### Childhood absence epilepsy

Childhood absence epilepsy (pyknolepsy) appears in the early and middle years of childhood (peak age 6–7 years), more commonly in girls than in boys and usually in children without learning disability or other neurological problems. It accounts for between 1 and 3% of newly dia-gnosed epilepsies and up to 10% of childhood epilepsies. The absence seizures (see p. 7) usually last 10–15 seconds, and are so brief that in many cases they pass unrecognized for long periods. Many can occur in a day, and the seizures

**Table 1.14** Subdivisions of idiopathic generalized epilepsy.

Benign neonatal convulsions
Benign myoclonus epilepsy of infancy
Myoclonic-astatic epilepsy
Epilepsy with myoclonic absences
Childhood absence epilepsy (pyknolepsy)
Juvenile absence epilepsy
Juvenile myoclonic epilepsy (impulsive petit mal)
Epilepsy with grand mal seizures on awakening
Absence epilepsy with peri-oral myoclonia

**Table 1.15** Clinical features shared by different subdivisions of idiopathic generalized epilepsy (IGE).

Onset in childhood or early adult life
Positive family history
Generalized seizure types—myoclonus, generalized absence (petit mal) and generalized tonic–clonic seizures
Normal EEG background
Paroxysms of generalized EEG discharges, either 3 Hz spike and wave or polyspike bursts, often exacerbated by over-breathing and photosensitivity
A diurnal pattern of seizure recurrence, with seizures especially on waking and during sleep
Normal intellect and low co-morbidity
Absence of identifiable underlying structural aetiology
Excellent response to therapy with sodium valproate

tend to cluster. The loss of consciousness is usually com-plete, and the patient is unaware that a seizure has occurred. Eyes, if closed at onset, open after 2–3 seconds. The seizures can be induced by hyperventilation. The classical EEG pat-tern is monotonous, generalized 3 Hz spike-wave. In a series of 194 patients with typical clinical features and EEG, approximately one-third also had generalized tonic–clonic seizures (GTCS) at some point and absence status occurred in 15%. The prognosis is good, and rapid remission on therapy is expected in 80% or more of patients. When followed up after 18 years of age, only approximately 20% of previously diagnosed patients are still having seizures. Prognosis is better in those with onset of seizures before 12 years of age, who have a more rapid response to therapy, a low chance of GTCS and a high remission rate. GTCS can develop, usually after years of exclusively absence seizures and usually in those whose response to therapy is incomplete. The nosological boundaries between this and the other syndromes of IGE are indistinct, and how often tonic–clonic seizures occur depends on the inclusiveness of the diagnostic criteria; the frequency is reported to be between 3 and 35%. The genetic basis is unknown in spite of serious attempts to identify susceptibility genes.

*Phantom absence* is a term used to describe the phenom-enon of short-lived EEG bursts of spike and wave without any obvious clinical sign. These may be quite common in some IGE syndromes and also seem to be associated with a relatively high incidence of absence status. There may be very subtle clinical signs, but sometimes even quite pro-longed EEG bursts seem to occur without any noticeable clinical change. It is considered by some that *phantom absences* are particularly common in patients with the syndrome of epilepsy with grand mal seizures (GTCS) on awakening (see p. 19) and others that the occurrence of phantom absence and tonic–clonic seizures is itself a separate syndrome (IGE with phantom absences).

### Juvenile myoclonic epilepsy

Juvenile myoclonic epilepsy (JME; also known as impulsive petit mal and Janz syndrome) is the most common subtype of idiopathic generalized epilepsy, and accounts for up to 10% of all epilepsies. The characteristic seizures are brief myoclonic jerks, occurring in the first hour or so after waking, and usually in bursts. These are sudden, shock-like jerks, affecting mainly the shoulders and arms, usually but not always symmetrically. It may not be clear whether consciousness was retained or lost. In 80% of cases, the myoclonus develops between the ages of 12 and 18 years (and always between 6 and 25 years), but may be unrecognized initially and taken to be early morning clumsiness. In about 80% of cases, GTCS also occur, usually months or years after the onset of myoclonus, and it is these that often lead to the diagnosis. It is worth enquiring specifically about myoclonus in anyone presenting with generalized epilepsy. The tonic–clonic seizures are usually infrequent (average two per year). About one-third of patients also develop typical absence seizures (usually very brief, lasting 2–5 seconds) and again usually on waking. Almost invariably, the absence seizures occur in patients with both myoclonus and tonic–clonic seizures. About 5% of patients exhibit strong photosensitivity, and the myoclonus (and other seizures) can be precipitated by photic stimuli. The seizures (myoclonus and GTCS) often have other clear precipitants such as lack of sleep, alcohol, hypoglycaemia and poor compliance with medication. Myoclonic jerks may evolve into myoclonic status, and the tonic–clonic seizures are also often preceded by increasing myoclonus. About 50% of cases show interictal abnormalities—3 Hz spike-wave or faster polyspike-wave at 4–6 Hz—which can be symmetrical or asymmetrical. The background EEG is normal. In about one-third of untreated cases, EEG shows a photo-paroxysmal response. Intelligence is normal and there is usually no other neurological or other co-morbidity. It has been claimed that patients show typical personality traits, but whether this is really the case is unclear. Complete response to treatment can be expected in 80–90% of cases, but lifelong therapy may be needed. Appropriate drug therapy is important (see p. 85) as carbamazepine, vigabatrin, tiagabine and phenytoin can exacerbate myoclonus. Imaging is normal, although there is an isolated unconfirmed report of quantitative MRI cortical volume change. The genetics of JME have been controversial. Initial reports of a linkage to chromosome 6 have not been substantiated consistently. Recently, a mutation in a gene for the γ-aminobutyric acid A (GABA-A) receptor has been reported in a family with autosomal dominant inheritance of JME, but JME is now generally assumed usually to have polygenic inheritance. A family history of epilepsy is found in about 25% of cases, and in about 5% of close relatives (of whom one-third have JME, and most of the others have other IGE subtypes). The risk of epilepsy in offspring is about 5%.

### Other IGE variants with myoclonus

Other types of myoclonic IGE subtypes are less well defined, and their nosological position less clear-cut. Myoclonic absences occur at a younger age, have a male predominance, an EEG initially at least indistinguishable from that of typical absence epilepsy, are associated with intellectual disturbance, and are much more resistant to drug therapy; other seizure types evolve in two-thirds of cases. Eyelid myoclonia with or without absence is a photosensitive IGE variant characterized by very short attacks comprising jerking of the eyelids and upward deviation of the eyes. There may or may not be associated absence seizures. The peak age of onset is 6 years, there is usually a strong family history and a marked female preponderance. Many attacks per day can occur, and the children may induce attacks, which are associated with a pleasurable sensation, by photic stimulation. Tonic–clonic seizures develop in adolescence or adult life. The EEG shows 4–6 Hz polyspike-wave which can be triggered by eye opening and also marked photosensitivity. Benign myoclonic epilepsy is a rare condition, occurring in infancy or early childhood, with spontaneous remission in most cases and without long-term sequelae.

Myoclonic-astatic epilepsy (myoclonic astatic petit mal) is an ill-defined syndrome with myoclonic and astatic (atonic) seizures, and an EEG signature of fast (> 3 Hz) spike-wave. Repeated episodes of non-convulsive status epilepticus are reported in severe cases, and usually associated with intellectual regression qualifying the condition as an epileptic encephalopathy. Young children often have seizures with falls, which can have serious consequences. The EEG changes reported in different series are also variable. The delineation of this symptom complex as a 'syndrome' is rather muddled, and cases that overlap with benign myoclonic epilepsy on the one hand and the Lennox–Gastaut syndrome on the other are reported. Idiopathic and symptomatic forms are proposed, and severity and outcome with respect both to epilepsy and to cognitive function are very variable. However, severe epilepsy with falls and episodes of non-convulsive status requires expert attention, and a 'syndrome' tag assists communication. Recently, mis-sense mutations on *SCN1A* and *GABRG2* genes have been described in children with a phenotype consistent with myoclonic-astatic epilepsy, and advances in an understanding of the genetic bases of the early childhood epilepsies may help clarify the basis of this syndrome.

### Epilepsy with grand mal seizures (GTCS) on waking

This condition overlaps considerably with other generalized epilepsies, especially with JME, in which most affected people also have GTCS on awakening. The EEG pattern is generalized spike-wave. Whether this syndrome represents a discrete entity or simply part of the spectrum of other forms of IGE has been the subject of discussion for several decades, without clear resolution.

## Benign partial epilepsy with centro-temporal spikes

Benign partial epilepsy with centro-temporal spikes (BECTS; also known as rolandic epilepsy or benign epilepsy with rolandic spikes) is the most common 'idiopathic' epilepsy syndrome, accounting for perhaps 15% of all epilepsies (Table 1.16). The peak age of onset is 5–8 years and over 80% of cases have onset between 4 and 10 years. It is likely that the condition is the result of an age-related genetically determined neuronal hyperexcitability in the rolandic area, resulting in characteristic giant EEG spikes and in seizures, although it is estimated that less than 10% of children with the EEG disturbance actually have seizures. The seizures are infrequent—25% of cases have only a single attack and 50% about five attacks in all. Less than 20% of cases have 20 or more seizures, and the total duration of seizure activity is 3 years or more in only 10%. About 50% of children have seizures only at night, about 40% both during the day and at night, and in 10% seizures occur exclusively during the day. The daytime seizures usually occur when the child is tired or bored (e.g. on a long car journey). The seizures are highly characteristic, usually beginning with spasm and clonic jerking of one side of the face and throat muscles. In many cases, the seizures sometimes evolve to secondarily generalized tonic–clonic attacks. The motor features may include speech arrest, a gurgling or guttural sound and profuse salivation. There are also often sensory symptoms involving one side of the mouth and the throat. The arm or rarely the legs can be involved. In most cases consciousness is preserved until the seizures secondarily generalize.

The EEG shows focal spikes which originate most often in the centrotemporal regions, although on repeated EEG recordings, the spikes often wander. The wave form and distribution are characteristic. In a small number of patients (probably less than 10%, although figures vary), generalized spike-wave is seen. There are no associated neurological disturbances and intellect is normal. The epilepsy remits in almost all cases, usually by the age of 12 years, without long-term sequelae. It is assumed that there is a genetic basis to the condition, although no genetic abnormality has been consistently described, and polygenic inheritance is likely. One family has been described with autosomal dominant inheritance and linkage to chromosome 15q14. The family history is positive for seizures of various types in 40% of cases. The treatment of BECTS is described on p. 84.

The prognosis of the typical condition is good and neurological development and cognitive function are generally normal and the seizures remit in more than 95% of cases. There are, however, children in whom the condition appears to evolve into other seizure syndromes and who develop intractable seizures and neuropsychological deficit.

The overlap even of BECTS, which seems a relatively specific symptom complex, and other syndromes is an illustration of the boundary problems that exist in all epilepsy syndromes. Transitional cases have been labelled atypical benign partial epilepsy (ABPE) or pseudo-Lennox–Gastaut syndrome, and some authorities consider BECTS, ESES and Landau–Kleffner syndrome to be part of a spectrum. Atypical features include bouts of status epilepticus, atypical absence seizures, atonic seizures, and cognitive and behavioural impairment combined with an EEG pattern of slow spike-wave. Similarly, although patients with BECTS are lesion-free, patients who manifest the same phenotype have been shown to have hippocampal atrophy, cortical dysplasia, lesions of corpus callosum, porencephalic cysts and toxoplasmosis.

## Other benign partial epilepsy syndromes

There are a number of other predominantly childhood syndromes with partial epilepsy, which are best divided according to anatomical origin of the seizures. Of these, the benign epilepsies arising in the occipital lobe are best delineated. Their treatment is described on p. 84.

### Childhood epilepsy with occipital paroxysms (benign occipital epilepsy; Gastaut type—idiopathic childhood occipital epilepsy)

This is a well-defined syndrome, with mean age of onset of 6 years, in which seizures occur with prominent visual symptomatology, including hemianopia and amaurosis, abstract and complex structured visual hallucinations, eye deviation and prominent postictal headaches with nausea and vomiting. There may be secondary generalization. The EEG shows prominent occipital epileptiform spike-wave activity which appears after eye closure and is suppressed by eye opening. The condition has an excellent prognosis with full remission in most cases. The condition needs to be differentiated from migraine and also from symptomatic occipital epilepsies, which include those due to mitochondrial disease (Alpers disease, MELAS), coeliac disease or cortical dysplasia. Seizures show a complete response to carbamaze-pine in over 90% of cases, and the prognosis is excellent. However, some patients require long-term treatment.

**Table 1.16** Benign epilepsy with centro-temporal spikes (BECTS).

15% of all childhood epilepsy
Age of onset 5–10 years
Simple partial seizures with frequent secondary generalization
Partial seizures involve the face, oropharynx and upper limb
Seizures typically during sleep and infrequent
No other neurological features; normal intelligence
Family history
EEG shows typical centro-temporal spikes
Excellent response to antiepileptic drugs
Excellent prognosis with remission by mid-teenage years

### Early onset benign occipital epilepsy (synonym: Panayiotopoulos syndrome)

This is another syndrome with age of onset between 1 and 14 years (mean 4–5 years). Estimates of prevalence have ranged from 0 to 0.6% of all children with epilepsy, and in one study it accounted for 28% of all benign focal epilepsies of childhood. Panayiotopoulos considers the condition to be due to diffuse maturation-related epileptogenicity activating emetic centres and the hypothalamus. The clinical presentation is distinctive. In the core syndrome, seizures take the form of eye deviation, nausea and vomiting, with subsequent evolution into clonic hemiconvulsions in some cases. They are often nocturnal and awareness may or nay not be altered. Other autonomic features occur including incontinence of urine, pallor, hyperventilation and headache. Typically, the seizures are prolonged, often lasting hours, and are therefore classified as episodes of status epilepticus (taking the form of absence or autonomic status epilepticus). Despite this high incidence of status, the prognosis of the syndrome is excellent and at least 50% of patients have only a total of 1–5 attacks. The interictal EEG shows occipital spikes, with a morphology similar to that in BECTS, and can be continuous. The EEG discharges are abolished by eye opening (the fixation-off phenomenon) and continue to be seen for years after the cessation of seizures. The boundaries of the syndrome are less well defined than in other syndromes. Some cases are included in which the prolonged seizures consist only of vomiting, or of syncopal symptoms, or prominent autonomic symptoms. This syndrome is often misdiagnosed as migraine, and also needs to be differentiated from other occipital epilepsies. The epilepsy usually remits over time without adverse sequaelae, although a minority of cases evolve to other forms of epilepsy. Usually, continuous antiepileptic drug treatment is not needed but a small night-time dose of carbamazepine, valproate or benzodiazepines will usually suppress all seizures. In the acute phase when seizures are prolonged, rectal diazepam should be given. Parents should be counselled about the condition and the acute management of the seizures.

### Other benign focal epilepsies

Epilepsy with occipital calcifications is an occipital epilepsy syndrome in which there is more severe epilepsy and a poorer outcome. Almost all cases are associated with coeliac disease, which may be demonstrable only on jejunal biopsy. Other rarer but interesting childhood benign focal syndromes have been described, sometimes in a handful of families only, and include: benign partial epilepsy in infancy, idiopathic photosensitive occipital lobe epilepsy, idiopathic frontal lobe epilepsy, familial temporal lobe epilepsy, autosomal dominant rolandic epilepsy with speech dyspraxia, and benign focal seizures in adolescents.

### Febrile seizures

Febrile seizures are defined as epileptic events that occur in the context of an acute rise in body temperature, usually in children between 3 months and 5 years of age, in whom there is no evidence of intracranial infection or other defined intracranial cause (Table 1.17). They are common. About 2–5% of children (7% in Japan and up to 14% in the Mariana Islands) will have at least one attack, and it has been estimated that between 19 and 41 per 1000 infants with fever will convulse. The first febrile seizure happens in the second year of life in 50% and in the first 3 years in 90%. Four per cent occur before 6 months and 6% after 6 years of age. Males are slightly more likely to have febrile seizures than females. In over 85%, the seizures are generalized and are usually brief, and never take the form of infantile spasm or myoclonic seizures. Febrile seizures are usually subdivided into simple and complex forms. Complex febrile seizures are those that last more than 15 minutes and have strongly unilateral features or those that recur within a single illness. Up to one-third of all febrile convulsions are classifiable as complex. The important risk factors seem to be an acute temperature rise, and viral infection is the underlying cause of the fever in 80%. The seizure usually occurs early, almost always within the first 24 hours, of the viral illness, and in about one-quarter of cases is the first recognisable sign of the illness. Seventy-five per cent of children affected have a temperature above 39º C. There is a family history of febrile convulsions in at least 25% of cases, and some families have an autosomal dominant pattern of inheritance. In these families, linkage to 8q, 2q23–24, 19p and 5q14–15 has been described. Similarly, one population study has shown an association between febrile convulsions and polymorphisms in the *SCN1A* gene, and similar abnormalities have been found in families with generalized epilepsy with febrile seizures (GEFS+). Other genes implicated in GEFS+ are *SCN1B* and

**Table 1.17** Febrile seizures.

| |
|---|
| 2–5% of all children |
| Peak age of onset 2–4 years |
| 10–20% of children have existing neurodevelopmental problems |
| Probably genetic basis to some cases |
| Tonic–clonic seizures |
| Usually at onset of fever |
| 35% children have a second febrile seizure and 15% a third (recurrence more likely with early age of onset, positive family history) |
| Prognosis worse in complex seizures (prolonged or focal; 30% of all febrile seizures) |
| May induce hippocampal sclerosis and subsequent temporal lobe epilepsy |
| Risk of subsequent epilepsy small (2–10%; more likely if onset < 13 months, complex convulsion or existing neurodevelopmental problems) |

*GABRG2* (see p. 27). The empirical risk for further offspring is 10–15% if there is one affected sibling, rising to 50% if a parent and sibling have a history of febrile seizures.

These essentially benign seizures need to be differentiated from the 5–10% of first seizures with fever in which the seizure is in fact due to viral or bacterial meningitis, and other cases where the fever lights up an existing latent predisposition to epilepsy. In neither of these situations should the term 'febrile convulsion' be used, as both carry significantly different clinical implications.

Obviously, in all cases, the aetiology of the fever should be established. Febrile seizures occurring before 6 months of age particularly raise the possibility of bacterial meningitis and urgent lumbar puncture is indicated. In older children, investigation depends on the clinical circumstances, but may include lumbar puncture or brain scanning.

The outcome of febrile seizures has been the subject of intensive study, which has concentrated on three aspects: the risk of recurrent febrile convulsions, the risk of neurological or developmental deficit, and the risk of subsequent non-febrile epilepsy. Although parents, on witnessing the first febrile convulsion, almost invariably feel that the child is about to die, the mortality risk due to febrile convulsions is negligible.

About 35% of susceptible children will have a second febrile seizure and 15% three or more. Recurrence is more common if the initial convulsion was at a young age, in those in whom the convulsion occurred at a relatively low temperature (below 39° C), and in those with prolonged initial convulsions. However, even in recurrent attacks, the outcome in relation to longer-term neurological function is usually excellent. In fact, the mental and neurological development of children after a febrile convulsion is usually entirely normal, providing there were no pre-existing developmental problems. In about 10–20% of children, subsequent neurodevelopment problems are noted, but these usually reflect pre-existing problems and are not due to the convulsions. There are, however, occasional exceptions after prolonged convulsions, which can sometimes result in acute cerebral damage (the HHE—hemiplegia, hemiatrophy, epilepsy—syndrome typically develops after febrile status). These effects are apparent in the immediate aftermath of the prolonged seizure, and the longer the duration of the attack, the more likely is cerebral damage. It is for this reason that seizures continuing for 15 minutes or more require emergency therapy.

The occurrence of febrile seizures is also associated with the later development of subsequent epilepsy. The risk of epilepsy is small—about 2–10% in children with a history of febrile seizures, compared with 0.5% in those who have not had a febrile seizure. The risk is higher in those with pre-existing neurodevelopmental dysfunction, and in some of these cases the febrile seizure is simply the first manifestation of an existing predisposition to epilepsy. It is also said, albeit on rather poor evidence, that the risk of subsequent epilepsy is somewhat higher after complex febrile seizures (4–12%), compared with single febrile seizures (2%).

It has been proposed that febrile convulsions cause hippocampal sclerosis and, by this mechanism, subsequent temporal lobe epilepsy. Certainly, at least 50% of those with temporal lobe epilepsy and MRI evidence of hippocampal sclerosis have a history of febrile convulsions, although distinguishing cause from consequence is difficult. However, several case reports exist in which serial MRI scanning after a febrile convulsion has demonstrated the development of hippocampal atrophy. There is also indisputable animal experimental data showing that focal status epilepticus induced in the hippocampus can result in subsequent hippocampal damage. There can be no doubt, therefore, that hippocampal damage (and subsequent temporal lobe epilepsy) can result from severe febrile convulsions, but how frequently this occurs is unknown.

However, because of the risk of immediate damage and the possible risk of late epilepsy, febrile seizures should be treated as a medical emergency. The principles of treatment are described on p. 82.

## West syndrome

West syndrome (Table 1.18) is a severe epileptic encephalopathy, with an incidence of 1–2 per 4000 live births, and a family history in 7–17%. The condition is defined by the occurrence of a typical form of epileptic seizure (infantile spasm) and EEG (hypsarrhythmia). The infantile spasms take the form of sudden, generally bilateral and symmetrical contractions of the muscles of the neck, trunk or limbs. The spasms grow in frequency as the condition evolves, and at its peak, seizures occur hundreds of times a day. The spasms show a strong tendency to cluster, with intensity waxing and waning during the cluster. In the most common type, the flexor muscles are predominantly affected, and the attack takes the form of sudden flexion with arms and legs held in adduction (the so-called salaam attacks). Extensor spasms are less common, and are rarely the sole type of seizure. Mixed flexor–extensor spasms commonly occur.

**Table 1.18** West syndrome.

| |
|---|
| 1–2 cases per 4000 live births |
| Age-specific epileptic encephalopathy |
| Variety of causes |
| Age of onset 4–8 months |
| Seizures take the form of infantile spasms (salaam attacks) |
| EEG shows hypsarrhythmia pattern |
| Response to corticosteroids or vigabatrin |
| Spasms remit on therapy or spontaneously |
| Prognosis poor. 5% die in acute phase. Learning difficulty and continuing epilepsy are common sequels |
| 20% cryptogenic, 80% symptomatic |

Severity is variable, and slight spasms consisting of head nodding and upward eye deviation or 'shrugging' of the shoulders are often overlooked, and it is a common experience to find that, when recorded on video-EEG, the actual number of attacks is usually far in excess of that reported by parents or carers. The stereotyped and repetitive nature is important diagnostically, and even mild but repetitive movements in an infant should raise diagnostic suspicion. About 5–10% of spasms are unilateral, and these are invariably associated with focal cerebral pathology.

The peak age of onset is 4–6 months, and the spasms rarely develop before the age of 3 months. Ninety per cent develop in the first year of life. The EEG shows the characteristic pattern of hypsarrhythmia in its fully developed form. Modified EEG forms frequently occur.

In the past up to one-third of patients who developed West syndrome were thought to have normal neurodevelopment prior to the onset of infantile spasms (idiopathic or cryptogenic cases). However, with advances in MRI, underlying dysplasia and congenital anomalies are found in increasing proportions of cases previously categorized as cryptogenic. Positron emission tomography (PET) studies furthermore show unifocal or multifocal abnormalities in over 95% of cases, which in the presence of normal MRI are claimed to be due to subtle dysplastic lesions. A wide variety of condition have been reported to cause this encephalopathy (Table 1.19), the most common of which are: tuberous sclerosis (7–25% of all cases), neonatal ischaemia and infections (about 15% of all cases), lissencephaly and pachygyria and hemimegalencephaly (about 10% of cases), Down syndrome and acquired brain insults.

The term 'idiopathic West syndrome' has been used to describe the condition in some patients who recover spontaneously following a brief course of infantile spasms. Probably less than 5% of patients with West syndrome have the truly idiopathic form. Other features include normal psychomotor development with preserved visual contact and tracking at the onset of the infantile spasm, symmetric hypsarrhythmia with absence of focal EEG abnormalities (spike- and-slow-wave focus) after intravenous diazepam; and reappearance of hypsarrhythmia between successive spasms in a cluster in an ictal record. Patients with truly idiopathic West syndrome can show normal subsequent neurological and cognitive development. It has been proposed that this subgroup represents a form of benign epilepsy of childhood. There is no relationship between the severity of the spasms and the prognosis.

Intellectual impairment is the second cardinal clinical feature of symptomatic West syndrome. There is often some evidence of developmental retardation before the onset of the spasms, and occasionally prior epilepsy, but as the spasms develop, the child's behaviour and responsiveness are rapidly impaired. Previously gained visual and social skills disappear and severe regression and autistic withdrawal are common.

West syndrome takes a terrible place among the childhood epilepsies because of its severe prognosis in terms of seizure recurrence and mental development, rapid deterioration of psychomotor status, resistance to conventional antiepileptic drug treatment and sensitivity to hormonal treatment. About 5% of children die in the acute phase of spasms, and the death rate was much higher before the introduction of adrenocorticotrophic hormone (ACTH) therapy. On treatment, the spasms remit in almost all cases, with few cases having attacks after the age of 3 years. However, both the development of the child and the ultimate neurological status are usually impaired. Of the survivors 70–96% have learning difficulty (which in over 50% is severe) and chronic epilepsy develops in 35–60%. The epilepsy can be severe, and evolve into the Lennox–Gastaut syndrome. The treatment of West syndrome is described on pp. 82–3.

## Lennox–Gastaut syndrome

This term denotes an ill-defined age-specific epileptic encephalopathy with a wide range of causes (Table 1.20).

**Table 1.19** Some causes of West syndrome.

Neurocutaneous syndromes (especially tuberous sclerosis, Sturge–Weber syndrome)
Cortical dysplasia (many types)
Congenital chromosomal disorders (many types)
Inherited metabolic disorders (many types)
Mitochondrial disease
Neonatal and infantile infections
Hypoxic–ischaemic encephalopathy
Tumours and vascular disorders
Trauma
Degenerative disorders

**Table 1.20** Lennox–Gastaut syndrome.

Epileptic encephalopathy—1–5% of all childhood epilepsies
Age of onset 1–7 years
40% cryptogenic, 60% symptomatic (identifiable underlying cause)
Learning disability, sometimes severe
Multiple seizure types—atypical absence, tonic, atonic, tonic–clonic, myoclonic
Episodes of non-convulsive status epilepticus common (75% of patients)
Seizures precipitated by sedation and lack of stimulation
Characteristic EEG pattern—slow spike-wave ($\leq$ 2.5 Hz), abnormal background, bursts of fast ($\geq$ 10 Hz) activity in non-REM sleep
Evolution over time
< 5% seizure remission
Poor response to antiepileptic therapy

It was first proposed in 1966 to describe the severe epilepsies of childhood in which multiple types of seizure are associated with slow spike-wave EEG discharges (2–3 Hz). Although some take the view that this is a specific syndrome, others disagree and view the clinical and EEG patterns as simply a reflection of severe epilepsy in childhood associated with learning disability. In favour of the latter view is the fact that there are many underlying causes, that there is no specific histopathological change nor specific treatment, and that it can evolve from other epilepsy syndromes (e.g. West syndrome, neonatal convulsions). This is a nosological jungle and the fine distinctions proposed by epileptologists are of largely academic interest only. There are few areas of more nosological confusion, even in epileptology (a subject blighted by esoteric and largely pointless argument about classification). Whatever else, the term has acquired wide currency and is used to denote a profoundly handicapping clinical symptom complex.

The Lennox–Gastaut syndrome accounts for between 1 and 5% of all childhood epilepsies, and occurs in up to 15% of institutionalized patients with mental handicap. The age of onset is usually between 1 and 7 years, although apparent adult-onset cases are recorded. It can develop from West syndrome, myoclonic astatic epilepsy or neonatal seizures. Many identifiable cerebral lesions can underlie the encephalopathy (Table 1.21) although in at least one-third no cause is identifiable (these cases are termed cryptogenic Lennox–Gastaut syndrome). About one-third of cases are due to malformations of brain development. About 20–30% of cases evolve from West syndrome, and when associated with frequent tonic seizures, these patients carry a particularly poor prognosis.

The epilepsy is very severe, with seizures usually occurring many times a day. These take the form of atypical absence, tonic, myoclonic, tonic and tonic–clonic seizures, and later complex partial and other seizure types develop. The most characteristic are tonic attacks, which occur most often in non-rapid eye movement (but not rapid eye movement [REM]) sleep and in wakefulness. They result in falls and the patients are prone to repeated head, facial and orthopaedic injury. Tonic seizures are said to occur in between 17 and 95% of cases, depending on the nosological

**Table 1.21** Underlying aetiology in symptomatic Lennox–Gastaut syndrome.

| |
|---|
| Cortical dysplasia (many types) |
| Neurocutaneous syndromes (tuberous sclerosis, Sturge–Weber, hypothalamic hamartoma, other forms) |
| Inherited metabolic disorders |
| Evolution from neonatal seizures or West syndrome |
| Ischaemic–hypoxic injury |
| Trauma |

inclusivity of the report. Atypical absence and tonic–clonic seizures are also universal, as are episodes of convulsive and more typically non-convulsive status. Indeed, non-convulsive status (atypical absence status) may last hours or days and be repeated on an almost daily basis. Consciousness may be little affected in these periods (which can be referred to by carers as 'off days') although the patients are usually obtunded to some extent, and there may be additional signs such as alteration of muscle tone, myoclonic jerks or increased sialorrhoea.

The EEG shows a characteristic pattern. The signature of the condition is the presence interictally of long bursts of diffuse slow (1–2.5 Hz) spike-wave activity, widespread in both hemispheres, roughly bilaterally synchronous but often asymmetrical. The spike-wave is not induced by hyperventilation and there is no photosensitivity. The background activity is abnormal with an excess of slow activity and diminished arousal or sleep potentials. Bursts of fast (> 10 Hz) activity, especially during non-REM sleep, sometimes without clinical manifestations and sometimes with tonic attacks, are also highly characteristic, and indeed are a diagnostic requirement by some authorities. The ictal EEG reflects the seizure type, although the ictal EEG during atypical absence attacks is often very similar to the apparently interictal EEG, and the distinction between ictal and interictal states, as alluded to above, can be difficult, with periods of non-convulsive status merging into the baseline state.

Learning disability is the other major feature of the condition. The intellectual impairment may be profound. At least 50% of cases have an IQ below 50. There may be a slow deterioration in skills, although progression is not particularly marked, and sometimes better control of the epilepsy results in intellectual improvement.

Subcategories of the syndrome have been proposed although these do not influence treatment strategies. Differentiation from the severe myoclonic epilepsies of childhood, and atypical or severe cases of 'benign partial epilepsy' can be problematic, but as the syndromic definition is vague, so inevitably is the syndromic differentiation. The prognosis for control of seizures and for the development of intellectual impairment is grave. According to some authors, long remissions from seizures or intellectual improvement occur in up to 15% of cases, although case definitions have not been uniform, and this seems optimistic. However, seizures do improve in adult life, and rarely is the epilepsy as ferocious as in early childhood. Persisting motor slowness and intellectual disability, however, are almost invariable. Many patients require institutional care in childhood and in adult life, and are dependent on carers for daily activities. Life expectancy has not been studied, but the encephalopathy is essentially static, and many patients live a stable adult life. Poor prognosis is associated with symptomatic aetiology, early age of onset, frequent tonic seizures and episodes of non-convulsive status, and a persistently slow EEG background. Conversely, a better outcome is found in those with onset after the age of 4 years, normal neuroimaging, EEG responsiveness to hyperventilation and faster spike-wave components (> 3 Hz). The treatment of the Lennox–Gastaut syndrome is described on pp. 83–4.

## Syndrome of electrical status epilepticus during slow wave sleep (ESES)

ESES (continuous spike-wave of slow sleep [CWES]; Table 1.22) refers to an epileptic encephalopathy characterized by the presence of generalized 1–3 Hz spike-wave discharges occupying 85% or more of the EEG of non-REM sleep. Of children with epilepsy, 0.5% show this EEG pattern. The condition is diagnosed during childhood (1–14 years) with a peak age of onset between 3 and 5 years. About 30% of children showing this pattern have identifiable brain pathology such as previous meningitis or brain anoxia, hydrocephalus and developmental lesions, and one pair of affected monozygous twins has also been reported. There are no specific clinical signs during sleep. Overt seizures occur in daytime and at night, and can take various forms, both focal and generalized. Episodes of status are common. The EEG pattern usually occurs in children with severe epilepsy and learning difficulty. Furthermore, many children exhibit the symptoms of the Landau–Kleffner syndrome, and some authorities consider the two conditions to be synonymous. However, ESES is also seen in cases of the Lennox–Gastaut syndrome and in some cases of BECTS. Indeed, whether this is a specific epileptic syndrome or simply a reflection of severe epilepsy is uncertain. ESES is a largely childhood phenomenon, and the EEG pattern usually disappears by the age of 16 years.

The EEG pattern is usually resistant to conventional antiepileptic therapy, and often long-term corticosteroids or ACTH are recommended, albeit without any clear evidence of efficacy. Intravenous immunoglobulin therapy has been used also. Oral antiepileptic drugs are given to control

seizures. Any first-line antiepileptic can be used and therapy follows conventional lines, although carbamazepine can exacerbate the nocturnal EEG disturbance. The EEG disturbance and seizures remit by the mid-teens. Cognition improves but most children do not gain normal functioning, especially in relation to speech and attention.

## Landau–Kleffner syndrome

The Landau–Kleffner syndrome is a childhood epileptic encephalopathy in which persisting aphasia develops in association with severe EEG abnormalities and epilepsy (Table 1.23). It is an uncommon condition with a male predominance and usually without a family history. Onset occurs at between 18 months and 13 years, in most cases between 4 and 7 years. The aetiology and pathogenesis of the syndrome, if indeed these are unitary, are unknown. The condition develops in children who were previously developmentally normal, and presents with a progressive aphasia, developing gradually over months or subacutely over weeks, although acute presentations are also encountered. Verbal comprehension and expressive speech both become severely affected. The children can become almost mute. Rather fruitless and inconclusive discussion has revolved around whether or not this is a true aphasia or an auditory agnosia, but the language disturbance seems particularly to involve the decoding of spoken words. The aphasia fluctuates, and indeed during the course of the condition speech can become quite normal, only to relapse again. Other inconsistent features include behavioural disorder, personality disturbance and intellectual decline. Overt epileptic seizures occur in about 75% of cases, and are usually mild, but 15% of cases have episodes of overt status epilepticus. The epilepsy, but not the EEG disturbance, is usually controlled by simple antiepileptic therapy. The EEG shows repetitive high-voltage spikes or spike-wave discharges in a generalized, focal/multifocal (temporal/ bitemporal) distribution, particularly affecting the speech areas of the brain. EEG studies have shown the origin of

**Table 1.22** Electrical status epilepticus during slow wave sleep (ESES).

Childhood epileptic encephalopathy
Age of onset 1–14 years
0.5% of children with epilepsy
EEG shows continuous epileptic activity during non-REM sleep (≥ 85% of time)
Overt seizures occur during wakefulness and sleep
Learning disability present in most cases
30% of children have an identifiable cause
Overlap with Landau–Kleffner and BECTS
Epilepsy often remits by age of 16 years

**Table 1.23** Landau–Kleffner syndrome.

Uncommon form of epileptic encephalopathy
Pathogenesis uncertain
Onset between 1 and 14 years (usually 4–7 years)
Dysphasia, fluctuating—often severe
Associated behavioural disorder and learning disability in some cases
EEG shows focal epileptiform patterns often amounting to electrographic status epilepticus. Also ESES
75% have overt seizures, often not frequent or severe, various types
Overlap with ESES and BECTS
Prognosis is variable
Treatment with antiepileptic drugs, ACTH/corticosteroids and/or multiple subpial transection

spikes to be over the dorsal surface of the superior temporal gyrus. The EEG abnormality is usually severe, and furthermore is activated by slow-wave sleep, and may become continuous, evolving into the ESES pattern. The pathophysiology of the speech disturbance is unclear. It is tempting to see this as a manifestation of continuous focal epileptic activity disrupting language (i.e. a functional disturbance, a form of non-convulsive status epilepticus), and there is a general correlation between the course of the speech disturbance and of the EEG changes, although this is not always very close. Imaging is usually normal, although cases with neurocysticercosis, polymicrogyria and cerebral tumour have been described. The long-term prognosis is variable. Some children make a complete recovery after years of aphasia, and others are left with permanent, sometimes severe, speech disturbance and mental impairment. The EEG changes usually recover, although ESES may persist. It is suggested that this syndrome is a form of BECTS, on the basis of EEG similarities, although its manifestations can certainly be very severe and its prognosis is more variable than that of the classic BECTS syndrome.

The treatment of the Landau–Kleffner syndrome is described on p. 84.

## THE CAUSES OF EPILEPSY

Epilepsy is often multifactorial. Even in the presence of a major aetiology, other factors (genetic and environmental) can play a part in its clinical manifestations. Lennox recognized this in the 1930s with his picturesque analogy of the reservoir or river. 'Causes may be represented as the sources of a reservoir. At the bottom is the already present volume of water, which represents the person's predisposition, a fundamental cause. But the reservoir is supplied also by streams which represent the contributory conditions, such as lesions of the brain acquired since conception, certain disorders of bodily function and emotional disturbances.' It is usual to differentiate the aetiology of epilepsy from factors that contribute to seizure precipitation in patients already with the propensity to epilepsy. Here, this convention will be maintained, albeit recognizing that this is a relative, not absolute, distinction.

The range of aetiology varies in different age groups, patient groups and geographical locations. Broadly speaking, congenital and perinatal conditions are the most common causes of early childhood onset epilepsy, whereas in adult life epilepsy is more likely to be due to external nongenetic causes, but this distinction is by no means absolute. In late adult life vascular disease is increasingly common. In certain parts of the world, endemic infections—including tuberculosis (TB), cysticercosis, human immunodeficiency virus (HIV) and viral diseases—are common causes. The specific 'epilepsy syndromes' are also highly age-dependent.

The approximate frequencies of different aetiologies in a typical Western population are shown in Table 1.2.

## EPILEPSY DUE TO GENETIC OR DEVELOPMENTAL CAUSES

Heredity plays a very important part in the production of epilepsy—a fact noted by Hippocrates 2000 years ago and only recently fully appreciated again. The idiopathic epilepsies are likely to have a strong genetic basis, usually polygenic or oligogenic in nature (although it has to be said that absolute proof of this is somewhat lacking). Gene expression can be variable and influenced by environmental factors, and the epilepsies are often also age-dependent. Single gene disorders probably underlie only 1–2% of all epilepsies, and usually in these conditions there are additional neurological or systemic features. It is useful to consider the 'pure' epilepsies separately from the epilepsies associated with other neurological defects, although this distinction, like most in medicine, is somewhat artificial and transitional cases occur in a grey area between categories. Epilepsies due to some developmental anomalies have genetic and acquired forms but are included here for the sake of convenience.

### The treatment of idiopathic and developmental epilepsy
The drug treatments of the idiopathic generalized epilepsies and also the childhood epilepsy syndromes have distinctive features. The drug treatment of the idiopathic partial epilepsy syndromes and most other genetic and developmental epilepsies, however, follows similar principles to that of the acquired epilepsies. This general lack of specificity of therapy is rather disappointing, but it is nevertheless important to identify cause as prognosis and response to therapy can differ widely. There are few cases of genetic epilepsy that can be treated by surgery, although occasional cases with epilepsy of developmental origin are amenable to a surgical approach. The principles of medical treatment are described in Section 2, and of surgical treatment in Section 5 of this book.

### Pure epilepsies due to single gene disorders
These are generally rare conditions, described in families (sometimes single families) but are potentially important for the mechanistic light they may throw on the more common polygenic epilepsies. Interestingly, almost all the genes identified which contribute to susceptibility to pure epilepsy are genes that code for ion channels and in this sense, epilepsy has been recognized in recent years to be one of a burgeoning group of neurological disorders with intermittent symptoms, which have underlying ion-channel genetic defects. Defects have been found in genes encoding the neuronal nicotinic acetylcholine receptor (*CHRNA4; CHRNB2*), GABA receptor (*GABARB3*), voltage-gated

potassium channels (*KCNA1, KCNQ2, KCNQ3*) and voltage-gated sodium channels (*SCN1A, SCN1B*).

### Benign familial neonatal convulsions

In this syndrome seizures start around days 2–15 of life (usually day 2 or 3). The seizures are clonic and occur during sleep. The seizures usually remit within weeks or months, and the ultimate prognosis is good, with about 10% of patients developing subsequent epilepsy, and 5% febrile convulsions. The condition is inherited in an autosomal dominant fashion and is due to mutations of voltage-gated potassium channel genes *KCNQ2* and *KCNQ3*. The abnormalities of these genes result in reduced potassium conductance and hence enhanced neuronal excitability. Why the effects are restricted to the first few weeks of life is unclear. One plausible hypothesis is that the mutated channels are replaced by other potassium channels that are upregulated early in life. The seizures are usually controlled by phenobarbital, phenytoin or valproate.

### Autosomal dominant nocturnal frontal lobe epilepsy (ADNFLE)

This was the first 'pure epilepsy' in which the causal gene was found. Various mutations in the $\alpha_4$ and $\beta_2$ subunits of the nicotinic acetylcholine receptor have been identified in families with this interesting condition. Typically, the condition is inherited in an autosomal dominant fashion with 75% penetrance. The patients suffer from purely nocturnal frontal lobe seizures—sometimes many each night—without daytime seizures and without other symptoms. The seizures are brief, lasting less than 1 minute, and are clustered around the onset and end of sleep. The seizures take the form of spasms with various motor and hyperkinetic features, and consciousness may be preserved. The onset is in childhood and the seizures persist, albeit with varying severity. The MRI is negative and the interictal EEG can show frontal abnormalities but is often normal. Because of their bizarre form, the seizures can be misdiagnosed as parasomnias or even pseudoseizures (in spite of the fact that pseudoseizures never arise from sleep!), and are not uncommonly resistant to therapy. There is a strong family history and, when investigated, even apparently unaffected members in a family can have subtle nocturnal events, mistaken as simply restlessness or normal sleep phenomena. Carbamazepine is the usual first choice drug therapy, and is often successful in controlling attacks. In more resistant cases, any of the conventional antiepileptic drugs can be used.

### Generalised epilepsy with febrile seizures plus (GEFS+)

This is a very heterogeneous form of epilepsy, inherited in an autosomal dominant fashion, with age-specific manifestations and variable penetrance (about 60% in the original families). Febrile seizures are the most common feature, and seizures precipitated by fever tend to occur throughout childhood. Afebrile seizures of varying types, generalised tonic–clonic, myoclonic, atypical absence, and less commonly focal seizures, develop later in childhood. Status epilepticus can occur. The severity during the active phase is very variable, but the condition often remits by late childhood or early adult life. The phenotype is so broad that it is arguable whether this condition really deserves the epithet 'syndrome'. Certainly, however, the families inherit epilepsy, and many different mutations in either the α or β subunits of the voltage-gated sodium channel genes *SCN1A* and *SCN1B*, and more recently the $\gamma_2$ subunit of the GABA-A receptor *GABRG2* gene have been identified, in families from many geographical locations. Functional studies have confirmed that these mutations confer abnormal membrane excitability. A really interesting question is how often sporadic mutations of sodium channel GABA receptor genes underlie sporadic febrile convulsions or even cryptogenic epilepsy, and this is a subject of active research. Another intriguing aspect of GEFS+ is its marked phenotypic variability, both within and across families. Digenic or oligogenic inheritance has been postulated to explain some of this variability. The seizures are treated along conventional lines for secondarily generalized epilepsy, and the prognosis is variable, with spontaneous remission of seizures in some cases and intractable epilepsy in others.

### Dravet syndrome (severe myoclonic epilepsy of infancy [SMEI]; polymorphic epilepsy of infancy)

Dravet syndrome is a severe form of epilepsy, developing in early life and with a poor prognosis. The frequency is about 1 in 20,000–40,000 live births. Twenty-five per cent of children affected have a family history of epilepsy, and interestingly many (but not all) cases have mutations in the *SCN1A* gene, the same gene that causes the more benign GEFS+, and indeed there are families in which both phenotypes co-exist. Furthermore, in spite of the frequency of a family history, curiously, the mutations are in the vast majority of cases *de novo*. Seizures develop between the ages of 2 and 9 months. These are often prolonged attacks, at least initially, taking the form of unilateral clonic or tonic–clonic seizures, and are precipitated by fever or even hot baths. Myoclonic seizures develop later (usually in the second year of life) are may not be a prominent feature. They take the form of massive myoclonia or of erratic (segmental) myoclonia and may be precipitated by photic stimuli. Focal seizures, atypical absence and episodes of convulsive and non-convulsive status epilepticus are common. Prolonged episodes of non-convulsive status can be mistaken for non-epileptic deterioration. Other motor signs and intellectual difficulties occur and the epilepsy is entirely intractable to treatment. The diagnosis, with seizures precipitated by fever, is highly characteristic. However, diagnostic confusion can occur with: febrile seizures (initially at least); immunization-encephalopathy as whooping cough immunization is given at a similar age; degenerative diseases; Lennox–Gastaut syndrome; myoclonic-astatic epilepsy. There are also transitional cases sharing features of Dravet syndrome and other childhood epileptic encephalopathies. The prognosis is very poor with intractable epilepsy, early death, severe retardation or institutionalization in all cases. Therapy follows conventional lines.

### Febrile seizures, temporal lobe epilepsy and hippocampal sclerosis

A research area of great current importance, and intensive investigation, is the study of the undoubtedly strong genetic influences on febrile seizures and thus on hippocampal sclerosis and temporal lobe epilepsy (TLE). Various strands of evid-ence exits. Families are reported with inherited TLE (mesial and lateral TLE and also epilepsy with variable EEG foci). Four foci have to date been found in linkage studies of febrile seizures. In cohort studies, polymorphisms in the interleukin-1β gene have been associated with TLE and hippocampal sclerosis. Associations with either TLE or hippocampal sclerosis have been reported in patients homozygous for the low-expression allele of the *PDYN* gene, a common polymorphisms of the *PRNP* gene and also the 1465G→A polymorphism of the GABA-A receptor 1 gene. These are intriguing data, but not definitive, but it is likely that the common and important genetic influences on febrile seizures and temporal lobe epilepsy will soon be identified.

### Other single-gene epilepsy syndromes

A rag-bag of other single-gene epilepsy syndromes have been described, in either single or a few families, and include: familial adult myoclonic epilepsy (in a few families from Japan), familial autosomal recessive idiopathic myoclonic epilepsy of infancy (in an Italian family), X-linked infantile spasms, benign familial infantile convulsions, familial partial epilepsy with variable foci (linked to 22q), autosomal dominant epilepsy with auditory features (linked to 10q), and autosomal recessive rolandic epilepsy with paroxysmal exercise-induced dystonia and writer's cramp. Autosomal dominant rolandic epilepsy with speech dyspraxia (ADRESD) is a rare condition, with an unknown genetic basis, but which exhibits anticipation, suggesting that it may be a triplet repeat syndrome.

### Pure epilepsies with complex (presumed polygenic) inheritance

These are far more common than the single-gene epilepsies. Categories of idiopathic and cryptogenic epilepsy exist, both focal and generalized, with a strong presumption of a polygenic genetic basis (i.e. with complex inheritance, which does not follow simple Mendelian rules). These conditions are divided into the idiopathic generalized epilepsies (IGE; see pp. 17–19) and the benign partial epilepsies of childhood (see pp. 20–1), and have been the subject of intensive genetic study, but to date no common susceptibility genes have been identified.

To what extent other cryptogenic epilepsies have a genetic basis is less clear (e.g. febrile convulsions [pp. 21–2]; cryptogenic West syndrome [pp. 22–3]; cryptogenic Lennox–Gastaut syndrome [pp. 23–5]). The conditions are probably best conceptualized as polygenic disorders in which the phenotype is the result of interactions between susceptibility genes and environmental effects. There is often no strong family history of epilepsy and genetic studies have to be conducted using case–control methodology in large populations. The phenotypes are wide, and the susceptibility genes also have widely varying polymorphism. In this context, the concept of epilepsy syndromes as discrete entities that are clinically homogeneous and biologically distinct cannot be sensibly sustained. More attractive is the concept of the neurobiological continuum, in which there are widely varying phenotypes with similar genetic defects and also overlapping phenotypes caused by differing gene abnormalities. To confuse the picture further, many of these phenotypes can be due to a range of identifiable acquired and congenital brain disorders (symptomatic cases). In this sense, the epilepsy syndrome can be thought of as a genetically determined response of dysfunctional brain tissue to an acquired insult.

### Epilepsies in other single-gene disorders

At least 240 single-gene and chromosomal disorders result in neurological disorders in which epilepsy is part of the phenotype. Most are rare or very rare, manifest initially in childhood, and present for diagnosis to paediatric neurological services rather than to an epilepsy specialist; a detailed description of these is beyond the scope of this book. In only a few of these conditions does epilepsy have distinctive features or is a predominant or consistent feature (exceptions are the progressive myoclonic epilepsies and epilepsy in the neurocutaneous syndromes). The conditions most commonly seen in epilepsy clinics, albeit usually for treatment rather than diagnosis, are shown in Table 1.24.

The inborn errors of metabolism are conditions in which biochemical defects are inherited, usually in autosomal recessive fashion, and in which the epilepsy is one symptom within a much broader spectrum of learning disability and neurological and systemic features. These include conditions with intermittent or persistent metabolic changes including hypoglycaemia, hyperammonaemia, hypocalcaemia, hyperglycinaemia, metabolic acidosis, ketoacidosis, abnormal amino acid or oligosaccharide profile, mucopolysaccharidosis or lipid storage disease. The most common conditions encountered in epilepsy practice are considered below. The progressive myoclonic epilepsies form another cluster of similar conditions in which a unifying feature is the occurrence of progressive myoclonus. Similarly, the so-called neurocutaneous syndromes have dermatological as well as neurological features, and most but not all have an identifiable neurogenetic abnormality. In a substantial number of cases presenting with epilepsy and learning disability on a congenital basis, no cause can be identified.

**Table 1.24** Some single-gene disorders causing epilepsy.

Agenesis of the corpus callosum
Acute intermittent porphyria
Alpers disease
Angelman disease
Argininosuccinicaciduria
Carnitine palmitoyltransferase 11 deficiency
Choreoacanthocytosis (neuroacanthocytosis)
Dentato-rubro-pallido-luysian atrophy (DRPLA)
Familial cavernoma
Glucocerebrosidase deficiency (Gaucher disease)
Hexosaminidase A deficiency
Huntington disease
Isovaleric acidaemia
Lafora body disease
Maple syrup urine disease
Menkes disease
Methylmalonic aciduria
Mitochondrial diseases (MERFF, MELAS, Leigh syndrome)
Mucopolysaccharidoses
Neuronal ceroid lipofuscinoses
Niemann–Pick disease
Ornithine transcarbamylase deficiency
Periventricular heterotopia
Peroxisomal enzyme deficiencies
Phenylalanine hydroxylase deficiency (phenylketonuria)
Porphyria
Pyridoxine deficiency
Pyruvate dehydrogenase deficiency
Rett syndrome
Sialidoses
Tuberous sclerosis
Unverricht–Lundborg disease
Urea cycle disorders
Wolf–Hirschhorn syndrome
Zellweger syndrome

MERFF, myoclonic epilepsy with ragged red fibres; MELAS, myoclonic epilepsy, lactic acidosis and stroke-like episodes. (List excludes the single gene disorders causing 'pure epilepsy'—see pp. 26–8)

## Alpers disease

Alpers disease (Progressive Neuronal Degeneration of Childhood with Liver Disease and Poliodystrophy) was a pathological diagnosis initially applied to patients with degenerative cerebral disease and characteristic autopsy findings of severe neuronal loss and vacuolation. Recent evidence suggests that the condition is a form of mitochondrial encephalomyopathy, with most cases due to mutations in the *POLG1* gene (and less often in the *COX 11* gene) causing a deficiency in mitochondrial DNA polymerase gamma (POLG) catalytic activity—similar to that in another mitochondrial syndrome MNGIE. It is a rare condition (<1 per 200,000 births) inherited in an autosomal recessive fashion, presenting usually in infancy or early childhood with intractable seizures and developmental arrest. Late-onset cases occa-

sionally occur, in childhood or early adult life, presenting typically with status epilepticus. Other signs include dementia, spasticity, peripheral neuropathy, optic atrophy and gastrointestinal disturbance. Liver dysfunction is usually evident and severe hepatic failure is common. The seizures in Alpers disease characteristically take the form of tonic-clonic status epilepticus or epilepsia partialis continua (EPC). Antiepileptic therapy follows conventional lines, but the seizures are invariably severe and intractable. The prognosis is poor with death usually within a short time of diagnosis.

## Angelman syndrome

This condition, with a frequency of about 1 in every 10,000–20,000 births, accounts for about 6% of all those with mental retardation and epilepsy. The condition usually presents with developmental delay apparent between 6 and 12 months of age. It is characterized by dysmorphic features, grave mental and motor handicap, severe epilepsy, a characteristic motor disturbance with 'puppet-like' movements due to truncal ataxia and titubation, a happy demeanour with a rather specific behavioural phenotype, and severe speech disturbance. There is a characteristic morphology with protruding jaw, occipital depression and blue eyes. Epilepsy is present in 85–90% of cases, and typically can include episodes of absence or myoclonic status, myoclonus, absence and tonic–clonic seizures. Partial seizures with occipital symptomatology also seem common. Jerky movements, additional to ataxia, can occur and can be due to unrecognized myoclonus or myoclonic status. Angelman syndrome is one cause of the Lennox–Gastaut syndrome. In about 80% of cases defects are present in the chromosome 15q11-q13 region, and involve a deletion, maternal disomy, imprinting defect or rarely translocation. This region contains a cluster of GABA receptor subunit genes. Iatrogenic mutations in the *UBE3A* gene are found in about 10% of cases. Diagnostic genetic testing is available. About 80% of cases can be identified via the methylation test, and mutation testing of the *UBE3A* gene can be used in cases where the methylation test is negative. The MRI is normal, the EEG usually shows large amplitude slow spike-wave. Life span is probably normal. Treatment of the epilepsy follows conventional lines, and has no specific features.

## Disorders of folate and B$_{12}$ metabolism

Various autosomal recessive enzyme defects occur, of which the most common is methylenetetrahydrofolate reductase deficiency. Epilepsy can be very prominent, with multiple seizure types, and associated with mental regression, motor deterioration, psychosis, stroke-like episodes and homocystinuria.

## Gaucher disease

Gaucher disease (glucocerebrosidase deficiency; glucosylceramidase deficiency) is caused by deficient activity of the lysosomal enzyme glucosylceramidase and the resultant accumulation of its undegraded substrate, glucosylceramide and other glycolipids. In the central nervous system glucosylceramide originates from the turnover of membrane gangliosides. There is a wide phenotypic range, and the condition is usually divided into five subtypes. The frequency is about 1 case per 50,000–100,000 live births. There is a marked founder effect in some populations and the condition is particularly common in Ashkenazi Jewish populations, the Swedish and the Jenin Arabs. Only types 2 and 3 are primarily neurological disorders. Type 2 has onset of disease before the age of 2 years, and presents as regression, profound psychomotor delay and a rapidly progressive course with death in the first 4 years of life. Type 3 has a more slowly progressive course, and death occurs in the second to fourth decades. Seizures occur and may take the form of progressive myoclonic epilepsy. The diagnosis of Gaucher disease relies on demonstration of deficient glucosylceramidase enzyme activity in peripheral blood leucocytes or other nucleated cells. Mutation analysis for the common mutations is available. Family studies can be carried out.

### Lysosomal disorders (lipidoses)

The most important lipidosis resulting in epilepsy is due to mutation of the hexosaminidase A (*HEXA*) gene. At least 90 different disease-causing mutations have been identified, of which six account for 98% of all cases in the Ashkenazi Jewish population but less than 50% in the non-Jewish cases. Defects in the enzyme result in a spectrum of disorders caused by the intra-lysosomal storage of the glycosphingolipid GM2 ganglioside. The diagnosis depends on the demonstration of deficient hexosaminidase A enzyme activity in the serum or white blood cells (with normal hexosaminidase B activity). The acute infantile condition Tay–Sachs disease presents in the first year of life with severe regression, visual deterioration, severe seizures and progressive enlargement of the head. An exaggerated startle response and startle-induced seizures occur. Death is inevitable by the age of 4 years. The condition is relatively common in Ashkenazi Jewish populations (91 in 3000 live births and carrier rates of 1 in 30), and 100 times less common in non-Jewish or Sephardic populations. The juvenile form begins with ataxia and then progressive intellectual decline with seizures and death by the age of 20 years. The adult forms do not commonly cause epilepsy.

### Menkes syndrome

This X-linked recessive disorder is the result of mutations in the ATP-ase copper transport gene *ATP7A*. A range of mutations have been found, which result in an abnormal ATP-ase transport protein and low copper concentrations in tissue. Classic Menkes disease presents around the age of 2 months with severe neurological regression and epilepsy, and other features including characteristic changes in the hair (kinky hair), autonomic and gastrointestinal dysfunc-

tion, and other abnormalities. Death occurs between 7 months and 3 years. A few patients have been described with a mild condition, with ataxia, tremor, weakness, mild intellectual impairment and seizures developing in mid to late childhood. Diagnosis is by measurement of copper and caeruloplasmin. Genetic testing is also available, including prenatal testing. Treatment of the underlying condition consits of subcutaneous injections of copper histidine or copper chloride (250–500 μg/day). If given within 10 days of birth, developmental outcome can be normalized.

### Neuroacanthocytosis

Neuroacanthocytosis (choreoacanthocytosis) is a progressive neurological disorder with prominent epilepsy, motor dysfunction, myopathy, cognitive and behavioural changes, and acanthocytosis of the red blood cells. The condition is inherited in an autosomal recessive manner. Seizures are observed in almost half of affected individuals, are often the initial manifestation, and can be very severe. Chorea and dystonia are common, particularly affecting the facial and buccal muscles, causing dysarthria and dysphagia with resulting weight loss. Habitual tongue and lip biting are characteristic. Progressive cognitive and behavioural changes have strong frontal lobe features. The mean age of onset is about 35 years of age, but the disease can present at any time between 10 and 70 years of age. The diagnosis of choreoacanthocytosis depends upon the presence of characteristic MRI atrophy of the caudate nuclei and T2-signal increase in the caudate and putamen. Acanthocytes are present in 5–50% of the red cells, and it is usually advised that acanthocytes are searched for on fresh smears on six separate occasions before the condition is excluded. Increased serum concentration of muscle creatine phosphokinase is observed in most cases. Acanthocytes also occur in McCleod syndrome and abetalipoproteinaemia with vitamin E deficiency. Muscle biopsy reveals central nuclei and atrophic fibres. Mis-sense, frameshift, nonsense, splice site and deletion mutations in the *VPS13A* gene are associated with some cases. Molecular genetic testing is currently available only on a research basis. Acanthocytosis needs to be differentiated clinically from Huntington disease, Lesch–Nyhan disease and pantothenate kinase-associated neurodegeneration (PKAN: Hallervorden–Spatz syndrome). There is no effective curative therapy and treatment is symptomatic and palliative. The disease runs a chronic progressive course leading to major disability within a few years and death after 10 years or more. Treatment of the epilepsy follows conventional lines, and has no specific features.

### Niemann–Pick disease type C

Niemann–Pick disease type C (NPC) is a lipid storage disease presenting in infants, children or adults. NPC is inherited in an autosomal recessive manner and has a frequency of about 1 in 150,000 persons. The classic presentation occurs in middle to late childhood with the insidious onset of ataxia, vertical supranuclear gaze palsy, dementia, dystonia and seizures. The seizures are partial or generalized, or both. The epilepsy is often refractory to medical therapy, but improves if survival is prolonged, presumably reflecting neuronal loss. About 20% of affected children have cataplexy induced by laughing. Dysarthria and dysphagia eventually become disabling, making oral feeding impossible. Adults are more likely to present with dementia or psychiatric symptoms. The diagnosis of NPC is confirmed by bone marrow biopsy which shows lipid-laden histiocytes, the biochemical demonstration of impaired cholesterol esterification and positive filipin staining in cultured fibroblasts. The diagnosis is often delayed substantially because 'routine' screening tests for metabolic disease, such as urine screens and lysosomal enzyme panels, are negative. In about 90% of cases NPC is caused by an identifiable mutation in the *NPC1* gene (and a handful of cases have been described with *NPC2* gene mutations). Molecular genetic testing is available.

### Organic acidurias and aminoacidurias

These are autosomal recessive conditions. The most common is phenylketonuria due to defects in phenylalanine hydrolase, and over 400 disease-causing mutations in the gene have been described. The prevalence shows marked geographical and racial differences, ranging between 1 in 2600 and 1 in 200,000 live births, and carrier rates between 1 in 26 and 1 in 225 (in Turkey and Finland, respectively). It can and should be detected by neonatal screening, and early dietary treatment will prevent any abnormalities. If the condition is missed, mental retardation, epilepsy, microcephaly, motor and behavioural disturbance occur. A less common cause of phenylalaninaemia is tetrahydrobiopterin deficiency. Other acidurias in which epilepsy occurs include argininosuccinicaciduria, tyrosinaemia and histidinaemia. They commonly result in epilepsy associated with learning disability and other neurological and systemic features. Diagnosis is made by screening blood and urine for abnormal amino acids.

Lactic acidosis is present in blood and urine in Leigh's syndrome. This is usually due to X-linked or autosomal recessive nuclear gene mutations of one of the mitochondrial respiratory chain complex I or IV enzymes or pyruvate dehydrogenase (X-linked *PDHA1* gene). About 30% are due to mutations in mitochondrial DNA, which have been identified in at least 11 mitochondrial genes. The diagnostic features are a subacute encephalopathy, seizures (myoclonic or tonic–clonic), and progressive dementia with cerebellar and brainstem signs. Motor abnormalities include hypotonia, spasticity, ataxia, involuntary movements and bulbar problems. Vomiting, hyperventilation and abnormalities of thermoregulation are common. Optic atrophy, pigmentary retinopathy, deafness and cardiomyopathy are sometimes present. On imaging, basal ganglia lucencies are highly characteristic, and proton magnetic resonance spectroscopy (MRS) can detect high cerebral lactic acid levels. High alanine levels are found in plasma. The condition typically presents in infancy after a viral disease, but less commonly can occur at any age. Leigh-like conditions also occur without the full complement of features, and the complex 'neurogenic weakness, ataxia and retinitis pigmentosa' (NARP) is considered to be part of the spectrum of this condition. Genetic testing is available.

### Peroxisomal disorders

At least 17 autosomal recessive disorders are described due to abnormalities of 11 genes coding for peroxisomal enzymes. These enzymes act as metabolic pathways in the oxidation of long-chain fatty acids, necessary for myelin production. Zellweger syndrome and neonatal adrenoleucodystrophy are examples, presenting as severe seizure disorders often starting in the neonatal period and including all seizure types including infantile spasm. Other features include poor feeding, severe intellectual regression, bony stippling (chondrodysplasia punctata), retinal dystrophy, hearing loss, hypotonia and dysmorphic features (including high palate, high forehead and shallow orbital ridges). The EEG is severely abnormal. In some cases polymicrogyria is present. The diagnosis is made by measuring serum long-chain fatty acids in plasma, and then fibroblast culture. Mutations in 11 different *PEX* genes—those that encode peroxins—have been identified. Mutations of the *PEX1* is the most common cause, and sequencing of exon 13 and 15 will reveal at least one mutation in about 50% of patients. Such testing is clinically available. Later in life, X-linked adrenoleucodystrophy is the most common peroxisomal disorder, but seizures are the presenting symptom in only a minority, and are sometimes secondary to hypoglycaemia associated with adrenal failure.

### Porphyria

Porphyria is a term used to describe a range of at least eight different diseases in which the hepatic production of haem is disordered. There is a marked geographical variation, and the highest frequency is in South Africa, where a founder effect has been traced to a Dutch orphan immigrant in 1688. Acute intermittent porphyria (AIP) is an autosomal dominant condition due to mutations in the porphobilinogen deaminase gene. Symptoms (the acute attack) occur only intermittently, and are precipitated by hormones, low carbohydrate diet, and drugs. The drugs precipitate porphyria by inducing P450 enzymes and this increases hepatic production of haem precursors. Certain antiepileptic drugs are quite unsafe in this regard in porphyria, and treatment of the epilepsy can be complicated by the risk of exacerbating symptoms (Table 1.25). In an acute attack, seizures occur with nausea, vomiting, pain in the back and limbs, urinary retention, muscle weakness, tachycardia, confusion and hallucinations. Diagnosis is by the finding of increased

**Table 1.25** Antiepileptic drug use in acute intermittent porphyria.

| |
| --- |
| *Drugs that are unsafe and should be avoided* |
| Carbamazepine and oxcarbazepine |
| Lamotrigine |
| Ethosuximide/methsuximide |
| Felbamate |
| Phenytoin |
| Phenobarbital and other barbiturates |
| Topiramate |
| Valproic acid |
| |
| *Drugs that can be used with care* |
| Clonazepam and other benzodiazepines |
| Gabapentin |
| Vigabatrin |

levels of delta-aminolevulinic acid (ALA) and porphobilinogen in urine, in an attack. These tests may be normal between attacks, and measurement of ALA levels in red blood cells is possible, as is genetic testing on a restricted basis. Variegate porphyria is the most common form in the South African white population, but less frequent elsewhere. Skin photosensitivity is common. The defective enzyme is protoporphyrinogen oxidase and the most sensitive screening test is a plasma porphyrin assay.

### Pyridoxine deficiency

Pyridoxine deficiency is due to a recessively inherited defect in glutamic acid decarboxylase. It presents in infancy with neonatal convulsions and EEG disturbance. It responds rapidly to pyridoxine, and is, rarely amongst the inborn errors of metabolism, entirely curable if the diagnosis is made in time. Indeed, pyridoxine should be given to any neonate with seizures if no other cause is clearly present.

### Rett syndrome

This is an X-linked dominant disorder, almost always presenting in females. The defect is in the *MECP2* gene, which controls RNA production. Birth and development in the first 6 months are normal. In the classic phenotype, the children then decline with severe mental regression with autistic features, motor disturbances with highly characteristic manual stereotopies and eventually total quadraparesis, apnoeic attacks, and a complex disturbance of breathing and a tendency for gastric regurgitation. Short stature, growth failure, wasting and microcephaly are typical. Language is severely affected and speech may cease altogether. Epilepsy occurs in over 50% of identified cases, and tends to develop when the disease has stabilized. The seizures take many forms and include episodes of convulsive status epilepticus. The latter can be precipitated by inhalation due to gastric regurgitation. Often, however, the epilepsy is not severe, and can be controlled by relatively small doses of conventional antiepileptic therapy. MRI does not show specific features, but the EEG is often severely abnormal with predominant slow activity, spikes and spike-wave, and frequent electrographic seizures. It has recently become clear that the phenotype is much wider than in the classic descriptions, and it is recognized that some adult women with only mild intellectual disability have the same genetic defect. Occasional male cases survive who have either a 47,XXY karyotype or somatic mosaicism (those with 47,XY and *MECP2* mutations die in the first years of life). Diagnostic genetic testing is available.

### Urea cycle disorders

Various autosomal recessive disorders of urea cycle enzymes occur, with a prevalence of about 1 in 30,000 live births, resulting in abnormalities of protein breakdown and consequential hyperammonaemia. There are five urea cycle enzymes and one co-factor, and defects in each are described. The severity of the conditions vary, with some rapidly fatal. Ornithine transcabamylase (OTC) deficiency is the most common deficiency, with a frequency of about 1 in 80,000 live births. It is an X-linked trait, with marked phenotypic variation. Male homozygotes usually present in infancy with severe neonatal hyperammonaemic encephalopathy, whereas female heterozygotes may be virtually asymptomatic. In mild or moderately affected cases, epilepsy is common, associated sometimes with ataxia, tremor and other motor abnormalities. A significant number of carrier females exist, presumably due to X-chromosome inactivation. These patients also can have epilepsy, and are at risk of hyperammonaemic crises precipitated for instance by pregnancy, drugs such as corticosteroids or valproate, or intercurrent infection. The hyperammonaemic episodes are characterized by encephalopathy, vomiting, lethargy, behavioural and psychiatric disturbances and sleep disorder. The encephalopathy is sometimes misdiagnosed as nonconvulsive status epilepticus, and this can be a disastrous if further valproate is given. The diagnosis can be made by the demonstration of a high serum ammonia, and valproate withdrawal and/or treatment of the intercurrent illness will reverse the clinical picture. Genetic testing is possible, by linkage analysis (with linkage established in the family before individual testing) and the disease can be confirmed by enzymatic testing on hepatic tissue.

### Wilson disease

Wilson disease is a disorder of copper metabolism with hepatic, neurological and psychiatric features. The condition is caused by abnormalities of the *ATP7B* gene and is inherited in an autosomal recessive manner. The prevalence is about 1 in 30,000 in most populations, with a corresponding carrier frequency in the general population of 1 in 90. Wilson disease presents at widely differing ages (3–50 years) and has widely varying symptoms. The liver disease includes recurrent jaundice, simple acute self-limited hepatitis-like illness, autoimmune-type hepatitis, fulminant hepatic failure, or chronic liver disease. The neurological features usually develop in teenage or early adult years and include tremor, pyramidal signs, poor co-ordination, loss of fine-motor control, chorea, choreoathetosis, rigid dystonia, gait disturbance and pseudobulbar features. Psychiatric symptoms include depression, neurotic behaviours, disorganization of personality and, occasionally, intellectual deterioration. Treatment with copper chelating agents or zinc can prevent the development of hepatic, neurological and psychiatric findings in asymptomatic individuals and can reduce findings in many symptomatic individuals. Epilepsy occurs in less than 10% of cases, and is usually easily controlled on conventional therapy. The epilepsy can be precipitated by the initiation of therapy. The major clinical sign is the Kayser–Fleischer ring, resulting from copper deposition in Descemet's membrane of the corneal endothelium. These may be evident on direct inspection, but a careful slit lamp examination is essential to exclude their presence. The diagnosis depends in part upon the detection of low serum copper and caeruloplasmin concentrations and increased urinary copper excretion. Molecular genetic testing is clinically available for both diagnosis and carrier detection.

Treatment is available, and needs to be lifelong. With adequate therapy, the disease manifestations can be prevented or arrested. Therapy is with copper chelating agents (e.g. penicillamine or trientine) which increase urinary excretion of copper, zinc used after initial 'decoppering', co-medication with antioxidants, such as vitamin E, to prevent tissue damage, particularly to the liver. Also, restriction of foods very high in copper (liver, brain, chocolate, mushrooms, shellfish, nuts) is prudent. Orthotopic liver transplantation (OLT) is reserved for individuals who fail to respond to medical therapy or cannot tolerate it due to serious adverse side-effects. Individuals with neurological symptoms may experience some deterioration in neurological status at the onset of treatment. Neurological deterioration is much more common with penicillamine than with trientine, and it appears to be uncommon with zinc. The deterioration is usually transient and can be avoided by starting the penicillamine at a low dose.

## Progressive myoclonic epilepsy (PME)

This is a rather specific phenotype, which can be caused by a variety of genetically determined neurological disorders (Table 1.26). In most parts of the world there are six common underlying conditions: mitochondrial disorders, Unverricht–Lundborg disease, dentato-rubro-pallido-luysian atrophy (DRPLA), Lafora body disease, neuronal ceroid lipofuscinosis, and sialidosis. The term progressive myoclonic epilepsy should be confined to those cases where the predominant clinical symptom is myoclonus. This needs to be differentiated from other progressive encephalo-

**Table 1.26** Causes of progressive myoclonic epilepsy (PME).

*Most common causes*
Baltic myoclonus (Unverricht–Lundborg disease)
Ceroid lipofuscinoses
Dentato-rubro-pallido-luysian atrophy (DRPLA)
Lafora body disease
Mitochondrial disease (myoclonic epilepsy with ragged red fibres, MERRF)
Sialidoses

*Rarer causes*
Alpers disease
Alzheimer's disease
Biotin-responsive progressive myoclonus
Coeliac disease
Gaucher disease
GM2 gangliosidosis (juvenile type)
Hexosaminidase deficiency
Huntington disease
Juvenile neuroaxonal dystrophy
Menkes disease
Non-ketotic hyperglycinaemia
Phenylketonuria
Tetrahydrobiopterin deficiencies

In a significant proportion of patients no cause can be identified.

pathies with myoclonus and from the so-called progressive myoclonic ataxias. The antiepileptic drug treatment of the various forms of PME is described on p. 80.

There are marked geographic variations in the frequency, but in most countries the condition is uncommon, accounting for less than 1% of all referrals to tertiary epilepsy services.

### Baltic myoclonus (Unverricht–Lundborg disease)

This is the most benign form of progressive myoclonic epilepsy. It is an autosomal recessive disorder due to mutations in the *EPM1* gene coding for the cystatin B protein, a protease inhibitor. The most common mutation is an unstable expansion of a dodecamer repeat. There is marked geographic variation, with the condition being especially common in Finland (where the incidence is in excess of 1 in 20,000 persons), Scandinavia and the Baltic regions, due to founder effects in these isolated populations. Myoclonic movements first develop usually between the ages of 6 and 15 years and the condition slowly progresses. Initially the myoclonus is easy to control, but eventually it becomes intractable and disabling. Other seizures are infrequent, although tonic–clonic seizures may be the presenting symptom, and usually easily controlled. Ataxia and tremor also develop and become major clinical features. There is a very slow intellectual decline, but this can be mild. Death used to occur between the ages of 30 and 40 years, but with improved treatment survival now is often into the seventh decade. The EEG has an interesting pattern, sometimes showing spike-wave on waking at 3–5 Hz and with photosensitivity. Diagnosis can be made by genetic testing.

## Dentato-rubro-pallido-luysian atrophy (DRPLA)

Dentato-rubro-pallido-luysian atrophy is inherited in an autosomal dominant fashion. It occurs with markedly varying frequency around the world, being particularly common in Japan (a frequency of 0.2–0.7 per 100,000 persons) and in northern Europe. It is a triplet repeat disorder involving the *DRPLA* gene, which is of uncertain function. The normal repeat number is between 6 and 35 and the condition is present with full penetrance when the repeat number is greater than 48. DRPLA is a slowly progressive disorder in which ataxia, choreoathetosis, dementia and behavioural changes, myoclonus, and epilepsy occur. In common with other triplet repeat disorders, significant 'anticipation' is exhibited, and there is marked phenotypic variation even within a family. Fifty per cent of cases present tonic–clonic seizures and myoclonus, some present with ataxia–athetosis–chorea, and others with dementia in a 'pseudo-Huntington' form. The condition can present at any time from infancy to late adult life, the mean age of onset being 30 years. The mode of presentation of the condition is age-dependent, and there is also an inverse relationship between the age of onset of symptoms and the number of repeats. Individuals with onset before age 20 years invariably have epilepsy and frequently present with PME, although other forms of generalized seizures (tonic, clonic, or tonic–clonic seizures) occur. Seizures are rare in individuals with onset after age 40 years. The diagnosis of DRPLA rests on positive family history, the characteristic clinical findings, and the detection of an expansion of a CAG/polyglutamine tract in the *DRPLA* gene. The CAG repeat length in individuals with DRPLA ranges from 48 to 93. Molecular genetic testing is widely available. Diffuse high-intensity areas deep in the white matter are often observed on T2-weighted MRI in individuals with adult-onset DRPLA of long duration.

## Lafora body disease

Lafora body disease, an autosomal recessive condition mostly reported from southern Europe, is characterized the presence of Lafora bodies, which are periodic acid–Schiff (PAS) positive intracellular polyglucosan inclusions found in neurones, sweat glands and a variety of other sites. The age of onset is between 6 and 19 years (usually 12–17 years), although many patients have a history of isolated febrile or non-febrile seizures earlier in childhood, and the disease presents with progressive myoclonic and associated tonic–clonic and partial seizures. The partial seizures often have occipital or visual symptomatology, typically with ictal blindness and visual hallucinations. The seizure disorder becomes progressively more severe, and status epilepticus is common.

There is also a rapidly progressive and severe dementia. Ataxia and dysarthria also occur. The condition is progressive, although often in a stepwise form, and death occurs within 2–10 years of the onset of the disease, by which time the myoclonus is severe and disabling. The EEG may show spike-wave initially at 3 Hz, with faster frequencies developing over time, and focal occipital spike discharges, although these are not a reliable diagnostic finding. The myoclonus is not associated with EEG change and this helps differentiate early cases from myoclonus in idiopathic generalized epilepsy. Later EEG signs include slowing of background activity and the loss of normal sleep patterns. Up to 80% of patients have a mutation in the *EPM2A* gene, which codes for laforin, a tyrosine phosphatase protein. A second gene, *EPM2B*, has been identified, which codes for malin, a ubiquitin ligase protein. A third locus has recently been described in one family. The diagnosis can be confirmed by histological examination of the skin (which should include ecrine glands) and liver or muscle biopsy, but genetic testing has now rendered this largely unnecessary.

## Mitochondrial cytopathy (myoclonic epilepsy with ragged red fibres [MERRF])

A range of point mutations or deletions of mitochondrial or nuclear DNA result in dysfunction of the mitochondrial respiratory chain. There are over 70 different polypeptides on the inner mitochondrial membrane which form the respiratory chain, of which 13 are encoded by mitochondrial DNA; defects have been described in all of these. Two classic pheno-types (MERFF and MELAS) occur in which seizures are a common and important symptom, although intermediate and transitional cases are not uncommon. In a third mitochondrial disorder, the Leigh syndrome and NARP continuum, seizures are also common, but not a predominant feature. The full range of the phenotypes of mitochondrially inherited defects is probably not known, and it certainly seems possible that some cryptogenic epilepsies will have mitochondrial defects as yet undetected. The inheritance, of course, is usually maternal. Mitochondrial disease can result in forms of epilepsy other than PME. Other forms of myoclonus are characteristic and can be either focal or multifocal, but partial seizures and tonic–clonic seizures are also not infrequently encountered. The genetic defects underlying epilepsy are varied as are the syndromes (which can include MERFF, MELAS, Alpers disease (p. 29) or MNGIE (mitochondrial neuro-gastrointestinal encephalopathy syndrome).

The mitochondrial cytopathy that typically causes progressive myoclonic epilepsy is the syndrome of myoclonus epilepsy with ragged red fibres (MERRF). This is a multi-system disorder with a very variable phenotype, in which myoclonic seizures are often the first symptom, followed by generalized epilepsy, myopathy, ataxia and dementia. Other features are short stature, deafness, optic atrophy, retinopathy, ophthalmoparesis and cardiomyopathy with

Wolff–Parkinson–White syndrome. The clinical features are variable, even within families. The EEG shows spike-wave at 2–5 Hz with a slow background. Ragged red fibres are found on muscle biopsy in 80% of cases, and biochemical analysis will show decreased activity in respiratory chain enzymes. MRI may show atrophy, T2 signal change and also basal ganglia calcification. In 90% of cases the genetic defect is an A-to-G transition at nucleotide-8344 in the tRNA$^{lys}$ gene of mtDNA, and some other cases are caused by *T8356C* or *G8363A* mutations. Genetic testing is available. Heteroplasmy is responsible for some of the phenotypic variation and can complicate genetic diagnosis.

### Neuronal ceroid-lipofuscinosis

The neuronal ceroid-lipofuscinoses (NCLs) are a group of inherited lysosomal-storage disorders which may present with progressive myoclonic epilepsy and mental and motor deterioration. These are the most common of the hereditary progressive neurodegenerative diseases, occurring generally in about 1 in 25,000 live births, but there is marked geographical variation with a particularly high frequency in Finland. The phenotypes are categorized by age of onset: infantile neuronal ceroid-lipofuscinosis (INCL), late-infantile (LINCL), juvenile (JNCL), adult (ANCL), and Northern epilepsy (NE). Myoclonic epilepsy is a feature of all types. Almost all cases are inherited in an autosomal recessive manner although an autosomal dominant form of adult-onset NCL has been described. Carriers show no symptoms. In Santavuori disease (INCL), infants are normal at birth and then develop retinal blindness and seizures by 2 years of age, followed by progressive mental deterioration, and usually death in the first decade (although longer survival is possible with some mutations). Jansky–Bielschowsky disease (LINCL) appears typically between 2 and 4 years of age, usually starting with myoclonic epilepsy, followed by developmental regression, dementia, ataxia, blindness, and extrapyramidal and pyramidal signs. Death is usually between 6 and 30 years of age. Batten disease (JNCL) develops between 4 and 10 years of age with rapidly progressing visual loss. Epilepsy, taking the form of tonic–clonic seizures, complex partial seizures, or myoclonic seizures typically appears between ages 5 and 18 years. Other features include dementia and extrapyramidal features, and behavioural disturbance and psychosis. Death occurs between the late teens and the fourth decade. Kufs disease (ANCL) usually develops around 30 years of age, with death occurring about 10 years later. There are two major phenotypes. In type A, patients present with progressive myoclonic epilepsy with dementia, ataxia, and late-occurring pyramidal or extrapyramidal signs. Seizures are often uncontrollable. In type B, behavioural abnormalities and dementia are the presenting signs, sometimes associated with motor dysfunction, ataxia, extrapyramidal signs, and suprabulbar signs. Visual failure does not occur. Northern epilepsy is

characterized by tonic–clonic or complex partial seizures, mental retardation and motor dysfunction. Onset occurs between 5 and 10 years of age. The diagnosis of an NCL is based on clinical findings, electron microscopy of biopsied tissues, and, in some instances, assay of enzyme activity or enzyme levels, and molecular genetic testing. MRI shows atrophy and sometimes T2 hyperintensity, and VEPs and ERG are abnormal. White cells are vacuolated. Election microscopy of white blood cells, skin, conjunctiva, or other tissues typically reveals lysosomal storage material manifest as fingerprint, curvilinear profiles or granular osmophilic deposits. The levels of enzyme products of each of the six genes can also be assayed. There are six causative genes—*PPT1*, *CLN2*, *CLN3*, *CLN5*, *CLN6* and *CLN8*—and over 140 mutations have been described. There is a marked geographic variation in the genetic abnormalities, with CLN8 abnormalities, for instance, found only in Finland. Genetic testing and prenatal testing for each are available.

### Sialidosis

Sialidosis is less common than the other causes of progressive myoclonic epilepsy. There are at least two variants. All cases are inherited in an autosomal recessive manner. Type I sialidosis (cherry-red spot myoclonus syndrome) is due to *N*-acetyl neuraminidase deficiency, which results in defective cleavage, and thus accumulation, of oligosaccharides, typically with inclusion bodies with vacuolation. It has a juvenile or adult onset and is characterized by action myoclonus and an intention tremor, gradual visual failure, and later tonic–clonic seizures. There is little in the way of mental deterioration. A gene has been mapped to chromosome 6p21.3. In type II sialidosis there are defects in β-galactosidosis activity in addition to those in *N*-acetyl neuraminidase. Timing of the onset is variable from infancy to the second decade, and clinical features include severe myoclonus, tonic–clonic seizures, dysmorphic features, coarse facies, corneal clouding, skeletal dysostosis, cardiac involvement, and organomegaly and dementia. One gene has been mapped to chromosome 20. The genetic basis of this disorder is complex and not completed elucidated, and involves both the gene for Neu1 and that for cathepsin A, which forms a complex with Neu1. Diagnosis is confirmed by finding elevated urinary sialyliloligosaccharides and by assaying enzyme activity in leucocytes and cultured skin fibroblasts.

## Epilepsies in neurocutaneous syndromes

The so-called neurocutaneous conditions often result in epilepsy. Tuberous sclerosis complex, Sturge–Weber syndrome and neurofibromatosis (type 1) are the most important, and are not uncommonly encountered in epilepsy clinics. Other rare conditions causing epilepsy include hypomelanosis of Ito, epidermal naevus syndrome, hereditary haemorrhagic telangiectasia, Parry–Romberg syndrome, midline linear naevus syndrome, incontinentia pigmenti, and Klippel–Trénaunay–Weber syndrome.

## Tuberous sclerosis

Tuberous sclerosis or tuberous sclerosis complex (TSC) is a common and important cause of epilepsy. The incidence may be as high as 1 in 5800 live births and there is a high spontaneous mutation rate (1 in 25,000). It is inherited in an autosomal dominant fashion, and is usually caused by mutations of the *TSC1* or *TSC2* genes, both tumour suppressor genes. Mutations of *TSC1* tend to result in a milder disease with less tubers, less severe epilepsy, renal and retinal disease, although there is a large overlap in the phenotypic manifestations of mutations in either gene. To date, about 300 unique *TSC1* or *TSC2* mutations have been identified in nearly 400 separate patients/families. The *TSC1* mutations are primarily small deletions, insertions or nonsense mutations; in contrast, *TSC2* mutations also include significant numbers of mis-sense mutations, large deletions, and rearrangements. Between 60% and 80% of patients with TSC enrolled in research studies have an identifiable *TSC1* or *TSC2* mutation. The condition is a form of cortical dysplasia, and the histological appearance of the tumours shows similar features to other forms of focal cortical dysplasia. There is considerable clinical variability in the manifestations of tuberous sclerosis, and the extent to which some other forms of cortical dysplasia represent 'form fruste' cases will no doubt be established by modern genetic studies.

Epilepsy is the presenting symptom in 80% or more of patients. It can take the form of neonatal seizures, West syndrome, Lennox–Gastaut syndrome or as adult onset partial or generalized seizures. About two-thirds of patients present with seizures before the age of 2 years, with motor seizures, drop attacks or infantile spasms. About 25% of all cases of West syndrome are due to tuberous sclerosis. The skin is abnormal in almost all patients, and skin lesions include: hypomelanotic macules (87–100% of patients), facial angiofibromas (47–90%), shagreen patches (20–80%), fibrous facial plaques, and subungual fibromas (17–87%). The facial angiofibromas cause disfigurement, but none of the skin lesions result in more serious medical problems. CNS tumours are the leading cause of morbidity and mortality. The brain lesions can be distinguished on the basis of MRI studies and comprise: subependymal glial nodules (90% of cases), cortical tubers (70% of cases), and subependymal giant cell astrocytomas (6–14% of cases). Linear streaks seen on MRI represent disordered neuronal migration. Subependymal giant cell astrocytomas progressively enlarge, causing pressure and obstruction, and result in significant morbidity and mortality. Psychiatric disorders are common and include autism, hyperactivity or attention deficit hyperactivity disorder, and aggression. At least 50% of patients have developmental delay or mental retardation. An estimated 80% of children with TSC have an identifiable renal lesion by the mean age of 10.5 years. Five different renal lesions occur in TSC: benign angiomyolipoma (70% of affected individuals), epithelial cysts (20%), oncocytoma (benign adenomatous hamartoma) (< 1%), malignant angiomyolipoma (< 1%), and renal cell carcinoma (< 1%). Cardiac rhabdomyomas are present in 47–67% of patients with TSC. Lymphangiomyomatosis of the lung is estimated to occur in 1–6% of cases and primarily affects women between the ages of 20 and 40 years. The retinal lesions are hamartomas (elevated mulberry lesions or plaque-like lesions) and achromic patches (similar to the hypopigmented skin lesions). One or more of these lesions may be present in up to 75% of patients and are usually asymptomatic. Status epilepticus, renal disease and bronchopneumonia are the leading causes of premature death.

Diagnostic criteria are shown in Table 1.27. Molecular genetic testing for diagnostic confirmation and prenatal testing of the *TSC1* and *TSC2* genes are available but complicated by the large size of the two genes, the large number of disease-causing mutations, and the high rate of somatic mosaicism (10–25%).

The epilepsy is treated with conventional antiepileptic drugs, but in at least one-third of cases is highly resistant to

**Table 1.27** Diagnostic criteria of tuberous sclerosis.

*Major features*
Facial angiofibromas or forehead plaque
Non-traumatic ungual or periungual fibromas
Hypomelanotic macules (three or more)
Shagreen patch (connective tissue naevus)
Multiple retinal nodular hamartomas
Cortical tuber
Subependymal nodule
Subependymal giant cell astrocytoma
Cardiac rhabdomyoma, single or multiple
Lymphangiomyomatosis
Renal angiomyolipoma

*Minor features*
Multiple randomly distributed pits in dental enamel
Hamartomatous rectal polyps
Bone cysts
Cerebral white matter radial migration lines
Gingival fibromas
Non-renal hamartoma
Retinal achromic patch
'Confetti' skin lesions
Multiple renal cysts

Definite TSC: Two major features or one major feature plus two minor features
Probable TSC: One major feature plus one minor feature
Possible TSC: One major feature or two or more minor features

**Table 1.28** Screening protocol for patients with tuberous sclerosis.

- Renal ultrasonography (1–3 yearly—and then renal CT/MRI, if large or numerous renal tumors are detected)
- Cranial CT/MRI (1–3 yearly)
- Regular neuro-developmental/behavioural evaluations
- Periodic ocular, cardiological, dermatological, ophthalmalogical evaluations
- Echocardiography, electroencephalography, chest CT (if symptomatic)

**Table 1.29** Diagnostic criteria for neurofibromatosis type 1 (NF1).

*Two or more of the following features (NIH criteria):*
Six or more *café au lait* macules over 5 mm in greatest diameter in prepubertal individuals and over 15 mm in greatest diameter in postpubertal individuals
Two or more neurofibromas of any type or one plexiform neurofibroma
Freckling in the axillary or inguinal regions
Optic glioma
Two or more Lisch nodules (iris hamartomas)
Bone lesion such as sphenoid dysplasia or thinning of the long bone cortex, pseudarthrosis
First-degree relative (parent, sib, or offspring) with NF1

Only about half of patients with NF1 with a known family history of NF meet these criteria for diagnosis by 1 year of age, but almost all do by age 8 years because many features of NF1 increase in frequency with age. Children who have inherited NF1 from an affected parent can usually be identified within the first year of life because diagnosis requires just one feature in addition to a positive family history.

treatment. It is claimed on the basis of uncontrolled studies that vigabatrin is especially helpful in infantile spasm due to tuberous sclerosis, and this is a niche indication for this drug. Occasionally, surgical resection of individual lesions is curative. Pre-surgical work-up follows the normal principles of epilepsy surgery, and outcome is best when data from different modalities of investigation are convergent, when there is a single seizure type and a single large tuber, and when one cortical tuber is larger or calcified. Anterior callosotomy is sometimes useful to alleviate drop attacks or severe generalized epilepsy.

There is no curative therapy for tuberous sclerosis. However, control of seizures and treatment of individual lesions can greatly improve quality of life. It is important to monitor patients regularly for the development of lesions—a screening protocol is shown in Table 1.28. Patients with retinal lesions seldom develop progressive visual loss, so regular ophthalmological evaluations are unnecessary. The skin lesions (with the exception of the facial angiolipomas), too, seldom require therapy. Early identification of an enlarging giant cell astrocytoma permits its removal before symptoms develop and before it becomes locally invasive, and is the rationale for regular neuroimaging of children and adolescents with documented subependymal nodules.

### Neurofibromatosis type 1

Neurofibromatosis type 1 (NF1) is a common, dominantly inherited genetic disorder, occurring in about 1 in 3000 live births. Almost half of all cases are new mutations. The mutation rate for the *NF1* gene is about 1 in 10,000, amongst the highest known for any human gene. It is a large gene, and many different mutations have resulted in the clinical manifestations. Although the penetrance is essentially complete, the clinical manifestations are extremely variable. In NF1, the incidence of epilepsy is about 5–10%. The epilepsy can take various forms and present at any age. Infantile spasms due to NF1 are said to have a more favourable outcome than other symptomatic types. MRI can show heterotopia, other dysplastic lesions and congenital changes, but epilepsy can occur even if there are no overt MRI abnormalities.

Diagnostic criteria are listed in Table 1.29. Multiple *café au lait* spots occur in nearly all patients with intertriginous freckling. Numerous benign cutaneous or subcutaneous neurofibromas are usually present in adults. Plexiform neurofibromas are less common but can cause disfigurement and may compromise function or even jeopardize life. Ocular manifestations include optic gliomas, which may lead to blindness, and Lisch nodules (innocuous iris hamartomas). Scoliosis, vertebral dysplasia, pseudarthrosis, and overgrowth are the most serious bony complications of NF1. Other medical concerns include vasculopathy, hypertension, intracranial tumours and malignant peripheral nerve sheath tumours. About half of those with NF1 have a learning disability. Many of the manifestations are age-related. Optic gliomas, for instance, develop in the first 4 years of life. The rapidly progressive (dysplastic) form of scoliosis almost always develops between 6 and 10 years of age, although milder forms of scoliosis without vertebral anomalies typically occur during adolescence. Malignant peripheral nerve sheath tumours (neurofibrosarcomas) usually occur in adolescents and adults. Neurofibromas can occur in almost any organ in the body. The total number of neurofibromas seen in adults with NF1 varies from a few to hundreds or even thousands. Additional cutaneous and subcutaneous neurofibromas continue to develop throughout life, although the rate of appearance may vary greatly from year to year. Many patients with NF1 develop only cutaneous manifestations of the disease and Lisch nodules, but the frequency of more serious complications increases with age. Cerebrovascular abnormalities in NF1 typically present as stenoses or occlusions of the internal carotid, middle cerebral or anterior cerebral artery. Small telangiectatic vessels form around the stenotic area and appear as a 'puff of smoke' ('moya-moya') on cerebral angiography. There is no curative treatment, but annual follow-up by a physician familiar with the condition is important. This should include annual ophthalmological examination in childhood, less frequent examination in adults, regular developmental assessment by screening questionnaire (in childhood), regular blood pressure monitoring, and other studies as indicated by clinically apparent signs or symptoms. Genetic counselling and testing are available, but are complex, and need to be carried out by units experienced in the condition.

The treatment of epilepsy follows conventional medical lines, and in most cases the epilepsy is easily controlled. Surgical therapy usually has no role in the management of the epilepsy.

### Sturge–Weber syndrome

This is an uncommon sporadic developmental disorder, of uncertain causation. The principal clinical features are a unilateral or bilateral port wine naevus, epilepsy, hemiparesis, mental impairment and ocular signs. The port wine naevus is usually but not exclusively in the distribution of the trigeminal nerve. It can cross the midline and spread into the dermatomal distribution of the upper cervical nerve. If it affects the lip or the gum these can be enlarged. In 15% of cases the naevus is bilateral.

The epilepsy can be focal or generalized. It is often the earliest symptom, and most patients with Sturge–Weber syndrome develop seizures within the first year of life (at least 70%) and almost all have developed epilepsy before the age of 4 years. Adult onset epilepsy, however, can occur occasionally. The early seizures are often triggered by fever. The seizures take the form of partial or multifocal attacks often with frequent and severe secondary generalization. Convulsive status occurs in over half of cases. Seizures developing in the neonatal period can be very difficult to control and carry a poor prognosis. The hemiplegia and mental impairment deteriorate in a step-like fashion following a severe bout of seizures, and in Sturge–Weber syndrome there is little doubt that brain damage can result directly from epileptic attacks, presumably by ischaemic or excitotoxic mechanisms. Severe learning disability is now less common due to better control of the epilepsy. Similarly, outcome is better in the few cases in whom epilepsy is absent. In addition to the seizures and motor disturbance, there can be other neurological features. Ophthalmological complications (80%) include increased intra-ocular pressure with glaucoma or buphthalmos. Homonymous field defects are common, particularly when the cerebral lesion is in the occipital region (as is frequently the case), and episcleral haemangioma, choroidal naevi and colobomas of the iris can occur. The underlying brain pathology is a cerebral angiomatosis (often occipital) sometimes with gyral calcification. The affected cerebral hemisphere is often atrophic

and gliotic. The lesion is probably due to abnormal persistence of embryonic primordial vascular plexus.

The epilepsy should be treated aggressively to prevent neurological deterioration. There are no specific features to the choice of drug or drug regime, but control of seizures is important to prevent neurological deterioration. High doses of antiepileptic drugs may be required. Status epilepticus should be vigorously treated, as failure to rapidly control the status often results in a permanent and significant worsening of the neurological deficit. Resective surgery (either lesionectomy, hemispherectomy or lobectomy) can greatly improve quality of life and seizures, and should be given early consideration in any patient in whom control of seizures is poor. Surgical resection of abnormal tissue is worthwhile, particularly if carried out early in life and early in the course of the condition.

## Epilepsies in disorders of chromosome structure

Epilepsy is a feature of two common chromosomal abnormalities, Down syndrome and fragile X syndrome. It also takes a highly characteristic form in the rare ring chromosome 20. Other uncommon chromosomal abnormalities in which epilepsy is found include: trisomies 12p, 8, 13, ring chromosome 14, partial monosomy 4p (Wolf–Hirschhorn syndrome), inverted duplication of pericentromeric chromosome 15, and Klinefelter syndrome (where epilepsy occurs in about 10% of cases). In all these conditions there are addition behavioural and intellectual disabilities, and characteristic dysmorphic features. The seizures often take multiple forms, including myoclonus, and are of variable severity. Genetic testing is available for most conditions.

### Down syndrome

The Down phenotype occurs in about 1 in every 650 live births. It is usually caused by trisomy of chromosome 21, and triplication of 21q22.3 results in the typical phenotype. In 95% of cases the cause is a non-dysjunction, and in about 4% an unbalanced translocation. About 1% of cases are due to mosaicism. The risk of trisomy increases with maternal age. Epilepsy is present in up to 12% of cases and EEG abnormalities in more than 20%. Epilepsy typically develops either in the first year of life, due to perinatal or congenital complications, or in the third decade, possibly due to the development of Alzheimer-like neuropathological changes. The epilepsy is very variable and can take multiple forms, reflecting the complex pathogenesis. West syndrome is common, and Down syndrome can also cause febrile seizures and Lennox–Gastaut syndrome. Usually the epilepsy is rather non-specific, although frequent, small, brief, partial seizures seem particularly common in adults. Startle-induced seizures, however, are a characteristic feature. Treatment follows conventional medical lines, and the prognosis and response to treatment vary with type and cause. Surgical therapy for epilepsy has no role in this syndrome. Genetic testing and prenatal screening are available.

## Fragile X syndrome

Fragile X syndrome is a condition due to an increased number of CGG repeats (typically more than 200) in the *FMR1* gene (at Xq27.3) accompanied by aberrant methylation of the gene. It is an X-linked condition in which the presenting symptom is usually mental retardation, which is moderate in affected males and mild in affected females. Fragile X syndrome occurs in about 1 in 4000 male births and is the most common identified cause of mental retardation. Carrier rates in females (CAG repeats of approx 50–200) may be as high as 1 in 250, with some geographical and racial variation. Developmental delay is noticed from infancy, and manifests with abnormalities of speech, abnormal behaviour typically with tantrums, hyperactivity and autism. Dysmorphic features include abnormal craniofacies, with typically a long face, prominent forehead, large ears and prominent jaw. After puberty macro-orchidism, strabismus and rather abnormal behaviour are evident. Heterozygotic females show a milder but similar phenotype. Seizures are present in one-quarter of cases and EEG abnormalities in half of cases. The seizures usually develop before the age of 15 years and often remit in the second decade of life, and can take various forms (both generalized or partial) with equally variable non-specific EEG findings. Repeat numbers vary, and mosaicism is common, and these may account for the variable clinical features. Genetic and prenatal testing are widely available. The methylation status of the gene can also be identified using Southern blot. Identification of the abnormal protein is not usually required. The epilepsy is treated by conventional medical means and is often easily controlled.

## Ring chromosome 20

This is a rare condition, but one in which epilepsy is the predominant feature and it has a highly characteristic phenotype. The locus of fusion between the deleted short and long arms of the chromosome is at p13q13, p13q13.3.3 or p13q13.33. Seizures begin between infancy and 14 years of age, typically with episodes of non-convulsive status epilepticus. These episodes are characterized by confusion, staring, perioral and eyelid myoclonus, can be very severe —occurring daily—and are drug-resistant. The prolonged seizures may be misdiagnosed as non-epileptic behavioural disturbance. The EEG during episodes shows high-voltage rhythmic notched slow activity waves. Mental regression and retardation are present in addition to epilepsy. This is a sporadic condition which can be identified by genetic testing. Mosaicism is common and at least 100 mitoses may need to be examined before excluding the condition. The seizures can be highly resistant to therapy, which follows conventional lines. The treatment of non-convulsive status epilepticus is outlined on pp. 22–4.

## Epilepsies due to developmental anomalies of cerebral structure (the 'cortical dysplasias')

Cortical dysplasia (also known as cortical dysgenesis or malformations of cortical development) is a term that is applied to developmental disorders of the cortex producing structural change. A minority of these conditions are caused by identifiable genetic abnormalities (Table 1.30). Others are caused by environmental influences such as infection, trauma, hypoxia, and exposure to drugs or toxins. In most cases the cause is unclear. The form of dysplasia consequent on environmental insults depends not only on the nature of the insult, but also on the stage of development at which it occurred. The classification of these syndromes is controversial, but a pragmatic and descriptive classification based on MRI appearance is widely used (Table 1.30). Cortical malformations can be due to abnormal neuronal and glial proliferation, abnormal neuronal migration or abnormal synaptogenesis, cortical organization or programmed cell death.

**Table 1.30** Types of cortical dysplasia.

*Abnormalities of gyration*
Agyria (lissencephaly), macrogyria, pachygyria spectrum (focal or diffuse) (*LIS1*, *RELN*, *ARX* and *DCX* genes)
Polymicrogyria
Cobblestone complex (*FCMD* gene)
Schizencephaly (*EMX2 gene*)
Minor gyral abnormalities

*Heterotopias*
Periventricular nodular heterotopia (*FLNA* gene)
Subcortical nodular heterotopia
Subcortical band heterotopia (*DCX* and *LIS1* gene)

*Other gross malformations*
Megalencephaly and hemimegalencephaly
Agenesis of corpus callosum
Anencephaly and holoprosencephaly
Microcephaly

*Cortical dysgenesis associated with neoplasia*
Dysembryoneuroepithelial tumour (DNET)
Ganglioglioma
Gangliocytoma

*Other cortical dysplasias*
Hypothalamic hamartoma
Focal cortical dysplasia
Tuberous sclerosis (*TSC1* and *TSC2* genes)

*Microdysgenesis*

This is an arbitrary classification, based largely on neuroimaging appearances; the categories overlap.

The true prevalence of these conditions, previously thought to be rare, has only become apparent with the widespread use of MRI imaging, which can detect cortical dysplasia in cases previously classified as cryptogenic epilepsy.

Epilepsy is a leading feature of these conditions, usually but not always in association with learning disability and other neurological findings. Drug therapy follows conventional lines (as for any focal epilepsy), but in many cases, the epilepsy can be refractory to treatment. Cortical dysplasia is the underlying cause of the epilepsy in up to 30% of children and 10% of adults referred to epi-lepsy centres for intractable epilepsy. At the other extreme, easily controlled epilepsy is not uncommon with mild forms of dysplasia. The surgical therapy of cortical dysplasia is described on pp. 257–9.

### Hemimegalencephaly

This term describes a gross structural abnormality which can be the end result of various cerebral processes and insults. One cerebral hemisphere is enlarged and is structurally abnormal with thickened cortex, reduced sulcation, and poor or absent laminar organization. Giant neurones are found throughout the brain and in 50% of cases balloon cells also. The condition can occur in isolation, associated with other cortical dysplasias or as part of other syndromes (notably tuberous sclerosis or other rarer neurocutaneous syndromes such as epidemal naevus syndrome, Klippel–Trénaunay–Weber syndrome, neurofibromatosis type 1 or hypomelanosis of Ito). The restriction of the abnormality to one hemisphere may be due to somatic mosaicism, and it has been suggested that the condition is due to defects in the process of programmed cell death (apoptosis) in early fetal life. Hemimegalencephaly always results in severe epilepsy presenting in early life, accompanied by learning disability, hemiplegia and hemionopia. The epilepsy can take the form of neonatal seizures, West syndrome, Lennox–Gastaut syndrome or other less specific focal forms. Status epilepticus is common and a frequent cause of death in the early years. Medical treatment follows conventional lines, but is often unsuccessful. Surgical therapy (hemispherectomy or hemispherotomy) can be curative, and this is an important condition to identify early, as early surgery will prevent seizures, mitigate cognitive decline, and improve social behaviour and adjustment (see pp. 260–3).

### Focal cortical dysplasia

This is a common form of dysplasia, important to identify because of its potential for surgical therapy. The term encompasses a variety of subtypes, with different histological appearances due, possibly, to formation at different stages of embryogenesis. In some the cortical lamination is normal but in others there may be associated widespread macrogyria and polymicrogyria. Focal dysplasia can occur in any part of the cortex, and vary greatly in size. There are often widespread minor dysplastic abnormalities associated with some forms of focal cortical dysplasia, although in the Taylor form, diagnosed by the histological presence of 'balloon cells', the dysplastic changes are more limited. Dysplastic tissue generates epileptic discharges directly and seizures have been recorded by depth electrodes within dysplastic areas, possibly due to deranged GABA-ergic inhibition. Epilepsy is the leading symptom, and other features depend on the extent of the lesion and include learning disability and focal deficits. Focal cortical dysplasia can underlies neonatal seizures, West syndrome, or Lennox–Gastaut syndrome, but more typically does not take a syndromic form and presents in childhood or adult life as less specific focal or secondarily generalized epilepsy. Episodes of epilepsia partialis continua or tonic–clonic or partial status epilepticus are common. Interictal EEG can show rather typical continuous focal slow-wave activity. The MRI signs are increased signal on T2 imaging and FLAIR, blurring of the grey–white junction and simplified sulcation in the Taylor type, and similar but often more widespread changes in other types. Some cases of focal cortical dysplasia respond well to conventional antiepileptic drug therapy but others are highly resistant. Therapy should conform to the usual principles and there is nothing particularly specific about drug choice or usage. Surgical resection is possible in restricted and particularly small lesions, and surgical work-up follows conventional principles. The Taylor form responds particularly well to surgery.

### Schizencephaly

This term refers to the presence of clefts in the cortex, stretching from the surface to the ventricle. The clefts are subdivided into open-lip schizencephaly, in which the walls of the cleft are separated, and closed-lip schizencephaly, in which they are not. The clefts can be unilateral or bilateral and are usually perisylvian in location. Schizencephaly is often associated with polymicrogyria and less often with other focal cortical dysplastic anomalies, corpus callosum agenesis or septoptic dysplasias. The cortex may or may not have normal lamination. The pathogenesis in some cases is a failure of migration and in others an environmental insult causing focal necrosis of developing cortex. The causes are heterogeneous, and include germline mutations of the homoeobox gene *EMX2* and environmental insults during development including radiation, infection and ischaemia. The clinical presentation can be very variable. Epilepsy is the most common symptom (over 90% of cases), associated usually but by no means always with learning disability or cognitive changes. Focal neurological deficit is common in extensive or bilateral cases. Medical therapy follows conventional lines and, generally speaking, surgical resection is not possible.

## Agyria- pachygyria-band spectrum (lissencephaly, pachygyria, agyria and subcortical band heterotopia)

These are descriptive terms denoting abnormalities of cortical gyration, and are grouped together as they show an interconnected genetic basis. In all the gyration is simplified and the cortex is thickened. Lissencephaly (literally, smooth brain) is the most severe form, in which gyration is grossly diminished or even absent. Subcortical band heterotopia (subcortical laminar heterotopia, band heterotopia or double cortex syndrome) denotes the presence of a band of grey matter sandwiched by white matter below the cortical grey matter. The band may be thin or thick, and can merge with overlying cortex, in which case the cortex takes a macrogryic form. When the bands are thin and clearly separated from the cortical ribbon, the ribbon itself may appear normal. Thicker bands are usually associated with macrogyria, which refers to thickened cortex and can occur as an isolated phenomenon, is variable in extent and, when focal, is indistinguishable on clinical or imaging grounds from some forms of focal cortical dysplasia.

Most forms of lissencephaly occur without other noncerebral malformations and are known as isolated lissencephaly sequence (ILS). Isolated lissencephaly is present in 12 per million live births. The lissencephalic abnormality can affect the whole brain, resulting in profound retardation, epilepsy and spastic quadraparesis. Stillbirth can occur, and few patients survive beyond the age of 10 years. In less severe cases, where the lissencephaly is restricted to one region of the brain (albeit usually bilaterally, with an anterior or posterior gradient), the epilepsy and learning disability may be mild. Epilepsy presents before the age of 6 months in 75% of cases, as neonatal seizures or infantile spasms, and persists as multifocal and generalized types. Depth recording has shown discharges arising in the heterotopic tissue. The EEG shows characteristic high-amplitude fast activity. Of cases of isolated lissencephaly, 60–80% are caused by identifiable mutations in the *LIS1* or *XLIS* (also known as the *DCX*) genes, on 17p13.3 and Xq22.3-q24, respectively, and in 40% the entire gene is deleted. *LIS1* lissencephaly is predominately posterior in location, and the condition occurs in both sexes and is sporadic. Conversely *XLIS* cases almost always occur in boys (X-linked dominant lissencephaly) and the brain anomaly tends to be anterior in location. Genetic testing is available for both forms. Typically, abnormalities of the *DCX* gene result in anteriorly predominant lissencephaly and *LIS1* in posteriorly predominant lissencephaly. Anterior lissencephaly also occurs with abnormalities in the *ARX* gene and a range of phenotypes including West syndrome, dystonia and mental handicap. Posterior lissencephaly can be due to abnormalities in the *RELN* gene sometimes associated with cerebellar hypoplasia.

Other forms of lissencephaly have more widespread associations. The best known is the Miller–Dieker syndrome, which is caused by large deletions of *LIS1* and of several other contiguous genes on 17p13.3 (e.g. 14-3-3E). In this syndrome lissencephaly is associated with epilepsy, facial dysmorphism, microcephaly, small mandible, failure to thrive, retarded motor development, dysphagia, and decorticate and decerebrate postures. Other organs, including the kidney and heart, may be affected. Survival varies from months to several decades, and epilepsy is usually profound and intractable. Genetic testing is available. Cobblestone lissencephaly (type 11) is found also in some patients with muscular dystrophy and ocular malformations.

Subcortical band heterotopia is caused in about 80% of cases by germline deletions in the *DCX* (*XLIS*) gene and almost always (but not exclusively) occurs in females. The pachygyria and bands are anteriorly predominant. The genetic anomaly in the other 20% of cases has not been identified. The rare cases of subcortical band heterotopia in boys are probably caused by mis-sense mutations in *DCX* or *LIS1*. Subcortical band heterotopia is a much more benign condition than lissencephaly. It can present in children or in adults, with epilepsy and learning disability. Epilepsy occurs in at least 80% of cases, and 50% of cases present with the Lennox–Gastaut phenotype. However, the manifestations of this anomaly can be slight, and occasional patients present with mild epilepsy and with normal intelligence. The clinical severity of the syndrome seems to correlate with the extent of the cerebral anomaly. In two-thirds of those with epilepsy, the seizures are intractable. Similarly, patients with pachygyria or macrogyria also have epilepsy and learning disability of variable severity, depending on the extent and location of the anomaly. The histological changes of lissencephaly, macrogyria, pachygyria and band heterotopia may merge into one another, and in many patients these conditions represent a continuous spectrum rather than distinct entities. The anomalies are caused by abnormal cortical migration, and the factors influencing extent or severity have not been clearly identified. The cytoarchitecture varies, but in the Miller–Dieker syndrome, for instance, the lissencephalic cortex is thickened and has four rather than six layers (type I or classical lissencephaly). The changes can be regional and there may be associated dysplastic lesions.

Drug treatment follows conventional lines. Resective surgical therapy is not indicated, even where the bands or lissencephalic changes seems relatively localized, but callosotomy may help the occasional patients with frequent drop attacks.

## Agenesis of the corpus callosum

Agenesis of the corpus callosum is a dysplastic anomaly that occurs in various genetic and congenital disorders. Epilepsy is an invariable association, and often a leading symptom. In Aicardi syndrome the corpus callosum agenesis is associated with periventricular heterotopia, thin unlayered cortex and diffuse polymicrogyria. It is observed only in females (the only exception being males with two X chromosomes) and is X-linked with male lethality. The causal gene has not yet been identified, but linkage to Xp22.3 has been reported. Epilepsy is the leading feature, with severe mental regression. It presents with West syndrome and with partial seizures particularly involving the face in addition to infantile spasms. The seizures remain resistant to therapy and life expectancy is reduced, with only 40% of affected individuals living beyond the age of 15 years. Other syndromes with agenesis of the corpus callosum exist, and this anomaly may co-exist with other dysplastic features. The L1 syndrome is associated with mutations in the *L1CAM* gene and presents as hydrocephalus, mental retardation, spasticity and epilepsy.

### Polymicrogyria

The appearance of small and prominent gyri separated by shallow sulci is known as polymicrogyria. It can be diffuse or localized, and varies in severity as well as extent. The underlying cortex is invariably thickened, and can be unlayered or show an abnormal four-layered structure. The conditions may be a migrational defect in weeks 13–18 of fetal life, or the result of ischaemia or perfusion failure between weeks 12 and 24 of fetal life. Epilepsy is the leading clinical feature, associated with learning disability and focal neurological signs. The severity of all of these depends on the extent of the dysplasia. At one extreme the child is severely retarded with profound epilepsy and quadraparesis, while at the other the epilepsy is mild, and presents in adult life. There are various anatomical patterns of distribution of polymicrogyria, which may or may not have clinical specificity. The distribution of the polymicrogyria can be patchy, bifrontal, unilateral or concentrated in the sylvian or central areas. Polymicrogyria is an invariable association of schizencephaly, and is often associated with other cortical dysplasias. Both ischaemic and genetic defects can cause bilateral perisylvian polymicrogyria (Kuzniecky syndrome), a condition in which there is severe upper motor neurone bulbar dysfunction and diplegia as well as severe epilepsy and mental retardation. The presenting phenotype is wide, varying from that of the Lennox–Gastaut syndrome to patients with mild adult-onset seizures. In familial cases of polymicrogyria, inheritance conforms to an X-linked or autosomal dominant pattern with reduced penetrance. Some cases are sporadic and in other families individuals with clinical symptoms but no MRI change. There is marked phenotypic heterogeneity. No gene has yet been discovered, but linkage has been reported to *X28p* in 22q11.2. Polymicrogyria can also occur in the presence of chromosomal abnormalities. The medical therapy of polymicrogyria follows conventional lines. Surgical resection is only occasionally possible if the polymicrogyria is well localized.

### Periventricular nodular heterotopia

The presence of subependymal nodules of grey matter, located along the supralateral walls of the lateral ventricles is known as Periventricular nodular heterotopia (synonym: bilateral periventricular nodular heterotopia [BPNH], subependymal nodular heterotopia [SENH] ). The heterotopia is usually bilateral, although not always. It is much more common in females and conforms to X-linked dominant transmission. One mechanism may be X-chromosome inactivation. The condition is usually lethal in affected males, and in surviving males there is a high incidence of premature death due to vascular or haemorrhagic complications. Almost all cases have shown mutations in the *FLNA* (filamin-1) gene. It is probably the most common of all the cortical dysplasias, and has a very wide phenotype. At one extreme, the heterotopia can be asymptomatic. It commonly presents in older children or young adults with mild epilepsy, and at the other extreme can account for severe infantile or childhood partial epilepsy. Other features reported include early stroke due to vasculopathy, abnormalities of gastric motility, short digits, strabismus and cardiac anomalies. Depth recordings show that the nodules generate intrinsic epileptiform discharges. Periventricular nodules are found in about 5% of all cases of hippocampal sclerosis. In the presence of heterotopic tissue, temporal lobectomy for hippocampal sclerosis—even with clinical and EEG features typical of mesial temporal epilepsy—will usually fail to control seizures. In patients being assessed for temporal lobectomy, therefore, it is essential to scrutinize preoperative MRI with great care to exclude the presence of these lesions. Treatment is along conventional medical lines, but resective surgery has been occasionally been performed in isolated lesions.

### Other dysplasias

Various other types of dysplastic lesion exist, including sheets of abnormal neurones forming linear streaks in the white matter, abnormal cortical patterning (including stellate-like gyral formations), isolated clusters of grey matter within white matter, and microdysgenesis. The latter term refers to abnormally placed microscopic clusters of heterotopic neurones often associated with abnormal lamination of the cortex. Normal brains have occasional heterotopic cells, and distinguishing the truly pathological from the normal is to an extent a subjective judgement. Because of this, widely varying estimates of the frequency of microdysgenesis have been made. At one extreme is a study showing microdysgenesis in 38% of post-mortem specimens in epilepsy compared with a frequency of only 6% in controls.

## EPILEPSY DUE TO ACQUIRED CAUSES

Epilepsy due to an acquired or developmental cause is sometimes known as symptomatic epilepsy. Almost any condition affecting the cerebral grey matter can result in epilepsy, but here only the more common forms of acquired epilepsy will be mentioned. Many of the so-called 'acquired' epilepsies have a genetic loading, and in some (e.g. hippocampal sclerosis) the genetic influences may be considerable. The seizures in symptomatic and acquired epilepsy usually take a partial or secondarily generalized form, and there are often no particularly distinctive features associated with any particular cause. In acute cerebral conditions—for example stroke, head injury, or infections—the epilepsies share a number of general features. The epilepsies are often divided into 'early' (i.e. seizures occurring within a week of the insult) and 'late' (i.e. chronic epilepsy developing later). There is often a 'silent period' between the injury and the onset of late epilepsy. Presumably, epileptogenic processes are developing during this period, and this raises the possibility of neuroprotective interventions to inhibit these processes and prevent later epilepsy. To date, however, no effective neuroprotective agent is available, although this is an area of intensive research. Antiepileptic drug therapy will prevent early epilepsy but does not reduce the frequency of late seizures. Early seizures are often not followed by late epilepsy—a fact that is important to emphasize to patients.

### The treatment of epilepsy due to developmental and acquired causes

As the form of epilepsy in different causes is often identical, it is perhaps not surprising (although admittedly rather disappointing) that the antiepileptic drug therapy for most forms of acquired epilepsy follows similar principles whatever the cause. Factors predicting response to therapy are also similar for all conditions. This lack of specificity implies that there are similar underlying processes of epileptogenesis in epilepsies of many different causes. The approach to drug treatment is similar to that of any focal or secondarily generalized epilepsy, and this is described in Section 2 of this book. Where specific therapy is indicated, this is listed in the sections below. Surgical therapy is appropriate in a number of acquired epilepsies, and the assessment for surgery is described in Section 5.

### Hippocampal sclerosis

Hippocampal sclerosis is the most common cause of temporal lobe epilepsy. It is found in over one-third of cases of people with refractory focal epilepsy attending hospital clinics in whom there is no other structural lesion, but is less frequent in population-based cohorts and in patients with mild epilepsy. Hippocampal sclerosis typically causes complex partial seizures, and the clinical features and symptom complex associated with the syndrome of mesial temporal lobe epilepsy are described on pp. 13–14.

The pathological changes are described on p. 236. The pathogenesis of hippocampal sclerosis is probably multifactorial and the histological changes may be the end point of a number of different processes. Known causes of hippocampal sclerosis include cerebral trauma, infection (encephalitis or meningitis), vascular damage, toxins (e.g. demoic acid) or raised intracranial pressure. Familial

genetic forms exist (p. 28), and interestingly, in some families, relatives report *déjà vu* episodes, which may represent undiagnosed epilepsy. There is a very clear association with a history of childhood febrile convulsions, and one postulation is that the febrile convulsions, especially if prolonged or complex, damage the hippocampus and result in hippocampal sclerosis. Serial MRI studies have demonstrated that status epilepticus also can result in hippocampal sclerosis and there is clear evidence from animal experimentation that prolonged partial seizures can cause hippocampal damage. There is also evidence that, in some cases, hippocampal sclerosis may be a congenital lesion, and its frequent association with forms of cortical dysplasia (particularly subependymal heterotopia, p. 42) adds some strength to the view that hippocampal sclerosis itself may sometimes be a form of cortical dysgenesis.

The medical treatment of hippocampal sclerosis follows conventional lines, similar to that of any focal epilepsy, and the seizures can often be well controlled on medical therapy. Hippocampal sclerosis is also the most common lesion resected in epilepsy surgical practice, and is the most common pathology referred for epilepsy surgery. The surgical therapy of hippocampal sclerosis is dealt with in detail on pp. 236–48.

### Prenatal and perinatal injury

Epilepsy has traditionally often been thought to occur owing to perinatal injury, although it is now recognized that in many such cases there are genetic or other prenatal developmental pathologies causing the epilepsy. In most children with epilepsy, minor perinatal problems are quite irrelevant to the subsequent development of epilepsy, or indeed are themselves the result of the underlying defects. In controlled studies only severe perinatal insults—for instance perinatal haemorrhage and ischaemic–hypoxic encephalopathy—have been found to increase the risk of subsequent epilepsy. Factors such as toxaemia, eclampsia, forceps delivery, being born with the 'cord round the neck', low birth weight or prematurity have only a very modest association, if any, with subsequent epilepsy. Factors reported in some studies are not confirmed in others, but in one large case–control study, early gestational age, vaginal bleeding during pregnancy, birth by caesarian section, and socioeconomic factors were found to confer a small risk of subsequent epilepsy.

### Cerebral palsy

This term encompasses many pathologies, both prenatal and perinatal, and both genetic and acquired. It therefore has little utility, although is in widespread use. Whatever the cause, cerebral palsy is indicative of cerebral damage, and thus is strongly associated with epilepsy. In the US National Collaborative Perinatal Project, a prospective cohort study of infants followed to the age of 7 years, epilepsy was found to occur in 34% of children with cerebral palsy, and cerebral palsy was present in 19% of children developing epilepsy. In the same cohort the risk of learning disability (associated with cerebral palsy) was 5.5 times higher among children developing epilepsy following a febrile seizure than in children with a febrile seizure alone. Learning disability (IQ < 70) was present in 27% of the children with epilepsy, and seizures were present in about 50% of children with mental retardation and cerebral palsy.

### Post-vaccination encephalopathy

The possible role of vaccination (particularly pertussis vaccination) in causing a childhood encephalopathy and subsequent epilepsy and learning disability has been the subject of intense study, with contradictory claims. The UK National Childhood Encephalopathy Study found that children hospitalized with seizures and encephalopathy were more likely to have received diphtheria–tetanus–pertussis (DTP) vaccination in the previous 7 days than control children. However, the potential methodological bias of this study has been severely criticized. A more recent large series of 368,000 children after immunization found no difference in rates of epilepsy when compared with controls. Similarly, suggestions that mumps–measles–rubella (MMR) vaccine increases the risks of autism and epilepsy are now thought to be unfounded. Most vaccines are now not prepared from infected live neural tissue and as a result there has been a significant reduction in post-vaccination encephalomyelitits. Conventional medical advice is now that vaccination is safe, and although a small number of children do develop encephalopathic reactions which result in later epilepsy, the risk of this occurring is considerably less than the risk of encephalopathy after the naturally occurring viral illnesses that vaccination prevents. Thus, for instance, the generally accepted rate of post-vaccination encephalomyelitis following measles vaccination is about 1–2 per million, compared with the risk of post-measles encephalomyelitis of about 1–2 per 1000. Currently, the vaccine with the greatest risk is the smallpox vaccine, with a rate of 10–300 cases per million of post-vaccination encephalomyelitis, although safer vaccines are under development. The vaccines known to be associated with post-vaccination encephalomyelitis are smallpox, measles, DTP, Japanese B encephalitis, and rabies.

### Degenerative diseases and dementia

Epilepsy is a common feature of degenerative neurological disease that involves the grey matter, but is seldom a leading symptom in pure leucodystrophy.

The most common neurodegenerative disorders are the dementias in late life. Six per cent of persons over the age of 65 years have dementia, and the rate increases exponentially as a function of age. Alzheimer's disease is the most common cause of dementia, and patients with Alzheimer's disease are six times more likely to develop epilepsy than age-matched controls. Partial and secondarily generalized seizures occur, and are usually relatively easily treated with conventional antiepileptic therapy. Myoclonus is another common finding in patients with Alzheimer's disease, occurring in about 10% of autopsy-verified cases, and is a late manifestation. Non-convulsive status epilepticus can occur, and is often overlooked. An EEG is helpful in diagnosis, and should be considered in any demented person whose condition acutely deteriorates. Seizures occur in the other common dementing illnesses also, and are particularly common in cerebrovascular disease (see p. 51). As the population ages, the number of individuals affected by Alzheimer's disease and other dementias is going to increase, and so will the proportion of epilepsy attributed to dementing disorders.

Five per cent of patients with Huntington disease have epilepsy, usually in the later stages. Epilepsy is more common in the juvenile form, and occasionally takes the form of a progressive myoclonic epilepsy. Epilepsy, and indeed status epilepticus, can be the presenting feature of Creutzfeldt–Jakob disease. Generalized tonic–clonic or partial seizures occur in 10% of established cases, and myoclonus in 80%, and they can be induced by startle or other stimuli. The EEG usually shows the repetitive periodic discharges. In the terminal stages of the condition, the myoclonus and the epilepsy usually cease.

### Post-traumatic epilepsy

Head trauma is an important cause of epilepsy. Estimates of frequency of injury and of the risk of post-traumatic epilepsy have varied widely in different studies, partly owing to different definitions and changes in diagnosis and management. The figures given below are best-guess estimates based on modern practice. It is customary to draw a distinction between open head injury, where the dura is breached, and closed head injury, where there is no dural breach. Post-traumatic seizures are traditionally subdivided into immediate, early and late categories. Immediate seizures are defined as those that occur within the first 24 hours after injury, early seizures are those that occur within the first week, and late seizures occur after 1 week.

Closed head injuries are most common in civilian practice, usually from road traffic accidents, falls or recreational injuries, and in different series have accounted for between 2 and 12% of all cases of epilepsy. If mild injury is included, the incidence of traumatic brain injury in the USA has been estimated to be as high as 825 cases per 100,000 per year, with about 100–200 per 100,000 per year admitted to hospital. Early seizures after closed head injury occur in about 2–6% of those admitted to hospital, with a higher frequency in children than in adults. Early seizures indicate a more severe injury, but have not been found generally to be an independent predictive risk factor of late seizures. Approximately 5% of patients—estimates have varied between 2 and 25%—requiring hospitalization for closed head trauma will subsequently develop epilepsy (late post-traumatic seizures). Mild head injury—defined as head injury without skull fracture and with less than 30 minutes of post-traumatic amnesia—is, in most studies, not associated with any markedly increased risk of epilepsy. Moderate head injury—defined as a head injury complicated by skull fracture or post-traumatic amnesia for more than 30 minutes—is followed by epilepsy in about 1–4% of cases. Severe head injury—defined as a head injury with post-traumatic amnesia of more than 24 hours, intracranial haematoma or cerebral contusion—is followed by epilepsy, in most studies, in about 10–15% of patients. Less than 10% of all head injuries admitted to hospital are categorized as severe and more than 70% as mild. The extra risk of epilepsy is highest during the first year, with onset of epilepsy peaking 4–8 months post-injury, and diminishes during the ensuing years. After 10 years only severe injuries still exhibit an increased risk of seizures. In one large study the incidence of epilepsy at 1 year post-injury was < 1% (but 3 times the population risk) after mild injury, < 1% (but 7 times the population risk) after moderate injury, and 6% (but 100 times the population risk) after severe injury. The 30-year cumulative incidence of seizures is 2.1% for mild injuries, 4.2% for moderate injuries and 16.7% for severe injuries. The risk of seizures after severe injuries is 30 times higher than that after mild head injury during the first year and 8 times higher by year 5.

Post-traumatic epilepsy is much more frequent after open head injury. This is particularly so in penetrating wartime injuries with between 30 and 50% of patients suffering subsequent epilepsy. Overall, the risk of late epilepsy, if early epilepsy is present, is about 25% compared with 3% in patients who did not have early seizures. The risk of epilepsy after open head injury is greatest if the extent of cerebral damage is large and involves the frontal or temporal regions. About 50–60% of cases have their first (late) seizure within 12 months of the injury, with most cases developing within 4–8 months after the injury, and 85% within 2 years.

Calculations of the risk of epilepsy in various circumstances following injury have been made. The presence of a dural breach (for instance with a depressed fracture), an intracranial haematoma and long post-traumatic amnesia (≥ 24 hours) have been found consistently to increase significantly the risk of subsequent epilepsy. In one series, the risk of seizures by 2 years was 27% in the presence of depressed skull fracture, 24% with subdural haematoma (and 44% if this was severe enough to need surgical evacuation), 23% with intracranial haematoma and 12% with long post-traumatic amnesia. In another study, risks of single and combined factors were calculated. The risk of late epilepsy following an intracranial haematoma alone was 35% and after a depressed fracture alone was 17%. If three factors were combined, the risk of post-traumatic epilepsy exceeded 50%. Conversely, in the absence of a depressed fracture, intracranial haematoma or early seizures, the risk of late epilepsy is less than 2% even if post-traumatic amnesia exceeds 24 hours. Other factors found in some studies only to increase the rate of late seizures include the presence of early seizures, prolonged coma, depressed fracture without dural breach, and the presence of an unreactive pupil at the time of injury.

The pathophysiology of post-traumatic epilepsy is complex and multifactorial. The kinetic energy imparted to the brain tissue produces pressure waves which disrupt tissue and lead to histopathological changes, including gliosis, axon retraction balls, Wallerian degeneration, neurological scars and cystic white matter lesions. In addition, iron liberated from haemoglobin generates free radicals that disrupt cell membranes and have been implicated in post-traumatic epileptogenesis. Iron and other compounds have also been found to provoke intracellular calcium oscillations. Hippocampal damage following head injury also seems common (over 80% in one series), and this may be due to enhanced excitability secondary to the death of inhibitory dentate hilar neurones. Such hyperexcitability can last for months following the trauma with reorganization of excitatory pathways such as mossy fibre sprouting.

Post-traumatic epilepsy can be difficult to treat, and in one series after open head injury 53% of patients still had active epilepsy 15 years after the injury. The risks of epilepsy are increased in those who have a family history of epilepsy, confirming the often multifactorial nature of epilepsy.

Antiepileptic drug therapy reduces the risk of early seizures. However, there has been controversy about the role of longer-term prophylactic antiepileptic drug treatment after head trauma. Early retrospective reports suggested that such prophylactic treatment reduced the incidence of subsequent epilepsy, although none of the subsequent large-scale prospective trials showed any protective effect on late seizures. Nevertheless, it is now usual to prescribe antiepileptic drugs after severe head injury for a period of 6 months or so.

There is typically a latent period between the head injury and the development of late epilepsy, usually of a few months but sometimes longer. Presumably, during this period, epileptogenic processes are occurring, and thus there is a clear potential for neuroprotective interventions to inhibit or abolish these processes. This is an area of intensive research, but currently no specific therapy has been shown to be effective. Trials of antioxidents, antiperoxidants, steroids and chelating agents have taken place, but none have been shown to have any protective effect.

### Epilepsy after neurosugery

Neurosurgery is in effect a form of cerebral trauma, and not surprisingly can cause epilepsy. It is obviously important to define this risk, as it can influence the indications for operation, and it is an important topic for pre-operative counselling. The risk of late post-operative seizures is greater in patients with younger age, early post-operative seizures, and severe neurological deficit. The incidence of seizures varies according to the nature of the underlying disease process, its site and its extent. A large retrospective study found an overall incidence of 17% for post-operative seizures in 877 consecutive patients undergoing supratentorial neurosurgery for non-traumatic conditions. The patients had no prior history of epilepsy and the minimum follow-up was 5 years. The incidence of seizures ranged from 4% in patients undergoing stereotactic procedures and ventricular drainage to 92% for patients being surgically treated for cerebral abscess. The risk of craniotomy for glioma was 19%, for intracranial haemorrhage 21% and for meningioma removal 22%. All these risks were greatly enhanced if seizures occurred pre-operatively. Among patients developing post-operative seizures, 37% did so within the first post-operative week, 77% within the first year and 92% within the first 2 years. If early seizures occurred (i.e. those occurring in the first week), 41% of patients developed late recurrent seizures.

Studies after unruptured aneurysm show an overall risk of developing epilepsy of about 14%. The risk of a middle cerebral aneurysm resulting in epilepsy is 19%, and anterior communicating aneurysms and posterior communicating aneurysms carry a risk of about 10%. If the aneurysm has bled, causing an intracranial haematoma, the incidence of epilepsy is much higher, as it is if patients have perioperative complications including hemiparesis or meningitis, implying parenchymal damage. The overall risk of developing epilepsy following shunt procedures is about 10%, although this depends on the site of the shunt insertion. As is the case following cerebral trauma, the risks of epilepsy following neurosurgery are greatest in the first post-operative year, although a substantial proportion of cases (perhaps 25%) experience their first seizures in the second post-operative year.

Whether or not the prophylactic use of anticonvulsants after neurosurgical procedures is worthwhile is highly controversial. The best studies seem to show no effect, although all investigations in this area have been open to criticism. More definitive investigations are required, but currently it is usual to prescribe prophylactic anticonvulsant drugs for several months after major supratentorial neurosurgery and then gradually to withdraw the medication unless seizures have occurred.

## Cerebral tumour

Brain tumours are responsible for about 6% of all newly diagnosed cases of epilepsy. The rate is greatest in adults, and about one-quarter of adults presenting with newly developing focal epilepsy have an underlying tumour, compared with less than 5% in children. Seizures occur in about 50% of all people with brain tumours. The frequency of seizures is high in tumours in the frontal, central and temporal regions, lower in posterior cortically placed tumours and very low in subcortical tumours. The surgical therapy of tumours is considered on pp. 249–50, 253–7.

## Glioma

Gliomas are the most common form of brain tumour causing epilepsy. Slow-growing low-grade well-differentiated gliomas are the most epileptogenic lesions. In the Montreal series of 230 patients with gliomas, seizures occurred in 92% of those with oligodendrogliomas, 70% of those with astrocytomas and 37% of those with glioblastomas. Overall, slow-growing or benign tumours account for about 10% of all adult epilepsies, and less in children. The history of epilepsy will often have extended for decades, sometimes even into infancy. In chronic refractory tumoural epilepsy, oligodendrogliomas account for between 10 and 30%, dysembryoplastic neuroepithelial tumours (DNETs or DNTs) for 10–30%, astrocytomas for 10–30%, gangliogliomas for about 10–20%, and hamartomas for between 10 and 20%. These tumours are sometimes associated, particularly if situated in the temporal lobe, with hippocampal sclerosis. The generation of epileptic discharges does not take place within the tumoural tissue (the exception is in the DNET—see below) but in the surrounding tissue, and this has implications for surgical therapy. The mechanisms of epileptogenesis in patients with brain tumours include impaired vascularization of the surrounding cerebral cortex, morphological neuronal alterations, changes in the excitatory and inhibitory synaptic mechanisms, and genetic susceptibility.

## Ganglioglioma

These are mixed tumours that are composed of neoplastic glial and neuronal cell types and comprise 10% of more of the neoplasms removed at temporal lobectomy. Seizures are the primary presenting symptom in 80–90% of patients with gangliogliomas, and can develop at any age. These tumours are typically frontal or temporal in location and the outcome for seizure control is good if the tumour can be resected.

## Dysembryoplastic neuroepithelial tumour

The dysembryoplastic neuroepithelial tumour is a pathological entity only recently differentiated from other forms of 'benign glioma'. They are in fact a relatively common cause of 'tumorous epilepsy', accounting for 10–30% of resected tumours in the temporal lobe. DNETs are developmental in origin and the tumours co-exist with other forms of cortical dysplasia, including focal cortical dysplasia, heterotopias and microdysgenesis. The tumours are most commonly situated in the temporal lobe (two-thirds), but can occur in any cortical region. They are benign tumours with only a slight propensity for growth, and epilepsy is usually the only clinical symptom. The epilepsy can present in children or in adults, and the seizures are usually partial in nature and vary considerably in severity. Surgical resection is indicated only if lack of seizure control warrants the risks involved. Surgical resection, or even partial resection, will usually control the seizures and they are thus an important pathology to identify (see p. 250).

### Hamartoma

These benign tumours account for 15–20% of tumours removed at temporal lobectomy; they are more common in children. Their pathological features include proliferation of glial and neuronal elements, and they can be associated with other types of cortical dysplasia. Indeed the distinction between cortical dysplasia, hamartomas and relatively indolent neoplasms, such as DNET, can be blurred. The classic clinicopathological finding in tuberous sclerosis complex (see pp. 36–7) is the periventricular glial nodule or subependymal tuber. Histologically, these lesions are hamartomas and consist of foci of gliosis, which include both glial cells and neurones. Surgical resection of isolated hamartomas is often curative. In tuberous sclerosis complex, however, individual tubers are usually only one part of a wider epileptogenic process, and only rarely can a seizure focus be localized to a single cortical tuber that can be successfully resected.

### Hypothalamic hamartoma (and gelastic epilepsy)

The hypothalamic hamartoma is a particular form of hamartoma. These are benign tumours, usually small and sometimes confined to the tuber cinerium. They are present in young children, and characteristically present with gelastic seizures, learning disability, behavioural disturbance, and later with precocious puberty. They are diagnosed by MRI scanning, but the lesions can be very subtle, especially if small, without mass effect, and isodense on both T1 and T2 sequences.

Gelastic seizures are highly characteristic of tumours of the floor of the third ventricle and particularly of hypothalamic hamartoma (although they do occur occasionally in temporal lobe epilepsy). The seizures start before the age of 3 years in most cases, and are often very frequent. The attacks are brief, and take the form of sudden laughter associated with other variable motor features (clonic movements, head and eye deviation). The laughter is 'mirthless', is not associated with any emotional feelings of joy or happiness, and occurs in situations that do not provoke humour. The combination of severe gelastic epilepsy, precocious puberty and intellectual impairment can be a devastating disability. The seizures do not usually respond to conventional drug therapy, but surgical resection of the tumours can be very successful, with complete seizure remission expected in about 50% of cases (see p. 259).

### Meningioma

Epilepsy is the first symptom of meningioma in 20–50% of cases. Meningiomas located over the convexity, falx or parasagittal regions or sphenoid ridge are especially likely to cause epilepsy. There is no relationship between the presence of epilepsy and histological type. Surgical resection can be expected to stop seizures in about 30–60% of operated cases.

## CNS infection

CNS infections are a major risk factor for epilepsy. Seizures can be the presenting or the only symptom, or one component of a more diffuse cerebral disorder.

### Meningitis and encephalitis

The risk of chronic epilepsy following encephalitis or meningitis is almost sevenfold greater than that in the population in general. The increased risk is highest during the first 5 years after infection, but remains elevated for up to 15 years. The risk is much higher after encephalitis (relative risk [RR] 16.2) than bacterial meningitis (RR 4.2) or aseptic meningitis (RR 2.3). The presence of early seizures (i.e. during the acute phase of the infection) greatly influences the risk of subsequent unprovoked seizures. As encephalitis and bacterial meningitis are more prevalent in childhood and early adult life, most cases of post-infectious epilepsy develop in young individuals.

#### Meningitis

The most common forms of bacterial meningitis are now due to *Streptococcus pneumoniae* (peumoccoal meningitis) and *Neisseria meningitides* (meningococcal meningitis). *Haemophilus influenzae* type b (Hib) used to be a leading cause but new vaccines have virtually eradicated the condition in Western countries. Meningococcal meningitis is the most serious common form. Its incidence varies, and in Europe, for instance, the highest incidence is in Scotland and Iceland. Ninety-five per cent of cases are due to serogroups B and C, and the case fatality rate is between 5 and 10%. Treatment is with penicillin or rifampicin, but antibiotic resistance is growing. Viral meningitis is common but is usually mild and rarely results in epilepsy.

#### Encephalitis

Encephalitis is most commonly due to viral infection, but other infectious agents can cause post-encephalitic epilepsy (Table 1.31). The most common serious viral encephalitis is due to herpes simplex virus type 1 (HSV-1). The incidence of severe HSV-1 encephalitis is about 1 per million persons per year, but it is possible that more minor infection occurs which escapes detection. It has indeed been postulated that many cases of epilepsy, currently considered cryptogenic, are due to occult viral infection—although hard evidence in support of this point of view is entirely lacking. Immunological studies show varicella virus also to be a common cause of CNS infection, but overt varicella encephalitis is less common than HSV-1 encephalitis. In the USA, St Louis virus (a mosquito-borne arbovirus) is common. In Asia, Japanese B viral encephalitis results in up to 15,000 deaths annually. Two recent viral encephalitides which are increasing in frequency are those due to West Nile virus and Nipah virus.

Seizures are a frequent symptom in the acute phase of severe HSV encephalitis, and many survivors are left with neurological sequelae including severe epilepsy. The seizures take partial and secondarily generalized forms, and status epilepticus is common. The prognosis for epilepsy (and other sequelae) is worse in those with delayed antiviral treatment and with a low Glasgow coma score at the height of the illness. Of the other viral encephalitides, enteroviral encephalitis is usually mild without sequelae and arboviral encephalitis has a variable prognosis (depending on viral type).

The clinical diagnosis can be confirmed by serological tests, from cerebrospinal fluid (CSF) and serum, and by

**Table 1.31** Causes of infectious encephalitis.

---

*Causes of infective encephalitis in the immune-competent patient*
Viral:
　　Herpes simplex virus (HSV) type 1, other herpes viruses (e.g. varicella, HSV type 2, CMV, EBV, HSV type 6), measles, mumps, rubella, rabies, arbovirus (e.g. Japanese B, St Louis, West Nile, equine and tick-borne viruses), adenovirus, HIV, influenza (A,B), enterovirus, poliovirus

Bacterial and rickettsial (uncommon):
　　*Bartonella* spp., *Borrelia burgdorferi*, *Brucella* spp., *Leptospira interrogans*, *Listeria monocytogenes*, *Mycobacterium tuberculosis*, *Mycoplasma pneumoniae*, *Rickettsia rickettsii*, Q fever and other Rickettsial infections, *Treponema pallidum*, leptospirosis, *Nocardia actinomyces*, *Salmonella typhi*, *Legionella*

Protozoal (uncommon):
　　Malaria (*Plasmodium falciparum*), *Toxoplasma gondii*, *Naegleria fowleri*, *Acanthamoeba* spp., cysticercosis, *Echinococcus* spp., *Trypanosoma* spp., schistosomiasis

Fungal (uncommon):
　　Blastomycosis, coccidioidomycosis, histoplasmosis, cryptococcus, aspergillosis, candidiasis

*Causes of infectious encephalitis in the immune-compromised patient*
Viral:
　　Enterovirus, cytomegalovirus, HSV types 1, 2, 6, JC virus, measles, rubella, varicella

Protozoal:
　　Amoebic meningoencephalitis, toxoplasmosis

Fungal:
　　*Cryptococcus neoformans*, coccidioidomycosis, blastomycosis, histoplasmosis, aspergillus, *Candida*

---

neuroimaging. Viral encephalitis needs to be differentiated from acute disseminated encephalomyelitis (ADEM), which can present with a very similar picture, and other causes of non-infectious encephalopathy. Precise diagnosis of viral encephalitis can be difficult. HSV may be isolated from CSF in up to 50% of cases of neonatal HSV infection but is rarely found in specimens obtained from older children and adults with HSV encephalitis. Serological testing during the acute and convalescent phases of illness is of little immediate value in the diagnosis of HSV or enteroviral encephalitis. In contrast, the presence of arbovirus-specific immunoglobulin M (IgM) in spinal fluid is diagnostic of arboviral encephalitis. Polymerase chain reaction (PCR) is much more sensitive, with a 95% sensitivity and 100% specificity for HSV DNA in patients with biopsy-proven HSV encephalitis. PCR techniques show excellent specificity and sensitivity in the diagnosis of enteroviral meningitis. An MRI scan may be normal early in the course of HSV encephalitis, but within days focal oedema and haemorrhage are usually evident. EEG is a useful complementary test for the diagnosis of HSV encephalitis, showing focal unilateral or bilaterial periodic discharges localized in the temporal lobes. Viral encephalitis should be treated with aciclovir or other antiviral therapies, and the earlier therapy is started the better the outcome. The epilepsy is treated along conventional lines.

Patients with AIDS and other immunocompromised states have a different range of pathogens (Table 1.31), and cerebral infection is a common feature of the condition; the most common opportunistic CNS infections are cryptococcal meningitis, toxoplasmosis, tuberculosis and cytomegalovirus (CMV) encephalitis. Seizures may also be a sign of progressive multifocal leucoencephalopathy in HIV, although usually it is a minor aspect of the clinical presentation.

### Cerebral malaria

Seizures and typically status epilepticus are particularly common in the acute phase of cerebral malaria. Convulsive and focal seizures can occur, but in young children in coma seizures can be subtle, taking minor forms such as eye deviation or changes in respiratory pattern or salivation. Prolonged convulsions are associated with increased mortality and also neurological deficits in survivors, so detection and emergency therapy are important. The benzodiazepines, particularly diazepam, should be used initially, and phenobarbital used as second-line therapy. Artemisinin derivatives should be given as antimalarials in the acute phase, combined with cinchona alkaloids such as mefloquine. Chronic epilepsy is common after cerebral malaria, particularly if seizures occurred in the acute phase, and one study has shown a 9–11 (confidence interval [CI]: 2–18)-fold increase in risk of epilepsy compared with children without malaria. This risk is at least double the risk of epilepsy after complex febrile seizures.

## Pyogenic cerebral abscess

Pyogenic brain abscess is an uncommon but serious cause of infective epilepsy. Abscesses range in size from microscopic foci of inflammatory cells to major encapsulated necrotic areas of a cerebral hemisphere exerting significant mass effect. Modern imaging has greatly improved the survival rate and management of brain abscesses but the mortality rate of acute cerebral abscess is still 5–10%. The estimated annual incidence of brain abscesses in the USA is 1 in 10,000 hospital admissions, and abscess surgery accounts for 0.7% of all neurosurgery operations. Brain abscesses occur at any age but are most common in young adult life. The abscesses develop in association with a contiguous suppurating process (usually otitis media, sinus disease or mastoiditis; 50%), due to haematogenous spread from a distant focus (25%), as a complication of intracranial surgery (15%), and due to trauma (10%). Brain abscesses related to middle-ear infection are the most commonly encountered and are often solitary, developing in the inferior portion of the ipsilateral temporal lobe. Brain abscess is a rare complication of bacterial meningitis in adults; it is, however, more common in infants, particularly those with Gram-negative meningitis. Haematogenous metastatic spread from distant parts of the body frequently leads to the development of brain abscesses. The most common site of origin is a pyogenic lung infection, such as lung abscess, bronchiectasis, empyema, cystic fibrosis or acute endocarditis. Other potential primary foci include osteomyelitis, wound and skin infections, cholecystitis, pelvic infection, and other forms of intra-abdominal sepsis. Brain abscesses from blood-spread infections are most likely to occur in the middle cerebral territory and at the grey–white matter junction, and are frequently multifocal. Brain abscess complicates approximately 3–15% of penetrating cranio-cerebral injuries, especially those caused by gunshot injuries.

The species of bacteria responsible for brain abscesses depends on the pathogenic mechanism involved. Commonly isolated organisms are streptococci, including aerobic, anaerobic and microaerophilic types. *Strep. pneumoniae* is a rarer cause of brain abscesses, which are often the sequel to occult CSF rhinorrhoea and also to pneumococcal pneumonia in elderly patients. Enteric bacteria and *Bacteroides* are isolated in 20–40% of cases and often in mixed culture. Anaerobic organisms have become increasingly important organisms and in many instances more than a single bacterial species is recovered. Gram-negative bacilli rarely occur alone. Staphylococcal abscesses account for 10–15% of cases and are usually caused by penetrating head injury or bacteraemia secondary to endocarditis. Clostridial infections are most often post-traumatic. Rarely *Actinomyces* or *Nocardia* are the causative agents of a brain abscess.

The diagnosis of brain abscesses has been greatly facilitated by modern imaging, and most cases can now be identified rapidly. Surgical resection (p. 260) is the treatment of choice. The mortality is about 10% and up to 50% of patients have permanent neurological deficit after brain abscesses. Epilepsy follows in between 30% and 80% of cases, and can sometimes develop years after the acute infection. All patients with preoperative seizures are likely to continue to have seizures postoperatively, and the risk remains high for several years after the acute infection. Epilepsy is more likely after frontal lobe abscesses. Epilepsy following cerebral abscess can be very difficult to control. Antiepileptic drug treatment follows the usual principles, but in severe cases resection of the abscess cavity can be considered. Severe secondarily generalized epilepsy following a frontal abscess can respond to corpus callosotomy (see p. 263). Given the high likelihood of development of seizures, all patients with supratentorial brain abscesses should routinely be placed on prophylactic antiepileptic drugs for at least 1–2 years. If no seizures occur at this stage, the drugs can be then withdrawn, but only if the EEG shows no epileptogenic activity.

## Neurocysticercosis

Worldwide, neurocysticercosis (NCC) is the most common parasitic disease of the CNS and a major cause of epilepsy in endemic areas such as Mexico, India and China. Epilepsy is the most common clinical manifestation and usual presenting feature of NCC. The condition is a helminthiasis caused by the encysted larval stage, *Cysticercus cellulosae*, of the pork tapeworm *Taenia solium*. In the first stage, the human (definitive) host ingests undercooked diseased pork containing viable cysticerci from within which the scolex (head) of the organism evaginates in the gut and attaches to the intestinal mucosa. Over 3 months, the tapeworm matures to a length of 2–7 m. Gravid segments containing eggs are released into the faeces, often unknown to the host. Following ingestion, eggs hatch and activate in the pig (intermediate host) small intestine and develop in the CNS and striated muscle. Humans become intermediate hosts by ingesting infected tissue, and the lifecycle is completed in the human CNS, skin and muscle. Parenchymal cysts usually lie dormant for many years and symptoms usually coincide with larval death and an intense inflammatory response caused by the release of larval antigens. The solitary cerebral parenchymal lesion is a common form of presentation, but lesions are often multiple. Over time, the cysts shrink progressively and then calcify or disappear completely. Seizures are the most common symptom and develop when a cyst is degenerating or around a chronic calcified lesion. In the racemose form of NCC, the cysts can obstruct CSF flow and present with mass effect, hydrocephalus or basal arachnoiditis (the treatment of these cases differs from those presenting simply with epilepsy and is outside the scope of this book).

Diagnosis is made by imaging and by serological tests. CSF and EEG are rather non-specific. Computed tomography

(CT) is particularly useful for showing calcified inactive lesions. MRI is superior for demonstrating subarachnoid or intraventricular cysts and for showing inflammation around a cyst. Cysts may be single or multiple and at different pathological stages at any given time. A classification system that corresponds to parasite viability has been proposed, with divisions into active, transitional and inactive forms. In the active stage the CT appearance is that of a rounded, hypodense area or there may be a CSF-like signal on MRI. The 'starry night' effect—the presence of multiple eccentric mural nodules—is characteristic of NCC, although it may also be seen in cases of *Toxoplasma* infection. The transitional stage is due to cystic degeneration. This appears on CT as a diffuse hypodense area with an irregular border which enhances with contrast. They usually appear as high signal areas on T2-weighted MRI. Lastly, when the cyst dies, the lesion either disappears or becomes a calcified inactive nodule of low intensity on proton-weighted MRI or homogeneous high density on CT scan. Standard enzyme-linked immunosorbent assay (ELISA) diagnostic techniques have proved less useful than hoped because of high false-negative and false-positive rates. Newer enzyme-linked immuno-electron transfer blot (EITB) assays on CSF or serum appear to have higher sensitivity (98%) and specificity (100%) in multiple cysticercosis. Its superiority to ELISA is due to its ability to detect up to seven glycoproteins specific to *T. solium*. It is visualized like a western blot, so that non-specific bands can be ignored thereby ruling out cross-reactivity. Recently, an antigen detection ('capture') assay specific for viable metacestodes in CSF has been designed. So far, this has proved to be perhaps the most reliable method of detecting active cases of NCC in epidemiological studies. Serology is a sensitive way of detecting exposure, but in endemic areas, where population exposure rates are high, positive serology in any individual does not necessarily imply that neurocysticercosis is the cause of the symptoms.

Cerebral tuberculoma is the main differential diagnosis, but there are imaging differences. Typically, the lesions of neurocysticercosis are well circumscribed, discrete, less than 20 mm in size, and superficially located; they enhance relatively little, may have visible scolexes and less peri-lesional oedema, and only occasionally cause midline shift. Multiple cysts have a 'starry sky' appearance.

The mainstay of treatment is the control of seizures with antiepileptic drugs. Seizures caused by a single cyst are usually easily controlled. It is not a general policy to use anticysticercal drugs, especially with single lesions, because the enhancing cysticerci shown on imaging are by definition dying away and will resolve spontaneously. Multiple lesions are generally treated with antiparasitic drugs, although these drugs are contraindicated in the presence of cerebral oedema. If needed, two anticysticercal drugs are in wide use in endemic areas—albendazole and praziquantel—although no controlled trials exist that establish specific indications, definitive doses and treatment duration. If anticysticercal drugs are to be used, steroids need to be given in co-medication to prevent a sudden rise in intracranial pressure and exacerbation of symptoms. The role of surgical biopsy in diagnosis is discussed below.

### Tuberculoma

Tuberculosis remains a major problem in developing countries and the incidence is also rising in industrialized countries with increasing migration and the spread of the human immunodeficiency virus (HIV). The most common form of tuberculosis is pulmonary infection, and the incidence of intracranial tuberculoma (tuberculous abscess) has decreased, particularly in Western countries, owing to the BCG vaccination programme. In the early 20th century tuberculomas accounted for about one-third of all space-occupying lesions. The incidence fell dramatically throughout the century, although recently it has started rising again, and today tuberculomas account for about 3% of all cerebral mass lesions in India, for instance, and 13% of all cerebral lesions in HIV infected patients. The diagnosis of intracranial tuberculoma depends on neuroimaging. While both CT and MRI are equally sensitive in visualizing the intracranial tuberculoma, MRI is superior in demonstrating the extent and maturity of the lesion, especially for brainstem lesions. A 'target lesion' in an enhanced CT scan is considered highly characteristic of tuberculoma, although this sign may also be produced by cerebral toxoplasmosis.

Tuberculomas present particularly with epilepsy, and therapy for the epilepsy follows conventional lines. Surgical resection of the tuberculoma was the usual procedure in the past, but increasingly a conservative approach is now initially taken. Surgery is still indicated in the initial stages in cases of diagnostic uncertainty and where larger, symptomatic mass lesions cause midline shift and severe intracranial hypertension. In patients presenting simply with epilepsy, it is now usual to treat with antitubercular and antiepileptic drugs (with a short course of adjunctive steroids), and to defer surgery. When medical therapy is initiated, without diagnostic confirmation from a biopsy, the patient should be carefully monitored, and if the mass does not decrease in size after 8 weeks of therapy, biopsy should be reconsidered. With early diagnosis and a balanced combination of surgical and medical management, tuberculomas are now potentially curable.

### *Acute seizures with CT evidence of a single enhancing lesion*

Newly developing seizures associated with a single enhancing lesion on CT are a common clinical problem in endemic areas such as India. The differential diagnosis includes neurocysticercosis, tuberculosis, gliomas and other tumours, toxoplasmosis and other infective lesions. Over 90% of the lesions in India are due to neurocysticercosis, and currently the usual management strategy is to screen the patient for other signs of tuberculosis, and if none are present not to give antitubercular therapy. CT is repeated in 12 weeks and if the lesion has not regressed, or has increased, a review of diagnosis including surgical biopsy is the preferred approach. Antiepileptic drugs are given.

## Cerebrovascular disease

Epilepsy can complicate all forms of cerebrovascular disease. Stroke is the most commonly identified cause of epilepsy in the elderly, and occult stroke also explains the occurrence of many cases of apparently cryptogenic epilepsies in elderly individuals. A history of stroke has been found to be associated with an increased lifetime occurrence of epilepsy (odds ratio [OR] 3.3; 95% CI, 1.3–8.5). Among the other vascular determinants, only a history of hypertension was associated with the occurrence of unprovoked seizures (OR 1.6; 95% CI, 1.0–2.4). The risk of unprovoked seizures rises to 4.1 (95% CI, 1.5–11.0) in subjects having a history of both stroke and hypertension.

### Cerebral haemorrhage

The reported risk of chronic epilepsy due to intracranial haemorrhage has varied greatly from series to series, but is generally in the region of 5–10%. The incidence of early epilepsy (seizures in the first week) is higher, up to 30% in some series with status epilepticus in about 10%. Early seizures do not necessarily lead to chronic epilepsy, although they increase the long-term risk, and about one-third of those with early seizures continue to have a liability to epilepsy. Epilepsy is common after large haemorrhages and haemorrhages that involve the cerebral cortex, less common in deep haematomas and rare after subtentorial haemorrhage. The epilepsy almost always develops within 2 years of the haemorrhage. The risk of seizures after subarachnoid haemorrhage is between 20 and 34%, and the risk of chronic epilepsy among survivors of subarachnoid haemorrhage is highest in those with early seizures, intracerebral haematoma or other persisting neurological sequelae.

### Cerebral infarction

After cerebral infarction, epilepsy occurs in about 6% of patients within 12 months and 11% within 5 years of the stroke. Epilepsy is more common in cerebral infarcts located in the anterior hemisphere, and involving the cortex. The standardized mortality ratio (SMR) for epilepsy after infarction has been found to be 5.9 (95% CI, 3.5–9.4), and the risk of developing seizures is highest during the first year, and higher if there is a history of recurrent stroke. There is an inverse correlation between age and risk of seizures with a peak in patients aged less than 55 years. In a multivariant analysis, early seizures and recurrent strokes were the only clinical factors shown to predict the occurrence of epilepsy after infarction.

### Occult degenerative cerebrovascular disease

Epilepsy can also complicate occult cerebrovascular disease. Patients with late-onset epilepsy are significantly more likely to have otherwise asymptomatic ischaemic lesions on CT than age-matched controls, and it has been estimated from such CT-based studies that overt or occult cerebrovascular disease underlies about half of the epilepsies developing after the age of 50 years. Late-onset epilepsy can be the first manifestation of cerebrovascular disease. Between 5 and 10% of patients presenting with stroke have a history of prior epileptic seizures in the recent past, and in the absence of other causes new-onset seizures should prompt a screen for vascular risk factors.

### Arteriovenous malformations (AVMs)

An AVM is a racemose network of arterial and venous channels that communicate directly, rather than through a capillary bed. Between 17 and 36% of supratentorial AVMs present with seizures, with or without associated neurological deficits, and 40–50% with haemorrhage. Smaller AVMs (< 3 cm diameter) are more likely to present with haemorrhage than large ones. Conversely, large and/or superficial malformations are more epileptogenic, as are AVMs in the temporal lobe. About 40% of patients with large AVMs have epilepsy, and epilepsy is the presenting symptom in about 20%. Irrespective of the initial presentation, a significant proportion of patients with cerebral AVMs will develop epilepsy after diagnosis. The risk of seizures seems to be higher the younger the patient at the time of diagnosis. In one study, among patients aged between 10 and 19 years, there was a 44% risk of epilepsy by 20 years of age. This risk declined to 31% for patients aged 20–29 years and to 6% for patients aged 30–60 years. The annual risk of bleeding of an AVM is in the region of 2–4% per year, irrespective of whether the malformation presented with haemorrhage, and the average mortality is about 1% per year. The risk is dependent on the size of the AVM, its growth, the presence of aneurysms, the type of feeding and draining vessels, and the anatomy. Arteriovenous malformations also show highly characteristic MRI appearances, with high signal on T2-weighted images often with a notch-like configuration, and areas of decreased signal intensity representing previous intralesional bleeding. Resective surgery and radiosurgery of large lesions are usually carried out with the aim of preventing haemorrhage rather than controlling epilepsy. However, the complete resections of small AVMs will usually control seizures.

### Cavernous haemangioma (cavernoma)

Cavernous haemangiomas are well-circumscribed hamartomatous lesions consisting of irregularly-walled sinusoidal vascular channels, located within the brain but without intervening neural tissue, with large feeding arteries or draining veins. Pathologically, they consist of endothelial-lined 'caverns' filled with blood and surrounded by a matrix of collagen and fibroblasts. They have the potential to haemorrhage, calcify or thrombose and are multiple in 50% of cases. They account for 5–13% of vascular malformations of the CNS and are present in 0.02–0.13% of autopsy series. The majority of these lesions present in the third and fourth decades of life, but 20–30% present earlier in childhood or early adult life. Cavernomas can increase in size and number over time, particular in genetically-determined cases and in those in whom cavernomas have developed after cerebral irradiation. However, in most cases, the factors influencing the development of new lesions or growth of existing lesions are unknown. At least 15–20% of patients remain symptom free throughout their lives. Patients present with seizures (40–70%), focal neurological deficits (35–50%), non-specific headaches (10–30%), and cerebral haemorrhage. The seizures are typically partial in nature and often brief, infrequent and minor in form. Cavernous malformation can lead to death from cerebrovascular accident, but because of their low flow characteristics, haemorrhage from cavernomas is generally less severe than haemorrhage from AVMs. Retinal, skin and liver lesions have occasionally been reported, presumably on a genetic basis. Familial clustering can be found in 10–30% of cavernous haemangiomas, and familial cases have been found to be linked to genes at three different loci: the *CCM1*, *CCM2* and *CCM3* genes. Forty per cent of familial cases are due to *CCM1*, with higher rates amongst Hispanic individuals. Genetic testing is available.

The lesions are usually diagnosed on CT or MRI, whereas cerebral angiography often shows no abnormality. Typical CT appearances are those of a well-circumscribed hyperdense area with moderate enhancement and variable mass effect. CT may also show previous bleeding, calcification, oedema or cystic areas associated with the lesion. MRI is the most sensitive investigation. On T2-weighted images the typical appearance of cavernomas is that of a reticulated core of mixed signal representing blood in various states of degradation surrounded by a hypointense haemosiderin halo. T1 images show a similar pattern but they are less sensitive. There is slight contrast enhancement in some cases.

Cavernous malformations are twice as likely to be associated with seizures as other vascular lesions, such as AVMs, or tumours with similar volume and location, and the seizures are probably produced by the deposition of blood breakdown products, notably iron, around the lesions during leaks or small haemorrhages. The risk of overt haemorrhage from a cavernoma is in the order of 0.5–2% per annum.

Medical therapy follows conventional lines, and seizures can often be controlled on relatively simple antiepileptic drug regimens. Surgical resection is useful in patients with single lesions and particularly in those with superficial, easily accessible cortical lesions. Focused beam radiation is an alternative therapy.

### Venous malformations

Venous malformations are congenital anomalies of normal venous drainage. They are the most commonly documented intracranial vascular malformation by either brain imaging or autopsy, with a prevalence as high as 3%. They can be associated with cavernous malformations or, more rarely, with AVMs. On MRI they appear as a stellate vascular or contrast-enhancing mass. Angiography typically shows a caput medusae appearance in the late venous phase. These lesions are thought neither to have a high risk of haemorrhage nor to cause epilepsy.

### Collagen vascular diseases and other cerebral vasculitides

The epilepsy can be due to the primary disease process and also to the secondary complications such as arterial hypertension, infarction, vasculitic changes, immunological reactions, and hepatic or renal failure. Epilepsy is a common symptom of all forms of cerebral vasculitis, and particularly in systemic lupus erythematosus (SLE). In SLE, seizures can be the presenting and only symptom, and occur during the course of the illness in about 25% of cases. Seizures are particularly common in severe or chronic cases and in lupus-induced encephalopathy. Epilepsy can also occur in Behçet disease, Sjörgren syndrome, mixed connective tissue disease, Henoch–Schönlein purpura and other forms of large, medium or small vessel vasculitis, sometimes on the basis of infarction.

### Other vascular disorders

Cortical venous infarcts are particularly epileptogenic, at least in the acute phase, and may underlie a significant proportion of apparently spontaneous epileptic seizures complicating other medical conditions and pregnancy. Seizures also occur with cerebrovascular lesions secondary to rheumatic heart disease, endocarditis, mitral valve prolapse, cardiac tumours and cardiac arrhythmia, or after carotid endarterectomy. Infarction is also an important cause of seizures in neonatal epilepsy. Epilepsy is also common in eclampsia, hypertensive encephalopathy, and malignant hypertension and in the anoxic encephalopathy that follows cardiac arrest or cardiopulmonary surgery. Unruptured aneurysms occasionally present as epilepsy, especially if large and if embedded in the temporal lobe—for instance a giant middle cerebral or anterior communicating aneurysm.

## Other neurological disorders
### Rasmussen's encephalitis

This is a rare progressive neurological disorder, of unknown cause, in which severe epilepsy co-exists with slowly progressive atrophy of one cerebral hemisphere. The condition usually begins in late childhood, but can start in adults and also in young children. Pathologically, there is severe atrophy of one hemisphere with histological evidence of perivascular lymphocytic infiltration, neuronal loss and microglial nodule formation. The pathological changes are strikingly unilateral, and where changes do occur in the opposite hemisphere they are usually minor. The cause is unclear, although viral and immunological factors have been implicated. The genomes of various viruses have been found in biopsy tissue, including the Epstein–Barr and herpes simplex viruses, and IgG, IgA and C3 have been found. Glu-R3 antibodies have been reported in the sera of some patients. None of these findings, however, appears to be consistently present.

Clinically, the condition is highly characteristic, with the slow development of severe epilepsy, a progressive hemiparesis and other signs of unilateral hemisphere dysfunction. The condition usually presents with partial epilepsy. This can take any form and typically progresses and is difficult to control. Episodes of epilepsia partialis continua are highly characteristic. Secondarily generalized seizures also occur. As the epilepsy worsens, the patients develop a slowly progressive hemiparesis, which evolves over months or years. Unilateral cognitive dysfunction and other neurological signs, such as aphasia (if the dominant hemisphere is involved), occur. Hemionopia occurs in 50% of cases eventually. Psychiatric disturbances are common. MRI demonstrates progressive cortical atrophy, typically beginning around the sylvian fissure and eventually extending to involve the whole hemisphere. Patchy white matter hyperintensity also occurs involving one hemisphere predominantly, and sometimes the contralateral cerebellum. The CSF is usually normal although it may show oligoclonal bands. The EEG shows multifocal epileptiform discharges predominantly, but not necessarily exclusively, over the affected hemisphere.

Treatment of the epilepsy is difficult. Conventional therapy is frequently ineffective, especially in the case of focal motor seizures or epilepsia partialis continua, which can persist in spite of massive antiepileptic therapy. Corticosteroids, plasmapheresis and antiviral agents (ganciclovir, zidovudine) have been given with some success but seem usually not to have major benefit. The best reported results are with high-dose intravenous immunoglobulin, and frequently repeated courses may be required. Hemispherectomy or large multilobar resection is recommended in a proportion of cases and will alleviate the epilepsy in most operated cases. The evaluation for hemispherectomy and its timing can be difficult, and should be carried out by an experienced unit. The condition tends to 'burn out' after a number of years, leaving the patient with permanent and severe unihemispheric dysfunction.

## Demyelinating disorders

Several clinical series have reported an association between epilepsy and multiple sclerosis (MS). In one small population-based study, patients with MS had a threefold but non-significant increase (SMR, 3.0; 95% CI, 0.6–8.8) in the risk of epilepsy compared with the general population. In another series the cumulative risk of epilepsy in patients with MS was found to be 1.1% at 5 years, 1.8% by 10 years and 3.1% by 15 years. The mean interval until the onset of epilepsy is about 7 years after the onset of MS. Convulsive status epilepticus has been reported more frequently in patients with MS. Epilepsy is more likely to occur in large lesions and lesions which abut on to the cortex, and occasionally MS presents with an acute mass lesion with seizures. Although in some patients epilepsy precedes MS by years or decades, there is no evidence of an increased risk of epilepsy prior to the onset of the symptoms due to MS.

Acute disseminated encephalomyelitis (ADEM) is an acute inflammatory demyelinating disorder which can follow systemic infections, and which is immunologically mediated. Epilepsy is a feature of the acute attack, and occurs much more commonly than in an acute attack of MS. ADEM can follow infections with many different viruses (notably measles, mumps, rubella, varicella, HIV, hepatitis A and B, Epstein–Barr, CMV) or other infectious agents (notably *Mycoplasma, Streptococcus, Borrelia, Campylobacter, Chlamydia leptospira, Legionella*). The incidence after measles infection is about 1 in 1000; after varicella infection about 1 in 10,000; and after rubella infection about 1 in 20,000.

## Inflammatory and immunological diseases of the nervous system

Epilepsy can be a complication of many inflammatory and immunological diseases affecting the central nervous system. The mechanisms of seizures can be due to the direct effect of immunological processes (for instance in Rasmussen's encephalitis) or an indirect effect due to vascular disease and cerebral infarction (for instance in the cerebral vasculitides). In many conditions the mechanisms are unknown.

Seizures are the most common neurological complication of the inflammatory bowel diseases (ulcerative colitis and Crohn's disease), occurring in one series in 6% of cases. The epilepsy may be a direct effect or caused indirectly by dehydration or sepsis. Neurological complications occur in about 10% of patients with Whipple's disease, and the condition presents neurologically in 5%. In a series of cases with neurological symptoms, myoclonus occurred in 25% and seizures in 23%. About 10% of patients with coeliac disease have neurological symptoms, and epilepsy is associated with several rather distinctive neurological presentations. Epilepsy in association with occipital calcification can be the presenting symptom of coeliac disease. Epilepsy, myoclonus and cerebellar ataxia or spino-cerebellar degeneration, and sometimes dementia, is another characteristic neurological syndrome. Coeliac disease may also cause cerebral vasculitis. A recent study, however, suggested that epilepsy was no more common in coeliac disease than in the general population.

Myoclonus and seizures are also a prominent feature of Hashimoto's thyroiditis, a relapsing encephalopathy associated with high titres of thyroid antibody. Epilepsy is also a feature, although often not prominent, of the primary granulomatous diseases of the CNS such as sarcoidosis.

Paraneoplastic disorders can cause seizures. Epilepsia partialis continua (EPC) can occur as a paraneoplastic phenomenon. This is usually in the context of a paraneoplastic 'cortical encephalomyelitis' due to various tumours (notably small cell lung cancer and breast carcinoma). The MRI scan can show non-specific T2 signal changes. Seizures also occur in limbic encephalitis of paraneoplastic origin —often associated with memory loss, psychiatric and behavioural changes.

Another increasingly recognized cause of limbic encephalitis is the presence of voltage-gated potassium channel antibodies. Epilepsy, memory disturbance and neuropsychiatric changes are the leading symptoms. The epilepsy takes the form of minor complex partial seizures and are often frequent and intractable to therapy. Secondary generalized seizures can occur. The diagnosis is made by measuring levels of the antibody, and treatment is by acetazolamide and immunosuppression.

## SEIZURE PRECIPITANTS

One of the worst aspects of having epilepsy is the lack of predictability of seizures. For many people, the fact that a seizure can occur without warning on a more or less random fashion is far more problematic than the actual seizure itself. If there were sufficient advanced notice of seizures, the negative impact of epilepsy would be greatly reduced. Why seizures occur when they do is one of the major unanswered research questions in epilepsy. Of some interest is the tantalizing demonstration that subtle alterations in the EEG occur in the minutes or even hours before a seizure in some patients, without any clinical sign or any conscious awareness. Unfortunately, currently, in spite of considerable research, there seems no reliable way of utilizing these changes in a clinical setting to provide advanced warning to a patient, although implanted deep brain stimulators triggered by EEG change and seizure onset are being investigated. An interesting and quirky development has been the claim that dogs can be trained to recognize that a seizure is about to occur. Such 'epilepsy dogs' are now available in a number of countries, but their clinical utility or general applicability has not been subjected to rigorous research.

In a small number of patients, seizures are not unpredictable, but are invariably triggered by an identifiable precipitant (defined as a factor that, in patients with pre-existing epilepsy, precedes the onset of the attack and is considered to be an explanation of why the seizure happened when it did and not earlier or later). A greater number (some claim 50–60%) of people with epilepsy claim that precipitants are sometimes but not invariably identifiable, and the most common factors are listed in Table 1.32. Attention to these factors can improve seizures in susceptible persons, and this is particularly true of avoidance of alcohol, sleep deprivation and stress. Where precipitants are invariable, their avoidance may obviate the need for antiepileptic drug therapy—this is usually only possible in patients with a history of mild epilepsy and infrequent seizures. In most other patients antiepileptic drugs are needed, although avoiding precipitants will lessen the propensity to seizures.

### Stress

Emotional stress is commonly thought to provoke attacks in many individuals, although attempts to define or quantify stress prove highly elusive. Where some measurement is possible, studies usually show a modest association between worsening seizures and stress, although this can be complex and stress reduction in many people has a disappointing lack of effect. A wide variety of often spurious psychic ex-planations have been made in this difficult area.

**Table 1.32** Factors that commonly influence the precipitation of seizures.

| |
|---|
| *Common factors* |
| Stress |
| Emotional disturbance |
| Sleep deprivation and fatigue |
| Sleep–wake cycle |
| Alcohol and alcohol withdrawal |
| Hypoglycaemia |
| Metabolic disturbances |
| Toxins and drugs |
| Menstrual cycle |
| Fever or ill health |
| Photic stimulation |
| |
| *Less common factors* |
| Startle |
| Fright |
| Dietary changes |
| Sexual intercourse |
| Pain |
| Fasting |
| Allergy |
| Hormonal changes |

## Alcohol

In people with pre-existing epilepsy, acute alcohol intoxication and, even more potently, acute alcohol withdrawal can precipitate generalized seizures. A 20-fold increase in the incidence of seizures is found in patients consuming large quantities of alcohol, and avoidance of alcohol is sometimes all that is required to prevent seizures. Antiepileptic drug treatment in alcoholic patients is often problematic, owing to interactions, systemic toxicity, poor compliance and psychosocial problems. Where possible the patient should abstain from alcohols, and drug treatment can probably be avoided. Seizures are also common in the 24 hours after acute alcohol withdrawal, taking the form of myoclonus and tonic–clonic convulsions, sometimes with photosensitivity. This period can be covered with benzodiazepine or clomethiazole therapy under medical supervision.

## Sleep and fatigue

The timing of seizures in relation to the sleep–wake cycle is intriguing. In the syndrome of idiopathic generalized epilepsy, all seizure types (absence, myoclonic and tonic–clonic seizures) are particularly likely to occur within an hour or so of waking or, less commonly, when drifting off to sleep or in the first 2 hours of sleep (most commonly in non-REM stage 2 sleep). About 60% of children with benign rolandic epilepsy have attacks confined to sleep. In autosomal dominant frontal lobe epilepsy, attacks occur only in sleep, and numerous attacks can occur each night without a single event during the day. Some patients with other forms of generalized or partial epilepsy also have attacks only in sleep, and it has long been recognized that focal EEG disturbances can be activated by light sleep. Seizures of frontal lobe origin have a particular propensity to occur during sleep. The EEG disturbances in ESES and in the Landau–Kleffner syndrome are also greatly enhanced by sleep.

Seizures occurring in sleep often have less serious social consequences than daytime attacks. Therapy may not need to be as intensive as in daytime epilepsy, and occasional patients prefer not to have any drug treatment. Drug treatment carries the risk of converting a pattern of regular nocturnal attacks into less frequent daytime seizures with catastrophic social consequences—an important consideration when changing therapy in a patient whose seizures are confined to sleep. It should not be forgotten, however, that nocturnal tonic–clonic seizures carry a particular risk of sudden death, especially if the patient sleeps alone and the seizures are unwitnessed. Advice about the choice of treatment should, therefore, be given on an individual basis.

Sleep deprivation and fatigue are undoubted precipitants of seizures in many people, and a few patients have attacks only when in these situations. Young adults with idiopathic generalized epilepsy seem particularly liable. EEG abnormalities, and therefore presumably also seizures, are also enhanced by sleep deprivation in many people with partial epilepsy. Fatigue can provoke attacks, although formal studies of why this should be are largely lacking. In susceptible individuals, the avoidance of fatigue or sleep deprivation greatly reduces seizures, and on occasions drug therapy can be averted.

## The menstrual cycle and catamenial epilepsy

The occurrence of seizures in females often fluctuates in relation to the menstrual cycle. About 10% of all women with epilepsy note a striking pattern, usually with seizures occurring during or just before menstruation. This may be due to factors such as the high oestrogen levels in the follicular phase of menstruation, premenstrual tension or water retention. Progesterone has a mild antiepileptic effect, and the rapid fall in progesterone levels just before menstruation may be relevant. Fluid retention has also been suggested to have a role, but diuretics are seldom helpful in therapy. Occasionally, seizures occur only around menstruation, and the epilepsy is then referred to as catamenial epilepsy.

Clobazam (10 mg/day; see p. 123) or acetazolamide (250–750 mg/day; see p. 200) can be given intermittently each month around menstruation (usually for periods of 3–5 days), or at other susceptible times during the menstrual cycle, to control catamenial epilepsy. In practice this approach is only occasionally effective, and there are very few women in whom intermittent therapy alone will control seizures, even where there is a striking catamenial pattern.

Perhaps surprisingly, even where the frequency of seizures is clearly related to menstruation, attempts to influence hormonal factors have proved equally ineffective. Trials of contraceptive therapy, progesterone, hormone replacement therapy, and even oophorectomy have been reported. None is generally effective.

## Fever and general ill health

Fever, general ill health and intercurrent illness are potent precipitants of seizures, and effective antipyretic therapy or treatment of intercurrent illness will lower susceptibility to seizure in many people. This relatively non-specific effect, in patients with existing epilepsy, should be differentiated from the phenomenon of childhood 'febrile convulsions' (see pp. 21–2).

Many patients consider that seizures are more likely to occur at times of general ill health, lowered mood or when feeling 'run down'. For these reasons taking vitamins or herbal remedies, regular exercise, adopting healthy lifestyles, and measures to improve general health are frequently advised. At an anecdotal level these can greatly improve epilepsy, although rigorous scientific evidence of effectiveness is lacking. Complementary and alternative therapies for epilepsy are outlined on pp. 110–112.

# THE REFLEX EPILEPSIES

The term reflex epilepsy is used to describe cases in which seizures are evoked consistently by a specific environmental trigger. In some cases the stimulus can be highly specific and in others less so. The term is not usually applied to patients whose seizures are precipitated by internal influences such as menstruation, nor to situations where the precipitating factors are vague or ill-defined (e.g. fatigue, stress), nor to patients with existing epilepsy where seizures are more likely to occur owing to specific precipitants (e.g. sleep deprivation, alcohol); transitional cases, however, occur in what can be a nosological grey area. The reflex epilepsies are sometimes subdivided into simple and complex types. In the simple forms the seizures are precipitated by simple sensory stimuli (e.g. flashes of light, startle) and in the complex forms by more elaborate stimuli (e.g. specific pieces of music). The complex forms are much more heterogeneous and the syndromes are less well defined than the simple reflex epilepsies. In hospital practice about 5% of patients show some features of reflex epilepsy. The stimuli most reported to cause seizures include flashing lights and other visual stimuli, startle, eating, bathing in hot water, music, reading, and movement.

## Visual stimuli, photosensitivity and photosensitive epilepsy

The most common reflex epilepsies are those induced by visual stimuli. Flashing lights, bright lights, moving visual patterns (e.g. escalators), eye closure, moving from dark into bright light, and viewing specific objects or colours have all been reported to induce seizures.

Photosensitive epilepsy is a form of simple reflex epilepsy. The term should be confined to those individuals who show unequivocal EEG evidence of photosensitivity, and differentiated from other, usually more complex, cases in which seizures can apparently be precipitated by visual stimuli but in whom EEG evidence of photosensitivity cannot be demonstrated. Photosensitivity (strictly defined) is present in the general population with a frequency of about 1.1 per 100,000 persons, and 5.7 per 100,000 in the 7–19 age range, and is very strongly associated with epilepsy. About 3% of persons with epilepsy are photosensitive and have seizures induced by photic stimuli (usually viewing flickering or intermittent lights or cathode ray monitors, bright lights or repeating patterns). The flicker frequency precipitating photosensitivity varies from patient to patient, but is most commonly in the 15–20 Hz range. The peak age of presentation of photosensitive epilepsy is 12 years, the male : female ratio is 2 : 3, and the propensity to photosensitivity declines with age. Most patients with photosensitivity have the syndrome of idiopathic generalized epilepsy, although photosensitivity also occurs in patients with focal epilepsy arising in the occipital region. In idiopathic generalized epilepsy, myoclonus, absence and tonic–clonic seizures can be precipitated by photic stimuli, and factors such as sleep deprivation or alcohol intake have additive effects—partying can involve all factors, and seizures are common the morning after the night before. Alternating patterns (such as in some video games, or when looking down large escalators) can precipitate seizures in photosensitive patients, as can disco lights or poorly tuned TV screens (which flicker at the mains alternating current frequency of 50 Hz in the UK and Europe, but not in the USA). Other common stimuli include bright light shimmering off moving water, or the flickering of light through trees from a moving vehicle, and the transition from relative darkness into bright light. Most photosensitive patients have non-photically induced seizures also, but photic seizures can be prevented or reduced by wearing glasses with tinted or polarized lenses, and by avoiding situations known to induce photosensitive responses. Photosensitivity also occurs in some patients with occipital lobe epilepsy and in some of the benign occipital focal epilepsy syndromes.

Television-induced seizures (and, far less common, seizures induced by video games or computer screens) can be reduced by taking the precautions listed in Table 1.33. In photosensitive persons with occipital lobe epilepsy, seizure discharges may also be caused by fixation-on or fixation-off stimuli.

Treatment with valproate, benzodiazepine drugs or levetiracetam usually completely abolishes photosensitivity, even at doses that do not provide complete seizure control.

## Startle-induced epilepsy

Startle can precipitate seizures in susceptible persons, and occasionally is the only precipitant. Startle-induced seizures usually occur in patients with a frontal or central focus and usually in lesional epilepsy. The seizures usually take a form similar to a tonic seizure, and the EEG is commonly normal

**Table 1.33** Tactics that can reduce the risk of television-induced seizures in susceptible individuals.

| |
|---|
| Use a small screen, or view screen from a distance, use a remote control for changing channels (thereby reducing the area of screen in the visual field) |
| View the screen from an angle |
| Use a 100 Hz television screen, a non-interlaced computer screen with a high refresh rate or a liquid crystal display |
| Close or cover one eye |
| Keep the screen contrast and brightness low |
| Avoid exposure when sleep deprived |
| Avoid looking at a fixed flickering pattern |
| Use polarizing glasses |

or shows rather non-specific changes. A susceptibility to startle is more common in late childhood and adolescence and may resolve as the patient get older. The most common stimulus is a loud noise, but touch, sudden movement or fright can also precipitate attacks. Startle-induced epilepsy must be differentiated from hyperekplexia, which has a very similar clinical form, but which is not a form of epilepsy. Treatment can be difficult although carbamazepine and the benzodiazepine drugs have been said at an anecdotal level to be most likely to control the attacks.

### Primary reading epilepsy

This is a specific rare epilepsy syndrome in which clonic jerking of the jaw or peri-oral muscles, which can evolve to a generalized convulsion, is precipitated by reading. The age of onset is usually 12–25 years. The condition has various forms. In some patients, the attacks occur only after prolonged reading. In individual cases, different aspects of reading seem to act as precipitating factors—content, comprehension, context. Reading difficult or unfamiliar passages, music, nonsense passages and foreign languages. In other patients, reading may precipitate jaw jerking after a few seconds. In some cases, there is evidence of focal onset of the epilepsy and others have features classifiable as a form of 'praxis-induced' juvenile myoclonic epilepsy (JME—see p. 19). The physiological basis of this curious syndrome is unclear, but there is a positive family history in about 25% of cases. The seizures can usually be aborted if reading is terminated as soon as the clonic jerking develops. Conventional antiepileptic drugs have been used with variable success. In the variants that resemble JME, therapeutic approaches are similar to those employed in JME and the prognosis is excellent.

### Other forms of reflex epilepsy

Other simple reflex epilepsies include cases with seizures induced by movement, touching or tapping. These should be differentiated from paroxysmal kinesogenic choreo-athetosis and stimulus-sensitive myoclonus. Hot-water epilepsy is a remarkable syndrome, common in parts of India but rare elsewhere, in which seizures are induced by pouring hot water over the head or immersion in hot water. The attacks take the form of tonic–clonic or partial seizures. Complex forms of a wide variety of other stimuli have been reported to induce seizures—and amongst the strangest are: telephones, noise of a vacuum cleaner, specific memories, writing and touch). These conditions are heterogeneous in terms of aetiology, EEG and seizure type. The mechanisms underlying these (and other) reflex epilepsies are uncertain and specific 'reflex arcs' have not been identified. Prevention of the precipitating cause is sometimes helpful, as is drug treatment along conventional lines.

## ACUTE SYMPTOMATIC SEIZURES

This unsatisfactory term is reserved for seizures that start in close temporal association to a sudden acute precipitant, in people who had not had prior seizures. If the epilepsy can be attributed to a pre-existing non-acute or static cause, it is referred to as remote symptomatic epilepsy, but clearly there is a grey area in which the distinction between acute and remote symptomatic epilepsies is rather arbitrary. The boundary is similarly blurred in some cases of reflex epilepsy or cases in which seizures have acute precipitants such as sleep deprivation or alcohol. Furthermore, if seizures continue after the acute phase, and if the cause remains present (e.g. post-stroke, post-trauma, tumoural, post-infectious epilepsy), seizures that were initially categorized as acute symptomatic are reclassified as remote symptomatic. This makes rather a nonsense of the classification scheme, the utility of which is best reserved for epidemiologically based incidence studies. Even in cases where the cause is reversible (e.g. acute metabolic disturbance or intoxication), there is a higher incidence of subsequent unprovoked seizures than in control populations, and classification as acute symptomatic even in these cases makes little sense. For all these reasons the term has fallen from common usage in research practice, although it remains useful shorthand to describe acute *de novo* seizures presenting in the context of sudden cerebral dysfunction, particularly where this is due to reversible factors such as metabolic or endocrine disturbance or exposure to alcohol, toxins or drugs (these factors are discussed below).

Acute symptomatic seizures usually take the form of tonic–clonic convulsions or tonic–clonic status epilepticus. Some causes of acute symptomatic seizures are given in Table 1.34. In epidemiological studies, the most common causes in a typical Western country are found to be: cerebral trauma (15%), cerebral infection (15%), cerebrovascular disease (15–30%), drugs, toxins and alcohol (15–20%), and metabolic disturbances (10%).

The age-adjusted incidence rate of symptomatic seizures, reported in an old study from the record-linkage system in Rochester, Minnesota, was about 40 per 100,000 person-years. In adults, acute symptomatic seizures are more common in men than in women (52 vs. 29 per 100,000 per year). The highest rate is in the first year of life due to metabolic, infectious and encephalopathic aetiologies. The rate decreases in childhood and early adulthood, with a nadir at 25–34 years, and then increases, producing a second peak at age 75 and older, accounted for mostly by cerebrovascular disorders. The cumulative incidence of acute symptomatic seizures has been estimated to be about 4% up to the age of 80 years.

The emergency treatment of acute seizures is described on p. 211.

**Table 1.34** Some causes of acute symptomatic seizures.

Acute cerebral infections—encephalitis, meningitis, abscess
Acute para-infectious encephalopathies—acute disseminated encephalomyelopathy
Acute metabolic disturbance—hypoglycaemia, hypocalcaemia, hyponatraemia, hypernatraemia, hypomagnesaemia
Acute hypoxia/ischaemia—stroke, cardiac arrest, acute hypotension, asthma, perinatal
Acute renal or hepatic failure, uraemic encephalopathy, dialysis disequilibrium syndrome and dialysis encephalopathy
Acute traumatic brain injury
Acute intoxication with drugs or toxins
Acute drug or alcohol withdrawal
Acute hypertension—hypertensive encephalopathy, eclampsia
Acute haemorrhage
Acute vasculitis—Henoch–Schönlein purpura, SLE, polyarteritis nodosa (PAN)

## Metabolic and endocrine-induced seizures

Many types of metabolic or endocrine disturbances can result in epilepsy. Hyponatraemia is the most common electrolyte disturbance to result in seizures, which typically occur if the serum sodium falls below 115 mmol/l. Seizures also routinely occur in the presence of hypernatraemia, hypocalcaemia, hypercalcaemia, hypomagnesaemia, hypokalaemia and hyper-kalaemia. Ten per cent of patients with severe renal failure have seizures, caused either by the metabolic disturbance, renal encephalopathy, dialysis encephalopathy or dialysis disequilibrium syndrome. Asterixis may develop into myoclonus and then epilepsy. Acute hyponatraemia and hypomagnesaemia are particularly likely to result in seizures, although chronic hyponatraemia does not cause seizures, and indeed is a common side-effect of carbamazepine and oxcarbazepine therapy.

Seizures are a common occurrence in hepatic failure. Hepatic encephalopathy may be overlooked and routine liver function tests can be relatively normal; hyperammonaemia is sometimes diagnostically helpful. Reye's syndrome should be considered in patients with liver failure, especially children, in whom it is associated with intake of aspirin.

Hypoglycaemia is a potent cause of seizures, which can occur if the blood sugar level falls below 2.2 mmol/l. This is commonly due to insulin therapy in patients with diabetes, but can also be due to insulinoma and to drugs such as quinine and pentamidine. Non-ketotic hyperglycaemia frequently causes seizures. Levels of blood sugar as low as 15–20 mmol/l can cause seizures if there is associated hyperosmolarity. The seizures in non-ketotic hyperglycaemia are focal and this implies the presence of cerebral pathology (usually cerebrovascular disease). Diabetic ketoacidosis does not frequently result in seizures.

Thyroid disease can result in seizures which are due either to immunological mechanisms, or directly to hormonal change or hormonally-induced metabolic change. Twenty per cent of patients with severe myxoedema have seizures. Hashimoto's encephalopathy, a steroid responsive encephalopathy associated with high levels of antithyroid antibody, is an immunologically-determined condition that results in altered consciousness, focal signs and other eatures of encephalopathy including myoclonus and tonic–clonic seizures.

## Alcohol- and toxin-induced seizures

Alcohol abuse is a potent cause of acute symptomatic seizures, and indeed of epilepsy, in many societies. There are various mechanisms. Binge drinking can result in acute cerebral toxicity and seizures. Alcohol withdrawal in an alcohol-dependent person carries an even greater risk of seizures. Withdrawal seizures are typically tonic–clonic in form, occurring 12–24 hours after withdrawal, and are associated with photosensitivity. Seizures can also be caused by the metabolic disturbances associated with binge drinking (notably hypoglycaemia, hyponatraemia and hepatic failure), the cerebral damage due to trauma, cerebral infection, subdural haematoma, the chronic neurotoxic effects of chronic alcohol exposure or to acute Wernicke's encephalopathy due to thiamine deficiency. It has been estimated that 6% of patients with alcoholism investigated for epilepsy have an additional identifiable causative lesion.

The risk of a first generalized tonic–clonic seizure in chronic alcoholics is sevenfold greater than in non-alcoholic controls, and in the USA, for instance, 15% of patients with epilepsy have alcoholism. The risk of seizures is only increased with a daily alcohol intake of 50 g/day or more, and the higher the intake the higher the risk. Odds ratios according to alcohol intake have been calculated to be 3.0 (95% CI, 1.7–5.4) for a daily intake of 51–100 g/day, 7.9 (95% CI, 2.9–21.9) for 101–200 g/day, and 16.6 (95% CI, 1.9–373.4) when the intake is more than 200 g/day.

Seizures can also be provoked by exposure to many different toxins. Potent causes include heavy metal poisoning and carbon monoxide poisoning (where carboxyhaemoglobin levels are above 50%). Although acute toxic exposure causes seizures, these are usually part of an acute encephalopathy. Whether low-level long-term exposure to carbon monoxide or to lead or other heavy metals carries any risk is quite unclear. This is a contentious and murky area in which claims are made without scientific backing, in which science is tangled up with legal processes, and in which much nonsense is perpetuated. To what extent organophosphate poisoning can result in seizures is equally contentious, and reliable data seem to be absent.

## Drug-induced seizures

A wide range of drugs, toxins and illicit compounds can cause acute symptomatic seizures and epilepsy, although seizures accounted for less than 1% of 32,812 consecutive patients prospectively monitored for drug toxicity. As many as 15% of drug-related seizures present as status epilepticus. In a population-based survey from Richmond, Virginia, drug overdose was the reported cause in 2% of children and 3% of adults with status epilepticus. Drugs can cause seizures due to intrinsic epileptogenicity, patient idiosyncrasy, antiepileptic drug interactions, impairment of the hepatic or renal drug metabolism, drug withdrawal phenomena, and direct cerebral toxicity (especially in intentional overdosage).

Almost any psychotropic drug carries a risk of inducing seizures. The risk is highest with the aliphatic phenothiazines (e.g. chlorpromazine [1–9% risk], promazine, trifluoperazine). The use of clozapine is associated with a 1–4% risk of seizures and with interictal epileptiform abnormalities. The piperazine phenothiazines (acetophenazine, fluphenazine, perphenazine, prochlorperazine, trifluoperazine), haloperidol, sulpiride, pimozide, thioridazine and risperidone are thought to have the lowest epileptogenic potential, although firm data are lacking. The risk of seizures with antidepressant drugs ranges between less than 1% and 4%, and varies with the drug category. Agents accompanied by a high risk of seizures include clomipramine and second-generation antidepressants, amoxapine, maprotiline and amfebutamone. The risk of seizures with tricyclic antidepressants (other than clomipramine), citalopram, moclobemide and nefazodone is thought to be lower. The seizure risk with the selective serotonin reuptake inhibitors (fluoxetine, sertraline, paroxetine), monoamine oxidase inhibitors (MAOIs), and trazodone is probably lower, although definitive data are lacking. All these drugs in overdose carry a significant (> 10%) risk of seizures. The narcotic analgesic meperidine is metabolized in the liver to normaperidine, a potent proconvulsant, which tends to accumulate after prolonged administration and renal failure. The monocyclic antidepressant amfebutamone, which is used to assist the cessation of smoking, provokes seizures in 1 in 1000 patients. Pethidine can also result in seizures, especially in the presence of renal impairment or in combination with MAOI drugs. Lidocaine-related neurotoxicity is common with intravenous use, especially with advanced age, congestive heart failure, shock, and renal and hepatic failure. The anaesthetics enflurane, propofol and isoflurane can be proconvulsant. Quinine and the other antimalarial drugs, especially mefloquine, can provoke acute seizures, and are relatively contraindicated in epilepsy. Various traditional remedies, including evening primrose oil and some Chinese and Indian herbal medicines, can provoke seizures.

Neurotoxic reactions may occur frequently with β-lactam antibiotics (semi-synthetic penicillins and cephalosporins), probably due to GABA-antagonist action. Benzylpenicillin, cefazolin and imipenem/cilastatin have the higher neurotoxic potential, and the risk is increased at higher doses, in the presence of renal failure, blood–brain barrier damage and pre-existing CNS disorders, co-medication with nephrotoxic agents or drugs lowering seizure threshold. Isoniazid can induce seizures by antagonizing pyridoxal phosphate (the active form of pyridoxine), which is involved in GABA biosynthesis. Seizures have also been reported, especially in elderly patients, due to aminoglycosides, metronidazole, quinolones and amantadine. Quinolones (nalidixic acid, norfloxacin, ciprofloxacin) probably enhance seizure activity by inhibiting GABA binding to membrane receptors. The tetracyclines seem to be less proconvulsant than these other antibiotics. Zidovudine and other antiviral agents have caused seizures in HIV patients. Seizures (and non-convulsive status epilepticus) have been reported after administration of intravenous contrast media, and the risk is as high as 15% in patients with brain metastases.

The anticancer chemotherapeutic agents can provoke seizures, especially chlorambucil (5%), and cyclosporin (1–3%), asparaginase, tacrolines and amfebutamone, but also the platin drugs, vinca alkaloids, bleomycin, anthracyclines and azathioprine.

Theophylline is a potent convulsant which can result in seizures or status epilepticus, possibly due to the anti-adenosine action. β-blockers and other antiarrhythmic agents have been reported to precipitate seizures, particularly in overdose. Cimetidine, levodopa, insulin, thiazide diuretics, lidocaine, salicylates, chemotherapeutic agents, L-asparaginase and baclofen have been reported to cause seizures. The non-steroidal analgesics also predispose to seizures (for example NSAIDs, tramadol, diamorphine and pethidine).

Seizures may be precipitated after sudden withdrawal of any antiepileptic drug but seem to be a particular problem in benzodiazepine, carbamazepine and barbiturate withdrawal.

Recreational drugs can cause seizures. The greatest risk is with the stimulant drugs such as cocaine, amphetamine and 'ecstasy' (3,4-methylenedioxymethamphetamine, MDMA). The hallucinogens such as phencyclidine ('angel dust') and lysergic acid diethlyamide (LSD) less commonly cause seizures. The opiates and the organic solvents are least epileptogenic, although past or present heroin use has been shown to be a risk factor for provoked and unprovoked seizures (OR 2.8; 95% CI, 1.5–5.7). Of the performance-enhancing drugs, erythropoietin has strong epileptogenic potential. By contrast, in one study, use of marijuana by men was shown to have a protective action against non-provoked seizures (OR 0.4; 95% CI, 0.2–0.8) and provoked seizures (OR 0.2; 95% CI, 0.1–0.8).

# 2 The principles of drug treatment

WHY TREAT EPILEPSY?

The treatment of epilepsy has a number of specific aims, and a balance needs to be drawn between the risks of epilepsy and the risks and benefits of therapy. This can be a complex equation, and here the aims of therapy, and the risks of epilepsy and its treatment, are briefly described. A rational approach to therapy needs to bear these in mind.

## The aims of drug treatment

As Hippocrates noted, the primary aim of medical treatment is the prevention of distress. Simple seizure control is only one aspect of this, and although important should not obscure other points. The general objectives of medical treatment can be summarized as follows.

### Seizure control

The antiepileptic drugs are remarkably effective in suppressing seizures. Population surveys have shown that between 80 and 90% of patients will gain 1–2 year remissions from seizures when therapy is started, and long-term remission is gained in about 70% of all patients treated with antiepileptic drugs. The physician should be able to make accurate prognostic estimates about the extent of seizure control by taking into account the type of epilepsy, its cause and its clinical context. In the remaining 30% of patients seizure control is less effective, and treatment more difficult; the art of therapy in these patients is to balance the adverse effects of drugs against their benefits, and to implement wider aspects of epilepsy management.

### Avoidance of side-effects

Side-effects can be generally classified as follows:
• Idiosyncratic reactions (immunologically determined, allergy, hypersensitivity). These are usually rare, but can be severe and occasionally life-threatening (pp. 63–4);
• Dose-related reversible side-effects. These are common, usually mild, typically CNS or gastrointestinal in nature, and are reversible when the dose is lowered. The occurrence of these effects depends on dose and rate of incrementation. The side-effects of individual drugs are described in Section 3 (p. 114);

• Long-term irreversible side-effects. These are not strictly dose-related, although they are more common in patients who have taken high-dose therapy for long periods. They can affect diverse body systems, and are usually but not always mild in nature. The side-effects of individual drugs are described in Section 3;
• Teratogenicity. The teratogenic effects of drugs are described on pp. 103–4.

The choice of drug should be tailored to the needs of the individual patient, and will depend greatly on the side-effect profile and an estimate of the likelihood of a side-effect and its risk. These are not easy estimates to make.

### Avoidance of social consequences of epilepsy and secondary handicap

Therapeutic endeavours should also be directed at minimizing the adverse effects of epilepsy within the broader context of the patient's life and experience. Epilepsy has a number of potential social consequences which can be more important than the immediate effects of individual seizures. 'Being epileptic' can be far worse than simply having seizures. These aspects require a holistic approach to therapy of which drug treatment is often only a small part. The establishment of a good patient–doctor relationship, counselling, psychological therapy and lifestyle advice are all important. The overall aim is to encourage as normal a lifestyle as possible, and to balance choices against the risks imposed by the epilepsy. The treatment decisions should be made ultimately by patients and carers. The role of the treating physician is to assist decision making by providing information and advice.

### Suppression of subclinical epileptic activity

Antiepileptic drug therapy as a rule should be aimed at suppressing seizures and not the reduction of EEG activity. However, in selected situations, therapy can be targeted at EEG disturbances where these are considered to be having adverse clinical effects ('subclinical activity'). These include: reduction of 3 Hz spike-wave paroxysms in children with absence seizures; abolition of EEG changes in the Landau–Kleffner syndrome (pp. 25–6); abolition of photosensitivity in photosensitive epilepsy; reduction in slow spike-wave paroxysms in patients with Lennox–Gastaut syndrome and others epileptic encephalopathies (pp. 23–4); and reduction of paroxysmal discharges where these cause clinical impairment.

### Reduction of mortality and morbidity
This is described below.

### Prevention of epileptogenesis
It has been postulated that epileptic seizures induce cerebral changes which lead to further seizures. Antiepileptic therapy, by controlling seizures, may thus theoretically lessen the chances of this happening. Although a protective effect has been demonstrated in animal experimentation, there is no good evidence for any such action in human epilepsy. It is likely that antiepileptic drugs merely exert a suppressive effect on seizures, and have no influence on the long-term natural course of the disease. Similarly, the use of antiepileptic drugs prophylactically does not seem to prevent epilepsy developing in individuals at high risk, for instance after head injury, neurosurgery, stroke or tumour. Furthermore, it is now generally agreed that continuous pharmacological prophylaxis in children over the age of 1 year after febrile seizures is ineffective. Neuroprotective strategies using other types of drug are in development, and this is an area of intensive research activity, but as yet no effective neuroprotective therapy is available.

### Improving quality of life
The efficacy of antiepileptic drugs (AEDs) is traditionally assessed by measuring their impact on seizure frequency, but in recent years the effect of drug therapy on quality of life has been the subject of intensive study. Not surprisingly, studies have consistently shown that complete freedom from seizures is by far the most important predictor of improved quality of life. However, even where freedom from seizures is not achieved, drug-induced reduction of seizure severity is beneficial as is the positive psychotropic effects of some drugs. These must be balanced against the side-effects, particularly the cognitive and neurological effects, of medication—a balance sometimes difficult to achieve.

## Risks associated with epilepsy
Active epilepsy is associated with significant risks in terms of both mortality and morbidity, and it is obviously important to know to what extent these can be alleviated by reducing seizures using antiepileptic drug treatment. These benefits also need to be set against the risks of the treatment itself.

## Mortality in epilepsy
Epilepsy is a potentially life-threatening condition, a fact that is often overlooked. The key question is the extent to which this could be avoided by adequate drug treatment. Deaths associated with epilepsy can be classified into three categories: (i) those caused directly by the seizures, such as accidental death and SUDEP; (ii) those related indirectly, or only partly, to epilepsy, for instance suicide; and (iii) those due to other factors, for example the underlying causes of the epilepsy. Successful AED therapy should prevent deaths in the first category, may prevent some deaths in the second category, but will have no preventive effect in the third category. The risk of death is best expressed as the standardized mortality ratio (SMR), which is defined as the ratio of deaths in patients with epilepsy compared with those in age- and sex-matched control populations.

### Newly diagnosed epilepsy
In one study 161 of 564 patients (29%) with newly diagnosed epilepsy had died within 6 years of the diagnosis. The rate of death was over three times that expected in an age-matched population. However, the excess mortality was due almost entirely to the underlying disease, and not the epilepsy itself, and antiepileptic drug treatment would be unlikely to have had much impact on mortality rates at this stage.

### Chronic active epilepsy in adults
In contrast to new-onset epilepsy, much of the excess mortality in patients with chronic active epilepsy is seizure- or epilepsy-related. Thus, in one study of 601 adult outpatients attending tertiary referral clinics and followed for 3 years, the SMR was 5.1 (95% CI, 2.9–3.1), with 24 deaths being recorded in 1849 patient-years of follow-up. Most patients in this population had long-standing intractable partial or secondarily generalized seizures. Of the 24 deaths, 14 were seizure-related, and 11 of these were classified as SUDEP. Because risk is much greater in convulsive seizures, and in patients with frequent seizures, successful AED therapy could have an important preventive role.

### Chronic active epilepsy in children
In a community-based study in Nova Scotia, mortality rates among 693 children followed up for 14–22 years were 0/97 for absence epilepsy, 12/511 (2%) for partial and primarily generalized seizures, and 9/36 (25%) or 4/49 (8%) for secondarily generalized seizures with onset before or after 1 year of age, respectively. Only one patient died from SUDED. In another paediatric community-based study, mortality rates associated with symptomatic epilepsy were 50-fold higher than in the general population, but there was no increased mortality in idiopathic epilepsy. Thus, in children, the risks of seizure-related deaths are less than in adults, and effective drug treatment therefore will have less impact.

## Causes of seizure-related deaths
There is an obvious potential for antiepileptic drug treatment to reduce the risk of seizure-related death, the main causes of which are as follow.

### SUDEP seizure- and epilepsy-related deaths

SUDEP is the most common seizure-related cause of death in epilepsy, and occurs after convulsive seizures. Patients at specific risk are those with high rates of convulsive seizures, symptomatic epilepsy, learning disability, seizures during sleep, and unwitnessed seizures. Suboptimal drug levels constitute another risk factor in some studies, as does death during drug changes, presumably owing to the increased incidence of convulsive seizures. SUDEP is probably usually the result of respiratory arrest in the aftermath of a convulsive seizure, although cardiac arrhythmias may be responsible for a proportion of cases. Respiratory effort after a seizure can be restarted by stimulation and arousal, and this is perhaps why SUDEP is rare in witnessed seizures. For this reason, it is important to come to the assistance of a person in a convulsive seizure and dangerous to leave the person unattended.

The rates of SUDEP in different populations largely relate to the frequency of tonic–clonic convulsions. Thus, in patients with largely controlled epilepsy the risk seems to be in the region of 1 case per 2500 patients per year, whereas in patients with severe intractable epilepsy the risk may be as high as 1–2 cases per 100 patients per year. Overall, in population-based studies, the risk has been found to be about 1 case per 1000–2000 persons on treatment for epilepsy per year. It has been estimated that—as a rough approximation—SUDEP will occur in 1 in every 2000–5000 tonic–clonic convulsions. SUDEP deaths would be potentially preventable if seizures were brought under control. The extent of this problem was demonstrated in a recent sentinel audit carried out by the UK Department of Health which found, on the basis of a case note review, that 39% of deaths in patients with epilepsy might have been prevented with more appropriate drug therapy.

### Status epilepticus

About 20% of patients with convulsive status epilepticus admitted to intensive care will not survive. Death is usually due to the underlying cause, but skilful therapy will lessen both morbidity and mortality rates. Status accounts for less than 2% of deaths among people with epilepsy, and it is comparatively more common in children, especially those with learning disabilities.

### Death in an accident

The SMR for accidental death has been found in one study to be 5.6 (95% CI, 5.0–6.3). Accidents occur in employment, outside and in the home, and the problem is worse if the seizures involve falls. Common causes of death are falling from heights, road traffic accidents, and accidents in domestic settings. Drowning in a bath was a leading cause, and in another study 58 of 2381 drowning deaths recorded in a 5-year period were seizure-related. Effective control of seizures will greatly lessen the risk of accidental death.

### Suicide

The suicide rate in epilepsy in one study was found to be considerably higher than in the general population (SMC 3.5; 95% CI, 2.6–4.6). In cases series, suicide is reported to account for between 2 and 10% of all deaths in epilepsy. The suicide is usually by drug overdose, and occurs usually in patients with depression and psychosis. The treatment of the psychiatric complications of epilepsy are discussed on p. 108, and effective therapy will lessen the risk of suicide.

## Morbidity of epilepsy

It is perhaps not surprising that epilepsy results in higher rates of morbidity. There are higher rates of fractures, head injury and burns, and the rates are highest in those with seizures with falls or loss of consciousness, and severe seizures. This is important because treatment, by reducing the frequency or severity of seizures, may lower morbidity rates.

### Accidental injury

Fractures of vertebral bodies are common in convulsive seizures (crush fractures), occurring in 15–16% of patients in two series. Neurological deficit due to cervical cord injury in a convulsive seizure is rarer, and only seven cases of serious paraparesis were observed in about 3500 patient-years of follow-up in a residential centre for patients with severe epilepsy, which corresponds to an incidence of about 1 case per 500 patient-years. Head injury is common in severe epilepsy but is usually relatively minor. In a 12-month survey of 255 patients with severe epilepsy in residential care, 27,934 seizures were recorded, of which 12,626 (45.2%) were associated with falls. There were 766 significant head injuries, 422 requiring simple dressing and 341 sutures, one skull fracture, one extradural hematoma and one subdural hematoma. Thus, 1 in 37 falls resulted in the need for sutures and about 1 in 6000 falls in a potentially life-threatening intracranial haemorrhage.

Fractures of the facial bones are also common, although there are no authoritative estimates of frequency or severity. In a population-based survey of patients with at least one seizure per year, 24% reported a head injury, 16% a burn, 10% a dental injury and 5% a fracture due to seizures in the previous 12 months. It has been estimated that in epilepsy fractures occur at a frequency of about one per person every 14 years, compared with a population risk of 1 per person every 50 years. Scalding and burning are also relatively common in people with epilepsy in all societies. The risk depends upon social habits. In some African villages, epilepsy is known as the 'burn disease' because of the frequency of seizure-related burns incurred by falling into open fires. In Western societies, burns due to falls against radiators, eating or drinking hot fluids, during showering or during cooking are among the most common of all injuries. In one survey of 244 outpatients, 25 (10%) reported having been burned seriously enough to warrant medical attention and 12 (5%) required hospitalization.

### Cerebral damage

Another contentious issue is the extent to which seizures can result in cerebral damage or produce progressive motor, sensorial or cognitive impairment. The consensus view currently is that cerebral damage from short self-limiting seizures is extremely unusual, and prospective studies have generally failed to demonstrate any significant brain damage. The risk after prolonged seizures (e.g. status epilepticus) is quite a different matter, and severe status can result in significant cerebral damage and consequent cognitive decline. This is partly owing to the underlying cause, but there seems little doubt that the epileptic activity itself results in neuronal death and gliosis. The risk is probably greatest in children, and the longer the convulsive phase, the higher the risk of brain damage.

In some of the childhood epilepsy syndromes there is evidence that ongoing epilepsy results in cerebral damage, for instance in the Sturge–Weber syndrome, in West syndrome due to tuberous sclerosis, in callosal agenesis, and in Rasmussen syndrome. However, in most of the epileptic encephalopathies in which there is marked cognitive decline (e.g. West syndrome, Lennox–Gastaut syndrome, myoclonic-astatic epilepsy, ESES), it is not clear to what extent, if any, the epilepsy contributes to the decline. There is certainly no evidence that therapy improves longer-term outcome. Finally, it is possible that hippocampal sclerosis—the pathology commonly underlying temporal lobe epilepsy—is caused by childhood febrile seizures.

### Psychosocial morbidity of epilepsy

The diagnosis of epilepsy also carries psychosocial morbidity. In all large studies, a high proportion of patients with epilepsy had difficulty accepting the diagnosis, significant fears about the risks of future seizures, anxiety about the effect of stigma and the effects on employment, self-esteem, relationships, schooling and leisure activities. Patients with epilepsy carry higher rates of anxiety and depression, social isolation and unmarried status, and are more likely to be unemployed or registered as permanently sick (these aspects are covered in subsequent sections). The psychosocial morbidity of epilepsy can be greatly ameliorated if seizures are brought under control.

### Psychiatric morbidity

This is outlined on p. 108.

### The effect of seizures on the long-term prognosis of epilepsy

It has been repeatedly suggested that the failure to control early seizures may lead to higher levels of treatment resistance later in the epilepsy. If this were the case, aggressive early therapy would be of great importance. However, there is little evidence to support this view (with exceptions, for instance in the case of West syndrome or Sturge–Weber disease), and the currently predominant opinion is that the longer-term outcome of most forms of epilepsy is determined primarily by intrinsic factors (e.g. aetiology, syndromic classification, severity) irrespective of whether early control of seizures was achieved.

### Prevention of epilepsy

To date, there is no evidence that AEDs can prevent the development of epilepsy in patients at risk.

## Risks associated with antiepileptic drug therapy

Antiepileptic drug therapy itself carries risks, and these can be summarized as follows.

### Life-threatening side-effects—antiepileptic drug hypersensitivity

Life-threatening adverse effects are rare, and result from idiosyncratic or hypersensitivity reactions affecting the bone marrow, liver, skin or other organs.

### Acute marrow and hepatic failure

The risk of marrow and/or hepatic failure has been calculated for various drugs. The risk for carbamazepine, for instance, is about 1 in 200,000 for aplastic anaemia, 1 in 700,000 for agranulocytosis and 1 in 450,000 for death associated with these events. Felbamate is the only antiepileptic drug where the risk of bone-marrow suppression is so high as to restrict severely its clinical use. The incidence of aplastic anaemia is estimated to be between 1 in 2000 and 1 in 37,000. The overall incidence of hepatotoxicity has been estimated at 1 in 26,000 to 1 in 34,000. There is a risk of fatal hepatotoxicity with valproate, which varies with age and clinical context. The highest risk (1 in 600) is found in children under 2 years of age with complex neurological disorders receiving polytherapy. In older patients the incidence is no more than 1 in 37,000 for monotherapy and 1 in 12,000 for polytherapy, and fatalities beyond 20 years of age are exceedingly rare (it has been estimated that 132 patients have died of valproate-induced liver failure and/or pancreatitis). There is some evidence that the children at risk may suffer from undiagnosed urea cycle enzyme disorders or Alpers disease. Early recognition of liver failure is important in improving outcome, and blood measurements of liver enzymes, ammonia and prothrombin time are essential if vomiting or somnolence occurs.

### Anticonvulsant hypersensitivity syndrome

The arene oxide producing drugs—phenytoin, carbamazepine, phenobarbital, primidone and lamotrigine—can all cause acute hypersensitivity. This is a potentially fatal reaction and occurs in between 1 in 1000 and 1 in 10,000 exposures. The main manifestations include fever, rash and lymphadenopathy accompanied by multi-organ system abnormalities. The reaction is genetically determined and siblings of affected patients may be at increased risk. A recent study of the Han Chinese in Taiwan showed a very strong association between the HLA-B*1502 allele and carbamazepine-induced Stevens–Johnson syndrome (see p. 119). This severe reaction needs to be differentiated from commonly occurring minor hypersensitivity reactions due to the same drugs (see below).

Stevens–Johnson syndrome and Lyell syndrome are related severe cutaneous reactions. The risk is highest (1 in 50 to 1 in 300) with lamotrigine in paediatric practice, particularly when a high starting dosage is used or when the child is co-medicated with valproate. This limits the use of lamotrigine in young children, and the risk should be clearly mentioned to all patients initiating lamotrigine therapy. In adults, the incidence of lamotrigine-induced Stevens–Johnson syndrome is in the order of 1 in 1000. The frequency of Stevens–Johnson syndrome on carbamazepine is about 14 cases per 100,000. The risk of Stevens–Johnson syndrome can be greatly reduced if a drug is introduced at a low dose and if the dose is slowly increased—and the widespread adoption of this practice has greatly reduced the frequency of this severe reaction.

At least for skin reactions, there is considerable cross-reactivity among these drugs: in one study, 20 of 42 patients (48%) who had a rash from phenytoin or carbamazepine also developed a rash after switching to the other drug. Of 51 patients who had a rash from carbamazepine, 14 (27%) also had a rash from oxcarbazepine. It is therefore wise to avoid, if possible, the use of antiepileptic drugs with a potential for cross-reactivity. Valproate or clobazam seem to be safe alternatives in patients who had a rash from aromatic anticonvulsants. Other AEDs associated with a low risk of hypersensitivity reactions include gabapentin, levetiracetam, pregabalin, topiramate, tiagabine and vigabatrin.

The outcome of hypersensitivity reactions depends on rapid recognition and discontinuation of the offending agent. If the drugs are continued, in spite of developing reactions, mortality rates rise steeply. Steroids can be given, and care of conjunctival and skin lesions is important. Immediate hospitalization is recommended, and some patients require intensive care.

### Other life-threatening side-effects

These include severe bradyarrhythmias after intravenous phenytoin, aspiration pneumonia with nitrazepam in young children, and respiratory arrest following high-dose intravenous benzodiazepines. Deaths have also been recorded owing to drug–drug interactions in patients treated with warfarin.

### Other long-term irreversible side-effects

Other long-term side-effects can occasionally be severe and result in misery and distress, but are not fatal. The long-term effects of each individual drug are listed in Section 3. Common serious examples include the coarsening of facial features and cosmetic changes following long-term treatment with phenytoin, and visual-field defects with vigabatrin.

### Reversible side-effects

Hypersensitivity reactions range from mild maculo-papular rashes (affecting up to 15% of patients started on carbamazepine, lamotrigine or phenytoin) to serious but fortunately rare immune-mediated disorders such as systemic lupus erythematosus. It is not clear whether the mild hypersensitivity reactions and the Stevens–Johnson syndrome are part of the same spectrum or whether there is a distinctive pathogenesis. It is usual to recommend discontinuation of the drug if a rash develops, but some paediatricians particularly give a short course of steroids when a rash appears and continue the drug if the rash does not recur on steroid withdrawal.

In chronically treated patients, the most common side-effects involve the central nervous system (CNS) and include cerebello-vestibular and oculomotor symptoms (ataxia, dysarthria, dizziness, tremor, diplopia, blurred vision and nystagmus), drowsiness, fatigue, impairment of cognitive function, and disorders of mood and behaviour. Chronic non-CNS side-effects include weight gain with valproate and vigabatrin, nephro-lithiasis with topiramate, and endocrine disturbances with a variety of AEDs. It has been suggested that some of the newer AEDs are overall better tolerated than older agents, but this claim should be regarded cautiously because in many comparative studies the choice of titration schedules or dosing regimens was biased in favour of the innovative product. Moreover, clinical exposure to the newer drugs is still relatively limited and experience shows that it may take many years for important adverse effects to be discovered (see Table 2.11).

### The risk of antiepleptic drug prescribing in co-morbid disease

#### Liver disease

Although many AEDs undergo hepatic metabolism, their clearance is seldom affected to an extent that it influences the risk–benefit ratio, except for severe hepatic failure. Similarly, decreased protein binding of phenytoin and valproate has little bearing on risk assessment, even though it is relevant for a correct interpretation of total serum drug concentrations. Valproate should be avoided if possible in patients with liver dysfunction owing to its potential hepatotoxic effects. Phenobarbital and benzodiazepines should be avoided in advanced stages of hepatic failure because of the risk of induction or aggravation of hepatic encephalopathy. Although theoretically non-metabolized drugs such as gabapentin and vigabatrin are attractive options for treating patients with hepatic impairment, pharmacodynamic changes can occur in advanced hepatic disease.

### Porphyria

Seizures may be a component of an attack of acute intermittent porphyria. Prescribing can be difficult as the enzyme-inducing antiepileptic drugs can precipitate acute attacks. A list of safe drugs is given on p. 32.

### Renal failure

Renal failure is associated with a decreased protein binding of phenytoin and valproate. The clearance of gabapentin, levetiracetam, pregabalin and vigabatrin will be reduced in severe renal failure, necessitating dose adjustments.

### Cardiac disease

Uncontrolled generalized tonic–clonic seizures are likely to be hazardous in patients with severe heart disease. The antiepileptic drugs that act on membrane ion channels can induce cardiac arrhythmias in predisposed patients. Studies have concentrated on carbamazepine, which should generally be avoided in patients with pre-existing disturbances in the cardiac conduction system or cardiomyopathies. There may also be a risk also with phenytoin, lamotrigine, oxcarbazepine and topiramate. Routine electrocardiography ECG should be obtained to exclude cardiac disease before starting treatment with these drugs, especially in elderly patients and in those with a history suggestive of heart disease. Intravenous administration of phenytoin should be made only with caution in patients with cardiac disturbances.

**Table 2.1** Pharmacokinetic parameters of antiepileptic drugs.

| | Oral bio-availability (%) | Time to peak level (h) | Metabolism | Half-life† (h) | Protein binding (%) | Active metabolite | Drug interactions |
|---|---|---|---|---|---|---|---|
| Carbamazepine | 75–85 | 4–8 | Hepatic | 5–26[1] | 75 | CBZ-epoxide | ** |
| Clobazam | 90 | 1–4 | Hepatic | 10–77 (50[2]) | 83 | N-desmethyl clobazam | * |
| Clonazepam | 80 | 1–4 | Hepatic | 20–80 | 86 | None | * |
| Ethosuximide | < 100 | < 4 | Hepatic | 30–60[1] | < 10 | None | ** |
| Gabapentin | < 65[3] | 2–3 | None | 5–7 | None | None | None |
| Lamotrigine | < 100 | 1–3 | Hepatic | 12–60[1] | 55 | None | ** |
| Levetiracetam | < 100 | 1–2 | Non-hepatic | 6–8 | None | None | None |
| Oxcarbazepine | < 100 | 4–6 | Hepatic | 8–10[1,2] | 38[2] | MHD | ** |
| Phenobarbital | 80–100 | 1–3 | Hepatic | 75–120[1] | 45–60 | None | ** |
| Phenytoin | 95 | 4–12 | Hepatic | 7–42[1,4] | 85–95 | None | ** |
| Pregabalin | 90 | 1 | None | 6 | None | None | None |
| Primidone | < 100 | 3 | Hepatic | 5–18[1] (75–120[2]) | 25 | Phenobarbital | ** |
| Tiagabine | < 96 | 1–2[5] | Hepatic | 5–9[1] | 96 | None | ** |
| Topiramate | < 100 | 2–4 | Hepatic | 19–25[1] | 15 | None | ** |
| Valproate | < 100 | 0.5–8[6] | Hepatic | 12–17[1] | 85–95 | None | ** |
| Vigabatrin | < 100 | 0.5–2 | None | 4–7 | None | None | None |
| Zonisamide | < 100 | 2–4 | Hepatic | 49–69[1] | 30–60 | None | ** |

†, Half-life in healthy adult.

[1], Half-life varies with co-medication; [2], value for active metabolite; [3], absorption of gabapentin is by a saturable active transport system, and rate will depend on capacity of the system; [4], phenytoin has non-linear kinetics, and so half-life can increase at higher doses; [5], absorption of tiagabine is markedly slowed by food, and it is recommended that the drug is taken at the end of meals; [6], the time to peak concentration varies according to formulation (0.5–2 h for normal formulation, 3–8 h for enteric coated).

**, Many interactions, frequently of clinical relevance and many require dose modification; *, minor interactions common, but not usually of much clinical relevance; MHD, the monohydroxy metabolite of oxcarbazepine.

## PHARMACOKINETIC PRINCIPLES OF ANTIEPILEPTIC DRUG TREATMENT

To use drugs effectively, the reader should be aware of certain pharmacokinetic principles, some of which are enumerated here (Table 2.1); ignorance of these aspects of simple pharmacology will expose a patient to risks and inefficiencies.

## Drug absorption
### Oral absorption
This process depends both on the physical and pharmacological properties of the drug and biological properties of the person ingesting it. Physical properties include the formulation of the tablets, the lipid solubility, the binding and the degree of ionization at the pH levels in the gastrointestinal (GI) tract. Solutions are usually rather more quickly absorbed than tablets or capsules. The movement from GI tract to plasma for most drugs is a passive process which depends on factors including:
- the concentration gradient across the gut membrane;
- the lipid solubility of the drug. As the non-ionized form of the drug is generally the most lipid soluble, absorption is quickest of drugs that are not ionized at physiological pH level; and
- the absorption area and time in contact with the absorption surface. Although acidic drugs are less ionized in the stomach than the small intestine, most orally administered drugs, whether acidic or basic, depend largely on the small intestine for absorption because of its large absorptive area.

Several antiepileptics are absorbed by an active transport system (e.g. gabapentin, pregabalin and possibly phenytoin). The gabapentin absorption mechanism has a limited capacity, and higher doses may saturate the system. At saturated levels, increases in dosage do not greatly increase drug uptake. P-glycoprotein (see below) is widely distributed in the GI tract and it may have an important role in the absorption of antiepileptic drugs. The expression of the drug can be induced and inhibited by other drugs, many of which are also inhibitors or inducers of CYP3A4, and some of the so-called hepatic enzyme effects may in fact be due to alterations of oral absorption.

The following parameters are important to know for any drug being administered orally (see Table 2.1):

### pKa
The pH at which there is maximum ionization. The equation pH = pKa + Log [ionized/total drug] will provide the concentration of drug available for absorption in the GI tract environment with its varying pH levels. Some drugs have different structural properties at different pHs and may have different pKa values for each structural subtype (e.g. clonazepam, gabapentin).

### Oral bioavailability
This is the proportion of the oral dose that is absorbed and therefore available for use by the body. It is important to know to what extent such factors as age, gender or food taken with the drug alter its bioavailability. For drugs requiring an active system for absorption, the bioavailability may be reduced at higher doses as the system becomes saturated (e.g. as for gabapentin). Because of the dependence of absorption on gut motility, drugs with a low bioavailability tend to show high dose to dose variability of absorption. Motility is also reduced in some gastrointestinal diseases and in acute illness. Certain drugs interact with antiepileptics to reduce absorption, an example being the interaction of antacids and phenytoin. Several hours should elapse be-tween dosing with individual drugs that have the potential to interact. Food has an effect on the absorption of a number of antiepileptic drugs, but is only clinically important routinely in the case of tiagabine (which should always be taken at the end of a meal—it is important to advise patients about this).

The oral bioavailability of most antiepileptics approaches 100%. The exceptions are carbamazepine (75–85%), clonazepam (80%) and gabapentin (dependent on saturation and sometimes below 60%). These drugs are particularly subject to variable absorption. Different formulations of phenytoin have slightly different bioavailability and this too is occasionally clinically important.

### $T_{max}$
The time taken for peak serum levels to be reached following oral ingestion. This reflects a balance of absorption, distribution and elimination, and is in effect the beginning of the time when elimination exceeds absorption. For practical purposes, for most drugs the rate of absorption is, however, the major factor. At steady state, for drugs that are subject to auto-induction, $T_{max}$ is reached earlier than after the initial phase of drug therapy. The importance of this is shown in the case of carbamazepine, where initial $T_{max}$ can be 4–8 hours and the $T_{max}$ at steady state 1–3 hours.

### Modified-release formulations
The absorption of the standard preparation of many antiepileptics is relatively fast. Modified release formulations can be used to slow down absorption for more prolonged effect or to produce less fluctuation in serum levels. The slow (or controlled) release formulations are modified by such devices as coating the tablets in an acid-insoluble covering, increasing the size of the drug particles or embedding the drug in a matrix. The bioavailability of such preparations can differ from that of the unmodified parent. The slow-release formulation of carbamazepine, for example, can have lower bioavailability than the standard preparation.

### Generic formulations
Generic formulations of a compound are required to have a bioavailability that is approximately similar to the

proprietary compound. Rates of absorption, however, do vary somewhat, even if the extent of absorption does not. For all but the occasional patient, generic formulations are perfectly acceptable, and the reader is advised to ignore commercially driven research that purports to show otherwise. Only in the case of phenytoin, at levels close to saturation, do generics pose any particular problem in epilepsy, and even then serum-level monitoring can guide dosage.

### Rectal administration

Some drugs are readily absorbed by the rectal mucosa. This is an important mode of administration in emergency practice, as the rate of absorption is often very rapid. Solutions are better absorbed than lipid-based suppositories. The conveniently packaged Stesolid® preparation of diazepam is a good example of a valuable liquid formulation that has greatly improved the therapy of febrile seizures, in contrast to the wax-based diazepam suppository, which is absorbed rectally much too slowly.

### Parenteral administration

Parenteral formulations are needed in acute situations (e.g. status, acute seizures) and for temporary substitution of oral administration (e.g. in acute illness, or peroperatively). Most antiepileptics cannot be given by intramuscular administration, as the extent and rate of absorption are inadequate. Only phenobarbital or midazolam—for emergency therapy—can usefully be given intramuscularly. Phenytoin, which crystallizes at tissue pH, can result in muscle necrosis. Intravenous administration is possible for many antiepileptics and special formulations are available to minimize thrombophlebitis and other local complications (e.g. the Diazemuls® formulation of diazepam and fosphenytoin formulation of phenytoin).

### Buccal and intranasal administration and inhalation

There has been recent interest in these forms of administration for acute seizures. Midazolam has been assessed rigorously by buccal and intranasal instillation, and absorption is excellent. The inhalation of antiepileptic drugs to obtain immediate effect in acute situations is currently under investigation.

## Drug distribution

Once in the plasma, drug molecules are available for transfer to other body areas (compartments); the resulting drug concentrations at different sites are determined by the process of distribution. Drug distribution is complex, depending on diverse factors, some of which differ over time in the same individual. Distribution to most sites is by concentration-driven passive transfer across lipid membranes. Lipid solubility is an important determinant of this. The more lipid-soluble the drug, the greater its penetration into tissue. The blood–brain barrier has particularly tight intercellular junctions and only lipid-soluble drugs are able to cross it to enter the brain.

### Drug transport systems across the blood–brain barrier—'drug resistance' proteins

Many drugs have been shown to be actively removed from the brain by transport systems (some referred to as 'drug resistance' systems), and the relevant genes and transporter proteins have been identified. Genes for the latter include MDR1 (p-glycoprotein; multiple drug resistance protein) and MRP1. Their importance has long been known in cancer therapy, but recent interest has focused on antiepileptic drugs. P-glycoprotein mediates the absorption of drugs such as phenytoin, phenobarbital, lamotrigine and felbamate across the blood–brain barrier and over-expression may be one mechanism of drug resistance. While this is an obviously attractive idea, there is little evidence currently to support it. Another attractive postulate is that genetic variations in these drug-resistance proteins can affect concentrations of antiepileptics in the brain and thus their efficacy, and this is an area of active research. P-glycoprotein is also found in the gastrointestinal tract, but its effect on antiepileptic drug absorption has not been studied.

Some antiepileptics, for instance vigabatrin, appear to have an active transport system bringing the drug into the brain.

### Other factors influencing drug distribution

Other lipid tissues (e.g. muscle and fat) compete with brain for lipid-soluble drugs, and the concentration of a drug in any one compartment will depend on equilibrium with the others. The distribution of less lipid-soluble drugs may depend on blood flow through an organ (e.g. IV phenobarbital into brain during status epilepticus). Mathematical modelling of drug concentrations in the various compartments is possible in chronic oral and acute IV therapy, and an appreciation of IV drug distribution is necessary in the emergency therapy of status epilepticus (p. 225). The amount of drug available for distribution is the free fraction in the plasma, which is considerably lower than total plasma concentrations for protein-bound drugs (e.g. valproate, phenytoin).

### *Apparent volume of distribution ($V_d$)*

This is a proportionality constant that provides an estimate of the extent of distribution of the drug in tissues (Table 2.2). It is defined as the volume of fluid that would be required to contain the drug if a single compartment were assumed. The larger the volume of distribution, the greater the distribution in tissues (and the greater the risk of accumulation). Thus, if $V_d$ is approximately 0.05 l/kg (5% of body volume) the drug is confined to the vascular compartment; if it is 0.15 l/kg the drug is confined to the extracellular water; and if it is 0.5 l/kg the drug is distributed throughout the total body water. Higher values indicate that the drug is concentrated in tissue. $V_d$ can also be used to make a rough estimate of peak plasma level after the initial dose (very approximately equal to dose/$V_d$).

**Table 2.2** Volume of distribution ($V_d$) of common antiepileptic drugs.

---

*Drugs with very low $V_d$*
Nil

*Drugs with low $V_d$ (0.15– < 0.5 l/kg)*
Valproate

*Drugs with moderate $V_d$ (0.5–0.8 l/kg)*
Ethosuximide
Felbamate
Levetiracetam
Oxcarbazepine
Phenobarbital
Phenytoin
Pregabalin

*Drugs with a high $V_d$ (> 0.8 l/kg)*
Carbamazepine
Clobazam
Clonazepam
Gabapentin
Lamotrigine
Primidone
Tiagabine
Topiramate
Vigabatrin
Zonisamide

---

### Protein binding

The protein binding of a drug is expressed as a percentage, denoting the proportion of the total plasma concentration that is bound chemically to plasma proteins. The bound portion is not available for distribution. Plasma protein binding may alter in disease states (e.g. hepatic or renal disease), and tends to fall with age. There can be competition for binding sites between drugs. The effects of mild alterations in protein binding are often complex, but usually have few practical clinical implications. The most important in epilepsy is the displacement of bound phenytoin by valproate, and this can account for the signs of phenytoin toxicity on co-medication with valproate, with 'normal' total phenytoin blood levels. Tiagabine is also displaced by valproate, and this may also be an important effect.

### Total and free antiepileptic serum level

The total serum level refers to the total plasma concentration of a drug, i.e. both its bound and unbound fractions. The free serum level is the amount of unbound drug, i.e. that available for distribution.

## Drug elimination (metabolism and excretion)

A drug is cleared (eliminated) from the body by the processes of metabolism and excretion.

### Drug metabolism (biotransformation)

Most antiepileptics are metabolized in the liver by hepatocyte microsomal enzymes. Metabolism is frequently in two phases. Phase one is usually a process of oxidation, reduction or hydroxylation. Most of these metabolic reactions are mediated by the microsomal cytochrome P450 and glucuronyl transferases (see Tables 2.3 and 2.4). The metabolites are usually less biologically active, although this is not always the case (e.g. phenobarbital from primidone, desmethylclobazam from clobazam). Most oxidation process are carried out by the cytochrome microsomal P450 enzyme system, although there are exceptions, for instance the oxidation of valproate via a non-microsomal branched-chain fatty acid enzyme system involving monoamine oxidase, and the hydrolysis of levetiracetam by enzymes in red blood cells and other tissues. In phase two reactions the resulting metabolites are conjugated, usually by glucuronidation. The conjugates are almost always biologically inert and more polar (therefore more easily excreted) than the parent drugs. Biotransformation rather than renal excretion of unchanged drug is the main route of elimination for most antiepileptics.

### Drug interactions due to induction/inhibition of hepatic enzymes

The most important antiepileptic drug interactions are those mediated by changes in the P450 enzyme system. These metabolic processes can be induced or inhibited by antiepileptic drugs, and also auto-induced (induction of the drug's own metabolism). In fact carbamazepine, phenytoin, and phenobarbital are among the most potent enzyme-inducers in the pharmacopoeia. Pharmacokinetic interactions between antiepileptics (and other drugs) are therefore very common and can have a serious impact on clinical therapeutics. In recent years the characterization of the isoenzymes involved in antiepileptic drug metabolism has greatly improved our understanding of drug interactions. There are two main families of enzymes. The P450 enzyme system is involved in the phase 1 metabolism of a number of antiepileptic drugs (Table 2.4). Five of the isoenzymes (CYP3A4, CYP2C9, CYP2C19, CYP2E1 and CYP1A2) are the most important from the point of view of the antiepileptic drugs. Phase two reactions (conjugation) are usually mediated by the uridine glucuronyl transferase enzyme families (UGTs) of which 16 subtypes are recognized.

Examples of the most common and important interactions between antiepileptic drugs in routine epilepsy practice are as follow:

• The inducing effects of carbamazepine, phenytoin, phenobarbital and primidone on P450 and UGT enzymes, which commonly result in a clinically significant reductions in levels of carbamazepine, ethosuximide, lamotrigine, oxcarbazepine, tiagabine, topiramate, valproate and zonisamide. For instance, in one study, valproate concentrations were reduced

**Table 2.3** Some of the known interactions of antiepileptic drugs with hepatic enzyme systems.

| Enzyme | Antiepileptic drugs metabolized by the enzyme | Antiepileptic drugs that induce enzyme | Antiepileptic drugs that inhibit enzyme | Other drugs that induce enzyme* | Other drugs that inhibit enzyme* |
|---|---|---|---|---|---|
| CYP3A4 | Carbamazepine Clonazepam Ethosuximide Midazolam Phenytoin Tiagabine Zonisamide | Carbamazepine Felbamate Oxcarbazepine Phenobarbital Phenytoin Primidone Topiramate | | Glucocorticoids Rifampicin | Many others including: Cimetidine Ciclosporin A Diltiazem Erythromycin Fluconazole Fluvoxamine Verapamil Grapefruit juice |
| CYP2C9 | Phenytoin Phenobarbital Valproate | Carbamazepine Phenytoin Phenobarbital Primidone | Valproate | Rifampicin | Amiodorone Chloramphenicol Fluoxetine Fluoxamine Miconazole |
| CYP2C19 | Diazepam Phenytoin Phenobarbital Valproate | Carbamazepine Phenytoin Phenobarbital Primidone | Felbamate Oxcarbazepine Topiramart | Rifampicin | Cimetidine Fluoxamine |
| CYP2E1 | Felbamate Phenobarbital | | | Alcohol Isoniazid | |
| UGT1A4 | Lamotrigine Oxcarbazepine (MHD derivative) Phenobarbital Valproate | Carbamazepine Lamotrigine Oxcarbazepine Phenytoin Phenobarbital | Valproate | | |

*, A selection of drugs known to interact commonly with the antiepileptic drugs.

by 76%, 49% and 66% by co-medication with phenobarbital, phenytoin and carbamazepine, respectively.

• The inhibiting effects of valproate (on CYP2C9, CYP2C19 and UGT1A4) can elevate levels of phenobarbital and lamotrigine, sometimes by as much as 80%, and almost always necessitate dosage modification. Lesser effects of valproate occur on phenytoin and carbamazepine-epoxide concentrations.

• Other inhibiting effects occur, but are generally less important. These include the effects of phenytoin and phenobarbital on the metabolism of each other, and the inhibiting effects of carbamazepine and oxcarbazepine on phenytoin metabolism.

• Felbamate is by far the strongest inhibitor of CYP enzyme activity and has been shown to result in clinically significant elevations of the levels of phenytoin, valproate, phenobarbital, carbamazepine-epoxide and N-desmethyl clobazam.

Other non-antiepileptic drugs are also involved in interactions at the level of hepatic enzymes, including: many antipsychotic drugs; many antidepressants; many antibiotics (including rifampicin, erythromycin, clarithromycin); theophylline; warfarin; antifungal drugs; antihypertensive drugs (e.g. verapamil, diltiazem); and many cardiovascular drugs. The list of known interactions is very long, and before any co-medication is considered the potential for drug interaction should be checked.

### Drug excretion

Most drugs and their metabolites are excreted via the kidney. Nearly all the various processes of renal excretion are mediated by concentration-dependent passive transfer, although acidic molecules, including the glucuronide conjugates, are also actively pumped into the proximal renal tubules. The more polar the molecule the less resorption occurs in the distal tubule. Severe renal disease affects this process and can result in impaired excretion and greater drug accumulation. Mild renal disease rarely has any practically important effects on antiepileptic drug handling. Some antiepileptics are excreted without prior hepatic metabolism (e.g. gabapentin, levetiracetam, piracetam, pregabalin

| Drug | Phase 1 reactions | Phase 2 reactions[1] | P450 enzymes identified in the phase 1 reactions[2] |
|------|-------------------|---------------------|---------------------------------------------------|
| Carbamazepine | Epoxidation, hydroxylation | Conjugation | CYP3A4 CYP2C8 CYP1A2 |
| Clobazam | Demethylation, hydroxylation | Conjugation | |
| Clonazepam | Reduction, hydroxylation | Acetylation | CYP3A4 |
| Ethosuximide | Oxidation | Conjugation | CYP3A4 |
| Gabapentin | Renal excretion without metabolism | | |
| Lamotrigine | No phase 1 reaction | Conjugation | |
| Levetiracetam | Hydrolysis by non-hepatic enzymes | | |
| Oxcarbazepine | Reduction | Conjugation | CYP3A4 CYP2C8 |
| Phenobarbital | Oxidation, glucosidation, hydroxylation | Conjugation | CYP2C9 CYP2C19 CYP2E1 |
| Phenytoin | Oxidation, glucosidation, hydroxylation | Conjugation | CYP2C9 CYP2C19 CYP3A4 |
| Pregabalin | Renal excretion without metabolism | | |
| Primidone | Transformation to phenobarbital and a phenylethyl derivative, then metabolized as per phenobarbital | | |
| Tiagabine | Oxidation | Conjugation | CYP3A4 |
| Topiramate[3] | Hydroxylation, hydrolysis | Conjugation | |
| Valproate | Oxidation, hydroxylation, epoxidation, reduction[4] | Conjugation | CYP4B1 CYP2C9 CYP2A6 CYP2B6 CYP2C19 |
| Vigabatrin | Renal excretion without metabolism | | |
| Zonisamide | Acetylation, reduction | Conjugation | CYP3A4 |

**Table 2.4** Metabolic pathways of antiepileptic drugs.

[1], Conjugation (phase 2) is always by glucuronidation involving the UDPGT family enzymes; [2], this lists known enzymes. Other enzymes, not yet fully characterized, play a part in the metabolism of many of these drugs; [3], in non-induced patients, most topiramate is excreted renally without metabolism; [4], some of the biotransformation of valproate is via non-P450 enzyme systems.

and vigabatrin) and doses have to be reduced in severe renal disease. Alkalinization of the urine will reduce the absorption of acidic drugs from the renal tubules and this is an interaction that can effect the blood levels of phenobarbital (and is used therapeutically in barbiturate overdose).

Drugs can also be excreted through the lungs, sweat, tears and maternal milk, but with the exception of the pulmonary excretion of gaseous anaesthetics used in status, these routes of excretion are generally of no importance in regard to the antiepileptic drugs, although excretion in maternal milk does have implications for prescribing in breast-feeding women (see p. 107).

### Elimination half-life

This is the period of time after absorption over which half of the drug is eliminated from the body. For most drugs this depends primarily on their metabolism. There can be marked inter-individual variation as well as intra-individual changes over time. Drug interactions can also have marked effects on elimination half-life. Three-quarters of a drug is eliminated within two half-lives, and approximately 93% within four half-lives. Once a steady state has been reached, at a very rough approximation, dosing a drug at intervals equivalent to one half-life will keep trough levels within 50% of peak concentrations.

### Fraction (of dose) excreted unchanged in urine ($Fu_{(x)}$)

After a drug is given intravenously and the subject's urine is collected for seven half-lives, the proportion of the drug present in an unchanged form ($Fu_{(x)}$) measures the contribution of renal excretion to total drug elimination (the rest being eliminated by metabolism). If this fraction ($Fu_{(x)}$) is high, renal impairment may require drug doses to be lowered; if it is low, renal impairment is unlikely to seriously affect drug kinetics. Similarly, high values of $Fu_{(x)}$ imply that modification of drug dosage will be unnecessary in hepatic disease, and low $Fu_{(x)}$ values that such modification may be necessary. In the elderly, because renal excretory capacity falls, it is wise to consider lower than average doses of drugs with high $Fu_{(x)}$ values. Antiepileptic drugs with a high $Fu_{(x)}$ value include gabapentin, levetiracetam, piracetam, pregabalin and vigabatrin.

### Clearance

This is defined as the amount of drug excreted over a unit time. Plasma clearance is a measure of the amount of drug removed from the plasma. Renal clearance is a measure of the amount of drug removed by the kidneys. As a general rule, if $Fu_{(x)}$ is low, then clearance is largely dependent on hepatic metabolism; conversely, if $Fu_{(x)}$ is high, clearance is largely dependent on renal excretion. When drugs are avidly taken up by the liver, clearance values can be as high as 1.4 l/kg/h (i.e. the rate of hepatic blood flow).

### Kinetics of biotransformation

Metabolism is an enzyme-catalysed process that is potentially saturable, described by the Michaelis–Menten equation: $V = V_{max} \times C/(Km + C)$, where $V$ = velocity of the process, $V_{max}$ = the maximum velocity possible, $Km$ = the Michaelis–Menten constant, and $C$ = the concentration of the drug. For most drugs, the required serum concentrations are well below their $Km$ values, and in these circumstances $V$ is virtually equal to $V_{max}$ (i.e. metabolism is not saturated). These drugs have a linear relationship between drug dose and serum level in the ranges that are clinically useful, so-called 'first-order kinetics'. A few antiepileptic drugs, however, have levels close to saturation (e.g. phenytoin, thiopental). When concentrations reach levels that overwhelm the capacity of the system (i.e. where $V$ is close to $V_{max}$), the velocity of metabolism cannot be increased. In this situation, small increases in dose may result in large and unpredictable rises in the level in the blood.

**Table 2.5** Factors influencing levels of antiepileptic drugs.

*Drug factors*
Formulation
Interactions

*Patient factors*
Genetic/constitutional factors affecting pharmacokinetics (absorption, metabolism, excretion)
Disease states affecting pharmacokinetics (renal, hepatic, changes in plasma proteins, GI disturbance)
Pregnancy, nutritional status, body weight changes

### Steady-state values

Steady-state values are those that are achieved when, for any particular drug dose, the pharmacokinetic processes reach equilibrium. The time to steady state (Tss) is dependent on many factors, but as a rule of thumb it is equal to 5 times the elimination half-life of the drug. In long-term treatment, steady-state values (e.g. for serum levels, clearance, $V_d$, half-life, $T_{max}$) are generally of greater use to clinicians than values at initial dosing.

## Blood level measurements

When a steady state has been reached, there is a fairly consistent relationship between plasma concentration of any drug and the concentration in brain or other tissues. It should therefore be possible to define those plasma levels that are associated with optimal clinical effects (i.e. an optimal balance between effectiveness and side-effects). Because of biological variation, such levels vary from individual to individual (Table 2.5), but nevertheless a range can be developed which is based on statistical or population parameters. This is the 'target range' (also known as the 'therapeutic range' or the 'optimal range').

In practice, skill is needed to interpret serum drug concentrations wisely. The clinician should know when to ignore as well as when to heed blood level information.

### Timing of blood samples

Generally, blood samples should be taken at steady state, i.e. at a period after any dose change that is greater than 5 times the drug elimination half-life. Steady-state serum levels of drugs with short half-lives fluctuate through the day in patients on oral medication, and thus blood sampling should be taken at a similar time (the trough level—that taken before the morning dosing—is a conventional preference) to assess blood level changes. For drugs with a long half-life (e.g. phenobarbital), there is little diurnal fluctuation and timing is unimportant.

### Rapid assay

Technology exists for rapid assay of the commonly used drugs. It can be extremely helpful to have blood level data available before a consultation and in large clinics it is cost effective to offer an immediate assay service (equivalent to having the blood sugar results during a diabetic clinic).

### Salivary vs. serum concentrations

The salivary concentration of certain drugs (e.g. ethosuximide, carbamazepine, phenytoin) correlates well with the unbound (free) serum concentration. Salivary measurements avoid the need for venepuncture and so are particularly acceptable in children. However, measurement is more difficult and more prone to error than serum measurements, and can be complicated by gingivitis and dose residues in the mouth, and so have therefore not been widely adopted. It should also be noted that the relationship between unbound drug concentration in plasma and drug concentration in saliva is not the same for all drugs. The salivary concentration of phenobarbital, for instance, varies with salivary pH, and meaningful results must account for this. Similarly, valproate salivary concentrations, for various pharmacological reasons, have no consistent relationship with plasma concentrations.

### Target range

The target range is an estimate derived largely from hospital studies with a bias towards relatively severe cases. In fact there are many individuals whose epilepsy is well controlled at 'suboptimal' levels—at least one-third of patients treated with phenytoin for instance. There are also others whose seizures are only controlled, without side-effects, at 'supra-optimal' levels. Epilepsy is very heterogeneous, and generally speaking the more severe the epilepsy, the higher are the required blood levels. Thus, patients with frequent seizures or those with partial epilepsy often have higher 'therapeutic ranges' than those with less severe forms of epilepsy. The effectiveness and side-effects will vary in individuals due to genetic, constitutional and exogenous factors, which may not be well correlated with blood levels. For all these reasons, too rigid an adherence to the 'range' is quite inappropriate, and in all cases treatment must be tailored to individual requirements —the patient should be treated, not his/her blood level.

The concept of a 'target range' has most utility in the case of drugs that have a moment-by-moment action on cellular membrane function; phenytoin, carbamazepine, ethosuximide and lamotrigine, drugs acting at membrane ion channels, are the best examples of this (Table 2.6). Where drugs have more indirect antiepileptic actions, or multiple actions, blood level may be less well correlated with effect—for instance in the case of gabapentin, vigabatrin and topiramate. Also, the concept of a therapeutic range is undermined where pharmacological tolerance develops, as, for instance, with barbiturates or benzodiazepines.

### The 'individualized' therapeutic range

It is sometimes feasible to establish empirically a plasma concentration range for an individual patient in which the best therapeutic response is obtained. The measurement of blood levels during periods of optimal response will provide a useful reference. As emphasized above, the individualized therapeutic ranges may differ markedly from the published population-based ranges.

### Total vs. free serum drug concentrations

Routine analytical methods measure the total drug concentration (i.e. the protein-bound and unbound [free] fractions), whereas it is actually the free fraction that is available for biological action. Measurement of the total level is satisfactory as there is usually a consistent relationship between the free and the total levels. However, in certain states this relationship can be altered—for instance in low protein states, severe renal disease, severe hepatic disease, pregnancy, old age and in the neonatal period. In these situations the free levels may be higher than would be predicted from the total concentration, and reliance on total concentration may be misleading. Some advocate the routine direct measurement of free levels in all these situations. However, assay techniques are difficult, and the results are less accurate, and in routine practice free level estimations are rarely required.

### Active metabolites

Some drugs are converted into active metabolites, and interpretation of parent drug level measurements without accounting for the potential contribution of the active metabolite can lead to therapeutic errors. Carbamazepine is metabolized to a 10,11-epoxide which can cause side-effects similar to those of the parent drug. Measurement of the concentration of the parent drug alone may be misleading, especially as the proportion of carbamazepine converted to carbamazepine 10,11-epoxide can vary markedly (for instance in the presence of enzyme-inducing co-medication). In the case of clobazam and primidone, the concentrations of the active metabolites at steady state are much higher than that of the parent drug, and in this situation measurements of the level of the metabolites are more informative.

### When is blood level measurement required?

There is no doubt that the practice of monitoring plasma drug concentrations has improved the quality of epilepsy care. It has led to an appreciation of variability of drug levels, kinetic principles, drug interactions and the value of tailoring doses to individual patient needs. Feedback from blood level measurement improves a clinician's experience and clinical acumen and, as a result, effective therapy can often be chosen now on purely clinical grounds, as shown in a recent study in which there were no differences in outcome between patients randomized to have their regimens adjusted empirically and those in whom dosage was tailored based on drug concentration measurements.

The situations in which blood level measurements are most often required are shown in Table 2.7, and it will be

**Table 2.6** Value of measurement of blood levels of antiepileptic drugs.

| Drug | Target level (μmol/l) | Value of blood-level measurements in routine practice | Comments |
|---|---|---|---|
| Carbamazepine | 20–50 | *** | Measurements useful because response is closely linked to blood level, although kinetics are linear and often dose change can be made simply on a clinical basis. Measurements useful also to monitor the effects of drug interactions and because both the parent drug and the active metabolite contribute to clinical effect |
| Ethosuximide | 300–700 | *** | Measurements useful because response is closely linked to blood level, although kinetics are linear and often dose change can be made simply on a clinical basis |
| Lamotrigine | 10–60 | ** | Response is only partially correlated with blood level. However, measurement is useful where lamotrigine levels are affected by antiepileptic drug interactions, interactions with the contraceptive pill, and pregnancy |
| Oxcarbazepine | 50–140[1] | * | Measurements of limited usefulness only as response is not broadly linked to blood level. However, as parent drug and active metabolite contribute to clinical effect, it is sometimes useful to monitor changes |
| Phenobarbital | 50–130 | ** | Measurements have moderate utility, but tolerance complicates assessment, and the upper limit is imprecise because of the sedative effects |
| Phenytoin | 40–80 | *** | Measurements useful because response is closely linked to blood level, and because it is hazardous to alter dose without measurements owing to non-linear kinetics |
| Primidone | 25–50[2] | ** | Measurement of the derived phenobarbital levels of moderate utility (see above) but measurement of primidone level is of only limited usefulness |
| Topiramate | 10–60 | * | Measurements of limited usefulness only as response is not broadly linked to blood level. However, serum level measurement useful to monitor effects of drug interactions |
| Valproate | 300–700 | ** | Measurement is of only limited usefulness, as response is only partially correlated to blood level and these vary widely through the day. However, serum level measurement is useful to monitor effects of drug interactions |
| Zonisamide | 30–140 | * | Measurements of limited usefulness only as response is not broadly linked to blood level. More experience with blood-level monitoring in this drug may lead to reassessment of value |
| Benzodiazepines | — | | There is no consistent relationship between blood levels and clinical response |
| | — | | The usefulness of routine measurements of these drugs has not been established |
| Vigabatrin | — | | Blood level not correlated with pharmacological effect (irreversible enzyme inhibition) |

Felbamate, gaba pentin, levetiracetam, pregabalin and tiagabine: target blood levels have been quoted, but their usefulness in routine practice is doubtful. The measurements are usually currently required only in exceptional circumstances or to check compliance.

***, Very useful, measurements should be made frequently; **, useful, measurements required often; *, limited usefulness, measurements occasionally required; —, no general utility, measurement only required in exceptional circumstances (or to check compliance); [1], MHD derivative; [2], primidone levels—measurement of derived phenobarbital levels is more useful.

apparent that these are relatively restricted; the variability of phenytoin levels is one example (Figure 2.1). In many clinical situations drug-level monitoring is wrongly relied upon, and measurements made unnecessarily or interpreted incorrectly. The most common mistake is to adhere too closely to the 'therapeutic range', and it is incorrect for instance to: (i) increase drug doses in patients fully controlled simply because the serum level is below the therapeutic range; (ii) lower drug doses in patients without side-effects because the serum level is above the therapeutic range; or (iii) ignore adverse effects because the levels are within the therapeutic range. The importance of 'treating the patient, not the serum level' cannot be overstated.

## CHOICE OF DRUGS FOR DIFFERENT SEIZURE TYPES

The efficacy and side-effects of individual drug are covered in Section 3. Here, a few general points will be made.

The original goal of the 1971 *Seizure Type Classification* was, at least in part, to divide seizures into categories on the basis of their response to different drugs. However, since then the number of available drugs has grown, and the role of therapy has become better understood, and it is now apparent that there is relatively limited specificity. A few general rules can, however, be discerned. Partial-onset (and

**Table 2.7** Indications for blood level monitoring.

- To assess blood levels where there is a poor therapeutic response in spite of adequate dosage. The measurement of levels of the parent drug and active metabolites may be necessary
- To identify the cause of adverse effects where these might be drug-induced. The measurement of levels of the parent drug and active metabolites may be necessary
- To monitor phenytoin dose changes in view of the non-linear kinetics and lack of predictability of the phenytoin dose–blood level relationship
- To measure pharmacokinetic changes in the presence of physiological or pathological conditions known to alter drug disposition (e.g. pregnancy, liver disease, renal failure, gastrointestinal disease, hypoalbulinaemic states)
- To identify and minimize the consequences of adverse drug interactions in patients receiving multiple drug therapy
- To identify which drugs require dosage changes to optimize therapy in patients on antiepileptic drug polytherapy
- To assess changes in bioavailability when a drug formulation has been changed
- To identify poor compliance

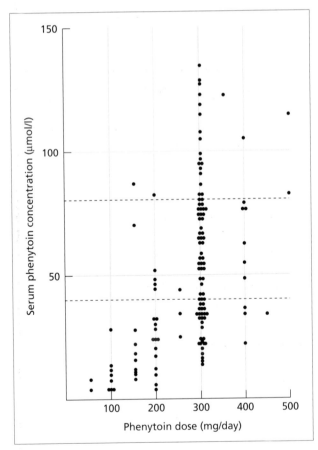

**Fig. 2.1** Distribution of steady-state serum phenytoin concentrations in 131 adult epileptic patients on admission to a residential centre. Note the large variability observed in patients receiving the same dosage.

secondarily generalized) seizures can be treated with almost any of the available drugs and show little specificity—perhaps a consequence largely of the fact that the required regulatory new drug trials are invariably carried out in partial-onset seizures. However, myoclonic and typical absence seizures have a more specific range of therapies, which overlaps but is not exactly co-incident with that of drugs effective in tonic, atonic and atypical absence seizures (Table 2.8).

Furthermore, the newer drugs have specific licences, which restrict their use even further. Although off-label prescribing is common in epilepsy, in a age of growing litigation and bureaucratic oversight, this carries risks and should be discouraged at least in non-specialist practice or without explicit justification. The European licensed indications of the newer drugs are shown in Table 2.9. The older drugs—clonazepam, ethosuximide, phenobarbital, primidone and phenytoin—were all licensed before stricter rules were imposed, and carry no regulatory age limitations or seizure-type restrictions.

Finally, it is, perhaps, a surprising fact that among the symptomatic epilepsies, drug choice seems to depend little, if at all, on the underlying aetiology. Thus, the therapy of epilepsy due to tumours, infection, vascular disease, head injury, congenital lesions, toxins or poisons is the same, regardless of cause. Symptomatic epilepsy causes largely partial-onset seizures, and virtually any of the antiepileptic drugs can be used in their treatment. Furthermore, there is considerable overlap between the range of drugs used to treat the generalized tonic–clonic seizures in idiopathic epilepsies and those used in symptomatic epilepsy. Whether advances in knowledge will help to differentiate therapy remains to be seen.

Various other clinical factors influence the choice of drugs (Table 2.10). Above all, treatment should be tailored to individual patients, and the relevance of any particular factor will vary from patient to patient. People differ, for instance, in their willingness to risk side-effects or to try new therapy. Patients' preferences depend on age, gender or comorbidity, co-medication, drug formulation, and dosing frequencies, and such factors as risks in pregnancy and a whole range of social aspects. Doctors' preferences and prescribing patterns also vary, and are dependent on such factors as prior experience, marketing pressures, the medical system within which they work, reimbursement patterns, and teaching and information sources. There is, however, only limited international consensus about drug choice. There are striking differences in the use of drugs in different countries. Phenytoin, for instance, is more widely prescribed in the USA than elsewhere, carbamazepine in northern Europe, and valproate in the Francophone world. The pattern of drug usage furthermore varies widely within countries and even within the same institution.

Another general point of importance is the length of time it has taken for some irreversible side-effects to be recog-

**Table 2.8** Choice of drug for seizure types.

| Seizure type | Drugs which show efficacy | Drugs that may worsen seizures |
|---|---|---|
| Partial seizures, secondarily generalized tonic–clonic seizures, primary generalized tonic–clonic seizures | Acetazolamide, carbamazepine, clobazam, clonazepam, felbamate, gabapentin, lamotrigine, levetiracetam, oxcarbazepine, phenobarbital, phenytoin, pregabalin, primidone, rufinamide, tiagabine, topiramate, valproate, vigabatrin, zonisamide | |
| Absence seizures (typical absence) | Acetazolamide, clobazam, clonazepam, ethosuximide, lamotrigine, levetiracetam, phenobarbital, topiramate, valproate | Carbamazepine, gabapentin, oxcarbazepine, tiagabine, vigabatrin |
| Myoclonic seizures | Clobazam, clonazepam, lamotrigine, levetiracetam, phenobarbital, piracetam, topiramate, valproate | Carbamazepine, gabapentin, oxcarbazepine, phenytoin, tiagabine, vigabatrin |
| Atypical absence, tonic, and atonic seizures | Acetazolamide, clobazam, clonazepam, felbamate, lamotrigine, phenobarbital, primidone, rufinamide, topiramate, valproate, zonisamide | Carbamazepine, gabapentin, oxcarbazepine, phenytoin, tiagabine, vigabatrin |

**Table 2.9** Licensed indications of the newer antiepileptic drugs (in Europe).

| Drug | Licensed indications | Monotherapy | Adjunctive therapy |
|---|---|---|---|
| Clobazam | Adjunctive therapy for epilepsy (no restrictions by seizure type) | Not licensed in monotherapy | ≥ 3 years (can be used in children over 6 months in exceptional circumstances) |
| Gabapentin | Adjunctive second-line therapy in partial and 2° generalized tonic–clonic seizures | Not licensed in monotherapy | ≥ 6 years |
| Lamotrigine | Partial and tonic–clonic seizures (1° or 2° generalized) seizures and Lennox–Gastaut syndrome | ≥ 12 years | ≥ 2 years |
| Levetiracetam | Adjunctive therapy in partial and 2° generalized tonic–clonic seizures | Not licensed in monotherapy | ≥ 16 years |
| Oxcarbazepine | Partial and tonic–clonic seizures (1° or 2° generalized) seizures | ≥ 6 years | ≥ 1 month |
| Piracetam | Adjunctive therapy in myoclonic seizures | Not licensed in monotherapy | ≥ 16 years |
| Pregabalin | Adjunctive therapy in partial and 2° generalized tonic–clonic seizures | Not licensed in monotherapy | ≥ 16 years |
| Tiagabine | Adjunctive second-line therapy in partial and 2° generalized tonic–clonic seizures | Not licensed in monotherapy | ≥ 12 years |
| Topiramate | Partial and tonic–clonic seizures (1° or 2° generalized) seizures and Lennox–Gastaut syndrome | ≥ 6 years | ≥ 2 years |
| Vigabatrin | Therapy-resistant partial and 2° generalized tonic–clonic seizures. Monotherapy in infantile spasms | No age limit specified | No age limit specified |
| Zonisamide | Partial seizures with or without secondary generalisation | Not licensed in monotherapy | ≥ 18 years |

Based on guidelines from the UK National Institute for Clinical Excellence (NICE).
1°, primarily; 2°, secondarily; indications in USA and other countries can differ slightly.

**Table 2.10** Factors influencing choice of treatment regimen in epilepsy.

*Personal patient-related factors*
Age and gender
Co-morbidity (physical and mental)
Social circumstances (employment, education, domestic, etc.)
Emotional circumstances
Attitude to risks of seizures and of medication

*Factors related to the epilepsy*
Syndrome and seizure type
Severity and chronicity
Aetiology (less important in chronic epilepsy)

*Factors related to the drug*
Mechanism of action
Strength of therapeutic effects
Strength and nature of side-effects
Formulation
Drug interactions and pharmacokinetic properties
Cost

This list illustrates the sort of factors that influence choice of drugs.
It is not comprehensive, and the importance of factors will vary from
individual to individual.

nized. Some examples are given in Table 2.11. In the light of this experience, it is wise, generally, to exercise caution when using newly licensed drugs, the full side-effect profile of which may yet not be completely apparent.

## Choice of drug for partial seizures and in secondarily generalized seizures

In most Western countries, newly introduced drugs for partial epilepsy are required to have specific licences for use as monotherapy and for use as polytherapy (i.e. as add-on therapy in refractory epilepsy—see Table 2.9). Regulations require a new antiepleptic to show proof of efficacy and safety separately for monotherapy and polytherapy indications, in spite of the fact that there are few, if any, examples of an AED that is effective in combination but not as

single-drug therapy. It is difficult to escape the cynical conclusion that the purpose of these regulations, partially at least, is to erect a bureaucratic hurdle to prevent the widespread and costly use of the newer drugs as first-line treatment. These trials take time and are expensive and to date, of the newer antiepileptics, only felbamate, gabapentin, lamotrigine, oxcarbazepine and topiramate have undergone sufficient monotherapy trials to have satisfied at least one of the major licensing authorities that monotherapy is appropriate. The older AEDs were introduced before this distinction between 'monotherapy' and 'polytherapy' licences was made, and are licensed for both indications.

### Drug choice in monotherapy

The landmark monotherapy study for traditional drugs was the double-blind multicentre comparison of phenytoin, carbamazepine, phenobarbital and primidone carried out by the American Veterans' Administration collaborative network. In this study 622 patients were randomized to treatment with one of the four drugs and followed for 24 months or until toxicity or lack of seizure control required a treatment switch. The patients were adults, and a mixture of newly diagnosed drug-naïve patients and patients who had been previously under-treated. Overall treatment success was highest with carbamazepine or phenytoin, intermediate with phenobarbital, and lowest with primidone, but the proportion of patients rendered free of seizures on the four drugs (between 48 and 63%) did not differ greatly. Differences in failure rates were explained primarily by the fact that primidone caused more intolerable acute adverse effects, such as nausea, vomiting, dizziness and sedation (in fact this was perhaps because too high a dose was used initially). This study confirmed the widely held view that—in terms of antiepileptic efficacy—there was little to choose between the four drugs, and that the main differences relate to their side-effect profiles. A follow-on study comparing carbamazepine and valproate in 480 adult patients showed no differences in the control of secondarily generalized seizures, although carbamazepine was more effective in complex partial seizures.

| Drug | Adverse reaction | Incidence of side-effects | Year of marketing | Year of discovery of side-effects |
|------|-----------------|--------------------------|-------------------|-----------------------------------|
| Phenobarbital | Shoulder–hand syndrome | Up to 12% | 1912 | 1934 |
| Phenytoin | Rickets and osteomalacia | Up to 5%* | 1938 | 1967 |
| Valproic acid | Hepatotoxicity | 1 in 600 to 1 in 50,000 | 1967 | 1977 |
| Vigabatrin | Visual field defects | 30% | 1989 | 1997 |

* Frequency in the 1960s, now lower.

**Table 2.11** Latency between the introduction of antiepileptic drugs to the market and the discovery of important adverse effects.

Two randomized open British studies, on the other hand, found no differences in efficacy when valproate and carbamazepine were compared in adults and children with newly diagnosed partial and/or generalized tonic–clonic seizures. In two additional randomized studies, carbamazepine, valproate, phenytoin and phenobarbital were compared as initial therapy in drug-naïve newly diagnosed children and adults. No differences in efficacy were noted, but phenobarbital was withdrawn more often in children because of side-effects. A similar comparative open monotherapy study in adults found no significant differences between carbamazepine, phenytoin or valproate in efficacy or side-effects. Similarly, the efficacy of valproate against absence seizures was found to be similar to that of ethosuximide. Taking these studies together, a few general conclusions can be reached. It seems clear that there are no major differences in efficacy between any of the drugs that are used for the treatment of focal epilepsy. Among these traditional drugs, carbamazepine may have slightly better efficacy in partial seizures than valproate, and both carbamazepine and phenytoin are better tolerated than phenobarbital in newly diagnosed epilepsy in children (Table 2.12).

As far as newer drugs are concerned, comparative monotherapy data are also limited. There have been a number of randomized studies in adults comparing lamotrigine with carbamazepine and phenytoin and no major differences in efficacy were found, even though lamotrigine showed some tolerability advantages, particularly in the elderly. Gabapentin has been compared with carbamazepine in one double-blind monotherapy study, which showed no

differences in efficacy at higher gabapentin doses. Topiramate has been compared in similar studies with carbamazepine and valproate, and oxcarbazepine with carbamazepine, valproate and phenytoin, and in none of these studies were significant difference in efficacy seen at comparable doses. In newly diagnosed epilepsy, topiramate 100 and 200 mg/day was found to be as effective as carbamazepine 600 mg/day or valproate 1250 mg/day. Oxcarbazepine and topiramate have both been shown to be superior to placebo in monotherapy (using an active control design). Monotherapy trials in which vigabatrin and gabapentin were compared with carbamazepine in patients with newly diagnosed epilepsy also failed to show any advantages in efficacy in favour of the newer drugs and, if anything, there was a trend for rates of freedom from seizures to be higher in the groups assigned to carbamazepine.

The most striking finding from all these studies is the similarity—not the difference—in responder rates among the various drugs in patients with partial-onset epilepsy. Because of this, choice in these patients will depend to a large extent on tolerability considerations, cost and other factors.

For all these reasons, carbamazepine or phenytoin is usually chosen as the drug of first choice in partial epilepsy. However, as emphasized above, the patient's preference should be paramount, not least because the newly diagnosed patient with epilepsy is likely to stay on the first antiepileptic drug chosen for many years. Detailed counselling is important, and the relative merits of each drug should be carefully explained. Factors such as cost, tolerability, safety, potential

**Table 2.12** Comparative monotherapy studies of standard antiepileptic drugs in partial and tonic–clonic seizures. The significance was measured by the hazard ratio; ND, no significant difference; †, difference 1.22 (CI, 1.04–1.44); ††, difference 1.97 (CI, 1.09–1.97); †††, difference 4.32 (CI, 1.77–10.6).

| | No. of studies | Treatment failure | 12-month remission | Time to first seizure |
|---|---|---|---|---|
| *Partial epilepsy* | | | | |
| Carbamazepine vs valproate | 5 | ND | ND | Slight advantage to carbamazepine† |
| Carbamazepine vs phenobarbital | 4 | | ND | ND |
| Phenytoin vs valproate | 4 | | ND | ND |
| Phenytoin vs phenobarbital | | Slight advantage to phenytoin†† | ND | ND |
| *Generalized epilepsy* | | | | |
| Carbamazepine vs valproate | 4 | ND | ND | ND |
| Carbamazepine vs phenobarbital | 3 | ND | ND | ND |
| Phenytoin vs valproate | 5 | ND | ND | ND |
| Phenytoin vs phenobarbital | | Advantage to phenytoin††† | ND | ND |

for teratogenicity, co-morbidity, convenience and ease of use are considerations that vary from patient to patient.

### Drug choice in combination therapy

As part of the Food and Drug Administration (FDA) rules, to be licensed, a new candidate antiepileptic drug is required to show a difference in efficacy and not simple equivalence. From the clinical (in contrast to the regulatory) perspective, this has had one serious disadvantage—all new drugs have been compared primarily with placebo, rather than with each other. Thus, the trials do not individually give much information to the clinician about the *relative* benefits of individual drugs. One way around this problem has been to carry out meta-analyses of trials, and to use meta-analytical statistical methods to compare and contrast drug therapies. Such analyses have obvious and well-known disadvantages, but at present provide the best information available for making choices about drugs. The first meta-analysis of antiepileptic drugs was carried out in Liverpool and has become justly influential. In a recent update, 36 randomized clinical trials were analysed in which one of eight new AEDs was tested against placebo as add-on treatment in patients with refractory partial epilepsy. The results are shown in Figure 2.2. This shows the mean odds ratio with their 95% confidence intervals of responder rates (i.e. having a ≥ 50% improvement in seizures on therapy compared with a baseline period). In this analysis, all drugs were found to be statistically superior to placebo (i.e. the means

and 95% confidence intervals are all greater than 1), and although there were striking (nearly twofold) differences between the mean odds ratios for different drugs, the confidence intervals were wide and overlapped, and thus these differences were not statistically significant.

One criticism of this method of display is that drugs are being compared at the dosages used in the clinical trials, and that higher doses of the seemingly less effective drugs might produce better odds ratios. Analysis at different doses certainly produces different mean values, and this effect is most clearly shown for topiramate and levetiracetam.

The rate of premature withdrawal from the randomized controlled trial is a commonly used measure of tolerability. Like all surrogate measures, this measure has limitations and, for instance, can be unduly influenced by transient initial side-effects and dose escalation regimens. Nevertheless, it is a useful measure of overall tolerability and it is susceptible to meta-analysis using the same statistical treatment as for comparisons of efficacy. Figure 2.3 illustrates the results of a meta-analysis of withdrawal rates of the eight antiepleptic drugs. The mean odds ratios show a nearly four-fold difference in tolerability, but again, as the confidence intervals overlap, the differences were not statistically significant. It is also noteworthy that the confidence limits for three drugs (lamotrigine, gabapentin and levetiracetam) overlap the placebo response, indicating no significant difference in withdrawal rate between placebo and active therapy.

Other analyses are possible from the same data set, including a 'number needed to treat' analysis which does

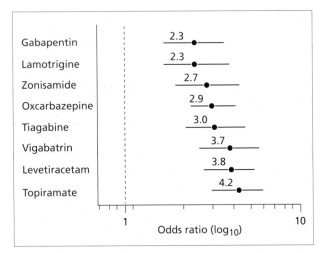

**Fig. 2.2** Odds ratios for 50% responder rates from placebo-controlled, adjunctive-therapy randomized controlled trials (RCTs) of eight recently introduced AEDs. This figure shows the summary odds ratios (overall odds ratio and 95% confidence intervals) of the RCTs of eight newly introduced AEDs. Note that the horizontal scale is logarithmic and that there are marked differences between the mean odds ratios. However, as the confidence intervals overlap, there is no statistical difference. Note also that, as the confidence intervals are all to the right of the vertical line, all drugs are significantly more efficacious than placebo.

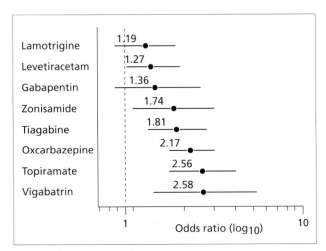

**Fig. 2.3** Odds ratios for rates of premature withdrawal from published placebo-controlled, adjunctive-therapy RCTs of eight recently introduced AEDs. This figure shows the summary odds ratios (overall odds ratio and 95% confidence intervals) of the RCTs of eight newly introduced AEDs. Note that the horizontal scale is logarithmic and that there are marked differences between the mean odds ratios. However, as the confidence intervals overlap, there is no statistical difference.

**Table 2.13** Tailoring antiepileptic drugs in partial-onset epilepsy to patient characteristics (based on preferences from the author's clinical practice).

| Patient characteristics | Drugs that are particularly suitable* | Drugs that should be particularly avoided |
|---|---|---|
| Patients with severe partial-onset seizures | Clobazam, carbamazepine, levetiracetam, oxcarbazepine, phenytoin, topiramate | |
| Patients with mild partial-onset seizures | Carbamazepine, gabapentin, lamotrigine, oxcarbazepine, valproate | |
| Patients who wish particularly to avoid cosmetic effects and weight gain | Carbamazepine, topiramate | Clobazam, gabapentin, phenytoin, valproate |
| Patients with prominent anxiety | Clobazam, carbamazepine, phenobarbital | Levetiracetam, tiagabine, vigabatrin |
| Patients with prominent depression | Carbamazepine, lamotrigine, valproate | Clobazam, clonazepam, phenobarbital, tiagabine, topiramate, vigabatrin |
| Patients with foreign tissue lesional epilepsy (e.g. tumour) | Carbamazepine, clobazam, phenytoin, tiagabine | |
| Patients at particular risk from allergy | Clobazam, gabapentin, levetiracetam, topiramate, vigabatrin | Acetazolamide, carbamazepine, felbamate, lamotrigine, oxcarbazepine, phenytoin |
| Patients at particular risk of heart disease | | Carbamazepine, lamotrigine, oxcarbazepine |

*, First-line drugs.

show statistical differences between the relatively weaker effectiveness of lamotrigine and gabapentin compared with levetiracetam, topiramate, vigabatrin or oxcarbazepine.

The validity of these meta-analyses has been the subject of wide-ranging criticism. Not least, all the studies used fixed doses, and different responses will occur at different doses. The overriding message from the analyses, however, is that none of the newer drugs has any unequivocal superiority in terms of efficacy or tolerability to any of the others.

## Tailoring drugs to different patient profiles

In spite of the disappointing lack of differentiation between drugs in the regulatory trials, it is absolutely clear that in routine clinical practice differences do exist. The art of therapy is to tailor the drugs to individual patient needs, and the recognition of drug differences is at the heart of skilful prescribing. On an empirical basis, among patients with partial-onset epilepsy, for instance, one can discern several distinctive patient profiles, commonly encountered in clinical practice, which require different approaches (Table 2.13). Clinical experience suggests that certain drugs convey certain advantages in these groups, either because of a lower risk of side-effects in susceptible persons or because of particular effectiveness. There are no controlled data on many of these points, and Table 2.13 summarizes the author's own preferences.

## Cost of drugs

The costs of drugs vary considerably, and furthermore differ in different countries and regions. The newer drugs are far more expensive than the older alternatives, and the following are typical UK prices charged to the National Health Service in 2004. The average 28-day cost of prescribing carbamazepine, phenytoin and valproate is between £2 and £12 (£9 and £15 for the controlled release formulations). The comparable costs of the newer drugs are: gabapentin 1800 mg, £82; lamotrigine 300 mg, £102; levetiracetam 2 g, £88; oxcarbazepine 900 mg, £34; tiagabine 30 mg, £76; topiramate 200 mg, £63; and vigabatrin 2 g, £50.

## Choice of drug for primary generalized tonic–clonic seizures

These seizures occur in various subcategories of idiopathic generalized epilepsy and are also the form of seizure in metabolic or drug-induced acute symptomatic seizures. Any of the drugs listed above for the treatment of secondarily generalized seizures can be used. There is a strong clinical suspicion, often voiced, that valproate is a better choice than carbamazepine for first-line therapy in this situation. Although this opinion is shared by a Cochrane review, there is in fact little if any conclusive evidence to support this proposition, and indeed most well-conducted studies show little difference in efficacy between any of the major antiepileptic drugs. However, on the basis that myoclonus and/or absence seizures often co-exist with tonic–clonic seizures in idiopathic generalized epilepsy, and as phenytoin and carbamazepine can worsen myoclonus or absence seizures, it seems reasonable to start therapy with drugs that have broad-spectrum effectiveness. Where valproate fails, however, any of the conventional antiepileptics can be tried. Among the newer drugs, lamotrigine, topiramate and levetiracetam have antiepileptic activity in primary generalized seizures.

## Choice of drug for typical absence seizures

Typical absence seizures ('petit mal' seizures) occur only in the syndrome of idiopathic generalized epilepsy. The traditional first-line treatment is with either ethosuximide or valproate. For many years ethosuximide has been standard drug therapy and it is highly effective and in general well tolerated. However, it is relatively ineffective in controlling generalized tonic–clonic seizures, which often co-exist with absence seizures, and has a number of troublesome adverse effects (p. 131). It has therefore been largely superseded by valproate as first-line therapy in drug-naïve patients. However, it still has a role, particularly in children where there is anxiety about the idiosyncratic effects of valproate. Valproate or ethosuximide can be expected to fully control absence seizures in over 90% of patients on initial therapy. Dosage should be titrated against response.

In patients in whom valproate is inappropriate, alternatives include phenobarbital and the benzodiazepine drugs. The newer drugs lamotrigine and topiramate have both shown clear evidence of effectiveness in absence epilepsy, and lamotrigine is occasionally used as first-line monotherapy. There is growing anecdotal evidence that levetiracetam is also effective in absence epilepsy. Currently this is an off-label indication, but if its promise is confirmed, levetiracetam may become a drug of first choice.

About 10–20% of absence seizures will be resistant to monotherapy with either valproate or ethosuximide, and the combination of both drugs may be helpful.

## Choice of drug for myoclonic seizures

Myoclonus is defined as a sudden brief involuntary muscle contraction arising from neuronal activity in the central nervous system. It can be non-epileptic in origin, arising from subcortical, brainstem or even spinal cord structures. Cortical myoclonus is a form of epilepsy, and this seizure type occurs in a variety of diverse clinical settings (Table 2.14). The effects of the seizures, the response to therapy and the outcome will vary in these different settings, but the principles of therapy are similar for all the myoclonic epilepsies. The myoclonus in idiopathic generalized epilepsy is generally well controlled on single drug therapy, whereas the myoclonus in the symptomatic generalized epilepsy, progressive myoclonic epilepsy or in the focal epilepsies are more difficult to treat, and drug combinations may be necessary.

The drug of first choice in all forms of generalized myoclonic epilepsy is valproate, which can be strikingly effective. Where valproate is not appropriate, alternative therapies include lamotrigine, phenobarbital, clobazam or

**Table 2.14** Epilepsies with myoclonus as part of the phenotype.

- Idiopathic generalized epilepsies (IGE)
- Benign myoclonic epilepsy syndromes
- Severe myoclonic epilepsy syndromes of childhood
- Symptomatic epilepsies with generalized myoclonus (especially due to metabolic disease (inherited and acquired), infections, drugs, toxins, poisoning)
- Partial epilepsies with focal myoclonus (occipital lobe and fronto-central epilepsy)
- Progressive myoclonic epilepsies (PME)

clonazepam, levetiracetam, topiramate, felbamate, zonisamide and piracetam.

Lamotrigine has a variable effect in myoclonus but can be tried especially in myoclonus in IGE and in focal epilepsy. Levetiracetam has not been subjected to controlled clinical trials and myoclonus is currently an unlicensed indication, but its excellent effect in myoclonus is clearly evident in routine clinical practice. Topiramate and felbamate are newer drugs for which there is anecdotal evidence of good antimyoclonic action at least in some patients. Zonisamide is also used as second-line therapy for intractable myoclonus, and can occasionally have a striking effect.

More complex myoclonic epilepsy can be treated with piracetam. This extraordinary compound is the only drug uniquely effective in myoclonus and that has no effect in other types of epilepsy. The doses required for myoclonus are extremely high, but the drug is very well tolerated. It is primarily effective in cortical myoclonus, but may also have some value in other myoclonic syndromes.

### Therapies for specific myoclonic syndromes

Specific therapy has been attempted in a number of the progressive myoclonic epilepsies, although none has an uncontested place in treatment regimens. Antioxidant treatments have been used for some years in the treatment of ceroid lipofuscinosis. N-acetylcystein has some advocates in Unverricht–Lundborg disease. Although often prescribed, it is doubtful whether these compounds have any major beneficial effect, and early claims have now been retracted. Alcohol has a beneficial effect on the myoclonus in Unverricht–Lundborg disease, as indeed it does in some forms of subcortical myoclonus.

### Drugs that aggravate myoclonus

The antiepileptic drugs vigabatrin and gabapentin frequently aggravate myoclonus and can indeed precipitate myoclonus for the first time in susceptible patients with other types of seizure. Phenytoin has been reported to worsen the myoclonus in Lafora body disease, although the evidence is not conclusive. Both carbamazepine and phenytoin can aggravate myoclonus in juvenile myoclonic epilepsy.

### Focal myoclonus

Focal myoclonus can be treated with any drug used for focal epilepsy. The treatment of epilepsia partialis continua can be fruitless and difficult, and this is discussed further on p. 222. Surgical therapy is sometimes effective for focal myoclonus due to focal cortical lesions, including focal cortical dysplasia and Rasmussen's encephalitis.

## Choice of drugs for atypical absence, atonic and tonic seizures

These seizure types occur largely in the context of the Lennox–Gastaut syndrome or the other severe epileptic encephalopathies. The drug treatment is essentially similar for each, although it is usually not possible to obtain full control of seizures.

### Drugs of choice

Valproate or lamotrigine are recommended by most as first-choice drugs. Traditional alternatives are the benzodiazepine drugs (e.g. clobazam or clonazepam), acetazolamide, phenobarbital or primidone. Phenytoin may be useful for tonic seizures, but may exacerbate atonic seizures.

Topiramate (target maintenance dose 6 mg/kg/day) has been shown to be effective in many open and controlled studies and zonisamide has been shown to be effective in all these seizure types. Felbamate also has a powerful effect in atypical absence, tonic and atonic seizures, and the drug still has a useful place in refractory cases where other medication has failed. Anecdotal experience with levetiracetam suggests that the drug has great promise in these types of epilepsy, but it has not yet been formally assessed.

### Drugs that exacerbate seizures

Carbamazepine and oxcarbazepine are frequently reported to exacerbate atypical absence and tonic seizures. Tiagabine can greatly worsen atypical absence seizures, sometimes resulting in non-convulsive status. It is likely that gabapentin and vigabatrin have similar effects. Benzodiazepine can exacerbate tonic seizures, and occasionally precipitate tonic status epilepticus.

## TREATMENT OF SPECIFIC EPILEPSY SYNDROMES

There are some specific aspects of therapy of some epilepsy syndromes, which can be considered here.

### Neonatal seizures

If the seizures are considered non-epileptic, antiepileptic drug treatment is not indicated. Indeed, medication may worsen the phenomenon by decreasing the level of cortical inhibition over subcortical structures. Whether genuine (cortical) but slight (subtle) epileptic seizures require treatment is uncertain, especially in infants who are not paralysed for artificial ventilation. Not uncommonly such seizure manifestations remit spontaneously after days or weeks and the usefulness of treatment in these situations is difficult to assess. Opinions vary about the need to treat infants with EEG evidence of seizure activity without overt clinical signs. There is also disagreement about the duration of therapy, although most would aim for as short a period as possible. Many neonatal seizures are self-limiting and overlong treatment carries its own risks.

For all other neonatal seizures, however, treatment is urgent. Management demands meticulous specialized paediatric care, usually on an intensive care unit. EEG monitoring is desirable and artificial ventilation often required; such critically ill infants should not be treated in non-specialist settings. The treatment should be directed primarily at the causal disorder where this is possible, and immediate investigation is required to ascertain the cause. Hypoglycaemia requires immediate correction with 2–4 ml/kg of a 20–30% solution of glucose intravenously. Hypocalcaemia requires the slow intravenous injection of 2.5–5% calcium gluconate with ECG monitoring. Hypomagnesaemia requires 2–8 ml of a 2–3% solution of magnesium sulphate intravenously, or 0.2 ml/kg of a 50% solution intramuscularly. Pyridoxine deficiency, although rare, responds dramatically to 50–200 mg pyridoxine. Infections, other metabolic disorders (e.g. hyperammonaemia, organic aciduria) and mass lesions require specific therapy.

Emergency antiepileptic drugs are indicated for all but isolated seizures. Traditional practice is to load the infant with either phenobarbital or phenytoin. Phenobarbital is given to obtain a blood level of 20 mg/ml, which requires a loading dose of 20 mg/kg followed by a maintenance dose of 3–4 mg/kg/day IV or IM. Phenytoin is a second-line drug, with a loading dose of 15–20 mg/kg administered intravenously at a rate not exceeding 1–2 mg/kg/min, and with a maintenance dose of 3–10 mg/kg/day to obtain a plasma level of between 15 and 20 mg/ml. It is mandatory to monitor blood levels in the first 2–3 weeks of life because of abrupt changes in half-lives of the drugs. Others tend to postpone the use of these long-acting antiepileptics until the diagnosis is clarified and/or after shorter-acting agents such as diazepam, lorazepam or clonazepam have failed. The shorter acting drugs are given for 24–48 hours and then withdrawn.

### Febrile seizures

The clinical features of febrile seizures are considered on p. 21, and genetic counselling on p. 112.

#### Emergency antiepileptic treatment

Prevention of prolonged seizures is the aim of therapy. Ninety per cent of seizures are self-limiting, but if a seizure continues for 5–10 minutes emergency therapy is needed. The standard treatment is the administration of diazepam solution at a dose of 0.5–1 mg/kg either by IV injection (at a rate not exceeding 2 mg/min) or, as is common in out-of-hospital settings, by rectal instillation. A convenient ready-made proprietary preparation for rectal instillation exists (Stesolid®). If there is no rapid effect, the same dose should be repeated. In an out-of-hospital setting, a maximum of two doses can be given. Diazepam should not be given by IM injection or via rectal suppositories as absorption by either method is too slow. Alternatives to diazepam in the out-of-hospital setting include IM or buccal midazolam 0.1–0.2 mg/kg.

In a hospital setting diazepam is given intravenously at 0.2–0.5 mg/kg up to a total (rectal plus intravenous dose) of 2–3 mg/kg over 30 minutes. A total dose of 20–30 mg diazepam is often required, but higher doses are usually not helpful. An alternative is lorazepam 0.05–0.1 mg/kg. It is rare for these measures not to terminate seizures, but if there is no rapid response an emergency infusion of phenobarbital can be initiated at a dose of 20 mg/kg at a rate no faster than 100 mg/min (with full ITU care).

Opinions differ about the value of cooling, but it is often recommended that the child should be cooled immediately using, for instance, cold water, cold flannels, tepid sponging, and removing clothes and bedcovers.

### Emergency prophylactic treatment

In susceptible children, prophylactic diazepam can be given rectally or orally as soon as a fever develops. Suitable twice or thrice daily doses, during the episode of fever, are 0.3–0.5 mg/kg rectally or 5 mg orally for children under 3 years of age and 7.5 mg orally for those over 3 year of age. Intranasal or buccal midazolam (0.2 mg/kg) are alternatives. Measures to lower temperature, including tepid sponging, removal of clothing and the administration of paracetamol, should also be taken to prevent a seizure. Unfortunately, as the seizure occurs before the fever is apparent in at least one-third of cases, prophylaxis is often not feasible.

Measures should also be taken to treat the underlying cause. Blood and urine culture and full haematological and biochemical screening tests should be carried out. CSF examination should be carried out whenever there is a suspicion of meningitis, in all children less than 18 months old at the time of presentation of the first seizure, and in any child with meningism. CT scanning should be performed before lumbar puncture in children with focal deficit after a prolonged convulsion or who do not recover consciousness. Serological and other investigations depend on clinical circumstances and it is difficult to provide general rules. Antibiotic therapy should be given as appropriate.

### Long-term prophylaxis

In the past, antiepileptics were commonly given for long-term prophylaxis in children with a liability to recurrent febrile seizures. However, with increasing concern about the risks to learning and development, long-term therapy is increasingly reserved for a very small number of children who are at a particularly high risk of frequent or complex febrile seizures. Typically, treatment is now given only to infants under the age of 1 year who have had episodes lasting 30 minutes or more, or who have had multiple seizures. The antiepileptic drugs used are either phenobarbital 15 mg/kg/day or valproate 20–40 mg/kg/day in two divided doses.

### Parental counselling

The occurrence of a febrile seizure is a profoundly distressing experience, and almost all parents at the time of a first febrile seizure think that the child is about to die. Parents should be reassured that the risk of brain damage is extremely small, that febrile seizures are common and harmless and are a presage of epilepsy in only a small percentage of cases. Information about the management of subsequent seizures should be given. The parents should be instructed in staying calm, placing the child on his/her side, not forcing anything between the teeth, and where appropriate administering emergency rectal (or intranasal/buccal) therapy. Parents should be instructed to call the emergency services if a seizure lasts more than 5 minutes, and the child should be brought immediately to the nearest medical facility.

## West syndrome

Infantile spasms are among the most serious and resistant of epilepsy syndromes, but opinions about management vary. Adrenocorticotropic hormone (ACTH) is usually the preferred first-line therapy in the USA and Japan. Vigabatrin is usually given first in most European countries and in Asia and Canada. In other countries steroids are only prescribed as second-line therapy after pyridoxine or high-dose valproate.

### ACTH and corticosteroid therapy

ACTH and corticosteroids have for many years been considered the standard therapy, in spite of limited controlled data and serious risks of medium-term toxicity. ACTH is usually preferred to oral corticosteroids. The usual initial recommended daily dose of ACTH is 40 IU (3–6 IU/kg), given for between 1 and 5 months. If seizures relapse either on therapy or after withdrawal, the ACTH should be recommenced immediately and doses of 60–80 IU may be needed. The incidence of adverse events is very high and almost all children develop cushingoid symptoms. Other common adverse effects include infections, increased arterial blood pressure, gastritis and hyperexcitability.

Oral steroids are less extensively prescribed, although they seem to be better tolerated than ACTH. In a prospective, randomized, blinded study, the efficacy of prednisone (2 mg/kg/day) was inferior to that of high-dose ACTH

(150 IU/day) given for 2 weeks, but no differences were found when ACTH was administered at lower doses. Spasms are immediately controlled in about 60% of children with spasms following therapy with ACTH or corticosteroids, but there is a relapse rate of about 20%. Uncontrolled evidence suggests that intellectual outcome in survivors is better with ACTH than oral corticosteroids.

### Vigabatrin

Vigabatrin is established as the drug of first choice for the treatment of infantile spasms in tuberous sclerosis. In this indication, controlled studies have demonstrated that vigabatrin (100–150 mg/kg/day) is both more efficacious and less toxic than steroid therapy. Vigabatrin therapy seems also to be associated with a better outcome in terms of intellectual function. However, in other aetiologies, there is much less consensus about the relative roles of ACTH and vigabatrin. There are no long-term data about the toxicity of vigabatrin, and no data on the effects on visual or intellectual function (there is no reliable method of visual field testing in children under the age of 6 years).

### Other drug therapies

The value of antiepileptic therapy in West syndrome is difficult to assess, but most conventional antiepileptic drugs are relatively ineffective. Valproate and clonazepam control 25–30% of cases, but relapse rates are high. Carbamazepine can worsen the spasms. Topiramate, lamotrigine, felbamate, and zonisamide have all been reported to help in small open-case series. Nitrazepam has been used but carries life-threatening side-effects. High-dose pyridoxine is often given and there are promising reports about IV immunoglobulin. The ketogenic diet and thyrotropin-releasing hormone have been reported to be occasionally helpful in refractory cases.

### Recommended treatment schedule

Chiron recommends the following treatment schedule. Initial therapy should be with vigabatrin 100 mg/kg/day for 1 week. If there is an incomplete response, the dose should be increased to 150 mg/kg/day. If there is still an incomplete response, hydrocortisone 15 mg/kg/day is added to 100 mg/kg/day vigabatrin for 2 weeks. If there is still an incomplete response, hydrocortisone should be replaced by ACTH. The duration of vigabatrin treatment in controlled patients should be determined by the balance between the risk of visual field defects and the risk of relapse of seizures. The persistence of EEG multifocal spikes is the best predictor of relapse of spasms, particularly in infants and in the case of cerebral lesions. It is therefore reasonable to stop vigabatrin monotherapy at around 2 years of age if the EEG is normal. Urgent treatment of the underlying cause is required where this is possible.

In the few cases of infantile spasms in which PET scanning shows clear-cut focal abnormalities, surgical resection can be performed with complete abolition of the spasm. The longer-term effects on neurological function of large surgical resection have not been fully established. Equally it is not clear to what extent cognitive development is affected by such radical treatment.

### Lennox–Gastaut syndrome

The clinical features of the Lennox–Gastaut syndrome are described on p. 24. It is a severe encephalopathy in which seizures are notoriously resistant to therapy. Complete control of seizures is rare, and almost all patients require polytherapy. A balance has to be drawn between optimum control of seizures and side-effects, a compromise often difficult to achieve. It is important to resist the tendency—in the face of severe epilepsy—to escalate treatment. Such an escalation is seldom effective, and high-dose polypharmacy may cause drowsiness, which is a potent activator of the atypical absence and tonic seizures and non-convulsive status epilepticus. In addition to control of seizures, some authorities recommend therapy to try to ameliorate inter-ictal EEG disturbances, on the basis that this may improve cognition and responsiveness. To what extent this is a valid approach is unclear.

Valproate remains the drug that is usually given initially, as it has broad-spectrum activity against all the seizure types experienced in the syndrome (notably tonic, atonic, atypical absence, myoclonic, tonic–clonic seizures, and status epilepticus). The drug has been reported to control seizures completely in 10% of cases, but this seems optimistic. It should be prescribed with caution in patients below 3 years of age in view of the risk of hepatic failure (p. 187).

Lamotrigine is an alternative initial therapy. In one double-blind randomized study of 169 patients, lamotrigine reduced the frequency of all major seizures from a weekly median of 16.4 at baseline to 9.9, and 33% of patients experienced at least a 50% reduction in seizures. It seems particularly effective in preventing falls. Lamotrigine has also been shown to improve cognition and quality of life ratings in the syndrome. Caution needs to be exercised, particularly when used in combination with valproate, in view of the risk of severe hypersensitivity reactions (see p. 139).

The benzodiazepine drugs are frequently used in Lennox–Gastaut syndrome in combination with other first-line agents. Clobazam, clonazepam and nitrazepam are all widely prescribed. Clobazam probably confers less drowsiness than clonazepam and is often combined with valproate. Small doses of nitrazepam can be helpful. Benzodiazepines can exacerbate tonic seizures.

Topiramate (at a target maintenance dosage of 6 mg/kg/day) was shown in a double-blind placebo-controlled trial to result in at least a 50% reduction in the frequency of seizures in 33% of patients, with a median reduction in the frequency of drop attacks of 14.8%. In the open-label extension (with a mean topiramate dosage of 10 mg/kg/day) there was a reduction in drop attacks of at least 50% in 55%

of the patients, and 15% of the patients had no drop attacks for at least 6 months.

Felbamate has a powerful effect in the Lennox–Gastaut syndrome. In a double-blind placebo-controlled study of 73 patients, felbamate therapy resulted in a 34% decrease in the frequency of atonic seizures and a 19% decrease in the frequency of all seizures. Quality of life was improved and the improvement was maintained for at least 12 months in subsequent open-label follow-up studies. However, severe hypersensitivity reactions (p. 205) now limit its use to patients not responding to other appropriate medication.

Zonisamide has a broad spectrum of antiepileptic activity, and was reported to reduce seizure frequency by 50% or more in 32% of 132 patients reported in open-label studies from Japan.

Phenytoin and carbamazepine are generally of little benefit in Lennox–Gastaut syndrome, and carbamazepine particularly can exacerbate atypical absence and myoclonic seizures. Barbiturates carry the potential for worsening hyperactivity and behavioural disorders and their sedative effects can exacerbate atypical absence and tonic seizures. Vigabatrin shows some effect in the Lennox–Gastaut syndrome but often exacerbates myoclonic seizures, as can gabapentin and tiagabine. The latter drug particularly has a propensity to induce non-convulsive status in some patients.

Other adjunctive treatments have been tried, in small studies, with very limited success. These include imipramine, amantadine, bromide, allopurinol and flunarizine. ACTH at doses of 30–40 IU/day is reported to be effective if started early but is now seldom used. Steroids can also be given in short courses to tide a patient over a bad patch. The ketogenic diet is often assumed to be an effective non-pharmacological treatment but evidence for its efficacy in the Lennox–Gastaut syndrome is in fact contradictory.

In small open studies, vagal nerve stimulation is reported to result in seizure-reduction rates of between 34 and 60% compared with baseline. Surgical therapy has included unilateral cortical resection and corpus callosectomy, which can reduce the incidence of drop attacks and tonic seizures. The underlying cause should be treated where possible (often it is not).

## Landau–Kleffner syndrome and ESES

The clinical feature of these conditions are considered on p. 25. In the Landau–Kleffner syndrome control of seizures is often possible with rather modest antiepileptic treatment. However, the EEG abnormalities may not disappear and the aphasia may not improve. If one accepts that the speech disturbance was caused by the EEG disturbance, then aggressive antiepileptic therapy to suppress the EEG disturbance is a logical approach even in the absence of overt seizures. All antiepileptic drugs have been tried in the syndrome, although vigabatrin and carbamazepine may worsen the EEG abnormalities and are therefore sometimes avoided. ACTH or high-dose corticosteroids are also commonly given for periods of several months. The relative benefits of these approaches are unclear, and no controlled trials have been carried out to assess them. Assessment of any therapy is made difficult by the fluctuating course of this curious condition. A fashion for surgical treatment using the technique of multiple subpial transection has also arisen, although results are very variable and even if there is improvement, it may be months or years after the operation. It seems quite unclear, to this author at least, whether the operation ever improves the long-term prognosis. All this is unsatisfactory, but until a better understanding of the underlying pathophysiology and of the prognostic determinants is gained, therapy can only be empirical.

The EEG pattern of ESES does not generally require specific treatment. Indeed, it is often not possible to abolish the spike-wave by oral antiepileptic therapy. If treatment is decided upon, ethosuximide, benzodiazepine drugs, ACTH, and corticosteroids as well as other conventional antiepileptic drugs (phenytoin, phenobarbital and valproate) have been used.

## Benign partial epilepsy syndromes of childhood

There are a variety of 'syndromes' of partial epilepsy at various stages of childhood which have an excellent prognosis. The clinical features of these conditions are considered on p. 20 and genetic counselling on p. 112.

### Benign epilepsy with centro-temporal spikes (BECTS)

In this common childhood epilepsy syndrome (p. 20), therapy is gratifyingly straightforward and indeed drug treatment is not necessary in all cases. If attacks are infrequent or mild, regular therapy seems inappropriate, especially as some children have only a few attacks before the epilepsy remits. Tonic–clonic seizures carry greater risks than the partial attacks and may tip the balance towards therapy. The partial seizures, when frightening and distressing, can warrant treatment, even if they are infrequent. If treatment is decided upon, over-medication and polypharmacy should be avoided. Both carbamazepine and valproate are highly effective, often at low doses. EEG disturbances in patients without seizures —a very common occurrence—do not require any treatment. Withdrawal of medication should be considered after 1–2 years free of attacks even if the EEG has not normalized.

### Other benign partial syndromes

The principles of treatment are similar to those for benign epilepsy with centro-temporal spikes. Where seizures are infrequent, treatment may not be necessary. Valproate may be the drug of choice before carbamazepine, and one has a strong clinical impression that the drug is particularly effective in seizures with occipital foci. Clobazam can be used in seizure clusters.

## Idiopathic generalized epilepsies (IGE)

The clinical features of this common and important syndrome (also known as primary generalized epilepsy) are described on pp. 18–20, and genetic counselling on pp. 17–18. The seizure types occurring in this condition are tonic–clonic, absence, and myoclonic seizures. On drug therapy, complete control of seizures can be expected in at least two-thirds of patients with generalized tonic–clonic seizures alone or in combination with absence or myoclonic attacks.

### Treatment of different seizure types in idiopathic generalized epilepsy

Treatment varies to some extent with the type of seizure, but some broad-spectrum drugs are available that treat all types.

### *Generalized tonic–clonic seizures in idiopathic generalized epilepsy*

As most antiepileptic clinical trials have been seizure- rather than syndrome-orientated, it is at present unclear whether the generalized tonic–clonic seizures of idiopathic generalized epilepsy respond to a different antiepileptic drug profile than the generalized tonic–clonic seizures in other types of epilepsy. The drugs most traditionally used include valproate, carbamazepine, phenytoin and phenobarbital. There is a clinical suspicion, held by many, that valproate is more effective in idiopathic generalized epilepsy than in other types, although there is little hard evidence from clinical trials to support this.

These seizures occur predominantly shortly after waking, when drowsy or while asleep, and the timing of some antiepileptic drug therapy can be varied to account for this. Sometimes avoiding sudden waking can prevent tonic–clonic seizures. Waking slowly, and drifting from sleep to wakefulness in a gradual fashion, can be very helpful. Sometimes tonic–clonic seizures occur after a prodromal period of increasing myoclonus. If this prodrome is long enough ($\geq$ 30 minutes) emergency clobazam or midazolam can prevent the seizure occurring. The use of prophylactic clobazam or lorazepam at other times of risk (e.g. after a late night, alcohol, fatigue or stress) can be useful.

Among the newer drugs lamotrigine, topiramate and zonisamide have proven efficacy in idiopathic generalized epilepsy. Uncontrolled studies of levetiracetam suggest that this may also be highly efficacious against tonic–clonic, absence and myoclonic seizures.

### *Absence seizures in idiopathic generalized epilepsy*

The absence seizures in idiopathic generalized epilepsy are usually well controlled on monotherapy with valproate, ethosuximide or lamotrigine. These are commonly used drugs of first choice and the benzodiazepines, phenobarbital and topiramate reserved for more resistant cases. The dosage required to obtain full control is usually only moderate.

### *Myoclonic seizures in idiopathic generalized epilepsy*

The myoclonic seizures in idiopathic generalized epilepsy are usually treated first with valproate. Alternative therapies of proven efficacy include topiramate, lamotrigine and benzodiazepine drugs (e.g. clobazam, clonazepam). Anecdotal experience with levetiracetam suggests a strong antimyoclonic effect, and with more experience the drug may turn out to be an alternative first-line therapy.

### Drugs that may exacerbate seizures in idiopathic generalized epilepsy

Vigabatrin and tiagabine can exacerbate primarily generalized tonic–clonic seizures, and have no role in the therapy of idiopathic generalized epilepsy. Gabapentin should also be avoided as it has little effect in generalized tonic–clonic seizures. Vigabatrin, tiagabine, gabapentin, carbamazepine and oxcarbazepine can also exacerbate absence and myoclonus.

### Other subcategories of idiopathic generalized epilepsy

The same principles apply to the various proposed subcategories of idiopathic generalized epilepsy, depending on the balance of seizure types. Eyelid myoclonia can be considered a type of myoclonus, and the syndromes with this as a predominant sign are treated in the same way as other myoclonic epilepsies (albeit with distinctive prognoses—see pp. 17–19).

### Lifestyle measures

Lifestyle manipulation can be very helpful in many cases of idiopathic generalized epilepsy, especially in adolescence. The avoidance of sleep deprivation, sleeping late after a late night, and excessive alcohol intake can be very beneficial. Many patients learn to recognize dangerous times, and take individual avoidance measures. Alternative or complementary medicine can be a useful adjunct to therapy (see pp. 110–12). Photosensitive patients should be counselled to avoid relevant stimuli (see p. 56). Occasionally, patients with established mild epilepsy can avoid drug treatment altogether with these simple measures. Patients with juvenile myoclonic epilepsy typically also have psychosocial problems which have been attributed to an 'unstable personality' (although this is unfair to most such patients) and in one series psychiatric difficulties were found in 14%. These should be addressed.

## PRINCIPLES OF TREATMENT OF NEWLY DIAGNOSED PATIENTS

The decision to initiate drug therapy has important implications for every person with epilepsy. In addition to its biological effects, therapy confers illness status, confirms the state of 'being epileptic', and can affect self-esteem, social relationships, education and employment. The decision to treat depends essentially on a balance between the benefits and drawbacks of therapy, and should be tailored to the requirements of the individual patient; there are no absolute rules (Table 2.15).

The balance is difficult to define. The benefits of therapy include the lower risk of recurrence of seizures, and thus of potential injury and even death, and the psychological and social benefits of more security from seizures. The drawbacks of therapy include the potential drug side-effects, the psychological and social effects, the cost, and the inconvenience. Chronic, long-term or subtle side-effects are not easily detected, and weigh heavily on the decision to treat. One example is the potential adverse effect on learning in children, and partly because of this paediatricians initiate therapy less early than neurologists treating adults.

Practice varies in different countries. In the USA, for instance, a higher proportion of patients are treated after a single seizure than in the UK and more often too by emergency loading therapy. Practice is also divided in Europe. The lack of consensus reflects more the differing social rather than medical contexts of therapy.

One proposition recently researched is that early effective therapy will improve long-term outcome, and thus that early antiepileptic drug therapy will prevent the establishment of chronic epilepsy. There is a striking lack of clear evidence to support this canard, and there seems to be no reason currently to modify the traditional approach.

## Factors influencing the decision to treat
### Diagnosis

It is essential generally to establish a firm diagnosis of epilepsy before therapy is started. This is not always easy, particularly in the early stages of epilepsy. There is almost no place at all for a 'trial of treatment' to clarify the diagnosis, as it seldom does. Rarely should treatment be started before a diagnosis is confirmed.

A good first-hand witnessed account is essential, as diagnostic tests are often non-confirmatory. In practice, the misdiagnosis rate is quite high. About 20% of all patients referred to a tertiary level epilepsy service, for instance, have psychogenic attacks. The diagnosis is also often delayed. In one study, in over one-third of patients,

**Table 2.15** Criteria that should be satisfied before initiating drug therapy.

- Risk of seizure recurrence should be sufficient
- Seizures must be sufficiently troublesome (this depends on seizure type, severity, frequency, timing and precipitation)
- Adequate compliance should be likely
- Patient has been fully counselled
- Patient's wishes have been taken account of fully

a firm diagnosis could be made only after 24 months after the onset of seizures.

### The risk of recurrence of seizures

The estimation of the risk of recurrence of seizures is obviously a key factor in deciding whether or not to initiate therapy. Most studied has been the risk of recurrence after a first isolated attack (i.e. the risk of a second seizure). Investigations have produced conflicting findings, largely owing to methodological issues, but most would now accept that between about 50 and 80% of all patients who have a first non-febrile seizure will have further attacks. The risk of recurrence is high initially and then falls over time. In a national UK study, the risk after the first seizure was 44% in the initial 6 months, 32% in the next 6 months, and 17% in the second year (Figure 2.4). It follows theefore that the greater the elapsed time since the first attack, the less likely is subsequent recurrence.

In many cases, by the time of presentation seizures will have already recurred. In a hospital-based study from the UK, the median number of tonic–clonic seizures occurring before the diagnosis was made was 4 (range 1–36) and the median number of partial seizures was 6 (range 1–180). If more than one spontaneous seizure has occurred, the risk of further attacks in the future without treatment is, in most clinical circumstances, over 80%, and generally speaking the more seizures that have occurred before therapy, the greater the risk of further attacks.

The risk of recurrence is influenced by the following factors.

### Aetiology

This is a most important factor. The risk is greater in those with structural cerebral disease, and least in acute symptomatic seizures provoked by metabolic factors or exposure to drugs or toxins. The risk of recurrence of idiopathic or cryptogenic seizures is approximately 50%, and lower after acute symptomatic (provoked) seizures, providing the provoking factor is removed. In those with pre-existing learning disability or cerebral damage, the risk approaches 100% (Figure 2.5).

### EEG

Informed opinion concerning the prognostic value of EEG is conflicting. While there is consensus that the risk of recurrence is high if the first EEG shows spike and wave discharges, the value of a normal EEG or an EEG with other types of abnormality after a single seizure—if there is any value at all—is slight.

### Age

The risk of recurrence is somewhat greater in those under the age of 16 or over the age of 60 years, probably because of the confounding effect of aetiology.

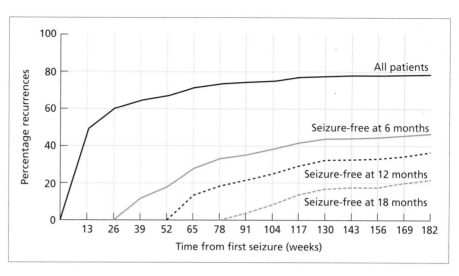

**Fig. 2.4** National General Practice Study of Epilepsy (NGPSE): actuarial percentage of recurrence after first seizure. A study of 564 patients followed prospectively from the time of diagnosis. Within 3 years of the first seizure, 78% of patients had a recurrence of their attacks. If attacks had not recurred within 6, 12 or 18 months, the chance of recurrence was substantially reduced, falling to 44, 32 and 17%, respectively.

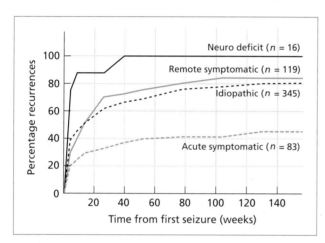

**Fig. 2.5** Actuarial percentage recurrences after first seizure by aetiological category.

### Seizure type and syndrome

Partial seizures are more likely to recur than generalized seizures, again because of the confounding effect of aetiology. In most of the childhood epilepsy syndromes, recurrent seizures are almost inevitable. The exceptions are the benign partial syndromes. Many patients with BECTS (p. 20) have a few seizures only, and patients with benign occipital lobe epilepsies (p. 21) often have a single attack only.

### The type, timing and frequency of seizures

Some types of epileptic seizure have a minimal impact on the quality of life; for example, simple partial seizures, absence or sleep attacks. The benefits of treating such seizures, even if they are happening frequently, can be outweighed by the disadvantages. If the baseline frequency of seizures is very low, the disadvantages of treatment can be unacceptably high. It would be unusual to treat a person

having less than one seizure per year, especially if this was confined to sleep, or it was a minor or partial seizure.

### Compliance

Antiepileptic drugs need to be taken reliably and regularly to be effective, and to avoid adverse events or withdrawal seizures. The decision to treat should be reconsidered in all circumstances in which compliance is likely to be poor (see Table 2.21).

### Reflex seizures and acute symptomatic seizures

Occasionally, seizures occur only in specific circumstances or with certain precipitants (e.g. photosensitivity, fatigue or alcohol). Avoiding these circumstances may obviate the need for drug treatment.

### The risks of mortality and morbidity in early epilepsy

The mortality rate of epilepsy in the early years after diagnosis is 2–3 times that in the general population. The excess mortality is due almost entirely to the underlying cause of the seizures (e.g. stroke, tumour) and risks due to other causes are slight. SUDEP, however, can occur in early epilepsy, and rarely indeed in the first seizure. Opinion is divided about whether a patient should be counselled about this risk on the first consultation—this will depend on clinical circumstances. Certainly, though, SUDEP should be discussed with most patients at some point early after diagnosis, and particularly if therapy is to be withheld. Accidental injury and the psychosocial and psychiatric morbidity of epilepsy are outlined on pp. 61–3.

### The risks of antiepileptic drug treatment

The benefits of treatment need to be balanced against the risk of adverse effects from the antiepileptic drugs (see pp. 63–8).

## The patient's wishes

This factor overrides all others. The role of the physician is to explain the relative advantages and disadvantages of therapy; the final decision must be left to the patient. Individuals differ greatly in their views about epilepsy and its treatment. For some, for instance, seizure control is paramount—for instance for driving or employment. Others have concerns about the concept of long-term medication or specific side-effects and would prefer to risk an occasional seizure, particularly if their attacks do not inconvenience them unduly.

The physician must explain the purpose and limitations of antiepileptic drugs. The points covered should include: the likelihood of success of therapy; the suppressant rather than curative role of therapy; the potential side-effects; the potential risks of withholding therapy; guidance in the event of idiosyncratic reactions; the need for regular medication; the importance of regular drug taking; guidance when a dose is missed; and the likely duration of therapy.

## A protocol for treatment in drug-naïve patients

It will be clear that there can be no absolute rules about when to start therapy and when not to do so. In general terms, if there is a risk of recurrence of convulsive seizures or seizures with risk of injury or death, treatment will be indicated. In other circumstances, however, the requirement to initiate therapy can be quite individual. Where seizures are infrequent and minor, where non-convulsive seizures occur exclusively at night, or in the benign syndromes of childhood epilepsy, treatment is often not indicated at all even in established cases. To reiterate, in all situations, the patient should be given advice based on the best available data and be allowed to make the final decision.

A protocol for the initial treatment of newly diagnosed patients is as follows (summarized in Table 2.16; the usual initial and maintenance doses and maximal incremental/decremental rates in routine practice are shown in Table 2.17).

1 Establish the diagnosis—there is little place for a 'trial of treatment'. Investigation will usually involve EEG, neuro-imaging, and other investigations as necessary. Neuro-imaging should be with magnetic resonance scanning in all patients with partial-onset epilepsy, patients with fixed neurological deficit, onset of seizures in the first year of life or after the age of 15 without good explanation.

2 Identify and counsel about precipitating factors—if these can be avoided, this occasionally obviates the need for drug therapy.

3 Decide upon the need for antiepileptic drug therapy. If therapy is needed, baseline biochemical and haematological parameters should be measured.

**Table 2.16** Principles of antiepileptic drug prescribing in patients with newly diagnosed epilepsy.

- Aim for complete control without adverse effects
- Diagnosis of epileptic seizures should be unequivocal
- Seizure type, syndrome and aetiology should be established
- Baseline haematological and biochemical investigations should be performed prior to initiation of drug therapy
- Use one drug at a time (monotherapy) at least initially
- Initial titration should be to low maintenance doses
- Further upward titration will depend on response and side-effects
- If first drug fails, alternative monotherapies should be tried
- Upward and downward titration should be in slow-stepped doses
- Polytherapy should be used only if monotherapy with at least the first three drugs chosen has failed to control seizures
- Patients should be fully counselled about goals, role, risk, outcome and logistics of drug treatment

4 Counsel about the topics listed in Table 2.18. Patients should be given clear instructions to seek immediate medical attention if signs of hypersensitivity or idiosyncratic drug reactions develop.

5 Start monotherapy with the chosen first-choice drug, initially at low doses, and titrating up slowly to a low maintenance dose (see Table 2.17). Emergency drug loading is seldom necessary except where status epilepticus threatens.

6 If seizures continue, titrate the dose upwards to higher maintenance dose levels (guided, where appropriate, by serum level monitoring).

*In about 60–90% of patients, these simple steps for initial therapy will result in complete control of seizures. In remaining patients:*

7 Alternative monotherapy should be tried with another appropriate first-choice antiepileptic drug. The second drug should be introduced incrementally at suitable dose intervals, and the first drug then withdrawn in slow decremental steps. The second drug should be titrated first to low maintenance doses and, if seizures continue, the dose increased incrementally to the maximal dose.

8 If the steps in 7 fail, a third alternative monotherapy should be tried in the same manner, or polytherapy used (step 10).

*If seizures continue, or recur after initial therapy with 2–3 drugs tried in monotherapy as above:*

9 The diagnosis should be reassessed. It is not uncommon in this situation to find that the attacks do not have an epileptic basis. Investigation should be considered to exclude the possibility of a progressive lesion. The possibility of poor compliance should be explored.

10 Alternative monotherapies or polytherapy should be considered.

11 The patient should be referred for specialist advice.

**Table 2.17** Usual dosing regimens and fastest routine incremental and decremental rates in adults (values in this table are based on the author's own practice, and may vary from those published elsewhere).

| Drug | Initial dose (mg/day) | Drug initiation: usual dose increment (mg/day) stepped up every 2 weeks | Usual initial maintenance dose on monotherapy (mg/day) | Usual maximum dose in monotherapy (mg/day) | Dosing intervals (per day) | Drug reduction: usual dose decrement (mg/day) stepped down every −2−4 weeks | Maintenance doses can be different when given as co-medication |
|---|---|---|---|---|---|---|---|
| Carbamazepine† | 100 | 100−200 | 400−1600 | 2000 | 2 | 200 | Yes |
| Clobazam | 10 | 10 | 10−30 | 30 | 1−2 | 10 | |
| Clonazepam | 0.25 | 0.25−0.5 | 0.5−4 | 4 | 1−2 | 1 | |
| Ethosuximide | 250 | 250 | 750−1500 | 1500 | 2−3 | 250 | Yes |
| Gabapentin | 300−400 | 300−400 | 900−2400 | 3200 | 2−3 | 300 | |
| Lamotrigine | 12.5−25 | 25−100 | 100−400 | 600 | 2 | 100 | Yes |
| Levetiracetam | 125−250 | 250−500 | 500−1500 | 4000 | 2 | 500 | |
| Oxcarbazepine | 600 | 300 | 600−2400 | 3000 | 2 | 300 | Yes |
| Phenobarbital | 30 | 30−60 | 60−120 | 180 | 1−2 | 30 | Yes |
| Phenytoin | 200 | 25−100 | 200−300 | 450 | 1−2 | 50 | Yes |
| Pregabalin | 150 | 50−100 | 150−600 | 600 | 2−3 | 150 | |
| Primidone | 62.5−125 | 125−250 | 250−1000 | 1500 | 1−2 | 125 | Yes |
| Tiagabine | 4−5 | 4−15 | 15−30 | 56−60 | 2−3 | 5 | Yes |
| Topiramate | 25−50 | 50−100 | 100−300 | 600 | 2 | 50 | Yes |
| Valproate | 200−500 | 200−500 | 600−1500 | 3000 | 2−3 | 200 | Yes |
| Vigabatrin | 1000 | 500 | 1000−2000 | 4000 | 2 | 500 | |
| Zonisamide | 100 | 50 | 200−400 | 600 | 1−2 | 100 | Yes |

†, Values are for the slow release formulation, which is the formulation of choice, particularly at high doses.

### Precipitating factors in early epilepsy

Avoiding factors that precipitate seizures can be very important. The common factors are listed in Table 1.32 (p. 54). Excess alcohol intake (or its abrupt withdrawal) was a predominant factor in 6% of first seizures in one UK series, and accounted for 27% of first seizures in those between the ages of 30 and 39 years. Sleep deprivation may also be a precipitating factor for seizures in susceptible individuals, and is often a contributory factor in those abusing alcohol. Photosensitivity is encountered mainly in adolescents with idiopathic generalized epilepsy, and is described on p. 56.

### Counselling and information provision

In addition to the topics listed in Table 2.18, it is sometimes important to offer counselling and information on a broader range of topics and lifestyle issues. The need for this will depend on individual circumstances. Most patients with newly diagnosed epilepsy enter rapid remission, and the epilepsy should not pose major problems, a fact that it is important to emphasize. The counselling required is not as intense or comprehensive as for chronic active epilepsy, where seizures are likely to persist. A balance is needed.

### Outcome of therapy

The outcome of therapy in newly diagnosed cases is generally good. In about 70% seizures will be brought under rapid control. If long remission occurs (say for 2–5 years), the risk of subsequent recurrence is low (approximately 10%) and most patients are eventually able to discontinue medication. About two-thirds of patients started on therapy will enter a 1-year remission within a year of initiating treatment, and three-quarters will be in 3-year remission at a point 5 years after starting therapy.

**Table 2.18** Topics for information provision and counselling in newly diagnosed epilepsy.

- Nature of epilepsy
- First aid management of seizures
- Avoidance of precipitating factors, including alcohol and sleep deprivation
- Purpose of medication and likely duration
- Nature of common adverse effects of medication
- Need to take medication regularly
- Risks of seizures (including SUDEP) and advice regarding common hazards
- Legal aspects of driving
- Interaction with other drugs, especially oral contraceptive pill (where relevant)
- Possibility of teratogenicity, where relevant

The presence of the following factors has been found to lessen the chance of achieving early remission: high frequency of tonic–clonic seizures before therapy; symptomatic epilepsy with structural cerebral disease; childhood epilepsy syndrome; partial or secondarily generalized seizures; and additional neurological handicap or learning disability.

## PRINCIPLES OF TREATMENT OF PATIENTS WITH ESTABLISHED ACTIVE EPILEPSY

The goal of drug therapy in newly diagnosed cases is the complete control of seizures, which is attained in about 60–70% of patients in the longer term. This means that about 30–40% of cases have continuing seizures, and the treatment of this 'chronic active' epilepsy is more complex and more difficult than that of a drug-naïve case. Different issues are raised, and the perspectives of therapy are different.

Complete seizure control in patients with chronic epilepsy can be obtained, even with skilful treatment, in only perhaps 30%, although it should be possible to lessen the frequency or severity of seizures in other cases. There remain a number of patients—perhaps 10% of all those developing epilepsy—whose seizures remain severe, frequent or intractable. Although small in number, these patients require a high level of medical input. The epilepsy often co-exists with additional learning disability, psychosocial problems or other neurological handicaps, and these factors complicate medical therapy further.

With active epilepsy there are high rates of morbidity and even mortality. The treatment should address both medical and social issues. Counselling on a wide range of topics is often required, and is best achieved via a team approach involving specialists, general practitioners, specialist nurses and counsellors. Issues vary in different patient groups, and the specific problems of women, the elderly and children are covered in later sections. A large population-based survey of patients on antiepileptic drugs was carried out in the UK, commissioned by the National Health Service; the areas in which epilepsy was considered by the respondents to be impacting on their lives are listed in Table 2.19.

### Treatment protocol for patients with established active epilepsy

When first seeing a patient with chronic uncontrolled epilepsy, a two-stage procedure should be adopted. First, an assessment of diagnosis and previous treatment history should be made; second, a treatment plan should be devised (Table 2.20).

This scheme can take a number of months to complete (the time depending largely on the frequency of seizures). It will require patience and tenacity. The procedure should be explained in advance to the patient to maintain confidence and compliance. It will require the expenditure of time and effort by the doctor, who should be available throughout for guidance and reassurance. Perseverance brings rewards, however, and the resolute will, following this protocol, become established on effective long-term therapy.

#### Assessment

• Review the diagnosis of epilepsy. An eye-witnessed account of the attacks should be obtained, and the previous medical records inspected. A series of normal EEG results should alert one to the possibility that the attacks are non-epileptic, although this is not an infallible rule.

• Establish aetiology. It is important at this stage to ascertain the cause of the epileptic attacks, and especially to exclude progressive pathology. This will often require EEG and MRI scanning (of sufficient quality; see pp. 237–8).

• Classify seizure type. This has some value in guiding the choice of medication.

• Review previous treatment history. This is an absolutely essential step, often omitted. The response to a drug is generally speaking relatively consistent over time. Find out which drugs have been previously tried, what was the response (effectiveness/side-effects), what was the maximum dose, and why the drug was withdrawn.

• Review compliance. This can be a reason for poor seizure control. A drug wallet, filled up for the whole week, can be of great assistance for patients who often forget to take the medication. Other methods for improving compliance are listed in Table 2.21.

#### Treatment plan

A treatment plan (schedule) should be formed on the basis of this assessment. The plan should take the form of a stepwise series of treatment trials, each to be tried in turn

**Table 2.19** Survey of the impact of epilepsy by age group (CSAG survey, 2001).

| Mild seizures | | Severe seizures | |
|---|---|---|---|
| **Impact** | **% of responders** | **Impact** | **% of responders** |
| *≤ 16 yrs (n = 33; impacts reported, 61)* | | *≤ 16 yrs (n = 54; impacts reported, 121)* | |
| School life | 36 | School life | 33 |
| Psychological | 27 | Psychological | 31 |
| Social life | 24 | Social life | 30 |
| Sports | 18 | Sports | 15 |
| Need to take tablets | 15 | Supervision | 11 |
| Sleep | 9 | Sleep | 11 |
| Learning difficulties | 9 | Play | 7 |
| None | 9 | Need to take tablets | 7 |
| | | | |
| *17–65 yrs (n = 568; impacts reported, 140)* | | *17–65 yrs (n = 347; impacts reported, 842)* | |
| Driving ban | 48 | Work | 51 |
| Work | 36 | Psychological | 35 |
| Social life | 19 | Social life | 32 |
| Psychological | 18 | Driving ban | 28 |
| Loss of confidence | 8 | Supervision | 10 |
| None | 11 | Independence | 9 |
| | | | |
| *> 65 yrs (n = 127; impacts reported, 191)* | | *> 65 yrs (n = 28; impacts reported, 57)* | |
| Driving ban | 32 | Driving ban | 39 |
| Psychological | 19 | Psychological | 29 |
| Work | 14 | Seizures | 21 |
| Bad memory | 9 | Work | 21 |
| None | 19 | Social life | 14 |
| | | Loss of self-confidence | 11 |
| | | Mobility | 11 |
| | | Supervision | 11 |

UK Survey of 3455 unselected persons with epilepsy and who were taking antiepileptic drugs. 1157 subjects had had a seizure in the past year and a seizure severity score (using the National Hospital Seizures Severity Scale) possible to assess, and completed a questionnaire about the impact of epilepsy on their lives. The results are summarized in this table.

(if the previous trial fails to meet the targeted level of seizure control).

The treatment plan is ideally devised to trial each available antiepileptic in turn, in a reasonable dose, singly or as two-drug therapy (or more rarely three-drug combinations). This will involve deciding upon which drugs to introduce, which drugs to withdraw, and which drugs to retain. Decisions will also be needed about the duration of each treatment trial. There is often nihilistic inertia in much of the treatment of chronic epilepsy which should be resisted, and an active and logical approach to therapy can prove very successful.

### Choice of drugs to introduce or retain

Generally these should be drugs that are appropriate for the seizure type and which have not been previously used in optimal doses or which have been used and did prove helpful. Rational choices depend on a well-documented history of previous drug therapy. Attention also needs be paid to drug interactions. The initial dose and maximum incremental increases in dose in routine practice are shown in Table 2.17.

### Choice of drugs to withdraw

These should be drugs that have been given an adequate trial at optimal doses and which either were ineffective or caused unacceptable side-effects. There is obviously little point in continuing a drug that has had little effect, yet it is remarkable how often this is done.

### Duration of treatment trial

This will depend on the baseline seizure rate. The trial should be long enough to differentiate the effect of therapy from that of chance fluctuations in seizures.

### Trials of therapy

It is usual to maintain therapy with either one or two suitable antiepileptic drugs. If drugs are being withdrawn, it

**Table 2.20** Principles of treatment in chronic active epilepsy.

*Assessment*
- Review diagnosis and aetiology (history, EEG, imaging)
- Classify seizures and syndrome
- Review compliance
- Review drug history:
  - Which drugs were useful in the past?
  - Which drugs were not useful in the past?
  - Which drugs have not been used in the past?
  - (also dose, length of therapy, and reasons for discontinuation)
- Review precipitants and non-pharmacological factors

*Treatment plan*
- Document proposed sequence of drug 'trials'
- Decide what background medication to continue
- Decide upon the sequence of drug additions and withdrawals
- Decide the duration of drug 'trials'
- Decide when to do serum-level monitoring
- Consider surgical therapy
- Consider non-pharmacological measures (lifestyle, alternative therapy, etc.)
- Recognize the limitations of therapy
- Provide information on above to patient

**Table 2.21** Methods for improving compliance with drug therapy.

Information about drug treatment:
- role
- limitations
- efficacy
- side-effects

Drug therapy:
- monotherapy
- simplify regimen
- introduce drugs slowly

Aide-memoire:
- drug wallet
- regular reminders
- cues

Reinforcement at regular clinic follow-up visits

is wise to maintain one drug as an 'anchor' to cover the withdrawal period.

## Drug withdrawal

Drug withdrawal needs care. The sudden reduction in dose of an antiepileptic drug can result in a severe worsening of seizures or in status epilepticus, even if the withdrawn drug was apparently not contributing much to seizure control. Why these happen is not clear. Experience from telemetry units suggests that most withdrawal seizures have physiological features similar to the patient's habitual attacks. It is therefore customary, and wise, to withdraw medication slowly. This caution applies particularly to barbiturate drugs (phenobarbital, primidone), benzodiazepine drugs (clobazam, clonazepam, diazepam), and to carbamazepine. Table 2.17 lists the fastest decremental rates that are recommended in normal clinical practice. In many situations even slower rates of withdrawal are safer. The only advantage of fast withdrawal is better compliance and the faster establishment of new drug regimens.

Only one drug should be withdrawn at a time. If the withdrawal period is likely to be difficult, the dangers can be reduced by covering the withdrawal with a benzodiazepine drug (usually clobazam 10 mg/day), given during the phase of active withdrawal. A benzodiazepine can also be given if clustering of seizures following withdrawal occurs.

It is sometimes difficult to know whether seizures during withdrawal are due to the withdrawal or simply the background epilepsy, and whenever possible a long-term view should be taken and over-reaction in the short term avoided. Sometimes the simple withdrawal of a drug will result in improved control of seizures by improving well-being, assuring better compliance and reducing interactions.

## Drug addition

New drugs added to a regimen should also be introduced slowly, at least in the routine clinical situation. This results in better tolerability, and is particularly important when adding benzodiazepines, carbamazepine, lamotrigine, levetiracetam, primidone or topiramate. Too fast an introduction of these drugs will almost invariably result in side-effects. It is usual to aim initially for a low maintenance dose, but in severe epilepsy higher doses are often required.

## Concomitant medication

Changing the dose of one antiepileptic (either incremental or decremental) can influence the levels of other drugs, and the changing levels of concomitant medication can contribute to changing side-effects or effectiveness.

## Limits on therapy

Drug therapy will fail in about 10–20% of patients. In this situation, the epilepsy can be categorized as 'intractable', and the goal of therapy changes to achieving the best compromise between inadequate seizure control and drug-induced side-effects. Individual patients will take very different views about where to strike this balance.

Intractability is inevitably an arbitrary decision. There are more than 10 first-line antiepileptic drugs, and far more combinations (with 10 first-line antiepileptic drugs there are 45 different two-drug and 120 different three-drug combinations). All combinations cannot therefore be tried. The chances of a new drug controlling seizures after five appropriate agents have failed to do so is small (less than 10%). At a pragmatic level, therefore, one can categorize an epilepsy as intractable when at least five of the major anti-epileptics have proved ineffective in adequate doses. There will, however, be occasional exceptions to this rule. A recent excellent suggestion is to define intractability by the number of ineffective drugs tried, thus second-level intractability is defined as the failure of two drugs, third-level intractability by the failure of three drugs, and so on.

### Counselling

Counselling should be offered for chronic patients, as for new patients, on the topics listed in Table 2.18. Those with chronic active epilepsy, however, have additional problems—fears about the risks of future seizures, anxiety about the stigmatizing effects of epilepsy, and its effects on employment, self-esteem, relationships, schooling and leisure activities. The areas in which the condition impacted were demonstrated in one large survey of 3455 persons on treatment for epilepsy in Britain, which are summarized in Table 2.19. Many of these could be ameliorated by appropriate counselling and these topics should be addressed. The issues depend on age and the severity of epilepsy.

### Monotherapy vs. combination therapy

Single-drug therapy will provide optimal seizure control in about 70% of all patients with epilepsy, and should be chosen whenever possible. The advantages of monotherapy are:
- better tolerability and fewer side-effects
- simpler and less intrusive regimens
- better compliance
- no potential for pharmacokinetic or pharmacodynamic interactions with other antiepileptic drugs.

Combination therapy is needed in about 20% of all those developing epilepsy, and in a higher proportion of those with epilepsy that has remained uncontrolled in spite of initial monotherapy (chronic active epilepsy). The prognosis for the control of seizures in these patients, even on combination therapy, is far less good. Nevertheless, skilful combination therapy can make a substantial difference by optimizing control of the epilepsy and minimizing the side-effects of treatment. The choice of drugs in combination has not been satisfactorily studied. It has been proposed, but without any substantial supporting evidence, that mixing drugs with differing modes of action has a synergistic effect. Patients need to be advised carefully about the implications of polytherapy in terms of drug interactions, teratogenesis and potential pharmacodynamic effects.

## TREATMENT OF PATIENTS WITH EPILEPSY IN REMISSION

Epilepsy can be said to be in remission when seizures have not occurred over long periods of time (conventionally 2 years or 5 years). At some point after the initiation of therapy 70–80% of patients will be in remission. Many cases of untreated epilepsy also remit and in the long term at least 50% of patients are in remission and off medication.

The clinical management of ongoing therapy in patients in remission is generally straightforward. In most cases little medical input is required, with appropriate care provided at primary care level and annual visits to the specialist. The seizure type, epilepsy syndrome, aetiology, investigations and previous treatment should be recorded. Routine haematological or biochemical checks are recommended on an annual basis in an asymptomatic individual. Inquiry should be made of long-term side-effects (e.g. bone disease in postmenopausal women) and counselling about issues such as pregnancy made where appropriate. At some point, however, the calm of this ideal situation is likely to be disturbed by the question of discontinuation of therapy.

### Discontinuation of drug therapy

It is often difficult to decide when (if ever) to discontinue drug treatment. The decision should be made by a specialist who is able to provide an estimate of the risk of re-activation of the epilepsy. This risk is influenced by the factors listed in Table 2.22, but it must be stressed that withdrawal is never entirely risk free. The decision whether or not to withdraw therapy will depend on the level of risk the patient is prepared to accept.

### Probability of remaining free of seizures after drug withdrawal

The best information comes from the Medical Research Council (MRC) antiepileptic drug withdrawal study, which included 1013 patients who had been free of seizures for 2 years or more (Figure 2.6). Within 2 years of starting drug withdrawal 59% remained free of seizures (compared with 79% of those who opted to stay on therapy). Other studies have had essentially similar findings.

#### Period of seizure freedom

The longer the patient is seizure free, the less is the chance of relapse. The overall risk of relapse after drug withdrawal, for instance, after a 5-year period of freedom from seizures is under 10%.

#### Duration of active epilepsy

This is probably an under-studied factor. There is a strong impression that the shorter the history of active seizures

**Table 2.22** Some factors that increase the risk of seizure recurrence after withdrawal of therapy in patients with epilepsy in remission.

- Short duration of freedom from seizures prior to drug withdrawal
- Age above 16 years
- History of myoclonic seizures or secondarily generalized seizures
- History of multiple seizure types
- Certain epilepsy syndromes (e.g. juvenile myoclonic epilepsy, childhood encephalopathies)
- Remote symptomatic epilepsy
- Prolonged period of active epilepsy before achieving seizure control
- History of seizures after treatment was initiated
- Seizure control requiring multiple drug therapy
- EEG showing generalized spike-wave discharges
- Presence of learning disability or associated neurological handicaps

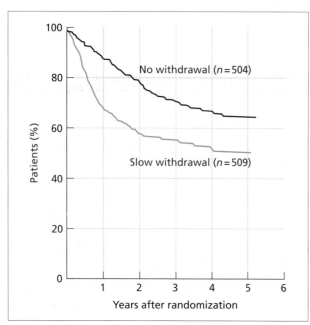

**Fig. 2.6** Actuarial percentage of patients seizure-free amongst those randomized to continuing or to slow withdrawal of antiepileptic drugs. A study of 1013 patients seizure-free for at least 2 years, randomized to either slow withdrawal of their antiepileptic drug therapy or to continuing drug therapy. Two years after randomization 78% of those who continued treatment and 59% of those who had treatment withdrawn were seizure-free, but thereafter the differences in recurrence rate between the two groups diminished.

(i.e. the duration of time from the onset of epilepsy to the onset of remission), the less is the risk of relapse.

### Type and severity of epilepsy

The type of epilepsy, and its aetiology, are important influences on prognosis. The presence of symptomatic epilepsy, secondarily generalized or myoclonic seizures, neurological deficit or learning disability greatly lessens the chance of remission, and also increases the chances of recurrence should remission occur. A higher number of seizures prior to remission, a greater number of drugs being taken to control the seizures, and the presence of two or more seizure types (a surrogate for severity of epilepsy) all increase the risk of relapse.

### EEG

The value of EEG in predicting the outcome of patients in remission is controversial, as it is in most other areas of prognostication. The persistence of spike-wave in those with primary generalized epilepsy is the most useful prognostic EEG feature, indicating a higher chance of relapse. Other EEG abnormalities have no great prognostic utility, and the presence of focal spikes or changes in EEG background are of little help in estimating the chances of remission or relapse after drug withdrawal. In general, the EEG has more prognostic value in children than in adults.

### Age

There is no clear overall relationship between age and the risk of relapse, although there are age-specific syndromes that have specific prognostic patterns. There is a low chance of relapse in the benign epilepsies of childhood or in generalized absence epilepsy. These data simply emphasis the obvious point that the overriding determinant of prognosis is the type and aetiology of epilepsy.

The risk factors are additive, and if two or more adverse factors are present, the risk of recurrence is over 70%. On the other hand, if positive factors exist such as a long duration of remission, a short history of epilepsy, mild epilepsy prior to remission, or idiopathic epilepsy with a normal EEG, the risks are lower than the mean relapse rate of 40% found in the MRC study. A predictive model has been developed on the basis of the study, which takes into account some of these features and provides useful estimates of relapse rate (Table 2.23).

### How to withdraw therapy—the importance of slow reduction

When a decision to withdraw therapy is made, the drugs should be discontinued one at a time slowly. Fifty per cent of patients who are going to experience a recurrence of seizures on withdrawal do so during the reduction phase, and 25% in the first 6 months after withdrawal; this should be explained carefully to the patient. Because of this, the UK driving licence authority recommends that driving be avoided during drug withdrawal and for 6 months afterwards; this (non-binding) advice should be given to patients.

The fastest recommended rates of withdrawal are given in Table 2.17, although in many instances there is no need to proceed so rapidly. In general terms, the slower the withdrawal, the less likely are seizures to recur. If seizures

**Table 2.23** Mathematical basis of model predicting risk of recurrence of seizures after drug withdrawal (from MRC drug withdrawal study).

| Starting score for all patients = −175 | Factor value to be added to score | |
|---|---|---|
| Age > 16 years | 45 | |
| Taking more than 1 AED | 50 | |
| Seizures occurring after the start of treatment | 35 | |
| History of any tonic–clonic seizure (generalized or partial in onset) | 35 | |
| History of myoclonic seizures | 50 | |
| EEG while in remission | | |
| not done | 15 | |
| abnormal | 20 | |
| Duration of seizure-free period (years), D | 200/D | |
| *Total score* | T | |
| *Exponentiate T/100* | | |
| $(Z = e^{T/100})$ | Z | |
| *Probability of seizure recurrence* | *by 1 year* | *by 2 years* |
| On continued treatment | $1 - 0.89^{Z}$ | $1 - 0.79^{Z}$ |
| On slow withdrawal of treatment | $1 - 0.69^{Z}$ | $1 - 0.60^{Z}$ |

do recur, the drug should be immediately restarted at the dosage that controlled the attacks.

A further issue, which must be emphasized to a patient before attempting drug withdrawal, concerns the longer-term prognosis if seizure relapse occurs after drug withdrawal. At least 10% of patients will not regain full remission even if the drug is replaced at the dosage that previously resulted in long remission. Why this should be the case is unclear but, in some patients at least, it seems that recurrence alters the risk of subsequent seizures.

## Counselling and decision making

The withdrawal of therapy can have marked psychological benefits. It often removes the stigma of a 'diagnosis' and may ameliorate 'illness behaviour'. Side-effects, sometimes not recognized on chronic therapy, may also be reversed. On the other hand, the recurrence of seizures can have both psychological and social consequences, and carries a risk of morbidity and even mortality. These issues demand careful consideration and discussion. It must be emphasized to the patient that there is no guarantee that withdrawal of treatment will be successful, and that if seizures do recur, there is no guarantee that a return to therapy will ensure future remission. An estimate of the risks of recurrence on with-

drawal from, and of further recurrence on return to, therapy should be given. The benefits of drug withdrawal should also be discussed. The decision to initiate withdrawal must be made by the patient—not the physician—and only after full appreciation of the issues involved. The role of the clinician is to provide information and to respond to queries and concerns; it is never appropriate to insist on drug withdrawal. The personal circumstances of the individual patient can be overriding. In adults, the avoidance of seizures is often of greater importance than in children, for instance in relation to holding a driving licence or employment. In women, the question of future pregnancy and of a drug-free pregnancy may be uppermost. In children, concerns about the effects of drugs on learning may encourage earlier drug withdrawal. It is not possible to make general recommendations, and the wishes of the individual patient should be paramount. One study has shown how poorly physician expectations are predictive of patients' decisions in this area.

## TREATMENT OF EPILEPSY IN CHILDREN

### General considerations

The treatment of epilepsy in infancy and early childhood differs in a number of ways from that in late childhood or adult life.

#### Clinical context

The aetiologies, clinical features and response to treatment of epilepsy are very different. Both seizures and antiepileptic drugs affect behaviour, learning, schooling, and social and emotional development. Special attention is needed to overall mental and neurological development. Approximately 20–30% of children with epilepsy have learning disabilities and, in many cases, attention to intellectual impairment takes precedence over epilepsy. Careful psychological and educational assessment is needed to identify problems and tailor treatment and educational programmes.

#### Social impact of epilepsy

The impact of epilepsy on the life of children can be very different from that in adults. Growing up with seizures affects the development of personality and can interfere with many aspects of everyday life, schooling and choice of career. Support for the child and his/her family is an important part of management. It is essential to spend time providing information and advice, and there are few areas where counselling is so important. Children with epilepsy should have a lifestyle that is as normal as possible, and the common tendency to over-protect ('cocoon') children should be discussed with parents and consciously avoided. Small increases in risk are to be preferred to extensive prohibitions.

*Epilepsy with falls*

Where epilepsy occurs with falls (e.g. drop attacks in the Lennox–Gastaut syndrome), special precautions are necessary. These epilepsies inevitably interfere with daily activities, and special schooling measures and protection of the head and face by wearing an adequate helmet are often required.

## Drug treatment

Drug regimens in young patients are often different from those in adults and also change with age through childhood. Absorption of antiepileptic drugs is usually faster in infants and young children than in adults. The half-lives of most antiepileptic drugs are prolonged in the first 1–3 weeks of life and shorten thereafter. The metabolism of antiepileptic drugs is faster during childhood and slows to adult rates during adolescence. Thus, higher doses per unit of weight are required by children, and dosage requirements can change over time.

The pharmacodynamic effects of antiepileptic drugs may also differ. The paradoxical effect of barbiturates and benzodiazepines causing excitation in children and sedation in adults is an example.

Side-effects are difficult to recognize in infants and in those with learning disability, and children may not be able to communicate their symptoms. These groups therefore require extra surveillance for side-effects.

In school-aged children, three times daily regimens (requiring dosing at school) should be avoided, as the middle dose is easily overlooked and can embarrass the child. Slow-release preparations of carbamazepine and sodium valproate have made it possible to maintain adequate plasma levels with twice-daily dosing.

The use of the newly marketed antiepileptic drugs in paediatrics has not been as extensively studied as in adults, and these drugs should generally not be used as first-line therapy except for special situations (e.g. vigabatrin in West syndrome associated with tuberous sclerosis).

Details of studies in children of individual drugs are found in Section 3.

## The ketogenic diet

The ketogenic diet is a high-fat and low-carbohydrate diet which was introduced into epilepsy therapy in the 1920s, and which in recent times has been the subject of a resurgence of interest. Its use is confined to the treatment of severe childhood epilepsy that has proved resistant to more conventional therapy. It has no role in adult epilepsy, where its use has proved difficult and dangerous.

The diet is high in fat and low in carbohydrate, with adequate protein, and provides nutrition with 1 g/kg of protein and 5–10 g of carbohydrate per day, the remainder of the calories (usually 75% of the recommended daily allowance) being in the form of long-chain triglycerides.

The diet must be followed strictly, an arduous and difficult task for the child and parent(s) alike.

Exactly how the diet exerts its undoubted antiepileptic effect is unknown. It mimics the biochemical changes of starvation (low carbohydrate intake) and this results in a switch from aerobic to ketogenic metabolism and the production of ketone bodies in the liver. These are transported into the brain by a monocarboxylic acid transporter, where they are utilized instead of glucose for energy production. This metabolic change has marked antiepileptic effects, as demonstrated in animal and human studies. To alter metabolism, however, requires dedication to a diet that is difficult to maintain and often unpalatable.

The diet is usually reserved for children with West syndrome, Lennox–Gastaut syndrome or other less-specific forms of severe epilepsy. Patients with gastrostomy tubes in place may be ideal candidates. A special indication is in children with glucose transporter protein (GLUT-1) deficiency and pyruvate dehydrogenase deficiency, where the diet is first-line therapy and can be life-saving. The diet is potentially dangerous, and should be avoided, in pyruvate carboxylase deficiency, porphyria, carnitine deficiency, fatty acid oxidation defects and in mitochondrial disorders.

The exact constitution of the diet must be calculated individually for each patient. The ratio of fats to carbohydrates and protein is based on the age, size, weight and activity level of the patient. A young child or infant is often prescribed a 3 : 1 diet to provide additional protein and older children a 4 : 1 diet. Obese children and adolescents are usually given a 3 : 1 diet. Calorie intake is generally about 75% of the recommended daily intake for age. Fluid intake must be rigorously maintained, and supplementation with magnesium, zinc, vitamin D, vitamin C, vitamin B complex and calcium is recommended.

The effects on epilepsy can be dramatic. Early studies in the 1920s and 1930s consistently showed impressive results, and these have been largely confirmed in more recent investigations carried out to modern standards. A recent study from Johns Hopkins University showed, at 1 year, a reduction in seizures of more than 50% in 50% of 150 treated children, and a reduction of more than 90% in 27%. At 3–6 years, 44% maintained the improvement. The use of the diet allows a reduction of adjunctive drug therapy, which is an added benefit. Other benefits of the diet include improvement in behaviour in those with and without autism. The diet can be given for months or years. A typical period of treatment is 1–2 years, if the diet proves initially successful. About 10% of children maintain the diet for 4 or more years, and one patient is reported who has maintained the diet for 15 years with no major side-effects. Discontinuation of the diet should take place gradually over 3–6 months.

Side-effects are not uncommon. Vomiting, dehydration and food refusal are common initially but are transitory.

Other minor side-effects include constipation, oesophageal reflux and acidosis. The effect of the diet on growth is a problem. A recent review of the diet in 237 children showed that the rate of weight gain decreased at 3 months but then remained constant for up to 3 years. There is also an effect on height. Renal stones occur in 5–8% of patients. Hypercholesterolaemia is common. Rare side-effects that have been reported include cardiomyopathy, pancreatitis, bruising, vitamin deficiency, hypoproteinaemia, Fanconi's renal tubular acidosis and prolonged QT interval. In adults, for whom the diet is not normally recommended, coronary heart disease and myocardial infarction have occurred, associated with hypercholesterolaemia.

### Treatment of epilepsy in patients with additional handicaps

Epilepsy in the context of learning difficulty is often severe and resistant to drug therapy. The usual principles of antiepileptic drug therapy apply, although certain points need specific emphasis (Table 2.24).

#### Side-effects

Vigilance for side-effects is particularly important. In the presence of cerebral damage, drug side-effects tend to be more frequent, occur at lower serum levels and to take unusual forms. Examples are confusion, neurological side-effects, behavioural change and mental deterioration, encephalopathy, and weight gain which may be attributed to neuroleptics or inactivity. Hypotonic children are hypersensitive to the muscle-relaxing effects of benzodiazepines, and dystonia and ataxia may occur in patients with pre-existent motor deficits. The individual with learning difficulty may not be able to communicate clearly the adverse consequences of drug therapy. It is an essential duty

**Table 2.24** Specific problems of diagnosis and management in handicapped patients.

*Problems of diagnosis*
- Communication
- Observation and interpretation of symptoms
- Distinguishing between epileptic and non-epileptic behaviours
- Identifying neuroleptic and other drug-induced symptoms
- Identifying non-epileptic seizures

*Problems of treatment*
- Communication
- Insidious side-effects (especially sedation, behavioural change)
- Sensitivity to medication and unusual side-effects
- Brittle epilepsy and tendency to status epilepticus
- Unusual seizure manifestations
- Attitude of family and carers
- Drug formulations

of the prescribing physician to maintain extreme vigilance for side-effects, to prevent distress or harm.

#### Serial seizures, clusters and episodes of status

These are common in patients with severe epilepsy and learning difficulty. They can be precipitated by seemingly minor problems such as intercurrent infections or trivial environmental changes. Emergency therapy (p. 211) is often needed earlier and more frequently than in a non-handicapped population. Drug regimens may need to be modified as handicapped individuals often show special sensitivities to the usual drugs. Tailored regimens for emergency intervention need to be defined for each individual, based on previous (often unfortunate) experiences. It is helpful to document these in writing, and to have them available to all carers and emergency medical services.

#### Over-medication

Over-medication in the face of intractable epilepsy is a particular problem in handicapped persons. The reasons are complex and include the severity of the epilepsy, the need for a third party to decide upon treatment on behalf of the individual, the difficulty in communicating side-effects, and the carer's tendency to over-protection. It is vital to resist this tendency. Great benefits (without loss of seizure control) are often gained by reducing the overall antiepileptic drug load.

#### Surgical therapy

Surgery can benefit a small number of individuals with epilepsy. The presence of handicap is not *per se* a bar to considering this. However, assessment should be carried out in experienced centres, and other issues such as quality of life gain and informed consent are often problematic.

### Institutional care

Overall, among individuals requiring long-term institutional care, between 30 and 50% have epilepsy. Epilepsy has been found to occur in 50% of those with IQ levels less than 20, and in 35% of those with IQ levels in the 35–50 range. Seizures are particularly common in those with post-natal cerebral damage. The frequency of handicap among those with epilepsy is difficult to ascertain. In a 1983 study of 223 adults with epilepsy in Finland, 30% had an IQ of less than 50, 20% were institutionalized and 15% were completely dependent. A more recent study, also from Finland, found handicap in 20% of children with epilepsy compared with 1% of controls.

The needs of individuals with multiple handicaps are often complex, and care is difficult to organize. In patients with severe epilepsy, the seizures usually pose the major problem but in others, the problems of epilepsy are secondary to the other handicaps. Epilepsy adds a dimension that care providers often find difficult to deal with. The responsibility of dealing with potentially life-threatening seizures is felt to be too great by many otherwise competent authorities. It is therefore often difficult to find suitable residential, daytime or vocational placements for people with epilepsy. A few specialized institutions provide expert epilepsy care, and although these provide a secure environment from the epilepsy point of view, they may be geographically distant, risking family estrangement. All institutions dealing with epilepsy require specialist medical input, and a failure to monitor the epilepsy is a dereliction of care. Team-work is needed, with facilities for outpatient and inpatient treatment and good communication between the different professional groups and also the family. Care can be shared between an institution and the family, and in both settings a balance has to be set between over-protection and neglect. This balance can be very difficult to define or achieve, and there is no one single correct position. Individuals deserve an individually tailored solution, and the issues involved (and the risks taken) should be explicitly agreed with the individual, the family and the professional carers.

## THE TREATMENT OF EPILEPSY IN THE ELDERLY

Epilepsy is a frequent and generally under-recognized problem in the elderly. Annual incidence rates in a recent study were 87 per 100,000 in the 65–69 age group, 147 per 100,000 of people in their 70s, and 159 per 100,000 of people in their 80s, and about 30% of new cases now occur in people over 65 years of age. The prevalence rate of treated epilepsy in those over 70 years is almost double that in children. Currently, about 0.7% of the elderly population are treated for epilepsy, and epilepsy in the elderly is now the third most common neurological condition after dementia and stroke. As the number of elderly people in the population is rising, the numbers of elderly people requiring treatment for epilepsy is also greatly increasing. The medical services must catch up to make adequate provision.

Cerebrovascular disease accounts for between 30 and 50% of cases (see p. 52), but this can be occult. Epilepsy is the first manifestation of previously silent cerebrovascular disease, and imaging evidence of cerebrovascular disease is found in about 15% of those presenting with apparently idiopathic late-onset epilepsy. The onset of seizures in the elderly can be a harbinger of future stroke, and in a recent study of 4709 individuals with seizures beginning after the age of 60 years, there was a 2.89-fold (95% CI, 2.45–3.41) increased incidence of subsequent stroke. In fact, the onset of seizures was a greater risk factor for stroke than either elevated cholesterol level or hypertension. Seizures also follow stroke, with a frequency of about 5% in the acute phase after stroke and 10% in the first 5 years after ischaemic

stroke (see p. 51 for further description of vascular causes of epilepsy). Subdural haematoma are another under-diagnosed cause of epilepsy in the elderly, and cerebral tumours account for between 5 and 15% of all late-onset epilepsies (p. 46). Ten per cent of the late-onset epilepsies are due to metabolic causes, such as alcohol, pyrexia, dehydration, infections, and renal or hepatic dysfunction. Drug-induced epilepsy (pp. 58–9) is common in the elderly both because drugs are given more frequently and also because of the complex pharmacokinetics in the elderly.

Seizures in the elderly have a serious impact. Postictal states can be prolonged. A confusional state lasting more than 24 hours has been found to occur in the wake of 14% of seizures in the elderly, and in some cases confusion lasted over a week. A postictal Todd's paresis is also more common than in the young, and seizures are commonly misdiagnosed as stroke. Fractures and head injuries are a potential risk. Falling in a seizure can mark a watershed in the older person's life, after which there is a sharp decline in functional independence. The loss of confidence and fear of further falls can render the person electively housebound. This loss of confidence can be compounded by other factors including the stigmatization of epilepsy, the assumption of impending death, the reaction of family and friends, the exclusion from activities, marginalization, loss of a driving licence, disem-powerment, and a perception of a shrinkage of life space.

### Diagnosis

It can be difficult to differentiate seizures from the abundance of other causes of 'funny turns' in the elderly. Syncope, hypoglycaemia, transient ischaemic attacks, transient global amnesia, vertigo and non-specific dizziness afflict up to 10% of the older population. Syncope can have cardiac causes or it may be due to blood pressure changes or impairment of the vascular reflexes linked to posture, and carotid sinus hypersensitivity is also common. Acute confusional states or fluctuating mental impairment can be ictal, postictal or due to non-convulsive status, but are frequently misdiagnosed as manifestations of functional psychiatric illness, dementia or vascular disease. The history may be less well-defined, and the differentiating features less clear-cut than in the younger patient, and pathologies may co-exist.

There are furthermore various EEG changes that are easily mistaken for epileptogenic patterns. Brief runs of temporal slow activity, especially on the left, become increasingly evident after the age of 50 years and should be considered a normal variant. Small sharp spikes during sleep and drowsiness also increase in frequency with age. Runs of temporal–parietal activity can occur in individuals over the age of 50 years (the subclinical rhythmic electrographic discharge in adults [SREDA] pattern) and are not associated with epilepsy. Cerebrovascular disease produces focal and bilateral temporal changes which are also commonly mistaken for epilepsy, and yet do not provide any assistance in determining which patients with vascular disease will or will not develop overt epileptic seizures.

## General aspects of management

Reassurance that seizures do not usually indicate cerebral tumour, psychiatric disorder or dementia, and that they can usually be controlled on medication, is of overriding importance.

Management often involves other professionals. Confidence needs to be rebuilt, mobility restored and the home circumstances reviewed. Advice and input from social services, remedial and occupational therapists are often needed. A home visit to identify sources of potential danger is helpful. A personal alarm can be very useful, as can counselling and written advice for friends and relatives. Factors known to precipitate seizures should be avoided, such as inadequate sleep, excess alcohol or hypoglycaemia.

Uncontrolled seizures are likely to be more hazardous in an elderly patient. Convulsive attacks carry greater risks in patients with cardio-respiratory disorders, and the elderly, fragile patient would be more susceptible to suffer fractures as a consequence of seizure-induced falls.

## Principles of antiepileptic drug therapy

The general principles of drug treatment in the elderly are similar to those in other adults. However, there are aspects that deserve special mention.

### Pharmacokinetic differences

The relationship between dose and serum level can be much more variable in the elderly than in young adults, and published pharmacokinetic values are often expressed as mean values which do not necessarily take into account the wide range in the older population. Protein binding may be reduced as albumin concentrations are lower in the elderly. Clearance is often lower in the elderly due to reduced hepatic capacity and lower glomerular filtration rates, and the volume of distribution for lipid-soluble drugs is often increased. For all these reasons, the half-life of many drugs is longer than in young adults. The interaction of the many medicaments taken by the elderly can greatly complicate the handling of drugs, by competition for absorption, protein binding, hepatic metabolism and renal clearance. In the USA, for instance, persons over the age of 65 years comprise 13% of the population yet receive 32% of prescribed medications, and in one study of epilepsy patients aged 75, a mean of three medications per patient were being taken in addition to the prescribed antiepileptic drugs.

### Pharmacodynamic differences

There are pharmacodynamic differences between the elderly and young adults. Anecdotal evidence suggests that the elderly are more sensitive to the neurological side-effects of drugs, and also that lower drug doses are sufficient to control seizures in the elderly compared with younger adults. The adverse effects of drugs in the elderly may take unfamiliar forms. Confusion, general ill health, affective change or uncharacteristic motor or behavioural disturbances can occur with many antiepileptic drugs. Thus, the 'therapeutic ranges' defined in younger age groups do not necessarily apply to the elderly, and should be generally adjusted downwards. Vigilance for unusual side-effects—both neurological and metabolic—should be maintained.

### Systemic side-effects

Membrane-stabilizing drugs (e.g. phenytoin, carbamazepine, lamotrigine) carry a risk of promoting arrhythmia and hypotension, which is increased in the elderly, although the extent of this risk is unknown. Other side-effects in the elderly include the dangers of loss of bone mass due to enzyme-inducing drugs such as phenytoin, carbamazepine or phenobarbital, a particular risk in post-menopausal women. Phenytoin and carbamazepine also pose potential problems and should be used cautiously in individuals with autonomic dysfunction, for instance in diabetes. Carbamazepine has an anticholinergic effect which can precipitate urinary retention.

### Compliance

Compliance with medication can be poor owing to memory lapses, failing intellect or confusion. In these situations, drug administration should be supervised. The provision of a weekly drug wallet can also be worthwhile. Other methods of improving compliance include using simple drug regimens, providing clear written instructions and clearly labelled medication, avoiding childproof bottles and blister packs, employing assistance from carers, relatives and others, and home visits or telephone contact by a specialist nurse.

### Drug dosing and regimens

For all the above reasons, therapy should generally be initiated with lower doses than in the young adult. Renal and hepatic function and plasma protein concentrations should be measured before therapy is started. Blood level measurements should be made at regular intervals, for relevant drugs, at least until stable regimens have been achieved. Drug combinations should be avoided where possible, and the advantages of monotherapy over polytherapy are greater in the elderly than in young adults.

## Antiepileptic drugs in the elderly

Annoyingly, most drugs have not been subjected to rigorous trials in the elderly, and as a result data on the use of antiepileptic drugs in the elderly are generally sparse. This is an area where more studies are urgently needed.

### Carbamazepine

Carbamazepine is the drug usually given initially in partial epilepsy. This preference is supported to a certain extent by evidence from a meta-analysis of individual data from 1265 elderly patients from five trials in which carbamazepine showed a non-significant trend towards superior control of seizures when compared with valproate. There is little information about age-related changes in the pharmacokinetics of carbamazepine—surprisingly, in view of its widespread use. One study of a small number of patients showed a 40% reduction in clearance in the elderly, and a longer half-life, compared with young adults, whereas a study in normal volunteers showed no age-specific changes in the area under the concentration–time curve, the elimination rate constants, or in carbamazepine 10,11-epoxide concentrations. Side-effects that are more common or more troublesome in the elderly include hyponatraemia and a small risk of drug-induced osteoporosis. Elderly patients are more vulnerable to AED-induced impairment of gait, as well as action and postural tremor, and possibly other subtle adverse neurological effects.

It is usual to initiate carbamazepine therapy slowly in individuals over 65 years of age, and only cautiously to increment the dosage. The slow-release formulation should always be used, as this causes fewer side-effects. A reasonable regimen would be to initial therapy on 100 mg/day, and to increase the dose by 100 mg increments every fortnight, to an initial maintenance dose of 400 mg/day. This can be then be increased as clinically indicated.

### Gabapentin

Gabapentin is absorbed by a saturable transport mechanism, and it is not known if this is affected by age. As it is not metabolized, and there is minimal protein binding, age-related changes in distribution or metabolism should not be expected. Age-related decreases in renal function significantly increase the renal clearance of gabapentin, thus the dose should be reduced in the elderly if renal function is impaired. For all these reasons, one would not expect age to modify gabapentin usage, providing renal function is unimpaired, and it should be a particularly safe drug in the elderly.

### Lamotrigine

Lamotrigine has been studied relatively extensively in the elderly. A double-blind randomized monotherapy comparison in elderly patients with new-onset epilepsy found lower rates of drop-out due to adverse events on lamotrigine (18%) compared with carbamazepine (42%). No difference in efficacy was found, but a greater percentage of patients treated with lamotrigine (71%) continued therapy than those treated with carbamazepine (42%). There are pharmacokinetic differences in the disposition of lamotrigine in the elderly. The plasma clearance of lamotrigine is reduced by about one-third when compared with young adults. The drug is about 55% bound to plasma proteins and undergoes extensive hepatic metabolism, and also interacts with other antiepileptic drugs, all of which can result in age-related irregularities.

It is wise to initiate therapy at lower doses than in young adults. Recommended maintenance doses are 100 mg in monotherapy, 50–100 mg when co-medicated with valproate alone, or 200 mg in patients co-medicated with other enzyme-inducing antiepileptic drugs. Drug-level measurements should be made regularly until a stable regimen is established.

### Levetiracetam

The lack of drug interactions, and the simple pharmacokinetics, of levetiracetam are advantages in the elderly, although detailed studies of its usefulness in this group have not been carried out. Anecdotal evidence suggests, however, that levetiracetam is useful and safe. Age-related changes in renal function can greatly affect the clearance of the drug, and doses should be reduced accordingly. An initial dose of 125 mg is recommended, with incremental steps of 125–250 mg until an initial maintenance dosage of 750–1500 mg/day is reached.

### Phenobarbital

Phenobarbital was once widely used in the elderly, but in recent years it has fallen from fashion, in recognition of the risk of adverse neurological and psychiatric effects. It is partly eliminated by the kidneys and as renal excretion declines with age, one might expect concentrations of phenobarbital to be higher per mg/kg dosage. Studies have shown significant changes in women but not in men. There have been surprisingly few comprehensive studies of metabolism or of absorption, metabolic or elimination parameters, and no studies of interactions, in elderly subjects. This is a galling omission as phenobarbital has been widely used for many years, and there are intensive pharmacokinetic studies in other age groups. Anecdotal experience suggests that the elderly are more sensitive to the sedative side-effects of phenobarbital, especially when co-medicated with benzodiazepine.

It would seem reasonable to use lower dosage than in young adults. The usual starting dose is 30–60 mg at night. Because of anxieties about the increase in sensitivity of the older person to the neurological side-effects of phenobarbital, dosage increments should be cautious and carefully monitored.

### Phenytoin

Phenytoin is commonly prescribed to the elderly, in spite of its complex pharmacokinetics. As it is metabolized by saturable processes, age-related declines in hepatic size and function might be expected to be of real significance. However, published studies are inadequate, and results have been conflicting. Early reports suggested that free phenytoin concentrations do indeed increase with age, although others showed increased clearance, partly attributable to the decreased albumin concentrations, and others showed no difference in the various elimination parameters between the young and the elderly. The metabolism of phenytoin can be saturated at lower levels than in younger persons. The picture is therefore rather confusing and advice is difficult to give. It would be wise to initiate therapy with phenytoin cautiously, at a relatively low dose (initial maintenance of 200 mg/day) followed by small dose increments (50 mg steps) as clinically indicated. Frequent measurements of phenytoin serum levels are essential. The measurement of free phenytoin concentrations is worthwhile in special circumstances (but not routinely), especially in ill or debilitated patients where serum albumin concentrations are low.

### Topiramate

Studies of topiramate in the elderly are very limited, but it has good efficacy and can be safely used. Clearance is reduced in the presence of hepatic or renal impairment. The incidence of central nervous system side-effects can be reduced with a slow-dose titration. For these reasons, dosage should be lower than in young adults. A recommended initial dose is 25 mg at night and dosage increments can be made in 25 mg steps to an initial maintenance dosage of between 50 and 150 mg/day in monotherapy.

### Valproate

Valproate is widely used in the elderly, particularly to control generalized tonic–clonic seizures. It is as effective as carbamazepine in this indication. There are pharmacokinetic differences in the elderly compared with young adults. Free valproate concentrations are increased and in one study the percentage of unbound valproate was found to be 10.7% in the elderly compared with 6.4% in younger persons. A 65% decrease in valproate clearance and a 67% increase in free valproate concentrations in old age was found in one study, and the half-life of valproate can be doubled in the elderly. Other studies have found lesser effects, and there is clear variability between patients. Valproate generally has few interactions at the hepatic level, and this is an advantage over other conventional antiepileptic drugs in older patients, who are often taking a cocktail of other drugs for various conditions. The drug should not be used if there is evidence of hepatic disease. There is an impression that encephalopathic side-effects of valproate are more common in the elderly and these should be carefully monitored.

For all these reasons, valproate should be initiated in the elderly at lower doses than those used in younger adults. A recommended starting dosage is 200 mg/day, and this should be increased in 200 mg increments to an initial maintenance dose of 600 mg. Whether the slow-release ('chrono') formulation has any real advantage is unclear.

## THE TREATMENT OF EPILEPSY IN WOMEN

There are aspects of therapy that are specific to women with epilepsy.

### Fertility

Fertility rates have been shown to be lower in women with treated epilepsy than in an age-matched control population. In one study of a general population of 2,052,922 persons in England and Wales, the overall fertility rate was 47.1 (95% CI, 42.3–52.2) live births per 1000 women with epilepsy per year compared with a national rate of 62.6. The difference in rates was found in all age ranges between the ages of 20 and 39 years (Figure 2.7). The reasons for these lower rates are probably complex. There are undoubtedly social effects: women with epilepsy have low rates of marriage, marry later, and suffer social isolation and stigmatization. Some avoid having children because of the risk of epilepsy in the offspring, and some because of the teratogenic potential of antiepileptic drugs. Other patients have impaired personality or cognitive development. However, there are other biological factors that could lead to reduced fecundity. These include genetic factors, and adverse antiepileptic drug effects. The latter are discussed below. It has been estimated that about one-third of menstrual cycles in women with temporal lobe epilepsy may be anovulatory, compared with 8% in control populations. The lowering of fertility is a worrying finding which is another and important source of disadvantage for women with epilepsy.

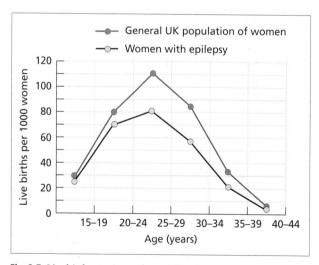

**Fig. 2.7** Live birth rates in mothers with epilepsy on treatment compared with general population (study of a UK population of over 2 million persons).

If there are potentially preventable causes, these should be sought.

Recently, one group of workers have found an association between valproate therapy and polycystic ovarian syndrome. This finding has become the subject of considerable marketing focus by other manufacturers, but the findings have not been widely duplicated and other workers have disputed the results; the evidence is therefore highly contradictory. Valproate can induce obesity, peripheral insulin resistance, hyperandrogenism and hyperinsulinaemia, and on theoretical grounds these could contribute to the induction of polycystic ovaries.

## Contraception

### Combined oral contraceptive

There is no reason why women with epilepsy should not take the combined oral contraceptive. However, drugs that induce hepatic enzyme activity (particularly CYP3A family enzymes—barbiturates, phenytoin, primidone, oxcarbazepine and carbamazepine) increase the metabolism of the oestrogen and progesterone components of the pill (sometimes by 50%) thereby reducing its efficacy. Topiramate lowers the level of oestrogen by 30% by a different mechanism. Patients co-medicated with these drugs therefore need higher doses of the pill to achieve contraceptive effect.

If women taking enzyme-inducing antiepileptic drugs wish to take the oral contraceptive pill, a preparation with at least 50 μg oestradiol should be safe in the majority of women, but not all. Breakthrough bleeding (mid-cycle bleeding) is a useful sign of inadequate oestrogenic effect, but it is not infallible, and contraceptive failure can occur without mid-cycle bleeding. Occasionally, 80 or even 100 μg oestradiol are needed for contraceptive effect. Alternatively, 'tricycling' a 50 μg oestrogen preparation can be employed, which entails taking three-monthly packets of the contraceptive without a break, followed by an interval of 4 days rather than the usual 7. Women should be advised that even using higher-dose preparations, there is a higher risk of contraceptive failure, and figures of three failures per 1000 women-years are quoted compared with the 0.3 per 1000 rate in the general population. It is also worth pointing out that the higher-dose contaceptives that are prescribed account for the increased metabolism, and the oestrogen levels attained are equivalent to those provided by lower-dose contraceptives in non-epileptic women. There is there-fore no excess risk of oestrogen-induced complications such as thrombosis.

There is no risk with non-CYP3A enzyme-inducing drugs (e.g. vigabatrin, valproate, clobazam, gabapentin, levetiracetam, pregabalin, valproate or vigabatrin). These drugs do not affect the metabolism of the combined pill and so a 30 μg oestradiol compound can be safely taken. However, the combined contraceptive pill tends to lower lamotrigine levels by 40–60%, so starting the pill in patients co-medicated with lamotrigine can result in poorer control, and higher drug dosage may be required. Lamotrigine can also reduce the effectiveness of the combined oral contraceptive.

In spite of the well-known risks of drug interaction, the inappropriate prescribing of low-dose contraceptives with enzyme-inducing drugs is widespread. In a large UK general practice survey, 17% (390/2341) of all women with epilepsy were on an oral contraceptive. Of these, 200 were co-medicated with an enzyme-inducing antiepileptic drug, and 44% (87 of the 200) were taking a contraceptive pill with less than 50 μg oestradiol. That this is a real problem is shown in one study which reported that 8.5% of pregnant epileptic women reported oral contraceptive failure.

### Progesterone-only preparation

The progesterone-only pill (the 'mini-pill') is affected in a similar manner, and patients should take at least double the usual dose or use alternative forms of contraception.

### Injectable contraceptives

Medroxyprogesterone acetate (Depo-Provera®) has no interactions with antiepileptics, as there is virtual 100% clearance on first pass through the liver, and enzyme induction should have no effect. The progestogen implant Implanon® is affected by enzyme-inducing drugs, and so should not be used in women with epilepsy.

### Post-coital contraception (the morning after pill)

The efficacy of this contraceptive is also affected by enzyme-inducing antiepileptic drugs, and so the first dose should be doubled and a second single dose given 12 hours later.

### Intra-uterine contraception (coils)

These are not affected by enzyme-inducing drugs.

## Menstruation and catamenial epilepsy

There is no doubt that in a sizeable proportion of women with active epilepsy, the pattern of seizures is related to the menstrual cycle. Oestrogen is mildly epileptogenic, and the high oestrogen concentration in the follicular phase of the menstrual cycle is a possible underlying cause for the greater propensity to seizures at this time. Premenstrual tension and water retention are other possible contributory factors.

Epilepsy in which the seizure pattern has a strong relationship to the menstrual cycle is referred to as catamenial epilepsy. There have been attempts to devise special treatment approaches to patients with catamenial seizures. Hormonal manipulation has been attempted with oral progesterone or norethisterone, with only marginal benefit. Attempts to abolish the menstrual cycle by hormonal means or even oophorectomy have had surprisingly disappointing results. In most patients seizures tend to continue at much the same frequency, albeit with some loss of pattern regularity. Intermittent antiepileptic therapy, taken around the risk period each month, has also been widely tried. Five to seven days' therapy with diuretics or acetazolamide has not proved generally successful. Clobazam, taken in the same manner, has shown more promise, with improvement noted in one study in 78% of women. This approach in routine clinical practice, however, produces a worthwhile effect in only a small number of women. Reasons for these disappointing results include irregularities of the cycle, the fact that the catamenial exacerbation is seldom reliably linked to any particular day of the cycle, and tolerance to the effects of clobazam.

## Teratogenicity of antiepileptic drugs

The first report of an antiepileptic drug-induced malformation was in 1963 (due to methphenytoin). In 1968, Meadows conducted a pioneering inquiry and concluded that congenital malformations were twice as common in children exposed *in utero* to antiepileptic drugs as would be expected in unexposed populations, and this has set the scene for numerous subsequent investigations, which have demonstrated conclusively that antiepileptics do increase the rate of malformations. Evidence includes: animal testing showing patterns of malformation similar to those seen clinically; drug-specific effects; malformation rates in the offspring of mothers with epilepsy on treatment are higher than those off treatment; mean antiepileptic drug levels are higher in the mothers of infants with malformations than in those without; and infants of mothers on polytherapy have higher malformation rates than those exposed to single-drug treatment. Factors complicating studies in this area, however, are the potential for seizures themselves to cause malformations, although this effect is probably small; social, dietary and socio-economic factors, resulting in greater maternal ill health; and maternal genetic factors that increase the risk of both epilepsy and malformations (particularly in idiopathic or cryptogenic epilepsy). Generally, however, carbamazepine and lamotrigine (at doses below, but not above, 200 mg/day) are amongst the safest drugs in pregnancy.

## Major malformations associated with antiepileptic drugs

The most common major malformations associated with traditional antiepileptic drug therapy (phenytoin, phenobarbital, primidone, benzodiazepine, valproate, carbamazepine) are cleft palate and cleft lip, cardiac malformations, neural-tube defects, hypospadias and skeletal abnormalities. Unfortunately, because most studies have been of women on multiple drug therapy, the risks of individual drugs are not fully established.

The risk of spina bifida has been particularly well studied. The background population risk of spina bifida is approximately 0.2–0.5% with geographical variation. Valproate is associated with a 1–2% risk of spina bifida aperta, a risk that is strongly dose-related. Carbamazepine carries a risk of spina bifida aperta of about 0.5–1%. It is instructive to note that the induction of neural-tube defects by valproate (and to a lesser extent carbamazepine) was not noticed in animal toxicology. The mechanism of production of drug-induced spina bifida may be different from that in unexposed populations. Both carbamazepine and valproate have been associated also with hypospadias.

The overall risk of malformations due to exposure with antiepileptic drugs are best studied using pregnancy registers. The UK register reports the following monotherapy malformations rates: overall 3.7%; carbamazepine 2.2%; valproate 6.2%; lamotrigine 3.2%; phenytoin 3.7%. The rates on valproate are lower at doses of < 100 mg; and at this dose approximate to rates on lamotrigine at doses > 200 mg. The major malformation rate on polytherapy was 6% overall, and 9% with combinations involving valproate and 4.5% with combinations involving carbamazepine.

One study purported to demonstrate smaller head circumference in babies of mothers on carbamazepine, but the statistical basis of this observation was not well founded. Small increases in rates of pre- and postnatal growth retardation have been found in controlled studies of mothers taking antiepileptics, but the growth differences had disappeared by the time the offspring were 5 years old.

It is not clear whether or not the benzodiazepines have any teratogenic potential, although there are case reports of facial clefts, and cardiac and skeletal abnormalities.

## Screening for fetal malformations

Some malformations can be detected in the prenatal phase. If therapeutic termination of pregnancy is acceptable, screening procedures should include, where appropriate, a high-quality ultrasound scan at 10, 18 and 24 weeks, measurement of alpha-fetoprotein levels, and amniocentesis. About 95% of significant neural-tube defects can be detected prenatally in this manner, as well as cleft palate and other midline defects, and major cardiac and renal defects. However, the mother should be informed that not all malformations are detectable even with the most sophisticated screening methods.

## Other developmental abnormalities

In addition to the major malformations, less severe dysmorphic changes ('fetal syndromes') have been postulated, although there is little agreement about their frequency or indeed even their existence. The problem is further complicated by the confounding influences of socio-economic and genetic factors. The fetal phenytoin syndrome was the first to be described, and is said to comprise a characteristic pattern of facial and limb disturbances (see Table 2.25). Most of these features, however, are minor and overlap with the normal variation seen in children born to healthy mothers. Recent prospective and blinded studies have shown that

**Table 2.25** Some features reported to occur in fetal anticonvulsant syndromes. This is a list of reported abnormalities, although many are uncontrolled observations and the frequency of the anomalies is unclear. The contribution of antiepileptic drugs is also unclear, and genetic, environmental and socio-economic factors may also have a role in their development.

*Growth*
- Pre- and postnatal growth deficiencies
- Microcephaly

*Craniofacial*
- Short nose, low cranial bridge
- Hypertelorism
- Epicanthic fold
- Strabismus and other ocular abnormalities
- Low-set ears and other aural abnormalities
- Wide mouth, and prominent lips
- Wide fontenelles
- Cleft palate and cleft lip

*Limbs*
- Hypoplasia of nails
- Transverse planar crease
- Short fingers
- Extra digits

*Cerebral*
- Learning disability
- Developmental delay

*General*
- Short neck, low hairline
- Rib, sternal and spinal anomalies
- Widely spaced hypoplastic nipples
- Hernias
- Undescended testicles
- Neuroblastoma and neural-ridge tumours
- Cardiac and renal abnormalities
- Hypospadias
- Neural-tube defects

only hypertelorism and distal digital hypoplasia occurred with any greater frequency, and even these associations are weak. Furthermore, the nail hypoplasia tends to disappear during childhood. Cases of a 'carbamazepine syndrome' are reported with craniofacial abnormalities, growth retardation, neural-tube defects and fingernail hypoplasia. Reports of primidone and phenobarbital 'syndromes' have been published, comprising facial changes and developmental delay. The complexity of the subject is shown by one report of four siblings with the classical 'hydantoin syndrome' born to a mother taking phenytoin and primidone for the first three pregnancies but only primidone during the fourth. A 'carbamazepine syndrome' has been claimed on the basis of a few case reports which are unconvincing. Finally, recent interest has focused on a 'valproate syndrome' said

to occur in up to 50% of infants born to mothers on valproate; again no blinded studies have been carried out and the true status of this syndrome is quite unclear.

Even greater controversy exists in relation to the question of whether maternal drug usage results in developmental delay and learning disability. While there is no doubt that these occur at a higher frequency among infants born to epileptic mothers (between a two- and sevenfold increase), the association could be due to genetic, environmental or socio-economic factors. A recent study showed that 41 children exposed to valproate monotherapy had significantly lower verbal IQ (VIQ) scores when compared with 52 children exposed to carbamazepine and 21 to phenytoin monotherapy. Low VIQ was also associated with the occurrence of five or more tonic–clonic seizures during pregnancy. There were also higher rates of dysmorphic features in the children exposed to valproate, and these were most common in those with low VIQ scores. Some caution needs to be exercised in interpreting these results. The study was a retrospective survey, the mothers were not randomized to different monotherapies, there was only a 40% response rate, and there are some inconsistencies, for instance, the fact that significant differences in VIQ rates were not found in fetuses exposed to valproate polytherapy, nor was there a significant dose response.

When considering the teratogenic potential of the newer antiepileptic drugs, three points from experience with the traditional therapies are worth making. First, even today, the full range of the teratogenicity has not been not established. Secondly, the risk of even major malformations was not noticed until the drugs had been in extensive use for decades. Thirdly, negative animal results are not a reliable indicator of safety. Any claims for safety for newer drugs should be taken in this context. Infants born to mothers taking vigabatrin with spina bifida, cleft palate, absent diaphragm, and conjoined twins have been reported. Topiramate, in animal models, causes right-sided ectrodactyly and rib and vertebral abnormalities, a pattern similar to that observed with acetazolamide, also a carbonic anhydrase inhibitor. No similar abnormalities have been reported in humans on carbonic anhydrase inhibitors, and none in the small number of topiramate pregnancies. Gabapentin causes hydroureter and hydronephrosis in rabbits, but there have been no reported human pregnancy abnormalities. Lamotrigine has not been associated with any consistent animal or human abnormalities, although human experience is limited. Currently the advice from the package inserts is to avoid the use of any of these drugs in pregnancy until more definitive advice can be given.

## Pregnancy
### Effects of epilepsy on pregnancy and delivery
About 3–4 live births per 1000 women of child-bearing age with epilepsy occur each year. Epilepsy has been reported

**Table 2.26** Complications of pregnancy that occur with increased frequency in women with epilepsy.

- Bleeding *in utero*
- Premature separation of the placenta
- Toxaemia of pregnancy and pre-eclampsia
- Miscarriage and stillbirth
- Intra-uterine growth retardation, low birth weight
- Perinatal mortality
- Premature labour
- Breech and other abnormal presentations
- Forceps delivery, induced labour, Caesarean section
- Precipitant labour
- Psychiatric disorders
- Seizures and status epilepticus

in retrospective (and therefore selected) series to increase by up to threefold the risks of various common complications (see Table 2.26). The perinatal mortality rate has been found to be twice that of the general population. No large-scale prospective investigation has been carried out, but there seems little doubt that these pregnancies require special consideration. The obstetrician may be more likely to recommend intervention and to manage the case in a distinctive manner. About 1–2% of all women with epilepsy will have tonic–clonic seizures during delivery and this can clearly complicate labour. The fetal heart rate can be dramatically slowed by a seizure, and fetal monitoring is recommended during vaginal delivery. Home birth should not generally be contemplated.

### Effect of pregnancy on the rate of seizures

Pregnancy has an unpredictable effect on the frequency of seizures. About one-third of women experience increased numbers of seizures, and this is especially likely in severe epilepsy. There are a number of potential causes including hormonal effects, non-compliance with medication, inappropriate dose reductions, changing drug disposition and serum levels, fluid retention, vomiting, stress, anxiety and sleep deprivation. A similar number of women have fewer seizures during pregnancy.

### The effect of seizures on the fetus

This is a controversial area. Clearly, in the latter stages of pregnancy, a convulsion carries the risk of trauma to the placenta or fetus, especially if the woman falls. However, most debate has revolved around the postulation that seizures damage the fetus through lactic acidosis or hypoxia. The hypoxia is usually very short-lived and the placenta is a well-buffered system, and these risks seem intuitively likely to be small. Fetal asphyxia manifested by prolonged bradycardia has been recorded after a maternal seizure, and one case of postictal fetal intracranial haemorrhage has

been recorded. However, these are probably exceptional, and in most situations isolated seizures are harmless. One study suggested that first-trimester seizures are accompanied by a higher risk of fetal malformation than seizures at other times, although methodological issues cloud the reliability of the conclusions. Stillbirth has been recorded after a single seizure or series of seizures, but this must be very rare. Partial seizures have no known effects upon a fetus.

Status epilepticus during pregnancy results in significant maternal and infant morbidity. A study of status epilepticus during delivery reported a 50% infant mortality and 30% maternal mortality.

### Folic acid supplementation

The fetus of an epileptic women is at a greater than expected risk of a neural-tube defect, particularly if the mother is taking valproate, but an association is also noted with exposure during pregnancy to other antiepileptics. A recent MRC trial of folic acid supplementation during pregnancy showed a 72% protective effect against neural-tube defects in women who had conceived a fetus previously with neural-tube defects, and a positive primary preventive action has also been demonstrated. Although there has been no specific study in epilepsy, it would seem reasonable for all epileptic women to be given folic acid supplementation during pregnancy, especially as many patients with epilepsy have low serum and tissue folate levels owing to enhanced drug-induced hepatic metabolism. This advice is given notwithstanding the weak evidence that folic acid may predispose to increased seizures. A dosage of at least 4 mg/day is recommended on an empirical basis, as lower dosage may not fully restore folate levels.

### Vitamin K

When the mother is taking enzyme-inducing antiepileptic drugs, the infant may be born with a relative deficiency of vitamin K-dependent clotting factors (factors II, VII, IX and X) and proteins C and S. This predisposes to infantile haemorrhage, including cerebral haemorrhage. The neonate should therefore receive 1 mg vitamin K IM at birth and at 28 days of life. Previous concern that IM vitamin K increased the risk of neuroblastoma has been dismissed, but there is possibly a slight increase in the rate of later acute lymphoblastic leukaemia. It is also sometimes recommended that the mother take oral vitamin K (20 mg/day) in the last trimester, although the evidence that this improves neonatal clotting is rather contradictory. If any two of the clotting factors fall below 50% of their normal values, IM vitamin K will be insufficient to protect against haemorrhage and fresh frozen plasma should be given intravenously. Similarly, if there is evidence of neonatal bleeding, or if concentrations of factors II, VII, IX or X fall below 25% of normal, an emergency infusion of fresh frozen plasma is required.

### New-onset epilepsy during pregnancy

The incidence of new-onset epilepsy at child-bearing age is about 20–30 cases per 100,000 persons, and so the development of epilepsy by chance during pregnancy is not uncommon. Occasionally, epileptic seizures occur only during pregnancy (gestational epilepsy) but this is a rare pattern.

Certain underlying conditions have a propensity to present during pregnancy. Some meningiomas grow in size faster during pregnancy owing to oestrogenic stimulation. Arteriovenous malformations are also said to present more commonly in pregnancy although evidence for this is weak. The risk of ischaemic stroke increases 10-fold in pregnancy. The underlying causes include arteriosclerosis, cerebral angiitis, moya-moya disease, Takayasu's arteritis, embolic disease from a cardiac or infective source, and primary cardiac disease. Haematological diseases can also present as stroke, including sickle cell disease, antiphospholipid antibody syndrome, thrombotic throbocytopenic purpura, and deficiencies in antithrombin, protease C and S, and factor V Leiden. There is also a higher incidence of subarachnoid haemorrhage and of cerebral venous thrombosis. Pregnancy can also predispose to cerebral infections due to bacteria (including *Listeria*), fungi (*Coccidioides*), protozoa (*Toxoplasma*), viruses, and HIV infection. Epilepsy can be the presenting symptom, or occur, in all these conditions. The extent of the investigation will depend on the clinical setting. X-radiation (including computerized tomography) should be avoided wherever possible. The risks of MRI to the developing fetus are unknown; nevertheless, MRI is the imaging modality of choice if urgent imaging is required. In the non-urgent situation, investigation should be deferred until the pregnancy is completed.

The treatment of new-onset epilepsy follows the same principles in the pregnant as in the non-pregnant person. The underlying cause may also need specific therapy.

### Eclampsia and pre-eclampsia

Most new-onset seizures in the late stages of pregnancy (after 20 weeks) are caused by eclampsia. Pre-eclampsia is characterized by hypertension, proteinuria, oedema, and abnormalities of hepatic function, platelets and clotting parameters. About 5% of cases, if left untreated, progress to eclampsia. The eclamptic encephalopathy results in confusion, stupor, focal neurological signs and cerebral haemorrhage as well as seizures. The epilepsy can be severe and progress rapidly to status. The incidence of eclampsia in Western Europe is about 1 in 2000 pregnancies, but it is more common in some developing countries with rates as high as 1 in 100. It carries a maternal mortality rate of between 2 and 5% and significant infantile morbidity and mortality.

Traditionally, obstetricians have used magnesium sulphate for the treatment of seizures in eclampsia, and the superiority of magnesium over phenytoin and/or diazepam has been clearly demonstrated in recent randomized controlled studies. Not only does magnesium confer better control of seizures, but there are fewer complications of pregnancy, and infant survival is better. Magnesium also seems to lessen the chance of cerebral palsy in low-birth-weight babies and has been shown to decrease secondary neuronal damage after experimental traumatic brain injury. The mechanism by which magnesium sulphate acts in eclampsia is unclear; it may do so via its influence on *N*-methyl-*D*-aspartate (NMDA) receptors or on free radicals, prostacyclin, other neurochemical pathways, or, more likely, by reversing the intense eclamptic cerebral vasospasm. It is possible that patients would benefit from magnesium and a conventional antiepileptic, but this has not been investigated. Magnesium sulphate should be administered as an IV infusion of 4 g over 5–15 minutes followed by an IV infusion of 1 g/hr for 24 hours. If seizures recur, an additional 2 g dose should be given by IV infusion.

### Management of labour

Regular antiepileptic drugs should be continued during labour. If oral feeding is not possible, IV replacement therapy can be given for at least some drugs. Tonic–clonic seizures occur in about 1–2% of susceptible mothers, and in patients at risk oral clobazam (10–20 mg) is useful when given at the onset of labour as additional seizure prophylaxis. Fetal monitoring is advisable. Most women have a normal vaginal delivery, but sleep deprivation, overbreathing, pain and emotional stress can greatly increase the risk of seizures. Elective Caesarean section should be considered in patients at particular risk. A history of status or life-threatening tonic–clonic seizures are an indication for a Caesarean section, and if severe seizures or status occur during delivery, an emergency Caesarean section should be performed. Intravenous lorazepam or phenytoin should be given during labour if severe epilepsy develops and the patient should be prepared for Caesarean section.

There is a maternal as well as infant mortality associated with severe seizures during delivery. The hypoxia consequent on a seizure may be more profound in gravid than in non-gravid women owing to the increased oxygen requirements of the fetus, and resuscitation facilities should be immediately at hand in the delivery suite.

### Puerperium

There is still an increased risk of seizures in the puerperium, and precautions may be necessary. It is sometimes helpful to continue clobazam for a few days after delivery to cover this period. If antiepileptic drug dosage had been increased owing to falling levels during pregnancy, the dosage should be returned during the first week to its previous levels; this is necessary as the pharmacokinetic changes of pregnancy are rapidly reversed in the puerperium. Drugs circulating in the mother's serum cross the placenta. If maternal antiepileptic drug levels were high, the infant may experience withdrawal symptoms (tremor, irritability, agitation, and even seizures) and neonatal serum levels should be measured in cases at risk.

### Breast-feeding

The concentration of most antiepileptic drugs in breast milk is less than 30% that of plasma; exceptions are concentrations of ethosuximide, gabapentin, lamotrigine, levetiracetam, phenobarbital and topiramate. Furthermore, even if a drug is present in significant concentrations in breast milk, the amount ingested by the infant is usually much less than would normally be considered necessary for clinical effects, and only in the cases of ethosuximide, lamotrigine, phenobarbital and primidone are significant doses absorbed. Thus, only with these drugs—and possibly levetiracetam, although data are sparse—are precautions necessary, at least at normal doses. The problem of lamotrigine is compounded if co-medication with valproate, which prolongs the half-life of the drug, is given. Particular caution is advised in the case of maternal phenobarbital ingestion, as in neonates the half-life of phenobarbital is long (up to 300 hours) and the free fraction is higher than in adults; neonatal levels can therefore sometimes exceed maternal levels. The neonatal half-lives of phenytoin and valproate are also increased (Table 2.27). Neonatal lethargy, irritability and feeding difficulties have also been attributed to maternal antiepileptic drug intake, although the evidence is slight, and these findings are not correlated with maternal drug dosage or serum level.

### Maternal epilepsy

A mother at risk from seizures with altered consciousness should not be left alone with a small child. There is a danger of dropping the child or leaving the child unattended, and maternal epilepsy probably poses a greater risk to infants and toddlers than to the fetus. Sensible precautions should be taken, such as avoiding carrying the child unaccompanied, changing and feeding the infant at ground level, and bathing the infant only when someone else is present.

## Reducing the risk of epilepsy in pregnancy to the mother and child
### Pre-conception review of drug therapy

The mother's antiepileptic drug regimen should be reviewed before conception, as most of the major malformations are established within the first trimester, many within the first 8 weeks. This is a counsel of perfection, often not realized, yet it is of great importance. Referral of a women for a review of drug therapy when she is 10 weeks' pregnant is thus too late to make changes which will minimize the teratogenic risks.

It is important to establish whether antiepileptic therapy is needed at all. This will be an individual decision, based on the estimated risk of exacerbation of seizures and their danger (remembering that tonic–clonic seizures can result in injury and occasionally death to both mother and fetus). The decision will balance the risks of teratogenicity against the risks of worsening epilepsy. Some women with partial or non-convulsive seizures will elect to withdraw therapy even if seizures are active or likely to become more frequent. Conversely, some women who are free of seizures will wish to continue therapy because of the social and physical risks of a recurrence of seizures.

In some patients it is reasonable to withdraw therapy for the first half of pregnancy and then to reinstate the drugs; this approach is based upon the fact that the teratogenic risk is greatest in the first trimester and the physical risk of seizures greatest in the later stages of pregnancy. The relative risks need to carefully assessed, however, and a specialist review is needed before embarking upon this unusual course.

**Table 2.27** Pharmacokinetic parameters of antiepileptic drugs transmitted to the fetus in breast milk.

| | Dose of antiepileptic drug acquired from breast milk (%)* | Breast milk : plasma concentration ratio | Elimination half-life (h) | |
| --- | --- | --- | --- | --- |
| | | | Adult | Neonate |
| Carbamazepine | < 5 | 0.3–0.4 | 5–26 | 8–28 |
| Ethosuximide | > 50 | 0.9 | 30–60 | 40 |
| Lamotrigine | > 50 | 0.6 | 12–60 | n/k |
| Phenobarbital | > 50 | 0.4–0.6 | 75–120 | 45–300 |
| Phenytoin | < 5 | 0.2–0.4 | 7–42 | 15–100 |
| Valproate | < 5 | 0.01 | 12–17 | 30–60 |

*, Amount of drug received in a fully breast-fed infant, expressed as a percentage of the lowest recommended daily therapeutic dose for an infant (personal communication from Dr M O'Brien); n/k, not known.

If the woman elects to continue therapy, the appropriate regimen in most cases is the minimally effective dose of the single antiepileptic that best controls the epilepsy. A few women with severe epilepsy will need combination therapy, but this should be avoided wherever possible.

It is useful to measure the serum drug concentrations that give optimal control of the epilepsy before contraception. These values form a starting point on which to base subsequent drug dosage adjustments.

### Drug dosage during pregnancy

If a pre-conception review has not been made, relevant drug adjustments should be made as soon as practicable, according to the principles listed above. However, it should be recognized that many of the major malformations are established within the first trimester, reducing the value of drug changes made after this. Once optimal therapy has been established, the use of antiepileptic drugs is relatively straightforward. It is important to emphasize the need for compliance. Dosage adjustments should be based upon serum levels, which should be monitored regularly (at least three monthly) during pregnancy. Dosage increases may be necessary as the serum levels of some antiepileptic drugs fall markedly especially in the last trimester. Levels of lamotrigine may be halved, and levels of phenytoin, phenobarbital, carbamazepine and valproate can be markedly reduced. Folic acid supplementation should be initiated in all patients who are or have recently been taking antiepileptic drugs and vitamin K should be given (see p. 105).

### Screening for fetal malformations

Some malformations can be detected in the prenatal phase. If therapeutic termination of pregnancy is acceptable, screening procedures should include, where appropriate, a high-quality ultrasound scan at 10, 18 and 24 weeks, measurement of alpha-fetoprotein levels, foetal MRI and amniocentesis. About 95% of significant neural-tube defects can be detected prenatally in this manner, as well as cleft palate, major cardiac kidney and midline defects, and thus ultrasound protocols such as these can almost (but not completely) eliminate the risk of a live birth with these malformations.

# THE TREATMENT OF PSYCHIATRIC DISORDERS IN EPILEPSY

There is a huge and contradictory literature on the psychiatric risks of epilepsy. In summary, most studies suggest, at a rough approximation, that about one-third to half of people with epilepsy have psychiatric difficulties, in a broad and vaguely defined sense. The precise incidence depends on the population studied and what conditions are included and what definitions are applied. Estimates have varied widely. In an influential study in the 1950s, 28% of 245 patients with epilepsy in a general population reported psychosocial difficulties, and overall psychiatric morbidity in epilepsy was estimated to range from 20 to 50%. In a reliable population-based study, the rate of psychiatric disorders among children with epilepsy was as high as 27%, compared with 7% in the general population. By contrast, in a more recent study in adults the prevalence of psychiatric disturbances was only mildly increased in patients with epilepsy (19% vs. 15%) compared with sex- and age-matched controls. In a study of 512 persons with epilepsy in Iceland, 7% had been psychotic at some point in time. The more chronic or more severe the epilepsy, the higher the rate of psychiatric disorders. The cause of psychiatric disturbances in epilepsy is probably multifactorial and includes the biological effects of seizures, the genetic and neurological context of the epilepsy, the effects of drugs, and social factors.

### Psychosis

Psychosis in epilepsy is usually differentiated into chronic, alternating and postictal categories.

#### Chronic psychosis

A grumbling interictal psychosis, with occasional exacerbation, is often seen in patients with severe epilepsy. Psychotic features may be quite mild, and complicated by irritability, anxiety, paranoia and dysphoria. In most cases antipsychotic medication is required. Sulpiride is a good drug for mild psychosis, and its additional anxiolytic effects can be helpful. During acute exacerbations of psychotic behaviour, risperidone, olanzapine or quetiapine may become necessary. Sometimes exacerbations of interictal psychosis are prolonged and non-responsive to treatment. In these cases clozapine can be used, but it can precipitate seizures and also carries a significant risk of leucopenia, and close monitoring of blood counts is necessary. Electroconvulsive therapy (ECT) has occasionally been used, and is often strikingly effective, but there is a theoretical risk of ECT-induced status epilepticus.

#### Alternative psychosis and forced normalization

In some patients periods of seizure control and normalized EEG appear to be associated with the development of psychoses, which is reversed when seizures recur (the phenomenon as applied to EEG is sometimes known as 'forced normalization'). However, the opposite pattern is also observed, and the true status of forced normalization is rather contentious. The exact mechanism of this pattern is unclear. Antipsychotics, antidepressants and anxiolytic drugs, as appropriate, can be used to treat these episodes. In some individuals the psychosis may be due in part to the introduction of an antiepileptic drug (associated with the remission of seizures), and the replacement of this drug by others is worthwhile. In exceptional cases it is deemed better to allow seizures to continue rather than risk psychotic breakdown.

### Postictal psychosis

This typically occurs, with a brief delay, after an exacerbation of seizures. Benzodiazepines are effective in controlling the psychosis in many cases, and it is possible that the psychotic manifestations relate to ongoing seizure activity (in effect status) in limbic structures. During the psychotic episode, lorazepam is the drug of choice, and is sometimes sufficient alone. In other cases, antipsychotic drugs are needed. Patients with postictal psychosis can show violent, aggressive or destructive behaviour, and admission to hospital is needed. After repeated episodes of postictal psychosis, some individuals develop a more chronic interictal psychotic state.

### Depression and anxiety

Conventional mood disorders are encountered in many patients with epilepsy, and these include anxiety, depression, dysthymia and panic disorders. Intermittent affective-somatoform symptoms are frequently present in chronic epilepsy and include irritability, depressive moods, anergia, insomnia, atypical pains, anxiety, phobic fears and euphoric moods. Some are present continually but others show marked variation in relation to seizure activity. Prodromal and peri-ictal dysphoria are common.

Both depression and anxiety in epilepsy respond to conventional antidepressant drugs. Tricyclic antidepressants and selective serotonin reuptake inhibitors (SSRIs) are routinely given. Fluoxetine is a widely prescribed drug, although it is a powerful CYP3A4 inhibitor and can interact with carbamazepine and other antiepileptics. Other SSRIs commonly used in patients with epilepsy include paroxetine and citalopram. Paroxetine does not interact with common antiepileptic drugs. Citalopram may be particularly beneficial in the subgroup of patients with mixed anxiety and depression. ECT is occasionally necessary in unremitting major depression. All the anti-depressant drugs have a mild proconvulsant action, and there is probably little difference between them in this regard. However, in patients with existing epilepsy, if depression is present to the extent that it requires anti-depressant therapy, the benefits of therapy generally greatly outweigh the proconvulsant risk.

It is a common practice to add an anxiolytic drug during the initial phase of treatment, before the antidepressant can produce its full therapeutic effects. The anxiolytic drug is slowly withdrawn when the action of the antidepressant becomes fully manifest, which may take between 4 and 6 weeks. This practice is particularly helpful because during the initial phases of therapy many antidepressants may provoke rather than control anxiety. Drugs such as clobazam and lorazepam are the drugs usually prescribed. Prophylactic antidepressants are sometimes given to patients with dysphoria around seizures. Clobazam can be used in short-lived dysphoria occurring around seizures, or in catamenial dysphoric disorders.

### Personality disorders

Much has been written on personality disorders in patients with epilepsy, much based on little firm evidence. Furthermore, the biological effects of the epilepsy, the effects of drug treatment, and the secondary handicap of living with epilepsy or growing up with epilepsy may all contribute to personality difficulties. It must also be stressed that most patients with epilepsy have perfectly normal personalities.

Specific patterns of personality disturbance have been postulated. These include a triad of disorders in temporal lobe epilepsy consisting of changes in sexual behaviour (usually a decreased interest in sexual matters), hypergraphia (compulsive writing) and hyper-religiosity (an expansive interest in religious matters). Laterality of the seizure focus is also reported to influence personality difficulties, although evidence here seems especially poor. Those with left-sided epileptogenic foci are said to be more ideative (i.e. to have philosophical interests, sense of personal destiny), with a tendency to have a poor opinion about themselves ('tarnish their own image'), whereas persons with right-sided foci have been described as being more emotional, with a tendency to alternate between periods of sadness and elation, and to have a high opinion of themselves ('polish their own image')—this has been referred to as the syndrome of temporal hyperconnection. This contrasts with the Klüver–Bucy syndrome of disconnection, which is associated with hypermetamorphosis (as opposed to viscosity and attention to detail), inappropriate hypersexuality (as opposed to hyposexuality), and placidity (as opposed to emotional intensity). It has also been pointed out that some of these personality traits in mildzforms have positive implications, in that they make these persons honest, reliable, dependable, and upstanding members of the community. Patients with juvenile myoclonic epilepsy have been reported as having a tendency to show immaturity and lability of mood and emotion, although again, evidence to support these propositions is poor.

The treatment of personality problems in epilepsy can be difficult. As in all other personality disorders, the mainstay of therapy is psychological treatments such as cognitive behavioural therapy, psychotherapy, counselling and supportive psychotherapy. These should be aimed at helping the individual and those in his/her environment to identify and to cope with the specific problem areas. A careful choice of antiepileptic drug could prevent or minimize disruption due to intermittent behavioural instability. Some patients require antidepressants or anxiolytic therapy. Antipsychotic agents are helpful in those prone to significant irritability, outbursts of temper and bouts of aggression. A low-potency antipsychotic such as sulpiride, administered continuously, can be a useful adjunctive therapy and prevent adverse behavioural exacerbations in some individuals.

### Disorders of sexual function

Hyposexuality has been long recognized as a feature of epilepsy in both men and women. Between 30 and 60% of men with epilepsy have reported lack of desire and impotence, and in one study 21% of men with chronic epilepsy had not experienced sexual intercourse. Among women, self reports of dyspareunia, vaginismus and arousal insufficiency are common, and also dissatisfaction with sexual experience. There are a number of potential mechanisms. Clearly the psychosocial difficulties encountered by people with epilepsy could play a part, including stigmatization, lack of self-esteem, restricted life styles, parental overprotection, and depression and anxiety. Biological changes including altered levels of sex hormones (especially free levels) are found in epilepsy, owing to the seizures and to the drug therapy; these too could contribute to sexual difficulties. Seizures involving limbic structures too might be expected to alter sexual behaviour, and there is evidence (albeit inconclusive) that those with temporal lobe epilepsy have a greater degree of sexual dysfunction than those with generalized epilepsy. Antiepileptic drugs can alter the metabolism of sex hormones and affect their protein binding. Epilepsy surgery can also profoundly change, usually lowering, sexual drive. Treatment should begin with a careful analysis of potential causes (some of which may, of course, be quite independent of the epilepsy or its treatment). Psychosexual counselling can be very helpful. Control of seizures and reduction of antiepileptic therapy (including the withdrawal of sedative drugs) may improve sexual functioning, as can individual or couple sexual therapy.

### Acute psychotic or depressive states induced by antiepileptic drugs

Although many antiepileptic drugs have a role in the management of bipolar disorder, virtually all these drugs have also been reported to precipitate severe adverse psychiatric reactions, notably acute psychosis or depression. The risk seems greatest in patients with a previous history of psychiatric disorders. How frequently this occurs is not clearly known, but levetiracetam, phenobarbital, topiramate and vigabatrin carry perhaps the greatest risk. These antiepileptic drugs should be used with caution in patients with concurrent psychosis, and carbamazepine or valproate might be preferred options.

Many of the drugs can also cause mild psychiatric symptoms, particularly feelings of depression, anxiety or irritation. Levetiracetam seems particularly to cause irritability and dysphoria (a 'short fuse') in a small number of patients, and vigabatrin and tiagabine can cause significant agitation. Barbiturate and benzodiazepine drugs can also cause agitation and behavioural changes, especially in children and those with pre-existing cerebral damage or learning disability.

### Psychiatric disturbance and personality change after epilepsy surgery

Epilepsy surgery carries a risk of precipitating psychiatric disturbance. The most common problems are mood swings, anxiety and depression. These are seen in 20–30% of people who undergo surgery for epilepsy. Although distressing, these are generally mild and remit within weeks or months, although some people may need antidepressant medication or counselling.

More severe psychiatric breakdown may also occur. In a recent study of subjects who had undergone epilepsy surgery in London, about 10% of patients undergoing temporal lobectomy suffered a depressive or psychotic episode after surgery of a severity that required hospitalization, and many more needed consultation and treatment. Compounding these problems is the fact that no pre-operative risk-factors have been identified that reliably predict post-operative psychiatric disturbance. The lack of pre-operative psychopathology does not seem to protect against post-operative anxiety or depression. There is also no clear relationship between psychiatric disturbance and either the lateralization of the operation or the nature of the pathological tissue.

The occurrence of personality change after surgery is a poorly studied subject, but one of great concern. Various changes have been well documented, but their frequency and the factors predictive of risk are largely unknown. Well recognized are changes in sexuality (usually hyposexuality), emotionality (flattening of emotional responses), impulsivity and obsessive–compulsive disorders. Anxiety, depression, personality change and psychotic breakdown can also occur after temporal lobe resections.

Counselling patients in this situation is difficult. In general patients, particular caution must be communicated to patients with a strong past or family history of psychopathology, as they have inherent biological vulnerability. While it is not clear if co-morbid psychopathology *per se* increases the risk of post-operative psychopathology, the burden of surgery is likely to be greater in someone who has an ongoing psychiatric illness. Also, candidates for surgery with poor psychosocial support, strained personal and familial circumstances, poor understanding of the process or unreasonable expectations are especially likely to develop post-operative psychopathology.

## COMPLEMENTARY AND ALTERNATIVE THERAPY IN EPILEPSY

A definition of complementary therapy is 'treatment that complements mainstream medicine by contributing to a common whole, by satisfying a demand not met by ortho-doxy, or by diversifying the conceptual frameworks of medicine'. One survey of 230 neurological outpatients found that 30% had used a non-conventional treatment in the previous year, and there is no doubt that many patients feel dissatisfied by conventional therapy and seek what they consider more natural and more gentle treatments. In epilepsy, a wide variety of techniques and therapies have been tried, although it has to be said that few have a sci-entific basis or have clearly established effectiveness by con-temporary scientific standards. Whitmarsh has provided a comprehensive and critical review, and this text borrows heavily from this. He has divided complementary therapies into psychological/behavioural therapies, exercise, herbal medicine, dietary measures, music therapy, exercise, homo-eopathy, acupuncture, transcranial magnetic stimulation and chiropractic therapy.

### Psychological therapies to reduce seizure frequency

These are known as 'countermeasures' and various differ-ent approaches have been attempted, including hypnosis, meditation, yoga, biofeedback, operant or classical con-ditioning, and changing arousal levels. Stress reduction techniques of various types are very commonly employed in epilepsy, and have undoubted benefit, although there are few controlled studies in this important area. There is a report of hypnosis that reduced Jacksonian seizures on one patient from 35·to 5 per week. Meditation (of various forms) and yoga (and similar techniques) are commonly em-ployed by patients with epilepsy, and have an enthusiastic following. There is at least one open study of meditation that showed a moderate benefit in reducing seizures and also changes in EEG parameters. Similarly, relaxation methods are widely practised and there are at least four controlled studies that show benefit. In one study a 29% decrease in the frequency of seizures occurred in those trained in progressive muscular relaxation techniques, which was significantly better than in a control group of those treated by 'sitting quietly'. EEG biofeedback has been extensively studied. This is an operant conditioning technique which aims to alter EEG rhythms of impend-ing seizures. There is quite clear experimental evidence in cats, as well as less clear human data, which show positive effects. In one combined analysis of 18 studies, 82% of 174 patients ·showed seizure reductions of at least 30% when biofeedback was employed. It has been claimed that most epileptic patients who show clinical improvement with EEG biofeedback also show contingency-related EEG changes and a shift towards EEG normalization. However, not all responders show EEG changes, and some patients who do show EEG changes show little clinical response. A few individual patients have been rendered seizure-free and have been able to withdraw from antiepileptic drug therapy.

### Other non-pharmacological therapies

Exercise has been clearly shown to improve the control of seizures in a number of studies, from institutions and outpatient clinics. A mean 40% reduction in seizures was observed in one study of aerobic dancing. Acupuncture has been used for thousands of years to treat epilepsy. There is some published animal experimental evidence of efficacy, and anecdotal accounts of long-term reduction of seizures and even status epilepticus. One study showed improvement in 89% of 98 cases treated with courses of scalp electro-acupuncture (30 minutes of electrical stimulation to the scalp at 2–3.5 Hz given daily for 15 days and repeated with a week-long break between courses). Well-conducted con-trolled studies, however, have failed to show benefit. There are case reports of chiropractic therapy reporting huge improvements in individual patients. Correcting 'upper cervical malalignment' in a 6-year-old, for instance, was reported to reduced the frequency of absence seizures from 25 per day to less than one per day. Another case report purported to show that chiropractic adjustment at the C6–C7 level aborted all seizure activity in a 21-year-old woman who previously had daily convulsive seizures. There is, however, a complete absence of published investigations with any controlled methodology. Finally, mention should be made of 'music therapy'. Normalization of the EEG in 23 of 29 epileptic patients listening to a Mozart sonata for two pianos (K448) for 10 minutes has been clearly demon-strated (the 'Mozart effect'), and there is one case report of an 8-year-old girl with Lennox–Gastaut syndrome whose seizures were greatly reduced by listening to the sonata for 10 minutes per hour. Other musical forms have had some success.

### Herbal medicine and homoeopathy

Herbal medicine is widely used in epilepsy in many parts of the world. In a recent review, 150 plants were said to be recorded as used in traditional medicines, and 10 were thought to warrant further investigation. The Chinese mixture *Saiko-Keishi-To* is made up of nine plants. In one recent open study, when given to 24 patients with frequent seizures, six became seizure-free and 13 improved in the frequency or severity of seizures, and in another study there was a reduction in seizures of at least 25% in 33% of patients. There are no controlled studies of homoeopathic remedies in epilepsy, but open-case series demonstrate some improvements. However, homoeopathic clinics, in the UK at least, do not on the whole make many claims for efficacious remedies in epilepsy.

### Special diets and nutritional supplements

The ketogenic diet is widely accepted now as main-line therapy for a few children with severe epilepsy (see p. 96). However, other diets are also used widely as complement-ary therapies. The Atkins diet (60% fat, 30% protein and

10% carbohydrate) has gained favour, no doubt because of its superficial resemblance to the ketogenic diet (typically 80% fat, 15% protein and 5% carbohydrate). In a small open study of six children and adults, 50% became seizure-free. The best results were seen in those who attained ketosis. Fasting also undoubtedly helps epilepsy, and on this basis, low carbohydrate diets have been attempted and have advocates. Oligoantigenic diets are widely used in paediatric practice, and have been the subject of limited scientific investigation. One interesting double-blind study in a 19-year-old woman with frequent seizures, a history of allergies and eosinophilia was carried out. She was found by an elimination diet to be sensitive to beef. Seizures occurred soon after taking capsules containing beef, but not chicken, and she remained free from seizures long term by avoiding any beef products, having stopped anticonvulsant medication. Diets are also commonly employed by patients with adult epilepsy. I have had one patient who was convinced that eating eggs stopped his seizures. Other patients have tried gluten-free diets with some success.

Nutritional supplements are very commonly used by patients, and all sorts of combinations of vitamins and trace elements are widely sold—and various spurious analytical procedures of hair and other tissue are available to try to ascertain 'deficiencies'. Vitamin E at a dosage of 400 IU/day has been formally studied in one double-blind study in which there was a responder rate of 83%. Vitamin D (at doses of between 4000 and 16,000 IU/day) has in open studies reduced the frequency of seizures by about 30%. However, at an anecdotal level in normal clinic practice, neither vitamin D nor E has proved at all efficacious. Supplements of selenium, zinc, manganese and magnesium have all been reported to improve seizure control in some patients and are widely used. Beta-hydroxybutyrate is a food supplement that has been the subject of a number of studies, and can induce ketosis in high doses.

## GENETIC COUNSELLING IN EPILEPSY

Hippocrates recognized over 2000 years ago that epilepsy was a 'genetic disorder', and in recent years the importance of genetic factors has been rediscovered. Counselling on this topic has become an important part of contemporary practice. Epilepsy, however, is a heterogeneous condition, and genetic influences will vary in different syndromes and aetiologies.

### Single-gene disorders
In Section 1 (pp. 26–42) some of the single-gene disorders underlying epilepsy are described, and counselling in these conditions should always be carried out. This will depend on adequate identification of the mutations, and this can involve genetic, biochemical or histochemical investigation. In general terms, genetic counselling depends on the mode of inheritance, although variations in penetrance, which may depend on other genes or environmental factors, complicate this. Furthermore, for some conditions (e.g. generalized epilepsy with febrile seizures [GEFS+]) there may be a large number of disease-producing mutations at different loci in different genes, and genetic analysis may be difficult or impossible in routine clinical practice. In this situation, counselling will fall back on careful examination of relatives and the pattern of inheritance.

### Autosomal dominant inheritance
If there is full penetrance, there is a 50% risk to offspring and siblings. Unaffected members of the family carry no risk of transmission. In conditions that are not fully penetrant, the siblings and offspring have a risk of carrying the gene without expressing the phenotype, the risk depending on the extent of penetrance. Examples of autosomal dominant 'pure epilepsies' are benign familial neonatal seizures (0.85 penetrance), autosomal dominant nocturnal frontal lobe epilepsy (ADNFLE; 0.9 penetrance), and GEFS+ (variable penetrance). Other autosomal dominant conditions with epilepsy include tuberous sclerosis, DRPLA, acute intermittent porphyria, and NF1.

### Autosomal recessive inheritance
The siblings of probands will have a 25% chance of being affected, a 25% chance of inheriting one disease-causing allele and being a carrier, and a 25% chance of inheriting both normal alleles and being unaffected. The normal siblings of a proband have a 2/3 chance of being a carrier. The offspring of a proband are all obligate heterozygotes. The chance of disease in subsequent generations depends on the frequency of the affected allele in the population and thus the rate of mating between two heterozygotes. Most inherited neurological conditions causing epilepsy are inherited in this manner, including Unverricht–Lundborg disease, sialidosis, neuronal ceroid lipofuscinosis, and many inherited enzyme deficiencies (pp. 28–35).

### X-linked inheritance
The mutations are usually transmitted from heterozygous healthy females (carriers) to 50% of their offspring. Male offspring will have the disease, because they lack the second normal copy of the gene (hemizygosity). Fifty per cent of male siblings will inherit the disease. Fifty per cent of female siblings will be carriers and 50% will be normal. Female offspring will be carriers. In most diseases female carriers will be healthy, although in some conditions minor signs of the disease can be detected (owing to inactivation of one X chromosome). There is no male-to-male transmission of the disease. Uncommonly, some X-linked genes show a dominant effect and heterozygous females express the

full phenotype and males do not survive. An example of a typical recessive X-linked condition with epilepsy is Rett syndrome. LISS1 lissencephaly and periventricular nodular heterotopia are examples of dominant X-linked conditions.

### Mitochondrial inheritance

The conditions are transmitted in the maternal line, and individuals with no clinical signs can transmit the disease. There is marked variation in the severity and manifestations of the disease. This is because the proportion of mutated mtDNA varies among different cells; in some cells all mitochondria carry the mutated mtDNA (homoplasmy), while in others only a fraction of mtDNA is mutated (heteroplasmy). Expression of the disease is strongly influenced by the amount and the tissue distribution of mutated mtDNA. The proportion of offspring affected also varies for the same reason, and the offspring or sibling risk of manifesting the disease cannot be predicted. An examples of an epilepsy inherited mitochondrially is progressive myoclonus due to MERRF.

### Complex inheritance

Most common disorders show a complex aetiology that includes genetic and environmental factors. In these disorders, the disease develops when several gene-producing mutations co-exist. There may be affected family members, but usually not very many. Affected members are more likely to be close relatives. The risk of recurrence for different degree relatives indicates the complexity of the genetic component. The higher the concordance rate among monozygotic twins, the stronger the contribution of genetic factors to the disorder. The lower the risk for relatives of probands, the higher is the number of genetic factors involved. Many forms of epilepsy show a complex inheritance, and recurrence risks can be estimated only from empirical data based on the number of affected members and the degree of relationship. Four epilepsy syndromes with complex inheritance have been specifically studied.

### Idiopathic generalized epilepsy (IGE)

For most sporadic cases, the risk of developing IGE in first-degree relatives is about 5–15%, and the risk to a second-degree or more distant relative is hardly elevated and close to that in the general population. A concordance rate of about 70–80% exists in monozygotic twins, increasing to 90% when EEG changes are considered. The Rochester study established the following risk estimates. The risk for siblings was 6%, increasing to 8% if photosensitivity is found in the proband or if a parent has epilepsy, to 12% when a parent also shows generalized EEG abnormalities, and to 15% when the sibling shows a generalized EEG trait. The risk to offspring of an affected individual was 4–6% (8.7% in female and 2.5% in male offspring).

An interesting feature of IGE is its clinical variability within a family. In a study of 74 families with at least three affected members, only 25% of the families were concordant for a specific IGE syndrome. In various studies, putative susceptibility loci have been localized on chromosomes 3p, 6p, 8p, 8q, 5p, and 5q. So far no genes or genetic mutations have been found that are clearly associated with the generality of cases.

Occasional large families are found with many affected members and these families have higher risks. Genes for rare autosomal dominant subsets have been mapped or identified for childhood absence epilepsy (CAE) (chromosome 8q) and for JME (chromosome 6p and the *GABRA1* gene on chromosome 5q).

### Benign epilepsy with centro-temporal spikes (BECTS)

The genetics of this condition are complex and ill understood. Concordance in monozygotic twins has varied from 0 to 100% in different studies. For most sporadic cases, the risk of developing epilepsy in first-degree relatives is about 15%, rising to 30% if centro-temporal EEG abnormalities are found. Rolandic epilepsy has also been found to segregate in association with other very rare Mendelian neurological conditions such as autosomal dominant rolandic epilepsy with speech dyspraxia, and autosomal recessive rolandic epilepsy with paroxysmal exercise-induced dystonia and writer's cramp.

### Severe myoclonic epilepsy of infancy (SMEI)

This sporadic condition is caused by mutations in the neuronal sodium channel gene *SCN1A* during gametogenesis. This explains its genetic but not inherited basis. Genetic analysis of the *SCN1A* gene is possible, and the identification of *de novo* mutations can exclude any increased risks for relatives.

### Febrile seizures

In monozygotic twins 35–70% clinical concordance has been found. Population-based studies have shown an increased risk for first-degree relatives ranging from 8% in Caucasians to up to 20% in Japanese. In most cases, inheritance seems likely to be polygenic, although there are a few reported large families with dominant inheritance. From the counselling point of view, it is therefore important to gain a detailed family history before estimating risk rates. There is also a two- to 10-fold increased risk of developing later afebrile seizures. Affected individuals in GEFS+ families have mutations on *SCN1A*, *SCN2A*, *SCN1B* and *GABRG2* genes, but these are not common in sporadic cases. One locus on chromosome 19p has also been found in a single family with apparently autosomal dominantly inherited febrile seizures.

# 3

# The antiepileptic drugs

## CARBAMAZEPINE

| | |
|---|---|
| **Primary indications** | Partial and generalized seizures (excluding absence and myoclonus). Also in childhood epilepsy syndromes. Adults and children |
| **Licensed for monotherapy/add-on therapy** | Both |
| **Usual preparations** | Tablets: 100, 200, 400 mg; chewtabs: 100, 200 mg; slow-release formulations: 200, 400 mg; liquid: 100 mg/5 ml; suppositories: 125, 250 mg |
| **Usual dosage—adults** | Initial: 100 mg at night<br>Maintenance: 400−1600 mg/day (maximum 2400 mg)<br>(Slow-release formulation, higher dosage) |
| **Usual dosage—children** | < 1 year, 100−200 mg/day<br>1−5 years, 200−400 mg/day<br>5−10 years, 400−600 mg/day<br>10−15 years, 600−1000 mg<br>(Slow-release formulation, higher dosage) |
| **Dosing intervals** | 2−3 times/day (2−4 times/day at higher doses or in children) |
| **Dose commonly affected by co-medication** | Yes |
| **Dose affected by renal/hepatic disease** | Severe hepatic disease |
| **Common drug interactions** | Extensive drug interactions; see p. 116 |
| **Serum level monitoring** | Useful |
| **Target range** | 20−50 µmol/l |
| **Common/important adverse events** | Drowsiness, fatigue, dizziness, ataxia, diplopia, blurring of vision, sedation, headache, insomnia, gastrointestinal disturbance, tremor, weight gain, impotence, effects on behaviour and mood, hepatic disturbance, rash and other skin reactions, bone marrow dyscrasia, leucopenia, hyponatraemia, water retention, endocrine effects |
| **Mechanism of action** | Inhibition of voltage-dependent sodium conductance. Also action on monoamine, acetylcholine, and NMDA receptors |
| **Main advantages** | Highly effective and usually well-tolerated therapy |
| **Main disadvantages** | Adverse effects, especially on initiating therapy; occasional severe toxicity |
| **COMMENT** | Well-established therapy. A drug of first choice in adults and children for many types of epilepsy |

Carbamazepine (CBZ) is the veritable work-horse of the antiepileptic drugs. Initial open clinical trials were carried out in the 1950s, and since then it has become established as the major first-line antiepileptic drug for partial and secondarily generalized seizures. It is the most commonly prescribed drug in Europe for epilepsy, and is very widely used worldwide. It was originally developed in the search for new antipsychotic compounds as an alternative to chlorpromazine. Disappointingly, no strong effect against psychosis was noticed, and then, as has been the case for many antiepileptics, its value in epilepsy was discovered largely by chance. Its analgesic effect in trigeminal neuralgia was later investigated, when it was shown in cat experiments to have a particularly strong effect on the trigeminal reflex. It is a tricyclic compound and is also widely used for the treatment of depression, other psychiatric syndromes, neuropathic pain syndromes, and trigeminal neuralgia.

### Physical and chemical characteristics

Carbamazepine (5H-dibenzyl[b,f]azepine-5-carboxamide, molecular weight 236.3) is a crystalline substance, which is virtually insoluble in water, but highly soluble in lipid and organic solvents. It is stable at room temperatures, but its bioavailability can be reduced by up to 50% by hot or humid conditions or when there has been absorption of moisture, and so care is needed in storage.

### Mode of action

Carbamazepine binds to the neuronal sodium channel, pre- and post-synaptically, and this binding results in a use- and frequency-dependent blockade of the channel. This is its main mode of action (an mode shared by phenytoin and lamotrigine), although a blockade of *N*-methyl-D-aspartate (NMDA)-receptor activated sodium and calcium flux may also be contributory. It has also been proposed that carbamazepine acts on other receptors including the purine, monoamine and acetylcholine receptors.

## Pharmacokinetics

### Absorption

As there is no IV formulation, bioavailability measurements can be estimates only, but it appears that generally speaking between 75 and 85% of the drug is absorbed following oral ingestion. Absorption, however, can be slow and erratic, there is a marked intra-individual variation, and different formulations may have different absorption characteristics. It does not appear to make any difference whether the drug is taken before or after food. Peak levels are reached between 4 and 8 hours after absorption. Preparations of carbamazepine in sorbitol do exist for rectal administration, but are not used in routine clinical practice. There is no parenteral preparation of carbamazepine currently marketed, although intravenous formulations are under development.

### Distribution

Approximately 75–80% of the drug is bound to plasma proteins. The free fraction of carbamazepine ranges from 20 to 24% of the total plasma concentration, and CSF carbamazepine levels vary in a range between 17 and 31%. The relationship between dose and plasma concentrations, in the normal clinical range, is linear, but there is a large inter- and intra-individual variability in the protein binding and the ratio of bound to unbound drug. Salivary levels bear a good and constant relationship to free blood levels, and can be a useful method of assaying drug concentrations. Hair concentrations are also reliably related to dose, and can also be used to monitor compliance. The apparent volume of distribution of carbamazepine is between 0.8 and 2.0 l/kg in adults, and of the 10,11-epoxide it is 0.59–1.5 l/kg. Brain levels are somewhat higher than plasma levels, for both CBZ-epoxide and parent drug, and there appears to be rather non-specific binding of carbamazepine to brain tissue, uninfluenced by gliosis.

### Biotransformation and excretion

Carbamazepine is extensively metabolized in the liver. The major pathway is first epoxidation to carbamazepine 10,11-epoxide (CBZ-epoxide) and then hydrolysis to carbamazepine 10,11-trans-dihydrodiol. There are also other conjugated and unconjugated metabolites and less than 1% of the drug is excreted unchanged in the urine. The main liver enzyme involved in carbamazepine metabolism is cytochrome P450 CYP3A4. The drug induces its own metabolism and there is a marked increase in clearance and a fall of about 50% in serum half-life during the first few weeks of carbamazepine therapy. This auto-induction is usually completed within a month. After a single dose, the elimination half-life is between 20 and 65 hours, but

---

**Carbamazepine**
Pharmacokinetics—average adult values

| | |
|---|---|
| Oral bioavailability | 75–85% |
| Time to peak levels | 4–8 h |
| Volume of distribution | 0.8–2 l/kg |
| Biotransformation | Hepatic epoxidation and hydroxylation, and then conjugation (cytochrome P450 enzymes CYPS3A4, CYP2C8m CYP1A2; UDPGT family enzymes) |
| Elimination half-life | 5–26 h (varies considerably with co-medication) |
| Plasma clearance | 0.133 l/kg/h (but very variable and affected by co-medication) |
| Protein binding | 75% |
| Active metabolite | Carbamazepine epoxide |

because of auto-induction, on chronic therapy the half-life is usually between 5 and 26 hours, but there is marked individual variation. In the post-induced state, a new steady state after changes in drug dosage will be achieved within 3 days. CBZ-epoxide levels are generally about 50% of carbamazepine plasma levels, although the ratio is subject to marked variation. The rate of metabolism varies both within and between individuals, and is affected by age, co-medication and dosing schedules. There is a relatively low extraction ratio (less than 10%), which reflects the limited ability of the liver to handle the plasma carbamazepine load. Because of the low intrinsic clearance and low extraction ratio, changes in hepatic blood flow do not alter carbamazepine clearance to any great extent. The mean clearance of carbamazepine is 0.133 l/kg/h but individual values are very variable.

Greater variations in serum levels are found during once-daily, than during two or three times-daily dosing regimens. One study showed a mean 79% change between peak and trough levels on twice-daily dosing, which was reduced to 40% on four times a day dosing. Peak-level side-effects are common in clinical practice, and these can be avoided by flattening out the diurnal blood level swings. This can be achieved by more frequent dosing, or the use of the controlled-release formulation of carbamazepine. There are no significant differences between the absorption and steady-state concentrations, efficacy or tolerability between conventional or chewable tablets, and the suspension, syrup and tablets have been shown to have similar pharmacokinetics.

There are no major differences between infants and adults in the absorption, protein binding or distribution of carbamazepine or CBZ-epoxide. The volume of distribution in children, however, is 1–1.5-times that of the adult level. The clearance of carbamazepine is higher in infants and young children, and the ratio of CBZ-epoxide to carbamazepine levels ranges from 16 to 66%. In older children, absorption, half-life and clearance show very marked intra-individual variations, although the mean population values are similar to those in adults. The diurnal variation in levels in children is greater than in adults, and to avoid peak dose side-effects it is often necessary to use 2 times or 3 times a day dosing and the slow-release formulation. In gastro-intestinal disease, the absorption of carbamazepine can be quite severely reduced, and drug levels require careful monitoring.

In the presence of severe liver disease, carbamazepine pharmacokinetics may be disordered and dose reductions needed, but moderate disease has little effect. Renal disease has no effect on carbamazepine kinetics, and dialysis does not have a marked effect on carbamazepine plasma levels. Severe congestive cardiac failure has been shown to result in abnormally slow absorption, and the drug is also cleared and metabolized at a slower rate. The water and sodium retention induced by the antidiuretic action of carbamazepine can also aggravate cardiac failure.

The absorption of carbamazepine is not modified during the first two trimesters of pregnancy. In the last trimester, the unbound levels of carbamazepine and CBZ-epoxide are not changed (nor is their ratio), but total levels fall as maternal plasma protein concentrations decline towards the end of pregnancy. Dose adjustments are only occasionally needed, and if clinically indicated, measurement of free levels can be useful. Breast-milk concentrations of carbamazepine are about 20–70% of those of maternal plasma.

Because of the wide variation in the dose–serum level relationship both at an inter- and intra-individual level, carbamazepine (and CBZ-epoxide) levels are commonly measured. There is a relationship between carbamazepine level and therapeutic effectiveness, but no universal 'therapeutic range'. Thus, although levels are useful as a guide, particularly in long-term therapy, there is little point in adhering to any pre-determined target range, and daily dosage should be tailored to individual need. Having said this, the maximum effect is usually observed between 10 and 50 μmol/l. The CBZ-epoxide has antiepileptic action and also contributes to the side-effects of carbamazepine, and for this reason it is often useful to measure the serum levels of both carbamazepine and CBZ-epoxide. The target range for the CBZ-epoxide is up to 9 μmol/l.

### Drug interactions

Drug interactions involving carbamazepine are common and often clinically important. The drug is a potent hepatic enzyme inducer of CYP3A4, CYP2C9, CYP2C19 and CYP1A2. It is itself also highly susceptible to enzyme induction (including auto-induction), and any drug which influences CYP3A4 (of which there are many) can have a marked effect on carbamazepine levels. The first metabolite of carbamazepine (carbamazepine 10,11-epoxide) itself has antiepileptic action, which complicates the clinical assessment of carbamazepine interactions.

### *The effect of other drugs on carbamazepine levels*

The levels of carbamazepine and CBZ-epoxide can be affected by co-medication with other drugs. The interactions with antiepileptic drugs are listed in Tables 3.1 and 3.2. The effects can be due to induction or competitive or non-competitive inhibition of both carbamazepine and CBZ-epoxide metabolism, and thus are complex and not easily predictable. Among the antiepileptic drugs, the most important interactions are the lowering of carbamazepine levels due to phenytoin (Figure 3.1), which can be so marked that carbamazepine concentrations cannot be raised to therapeutic levels without causing intoxication—presumably as a result of high CBZ-epoxide levels. Less commonly, similar effects can be due to felbamate, lamotrigine and phenobarbital. The effects of valproate depend on a balance of induction, inhibition and protein displacement. Even where carbamazepine levels are unchanged

**Table 3.1** The effect of carbamazepine co-medication on plasma levels of other antiepileptic drugs.

| Increased | Decreased | Variable | No effect |
|---|---|---|---|
| Phenobarbital (from primidone) | Clobazam | Phenobarbital | Lamotrigine |
| | Clonazepam | Phenytoin | Levetiracetam |
| | Ethosuximide | | Piracetam |
| | Felbamate | | Vigabatrin |
| | Lamotrigine | | |
| | Tiagabine | | |
| | Topiramate | | |
| | Valproate | | |
| | Zonisamide | | |

**Table 3.2** The effect of co-medication with other antiepileptic drugs on carbamazepine plasma levels.

| Increased | Decreased | Variable | No effect |
|---|---|---|---|
| Acetazolamide | Felbamate | Clobazam | Gabapentin |
| Vigabatrin | Lamotrigine | Clonazepam | Levetiracetam |
| | Midazolam | Ethosuximide | Piracetam |
| | Phenobarbital | Zonisamide | Oxcarbazepine |
| | Phenytoin | | Tiagabine |
| | Primidone | | Vigabatrin |
| | Oxcarbazepine | | Zonisamide |
| | Valproate | | Lamotrigine |

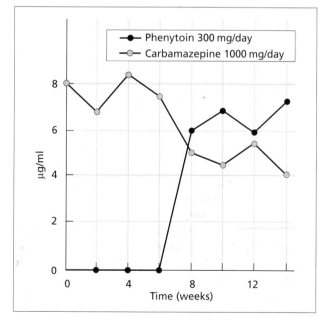

**Figure 3.1** The pharmacokinetic interaction between carbamazepine and phenytoin: 50% fall in plasma carbamazepine level following the addition of phenytoin as co-medication.

on valproate co-medication, CBZ-epoxide levels may be increased by as much as four times, an interaction due to valproate-induced inhibition of the enzyme epoxide hydrolase. The valproic acid prodrug, valpromide, is associated with an even greater inhibition, with up to eighfold increases in CBZ-epoxide levels. Serum carbamazepine levels in monotherapy have been shown to fluctuate by between 23 and 45% diurnally; this fluctuation will be greater in the presence of combination therapy, and the use of the slow-release formulation is advised in any patient on moderate doses of carbamazepine in combination with other drugs.

Various drugs and classes of drug inhibit the metabolism of carbamazepine, and this can result in marked increases in carbamazepine serum levels (see Table 3.2). These include: the macrolide antibiotics such as erythromycin, which can increase levels two- to three-fold; the calcium channel blockers diltiazem and verapamil, which can double levels (nifedipine has no effect); cimetidine, which can cause a 20–30% increase in carbamazepine levels (ranitidine has no effect); imidazole drugs such as nifimidone; propoxyphene, which increases concentrations by 30–60%; and the experimental antiepileptics denzimol and stiripentol, which can double carbamazepine levels; other drugs which have been shown to markedly increase levels include danazol, fluoxetine, fluvoxamine and viloxazine.

### The effect of carbamazepine on levels of other drugs

Carbamazepine induces the metabolism and hence lowers the concentration of a wide variety of concurrently administered drugs, although this is not usually a very marked effect. The most important are reductions in phenytoin, ethosuximide, felbamate, tiagabine, topiramate and valproate. The effects of carbamazepine on levels of phenobarbital and phenytoin are complex and variable.

Among the non-antiepileptic drugs where carbamazepine co-medication can compromise clinical effects are antidepressants, antipsychotic drugs, oral anticoagulants, beta-blockers, chemotherapeutic agents, and theophylline (and others). Carbamazepine also induces the metabolism of the oestrogen content of the oral contraceptive, carrying the risk of contraceptive failure (see p. 102). The levels of the common tricyclic antidepressants, clozepine, haloperidol, olanzapine, ciclosporin, nimodipine, doxycycline, vincristine and oral anticoagulants have been shown to be routinely reduced by as much as 30–60% when carbamazepine co-medication is prescribed; these are significant interactions which may have clinical effects. Carbamazepine can also increase the serum levels of other drugs by competing with or inhibiting their metabolism; the most common examples are listed in Table 3.3.

### Adverse effects

The reported frequency of side-effects in different studies has varied greatly, but overall between 30 and 50% of subjects

**Table 3.3** Common pharmacokinetic interactions involving carbamazepine and non-antiepileptic drugs.

*Effect of carbamazepine on levels of co-medication*

| *Increase* | *Decrease* |
| --- | --- |
| Chlorothiazides | Alprazolam |
| Lithium | Clozapine |
| Furosemide | Corticoteroids |
| Isoniazid | Ciclosporin |
| Monoamine oxidase inhibitors | Desipramine |
| Perphenazine | Doxicycline |
| Ketoconazole | Fluphenazine |
| Fluconazole | Haloperidol |
| Ritonavir | Itraconazole |
| Metronidazole | Propoxyphene |
| Danazol | Nortriptyline |
| Verapamil | Oral steroid contraceptives |
| Diltiazem | Praziquantel |
| Fluoxitine | Propranolol |
| Fluvoxamine | Trazodone |
| Viloxamine | Theophylline |
| Nefazodone | Vincristine |
| | Olanzopine |
| | Nimodipine |
| | Nifedipine |

*Increase in carbamazepine level caused by co-medication*

| | |
| --- | --- |
| Allopurinol | Haloperidol |
| Cimetidine | Isoniazid |
| Danazol | Ketoconazole |
| Desipramine | Miconazone |
| Dextropropoxyphene | Nefazodone |
| Diltiazem | Omeprazole |
| Erythromycin | Terfenadine |
| Fluoxetine | Verapamil |
| Fluvoxamine | Viloxazine |

taking carbamazepine will experience some side-effects (Table 3.4). These, however, are usually mild and often transient. Less than 5% of patients will need to withdraw the medication because of side-effects.

The dose-related side-effects are often exacerbated by fluctuations in serum level, and the use of the slow-release formulation of carbamazepine will greatly reduce these. There are few antiepileptic drugs where a slow-release formulation has such clear-cut advantages, and in clinical practice it has become common to recommend the slow-release formulation routinely in all patients taking doses of 800 mg/day or more, or in patients on co-medication. Most clinical studies of the drug were conducted using normal formulations, and this may explain why side-effects were more commonly reported than is the experience in routine clinical practice.

## Neuropsychiatric side-effects

These are common on initiating treatment with carbamazepine or when the dose becomes too high. Once a stable regimen has been established, however, adverse neurological effects are uncommon or mild. The most common side-effects on initiating therapy are sedation, headache, diplopia, dizziness and ataxia. These can be largely avoided by starting treatment at a low dose and incrementing the dose slowly. When the drug dose is too high, a highly characteristic side-effect pattern occurs with visual blurring or diplopia and unsteadiness, and sometimes dizziness. These side-effects tend to be manifest a few hours after dosing, and are due to peak blood levels either of the carbamazepine itself or of its 10,11-epoxide. Peak level side-effects can be reduced in frequency and intensity by switching to the slow-release formulation of the drug, or by increasing the frequency of dosing. These reversible transient neurotoxic side-effects are more common in patients taking combination therapy and also in the elderly. Carbamazepine-induced intermittent ataxia is particularly marked in infants after the intake of syrup formulations, which produce high post-absorptive peaks in serum drug concentrations, especially when high doses are ingested to compensate for the high drug clearance in this age group. The carbamazepine 10,11-epoxide to carbamazepine ratio is particularly high in infants and children, and this metabolite can contribute to adverse effects. For the same reason, carbamazepine intoxication in children is commonly caused by metabolic interactions with frequently prescribed co-medication, particularly macrolide antibiotics.

The only other common neurological side-effects due to carbamazepine are drowsiness, cognitive slowing and memory disturbance. Although these are frequently complained about in the clinic and blamed on drug therapy (including carbamazepine), a causative association can often not be established with certainty. Furthermore, formal testing of the drug in normal doses in normal volunteers has failed to show any marked sedative effect or change in cognitive ability.

Other rarer side-effects include headache, asterixis, dystonia, tremor, diarrhoea and nausea. Sporadic psychiatric disturbances have occurred in relation to carbamazepine therapy, but these are generally rare, and are less prominent with carbamazepine than with most of the other older or newer antiepileptic drugs. It was claimed when the drug was first introduced that the drug had a 'positive psychotropic action' owing putatively to its tricyclic structure. Such claims are now not made and, interestingly, similar claims were made for phenytoin and phenobarbital when they were introduced, and are now being made for lamotrigine and levetiracetam. These probably reflect over-ambitious marketing, placebo effect or simply over-optimism on the part of the doctor or patient. Carbamazepine can markedly

**Table 3.4** Frequency of adverse effects of carbamazepine monotherapy (VA study) therapy.

| Effect | Percentage of patients* (*n* = 231) | Percentage at 12-month visit** (*n* = 130) |
|---|---|---|
| Sedation | 42 | 8 |
| Weight gain | 32 | 9 |
| large weight gain | 8 | 3 |
| Nystagmus | 30 | 6 |
| Gastrointestinal symptoms | 29 | 6 |
| Gait problems | 25 | 4 |
| Change in affect or mood | 24 | 4 |
| Tremor | 22 | 5 |
| Cognitive disturbances | 18 | 3 |
| Rash | 11 | 1 |
| Diplopia | 10 | 0 |
| Impotence | 7 | 2 |

*, Percentage of patients in whom each type of adverse effect occurred at any time during the trial (mean follow-up, 36 months); **, Percentage of patients in whom each type of adverse effect was noted at the 12-month visit.

exacerbate atypical absence, tonic and myoclonic seizures, and has been said to worsen the aphasia in occasional patients with the Landau–Kleffner syndrome.

### Hypersensitivity, dermatological, hepatic and haematological side-effects

Carbamazepine may cause acute hypersensitivity. This most commonly affects the skin and bone marrow, although hepatic and renal hypersensitivity can occur.

When carbamazepine was first introduced, a number of serious skin reactions were recorded. These included fatal cases of Stevens–Johnson syndrome, Lyell syndrome and exfoliative dermatitis. It has been suggested that the rashes were due to the carbamazepine incipient in the early formulations, although there seems no doubt that carbamazepine itself can cause severe skin reactions. It has also been postulated that the lack of serious recent problems is due to the slow incrementation of dosage now recommended. Although the rate of severe skin reactions on carbamazepine has fallen, carbamazepine is still the third most common drug to cause Stevens–Johnson syndrome (14 cases per 100,000). In the Han Chinese in Taiwan, an exceptionally strong association has been noted with HLA-B*1502 allele and the occurrence of a Stevens–Johnson reaction. This allele occurs in 8% of Han Chinese and in 1–2% in Caucasians and is in linkage disequilibrium with a causative polymorphism which has not been identified. Identification of the polymorphism might allow a pre-

dictive test to be developed, and thereby the avoidance of carbamazepine in patients carrying this genotype.

Although a Stevens–Johnson or other severe skin reactions are rare, minor skin rash is common—occurring in about 5–10% of people in whom carbamazepine therapy is initiated. Discontinuation of the drug is usually recommended if a rash develops, but some paediatricians particularly give a short course of steroids when a rash appears. The rash fades with the steroids and if it does not recur on steroid withdrawal, the drug is continued. The rash is mediated by activation of the suppressor-cytotoxic subset of T cells, and successful desensitization carried out by the reintroduction of the drug at very low doses has been carried out without complications. Systemic lupus erythematosus has very rarely been induced by carbamazepine, although less often than with phenytoin. Isolated renal effects have occasionally been reported.

About 20 cases of carbamazepine hepatotoxicity had been reported by the 1980s, with a mortality rate of about 25%. This takes the form of either a hypersensitivity-induced granulomatous hepatitis or acute hepatitis with hepatic necrosis. Most cases had been taking carbamazepine for less than 1 month and the hypersensitivity was associated with rash and fever.

Severe haematological complications have also been recorded, including thrombocytopenia, aplastic anaemia, agranulocytosis and pancytopenia. During the first 25 years of clinical usage of CBZ, 31 cases of thrombocytopenia,

27 cases of aplastic anaemia, 10 cases of agranulocytosis, and 8 cases of pancytopenia were reported. The prevalence of aplastic anaemia is now estimated to be about 5 cases per million and the prevalence of agranulocytosis 1.4 cases per million. The overall risk of death due to marrow suppression is 2.2 cases per million. These hypersensitivity reactions usually develop in the first few months of therapy, and carry an appreciable mortality rate. They seem to be more common in the elderly.

In contrast to the rarity of severe hypersensitivity, carbamazepine frequently results in lowered total white blood cell and neutrophil counts. This is usually of no clinical significance. A white cell count below 5000 cells/mm$^3$ is encountered in between 10 and 30% of adults or children treated with carbamazepine, and does not seem to be dose-related. If the neutrophil count is below 1200 cells/mm$^3$, the patient should be monitored carefully but dose reduction is not necessary if the neutropenia is asymptomatic. If the neutrophil count falls below 900 cells/mm$^3$ the drug dosage should be reduced. In this situation restitution of the white count usually occurs within a few days. If red blood cell counts are also reduced in the presence of normal iron and low reticulocyte counts, the drug should be stopped.

### Hyponatraemia and other endocrine and biochemical changes

Carbamazepine has a dose-related antidiuretic effect, resulting in low serum sodium and water retention. This effect is dose-related and more frequent in the elderly. The mechanism is obscure, and evidence has been adduced for both a renal and a pituitary effect. Usually, the mild hyponatraemia and water retention are asymptomatic, and require no correction. Occasionally, a large fluid load (typically, pints of beer) will cause symptomatic hyponatraemia with nausea, weakness and dizziness. Caution is needed when prescribing carbamazepine to the elderly on low-sodium diets, and all patients should be monitored for symptoms of hyponatraemia. As a general rule, if the serum sodium is above 125 mmol/l in the absence of symptoms, no action is needed. If hyponatraemia becomes symptomatic, or where levels are repeatedly below 120 mmol/l, even in the absence of symptoms, the carbamazepine dosage should be reduced.

Elevated hepatic enzymes are found in up to 5–10% of patients taking carbamazepine, owing to induction of the hepatic enzyme systems, but these changes are without clinical significance.

Carbamazepine can induce a variety of changes in circulating pituitary and sex hormones, but the clinical significance of these effects is quite unclear. Free testosterone levels are reduced and hyposexuality and reproductive dysfunction have been attributed to carbamazepine therapy, but the effects are not clear-cut. Free cortisol levels can be increased. Complex effects on the biochemistry of thyroid function occur, but frank hypothyroidism is rare. T4

levels can be are reduced without hypothyroidism, owing to effects on binding, and the measurement of thyroid-stimulating hormone concentrations is a reliable way of assessing thyroid status. Mild hypocalcaemia and lowered vitamin D levels have been recorded, although frank osteomalacia has not. Although it has been suggested that antiepileptic drugs can contribute to osteoporosis, there is no evidence that carbamazepine can cause significant bone disease. Carbamazepine can have, usually minor, effects on testosterone (free, albumin bound, and sex hormone binding globulin [SHBG] bound), luteinizing hormone, and prolactin. Carbamazepine may alter cholesterol metabolism, leading to elevations of low-density lipoprotein (LDL) to total cholesterol ratio, apparently especially in women and children. The higher LDL to cholesterol ratio and low apolipoprotein A-I levels theoretically could increase the risk of atherosclerosis. Interestingly, elevated cholesterol concentrations also significantly decrease plasma carbamazepine concentrations by enhancing total-body clearance. Levels of IgG have been shown to be decreased in some patients on carbamazepine.

### Cardiac effects

Carbamazepine has occasionally induced bradyarrhythmia and atrioventricular conduction delay in susceptible subjects. Patients with underlying cardiac disease are most at risk, although heart block has been reported in otherwise healthy children and in patients with tuberous sclerosis. A few cases of cardiac arrest and death have been attributed to the initiation of carbamazepine therapy, and the drug should be used with caution in those with pre-existing heart disease and especially those with A–V conduction defects.

### Other side-effects

About 5–10% of subjects develop mild gastrointestinal side-effects such as nausea, vomiting or diarrhoea. Other rare side-effects that have been reported include colitis and stomatitis, and renal failure (usually in the context of acute hypersensitivity). A retinopathy and effects on the retinal pigment epithelium can occur owing to carbamazepine (as with other tricyclic compounds) causing usually asymptomatic alterations in colour vision. The teratogenic potential of carbamazepine is described on pp. 103–4.

### Overdose

Death can occur when very large quantities of carbamazepine are taken. The lowest known lethal dose is 69 g. In one series, two out of 23 cases died. The highest serum level reported was 65 µg/l and the patient survived, as did one patient taking 400 200-mg tablets. At levels above 170 µmol/l, coma and seizures occur. Overdose can be complicated also by cardiac arrhythmia, respiratory depression, anticholinergic effects and gastrointestinal effects. Gastric lavage is useful, as gastric emptying is delayed by the drug. Activated charcoal, dialysis, plasmapheresis and forced diuresis have been used although their effectiveness has been queried. Seizures should be treated with benzodiazepines.

## Antiepileptic effect

The drug was introduced on the basis of a number of open clinical studies before the introduction of current regulatory licensing regulations, which require strictly monitored randomized controlled studies, and such studies have not been carried out. The open studies, however, have uniformly shown great effectiveness in adults and in children, in monotherapy and in combination therapy. These studies were followed, after years of licensed experience, by a series of large-scale comparative studies, in which some element of randomization and control was introduced, and these too consistently showed superiority over placebo and valproate in partial epilepsy, and usually equal effectiveness when compared with phenytoin, valproate, phenobarbital, primidone, lamotrigine and clonazepam in generalized convulsive epilepsy. In some studies, carbamazepine was found to be more effective than phenobarbital. In the large comparative veterans study, for instance, 1-year remission rates were recorded in 58% and 44%, respectively, of patients with generalized and/or partial seizures. Complete freedom from seizures occurred with carbamazepine more frequently than with phenobarbital at 1, 2, and 3 years of follow-up (Figure 3.2). A second prospective randomized comparative study of 243 adults with previously untreated tonic–clonic or partial epilepsy with or without secondary generalized seizures has also been reported, with patients randomized to phenobarbital, phenytoin, CBZ or sodium valproate monotherapy. Complete seizure control was achieved in 27% and 1-year remission after 3 years of follow-up in 75%, with no difference between drugs. Adverse effects necessitating withdrawal were more common in phenobarbital-treated patients (22%) than patients with CBZ (11%), valproate (5%) or phenytoin (3%). In a similar study in 167 children, 20% became free from seizures and 73% had achieved a 1-year remission by 3 years of follow-up. Withdrawal of drug therapy required the phenobarbital arm to be discontinued, and of the remaining three drugs, phenytoin was more likely to result in withdrawal (9%) than carbamazepine (4%) or valproate (4%).

### Newly diagnosed epilepsy

A randomized comparison of carbamazepine and valproate in 300 adults with newly diagnosed generalized epilepsy was made in the open, multicentre EPITEG study. Overall control of primary and secondary generalized seizures was similar on both drugs, but adverse effects were more common with carbamazepine. In a similar paediatric study undertaken with 260 children randomized to either carbamazepine or valproate, equal efficacy was recorded and adverse effects were mild.

### Partial-onset seizures

Carbamazepine is generally considered the drug of choice for complex partial and secondarily generalized seizures in adults and children, and to be superior to other drugs in these patients. There is some evidence to support this. In one study, 51 patients with phenobarbital-resistant epilepsy were randomized to either CBZ or phenytoin. Patients who were administered CBZ showed greater improvement and fewer adverse effects than those on phenytoin, but the global evaluation by physicians and patients found no significant differences in efficacy or tolerability. In another randomized, double-blind study of 236 children aged under 6 years, 49% of the CBZ group and 47% of the phenytoin group remained seizure free for the 6-month study period. Carbamazepine has been found to be more effective than valproate in studies of complex partial seizures. In an open study of newly diagnosed or recurrent partial seizures with or without secondary generalization carbamazepine

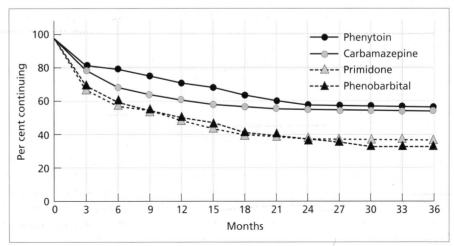

**Figure 3.2** The proportion of patients continuing on therapy with carbamazepine, phenobarbital, phenytoin and primidone. Patients were randomized to one of the four drugs and followed for 36 months. More than 50% of patients randomized to phenytoin or carbamazepine remained on therapy, significantly more than those on phenobarbital or primidone.

at a low dose of 600 mg was found to be as effective as lamotrigine 100 or 200 mg/day. Carbamazepine is also considered by many to be the drug of choice in benign childhood epilepsy with centro-temporal spikes (benign rolandic epilepsy), and other benign partial epilepsy syndromes.

### Generalized seizures

The use of carbamazepine in the generalized epilepsy syndromes of childhood, however, is more controversial. Some authors have reported benefit in the Lennox–Gastaut syndrome, but others consider carbamazepine contra-indicated, and it can certainly exacerbate myoclonus and the non-convulsive generalized seizures in this syndrome even when controlling the convulsive attacks. It can markedly worsen generalized absence and myoclonic seizures in idiopathic generalized epilepsy, and yet may control the tonic–clonic seizures of the same syndrome. Infantile spasms and febrile convulsions are also generally resistant to carbamazepine therapy.

## Clinical use in epilepsy

Carbamazepine is one of the most widely used antiepileptic drugs in the world, and certainly one of the most widely studied. It is the drug of first choice for partial and second-arily generalized seizures and is effective against the entire range of partial seizure types and in the cryptogenic and symptomatic partial seizure syndromes. In routine practice, it is often the first drug tried in these patients. Carbamazepine is also useful in generalized tonic–clonic seizures associated with idiopathic generalized epilepsy, but usually has little value against other forms of generalized seizure types or generalized epilepsy syndromes. It may exacerbate myoclonus, generalized absence seizures and other non-convulsive types.

Carbamazepine is available in 100, 200 and 400 mg tablets, chewable tablets for children at doses of 100 and 200 mg, slow-release formulations as 200 and 400 mg capsules, and as liquid and suppositories.

It is usual in adults to start at 100 mg/day and to double this dose every fortnight to a level of 400–800 mg/day in two divided doses. In adults, maintenance doses of between 400 and 1600 mg are commonly used, although higher doses (up to 2800 mg) are occasionally required and tolerated. Starting at a higher initial dose often results in acute nausea, diplopia, dizziness and drowsiness, and slow intro-

duction at a low dose reduces the risk of this reaction. Once the maintenance dose is reached, the slow-release formulation should be prescribed if the drug is poorly tolerated, and this formulation should be used anyway if the drug is taken at a dose of 800 mg/day or higher. It is usual to give the drug at a twice a day regimen, and the use of the slow-release formulation on a twice daily basis (equivalent to four times a day dosing of the conventional formulation in terms of blood-level fluctuations) is a far better option than a higher dosing frequency in most situations.

Measurements of plasma concentrations are advisable at the early stages of medication to establish baseline measures, when changes of seizure control or medication occur, or where toxic side-effects are suspected. The tolerability of carbamazepine is generally good, but side-effects can occur and the elderly particularly tolerate carbamazepine (and other antiepileptic drugs) less well. Blood count and serum sodium levels should be checked regularly (annually in patients on stable doses). Plasma carbamazepine and CBZ-epoxide measurements are moderately helpful in choosing regimens, but are only poorly correlated with clinical effects. Diurnal inter-individual and intra-individual variation, variability in plasma protein binding, and co-medication affect plasma concentrations of carbamazepine and CBZ-epoxide. Therefore, there is no universal 'therapeutic' level, although plasma concentrations are usually kept between 20 and 50 mmol/l. Having said this, low doses and low blood levels will completely control seizures in many cases, and some patients do not experience side-effects when the range is exceeded.

In children the same therapeutic principles apply. Children below 1 year of age require a maintenance dose of 100–200 mg, between 1 and 5 years of age a maintenance dose of 200–400 mg, between 5 and 10 years of age a maintenance dose of 400–600 mg, and between 10 and 15 years of age 400–1000 mg. As the clearance of carbamazepine in children is faster, three times daily dosing is often required.

In combination therapy, drug interactions are sometimes problematic. These can be complex and interactions of both carbamazepine and CBZ-epoxide metabolism can complicate their interpretation. In combination therapy, the blood levels are even more difficult to interpret.

Carbamazepine is considered one of the safest anti-epileptic drugs for use in pregnancy, and is classified as a category C teratogen by the Food and Drug Administration (FDA).

# CLOBAZAM

| | |
|---|---|
| **Primary indications** | Partial and generalized seizures. Also for intermittent therapy, one-off prophylactic therapy. Adults and children |
| **Licensed for monotherapy/add-on therapy** | Both |
| **Usual preparations** | Tablet, capsule: 10 mg |
| **Usual dosage—adults** | 10–20 mg/day; higher doses can be used |
| **Usual dosage—children** | 3–12 years: 5–10 mg/day |
| **Dosing intervals** | 1–2 times/day |
| **Dose commonly affected by co-medication** | No |
| **Dose affected by renal/hepatic disease** | No definitive clinical data |
| **Common drug interactions** | Minor interactions only |
| **Serum level monitoring** | Not useful |
| **Common/important adverse events** | Sedation, dizziness, weakness, blurring of vision, restlessness, ataxia, aggressiveness, behavioural disturbance, withdrawal symptoms |
| **Major mechanism of action** | GABA-A receptor agonist |
| **Main advantages** | Highly effective in some patients with epilepsy resistant to first-line therapy; fewer side-effects than with other benzodiazepines |
| **Main disadvantages** | Development of tolerance in up to 50% of patients |
| **COMMENT** | Excellent therapy for patients with partial and generalized epilepsy, given usually in patients resistant to first-choice therapy |

Clobazam is a remarkable drug whose role in epilepsy is underestimated. This is partly because it is a benzodiazepine, with all the encumbrance of this drug class, but there has also been a surprising lack of promotion by its manufacturers, in a market place not generally characterized by reticence. The drug has a 1,5 substitution instead of the usual 1,4 benzodiazepine structure. It is unique in this regard, and this structural change results in an 80% reduction in its anxiolytic activity and a 10-fold reduction in its sedative effects, when compared with diazepam in animal studies. The drug was introduced as an anxiolytic, its potent antiepileptic effects were demonstrated later, and its human antiepileptic effect was first reported a decade after its introduction. It has been licensed in Europe since 1975, Canada since 1988, but is unavailable in the USA. It is widely used in specialist epilepsy clinics, where this underdog of a drug has many champions.

## Physical and chemical characteristics
Clobazam (molecular weight 300.73) is relatively insoluble in water throughout the range of physiological pH, and therefore cannot be given by intravenous or intramuscular injection. It is a weak organic acid. It is also relatively insoluble in lipids, with a lipid solubility about 40% of that of diazepam.

## Mode of action
Clobazam acts at the benzodiazepine binding site of the γ-aminobutyric acid A (GABA-A) receptor complex, thus enhancing the inhibitory neurotransmitter action of GABA at the ligand-gated chloride ion channel. It enhances the conductance of the channel up to a concentration of 3 µmol. Quite why its action is distinct from those of other benzodiazepine drugs is not clearly known, but this could reflect differential binding to the various GABA-A receptor subunits (at least 16 have already been identified). The drug may also exert an action away from the GABA receptor, affecting voltage-sensitive calcium ion conductance and sodium channel function. An interesting speculation is that common polymorphisms in the benzodiazepine receptor will alter binding of drugs such as clobazam, and therefore their clinical effects, but the consequences of this clinically have not been explored.

## Pharmacokinetics

| Clobazam | |
|---|---|
| Pharmacokinetics—average adult values | |
| Oral bioavailability | 90% |
| Time to peak levels | 1–4 h |
| Volume of distribution | |
| Biotransformation | Hepatic demethylation and hydroxylation and then conjugation (cytochrome P450 system; UDPGT family enzymes) |
| Elimination half-life | 10–77 h (clobazam); 50 h (*N*-desmethylclobazam) |
| Plasma clearance | |
| Protein binding | 83% |
| Active metabolite | *N*-desmethylclobazam |

### Absorption

Clobazam has an oral bioavailability of about 90%. It is absorbed rapidly and the time to peak plasma concentrations ($T_{max}$) after oral dosing is 1–4 hours. Absorption is relatively unaffected by age or gender. The rate of absorption is reduced when the drug is taken with or after meals, but the extent of absorption is unaffected. For the epilepsy patient the timing of ingestion is seldom critical. It could be given rectally, and is rapidly absorbed, but this method of administration has not been adopted in clinical practice.

### Distribution

The plasma protein binding of clobazam has been found to be 83%, and the proportion of bound to unbound drug is independent of clobazam concentrations. There is a higher free (unbound) proportion, however, in situations where plasma protein concentrations are greatly lowered, for instance in advanced hepatic or renal disease, and dosage should be reduced in these situations. Clobazam is distributed widely, but the concentration in brain is proportional to the concentration of the unbound drug in the serum, as is the drug concentration in saliva. There is a good correlation between plasma concentration and dose in an individual patient, but there are large inter-individual variations. Concentrations in brain between 0.02 and 1.7 µmol/l—which equate in most people to maximum doses of about 30–40 mg/day—have been shown to be associated with a therapeutic response.

### Biotransformation and excretion

Clobazam is metabolized in the liver to *N*-desmethyl-clobazam (otherwise known as norclobazam). This is an important fact, as *N*-desmethylclobazam could be responsible for much of the antiepileptic effect of the drug (Figure 3.3). Arguing against this proposition are the fact that the lipid solubility of the metabolite is lower than that of the parent drug, and that its affinity for the benzodiazepine receptor is at least 10-fold less than that of clobazam. However, the half-life of norclobazam is very much longer, about 50 hours in healthy volunteers, but less in patients on other enzyme-inducing drugs, and its plasma concentration is considerably higher than that of the parent drug. This is swings and roundabouts, and the exact role of the metabolite has not been fully established. The elimination half-life of clobazam is variable, from 11 to 77 hours in one investigation. The longest half-lives are in the elderly. In patients receiving other antiepileptic drugs the half-life is reduced to approximately 12–13 hours, again greater in the elderly. Desmethylclobazam is itself conjugated in the liver and excreted in the bile as the glucuronide and in the urine as a sulphate. At normal clinical doses the plasma concentration of the metabolite is between 300 and 3500 ng/mL, about 10 times higher than the usual clobazam concentrations (20–350 ng/mL).

### Drug interactions

Clobazam has a potential for complex interactions, and it can cause either elevation or reduction in phenytoin, phenobarbital or carbamazepine drug levels, although usually these are clinically insignificant. However, some patients with high phenytoin levels develop phenytoin toxicity when clobazam is added. Carbamazepine epoxidation can also be enhanced by clobazam co-medication. A rare but

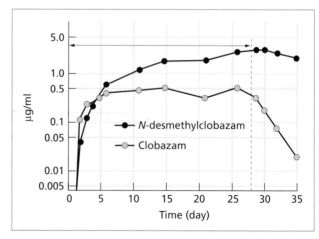

**Figure 3.3** Plasma concentrations of clobazam and *N*-desmethylclobazam after 28 days of therapy with clobazam 20 mg/day. Note that the *N*-desmethylclobazam levels at steady state are 10 times greater than those of clobazam. This explains why the active metabolite may be responsible for much of the pharmacological action of clobazam.

unpredictable increase in sodium valproate levels has also been reported, resulting in confusional states, and clobazam and valproate combinations should be carefully observed. Desmethyclobazam levels can be raised and clobazam levels lowered in patients on combination therapy with phenobarbital, phenytoin or carbamazepine. In the great majority of patients, however, the clinical effects of these interactions are slight and in normal practice problems are rare. However, the adverse effects occasionally observed when clobazam is added to polytherapy regimens can be caused by occult drug interactions.

## Adverse effects
### Neurotoxic effects

Because clobazam has been so widely used in psychiatric practice as an antianxiolytic, its side-effect profile is well known. The side-effects are essentially similar to those of other benzodiazepines, although sedation is much less common than on other drugs (Table 3.5). The frequency in clinical trials of its anxiolytic effect have been reported to lie between 20 and 85%, but in only 5–15% were the side-effects of a severity sufficient to change dose or terminate treatment. In clinical practice it must be said that side-effects are seemingly less common, possibly reflecting the different patient group. The most common are sedation and drowsiness, dizziness, dry mouth, nausea, headache and depression. Occasionally, behavioural disturbances, insomnia, irritability and disinhibition are reported, especially in institutionalized populations. Muscle fatigue and weakness occur, as with other benzodiazepines, owing to disorderly recruitment of motor units, and for this reason the drug should not be given to patients with myasthenia gravis. Of all these side-effects, sedation is the most important, but the measured effects of normal dosages of clobazam on cognitive tests has been shown to be very slight.

**Table 3.5** Summary of the reported side-effects of clobazam, diazepam and placebo from 70 double-blind studies of the anxiolytic effects of clobazam; percentage of patients reporting the effects.

| | Clobazam ($n = 1690$) | Diazepam ($n = 1084$) | Placebo ($n = 889$) |
|---|---|---|---|
| Drowsiness | 25.8 | 45.5 | 9.9 |
| Dizziness | 7.0 | 12.0 | 2.8 |
| Headache | 2.1 | 3.2 | 2.9 |
| Nausea | 1.6 | 1.5 | 2.1 |
| Dry mouth | 3.0 | 2.3 | 0.9 |
| Constipation | 2.1 | 3.4 | 0.3 |
| Depression | 1.7 | 2.2 | 0.3 |

### Tolerance and symptoms on withdrawal

Undoubtedly, clinically the most problematic phenomenon is the tendency for clobazam to lose its beneficial effect (the development of tolerance). This is a property shared by all benzodiazepines, but in animal studies tolerance developed more frequently with clobazam than with clonazepam. It is traditionally claimed that 30–50% of patients prescribed clobazam can expect to develop tolerance, although more recent studies show lower proportions, and this problem, in routine clinical practice, may have been exaggerated. Despite the importance of tolerance, the mechanisms are unknown, and the frequently quoted 'down-regulation of the GABA-A receptor' is descriptive rather than explanatory. Better news is that tolerance to the sedative effects is much more prominent than tolerance to the antiepileptic effects, and if a patient develops sedation on starting treatment, it is well worth while persisting with therapy, as the sedation usually wears off within a week or so. Tolerance is more common at higher doses and with continuous rather than intermittent therapy.

Withdrawal symptoms (irritability, restlessness or difficulties in concentrating) are noticeable in about 5–10% of patients during the first few weeks after withdrawal. Idiosyncratic allergic reactions are very rare, and as far as this author is aware, no fatal side-effects have been reported.

## Antiepileptic effect

The drug was introduced before double-blind placebo-controlled clinical trials had become a fundamental requirement. The first report was an open study by Gastaut in 1977, who became a great enthusiast of the drug, noting positive results in 76% of 140 patients with severe epilepsy, an effect, however, maintained in only 53% after a few months. Many other trials have followed. There have more recently been nine double-blind trials in refractory partial epilepsy, and all demonstrated striking benefit. In one study over 50% of patients showed a greater than 50% reduction of seizures, and in another the mean reduction was 30%. As the trials were all carried out in patients with long-standing chronic and previously refractory epilepsy, this is an impressive result—and certainly better than observed with many other currently available drugs. The patients in these clinical trials all had partial epilepsy, and all were taking other antiepileptic drugs.

The drug has also been the subject of numerous open studies, often with a wider range of patients, and some reported quite remarkable effects. A retrospective survey from Canada of 87 patients showed a greater than 50% response in 40% of patients, and 10–30% became seizure-free. It has been claimed, on an anecdotal basis, that patients with partial seizures but without widespread cerebral impairment obtain the most worthwhile benefit. Patients with secondarily generalized seizures also respond, however, as do those with absence seizures, myoclonus, the

Lennox–Gastaut syndrome, startle epilepsy, non-convulsive status epilepticus, electrical status during slow wave sleep (ESES), reflex epilepsies, alcohol withdrawal seizures, and those that accompany the benign childhood partial epilepsies.

There have been no large-scale trials of clobazam in monotherapy in adults, but in drug-naïve children with new-onset epilepsy, a recent multicentre Canadian study found the drug to be equally effective as monotherapy with phenytoin or carbamazepine.

No clear relationship has been found between serum level and seizure control, but this is confused by the development of tolerance. An optimum range of serum levels in chronic epilepsy has not been established.

### Clinical use in epilepsy

Clobazam should be considered as adjunctive therapy whenever treatment with a single first-line antiepileptic drug has proved ineffective. In my own practice, clobazam is often the first adjunctive drug to be tried. It is effective in a wide range of epilepsies, although perhaps best in those with partial seizures alone. It can be used in patients with Lennox–Gastaut and other primarily and secondarily generalized epilepsies. It is effective in a broad spectrum of other types of epilepsy and non-convulsive status syndromes. It is, in routine practice, very well tolerated,

with few side-effects. Its mild anxiolytic effect is also useful in some patients with epilepsy. The development of tolerance is the most prominent clinical problem. Manoeuvres such as drug holidays, initiation at very low doses or the use of very high doses have all failed to circumvent this problem.

Clobazam also has a particularly useful role as one-off prophylactic therapy on special occasions when it is particularly important to prevent a seizure (e.g. on days of travel, interview, examinations). Although there are no formal studies of the drug used in this way, the effect is often rapid and reliable, and the low incidence of side-effects makes it an ideal choice for such therapy. Clobazam can also be used in intermittent therapy (e.g. in catamenial epilepsy; see pp. 102–3) and is the best drug available for this purpose.

It is administered orally at a dose of 10–30 mg/day usually taken at night or in a twice daily regimen. The only available preparation is as 10 mg tablets. Higher dosages are seldom effective and should be avoided. The rectal administration of the drug has been explored experimentally, but is not used in clinical practice. There are no parenteral formulations. Withdrawal should be gradual (routinely, 10 mg per 1–2 months), and it is advisable to observe the same precautions with clobazam as with other benzodiazepine drugs.

# CLONAZEPAM

| | |
|---|---|
| **Primary indications** | Partial and generalized seizures (including absence and myoclonus). Also, Lennox–Gastaut syndrome, neonatal seizures, infantile spasms and status epilepticus. Adults and children |
| **Licensed for monotherapy/add-on therapy** | Both |
| **Usual preparations** | Tablets: 0.5, 1, 2 mg, liquid: 1 mg in 1 ml diluent |
| **Usual dosage—adults** | Initial: 0.25 mg at night<br>Maintenance: 0.5–4 mg/day |
| **Usual dosage—children** | < 1 year: 1 mg/day<br>1–5 years: 1–2 mg/day<br>5–12 years: 1–3 mg/day |
| **Dosing intervals** | 1–2 times/day |
| **Dose commonly affected by co-medication** | No |
| **Dose affected by renal/hepatic disease** | No definitive clinical data |
| **Common drug interactions** | Minor interactions only |
| **Serum level monitoring** | Not useful |
| **Common/important adverse events** | Sedation (common and may be severe), cognitive effects, drowsiness, ataxia, personality and behavioural changes, hyperactivity, restlessness, aggressiveness, psychotic reaction, seizure exacerbations, hypersalivation, tone changes, leucopenia, withdrawal symptoms |
| **Major mechanism of action** | GABA-A receptor agonist |
| **Main advantages** | Useful action especially in children; wide spectrum of activity |
| **Main disadvantages** | Side-effects are sometimes prominent, particularly sedation; tolerance and a withdrawal syndrome |
| **COMMENT** | Second-choice antiepileptic drug, with wide spectrum of activity, used particularly in children. Use limited by side-effects |

Clonazepam was one of the earliest benzodiazepine drugs used for epilepsy. It was licensed in Europe in 1975 and then in North America and throughout the world. It is a 1:4 substituted benzodiazepine, a structure shared with diazepam and all the other antiepileptic drugs of this class, with the notable exception of clobazam. It has in the past been widely used, although now it has largely been superseded by other drugs with fewer side-effects.

## Physical and chemical characteristics

Clonazepam is a crystalline powder (5-(2-chlorophenol)-1,3,dihydro-7-nitro-2H-1,4 benzodiazepin-2-one; MW 315.7) with pKa values of 1.5 and 10.5, and is virtually undissociated throughout the physiological pH range. It is highly lipid soluble.

## Mode of action

Clonazepam, like all other benzodiazepines, is an agonist at the GABA-A receptor. The benzodiazepines increase channel opening frequency at the GABA-A receptor, resulting in enhanced chloride conductance and neuronal hyperpolarization. Clonazepam has higher affinity binding to the benzodiazepine receptor than diazepam or other benzodiazepines, and furthermore clonazepam binds to subgroups of the GABA-A receptor that do not bind the other benzodiazepine drugs. In the rat, clonazepam alone binds in the spinal cord and striation and has a high concentration in the cerebellum. The drug also has some action on sodium channel conductance.

## Pharmacokinetics

| Clonazepam Pharmacokinetics—average adult values | |
|---|---|
| Oral bioavailability | 80% |
| Time to peak levels | 1–4 h |
| Volume of distribution | 1.5–4.4 l/kg |
| Biotransformation | Reduction, hydroxylation and acetylation (cytochrome P450 enzymes CYP3A4; UDPGT family enzymes) |
| Elimination half-life | 20–80 h |
| Plasma clearance | 0.09 l/kg/h |
| Protein binding | 86% |
| Active metabolite | None |

### Absorption

Clonazepam is well and reliably absorbed, with an oral bioavailability of 80% or more. It reaches a peak plasma level within 1–4 hours of oral administration in most people, although this may be delayed up to 8 hours. IV preparations are widely used for emergency therapy. Buccal or intranasal administration of a solution have been explored, but are not in common clinical usage.

### Distribution

Clonazepam is 86% bound to plasma proteins, with a volume distribution of between 1.5 and 4.4 l/kg reflecting its high lipid solubility. It rapidly crosses into the brain, where it is passively absorbed with a linear brain to plasma concentration ratio.

### Biotransformation and excretion

Clonazepam is metabolized in the liver first by reduction and then acetylation, both processes being greatly influenced by genetic factors (especially acetylator status). The acetylated compound is then nitrated. There are various metabolites, none of which has clinically important pharmacological activity. The clearance of clonazepam is slow, in adults approximately 0.09 l/Kg/H. Less than 0.5% of the parent drug is recovered unchanged in the urine. Because metabolism is influenced by individual genetic variation, the half-life of clonazepam is very variable, falling in most patients between 20 and 80 hours. In studies in neonates half-lives have been recorded of 20–43 hours and in children of 22–33 hours. There seems to be no correlation between antiepileptic efficacy and plasma level.

### Drug interactions

It is rare for clonazepam to alter levels of other drugs in any clinically relevant manner, although minor effects are common. Clonazepam levels are lowered by co-administration with carbamazepine or phenobarbital and presumably other enzyme-inducing drugs. Lamotrigine can raise clonazepam levels. However, these effects are seldom of clinical importance.

## Adverse effects
### Neurotoxic effects

The most common important side-effect of clonazepam is sedation. There is no doubt that, even at low doses, a significant number of patients experience unacceptable levels of drowsiness and this limits the value of the drug in normal clinical practice. This adverse effect seems to be less marked in children than in adults, and this might explain the greater popularity of clonazepam among paediatricians than neurologists treating adults. Other side-effects are much less troublesome and are typical of those of other benzodiazepine drugs. These include incoordination, hypotonia, blurred vision, hyperactivity, restlessness, irritability, short attention span, behavioural change, psychosis, depression and other neuropsychiatric effects. This list may be long, but the side-effects are not commonly dose-limiting. Behavioural changes seem to be more prominent in patients with psychiatric problems. The mixture of hypotonia, hypersecretion, somnolence and ataxia is characteristic and can be troublesome.

### Other side-effects

Hypersecretion and hypersalivation may be troublesome in infants and children. In infants too, cardiovascular and respiratory depression have been observed. Like other benzodiazepines, clonazepam may occasionally increase the frequency of certain seizure types (e.g. tonic seizures). Occasional idiosyncratic allergic reactions including marked leucopenia have been observed. The teratogenicity of clonazepam has not been well studied, although an increased risk of major malformations has been reported, as have growth retardation and dysmorphism.

### Tolerance and symptoms on withdrawal

Tolerance to the antiepileptic effects has been well described, and is common (although possibly less common than with clobazam) and troublesome. Cross-tolerance between benzodiazepine drugs is observed. Withdrawal symptoms can be prominent, and in one study in children symptoms occurred in over 50%. The symptoms most commonly reported on withdrawal include seizures, increased anxiety, insomnia, restlessness, confusion, and occasionally catatonia, and these are most marked in patients with psychiatric co-morbidity. Suddenly withdrawal carries a serious risk of seizure exacerbation and of status epilepticus. Gradual withdrawal minimizes these problems and, in routine practice, withdrawal at a decremental rate not exceeding 0.5 mg per month is strongly advised.

### Overdose

Benzodiazepine overdose produces respiratory depression and coma, and death is common if untreated. Supportive therapy is effective, and activated charcoal, exchange transfusions and flumazenil infusion can be used.

### Antiepileptic effect

Clonazepam is a potent antiepileptic drug. However, because of its potential to cause sedation and other side-effects, and the problem of tolerance, it is now not commonly used in routine practice, but is reserved as second-line adjunctive therapy in severe epilepsy. It has a wide spectrum of activity, although its main residual role is in the treatment of the generalized epilepsies. It is undoubtedly effective in absence epilepsy, and may work where other drugs have failed, and also has a useful effect against tonic–clonic seizures whatever their cause. It can be useful against all the seizure types in the Lennox–Gastaut syndrome. It is an effective therapy in myoclonic seizures, and is indeed one of the drugs of choice for this indication in primary generalized epilepsy and also the symptomatic secondary myoclonic epilepsies. It is frequently used by specialists in movement disorders for subcortical myoclonus. Early reports suggested that it was useful in partial seizures, although a recent literature review concluded that its effect is relatively modest. However, it is occasionally used in benign rolandic epilepsy and epilepsia partialis continua. Clonazepam has also been shown to be relatively safe in acute intermittent porphyria, and intravenous clonazepam is effective in controlling neonatal convulsions.

Clonazepam is still used widely in the treatment of various forms of status epilepticus. Its indications are exactly the same as those for diazepam, and its effectiveness is similar. It can be given intravenously or rectally in the emergency setting (see pp. 225–6).

### Clinical use in epilepsy

It is available as 0.5, 1 and 2 mg tablets and also as an intravenous solution. The initial dosage in adults is usually 0.25 mg and this is increased slowly to between 0.5 and 4 mg/day in a single or twice daily regimen. In children the dose is 1–3 mg/day.

# ETHOSUXIMIDE

| | |
|---|---|
| **Primary indications** | Generalized absence seizures. Adults and children |
| **Licensed for monotherapy/add-on therapy** | Both |
| **Usual preparations** | Capsules: 250 mg; syrup: 250 mg/5 ml |
| **Usual dosage—adults** | Initial: 250 mg<br>Maintenance: 750–2000 mg/day |
| **Usual dosage—children** | Initial: 10–15 mg/kg/day<br>Maintenance: 20–40 mg/kg/day |
| **Dosing intervals** | 2–3 times/day |
| **Dose commonly affected by co-medication** | Yes |
| **Dose affected by renal/hepatic disease** | Hepatic disease and severe renal disease |
| **Common drug interactions** | Extensive drug interactions; see p. 131 |
| **Serum level monitoring** | Useful |
| **Target range** | 300–700 µmol/l |
| **Common/important adverse events** | Gastrointestinal symptoms, drowsiness, ataxia, diplopia, headache, dizziness, hiccups, sedation, behavioural disturbances, acute psychotic reactions, extrapyramidal symptoms, blood dyscrasia, rash, lupus-like syndrome, severe idiosyncratic reactions |
| **Major mechanism of action** | Effects on calcium T-channel conductance |
| **Main advantages** | Well-established treatment for generalized absence seizures, without the risk of hepatic toxicity carried by valproate |
| **Main disadvantages** | Side-effects common |
| **COMMENT** | Useful drug for typical generalized absence seizures (petit mal) |

In the 1950s and 1960s a series of succinimide drugs were widely prescribed for the treatment of all types of epilepsy. Their toxicity limited their utility, and today only ethosuximide is in general use. Ethosuximide, introduced into clinical practice in 1958, has only one indication—the treatment of generalized absence seizures (petit mal seizures). It is still considered by some authorities to be first-line therapy for absence seizures, although more often now it is reserved for patients resistant to other more modern drugs.

## Physical and chemical properties

Ethosuximide (molecular weight 141.2) is a white crystalline racemate, freely soluble in water and alcohol, and it has a pKa of 9.3.

## Mode of action

The drug exerts a voltage-dependent blockade of low-threshold T-type calcium currents in the thalamus and this is almost certainly the mechanism of its effect against absence seizures. The drug also enhances post-synaptic GABA action and affects ATP-ase and membrane transport processes, but these effects are thought not to contribute to its antiepileptic properties.

## Pharmacokinetics

**Ethosuximide**
Pharmacokinetics—average adult values

| | |
|---|---|
| Oral bioavailability | < 100% |
| Time to peak levels | < 4 h |
| Volume of distribution | 0.65 l/kg |
| Biotransformation | Hepatic oxidation then conjugation (cytochrome P450 system, UDPGT family enzymes) |
| Elimination half-life | 30–60 h (varies with co-medication) |
| Plasma clearance | 0.010–0.015 l/kg/h |
| Protein binding | < 10% |
| Active metabolite | None |

## Absorption

Ethosuximide is rapidly absorbed, with an oral bioavailability of over 90%. Peak plasma levels are probably mostly reached within 4 hours of administration, although some studies have shown some delay with peak levels reached only after 7 hours. The syrup formulation tends to be more rapidly absorbed than the capsules, but both formulations are bioequivalent.

## Distribution

Ethosuximide is widely distributed. Concentrations in saliva, CSF, and tears are similar to those in plasma. The apparent volume of distribution following oral administration is 0.62–0.65 l/kg body weight in adults and 0.69 l/kg in children. There is negligibly plasma protein binding. The drug readily crosses the placenta and also readily crosses into breast milk (with a breast milk to serum ratio of 0.8–0.9) and the serum levels of a breast-feeding infant are approximately 30–50% of those of the mother.

## Biotransformation and elimination

Ethosuximide is extensively metabolized in the liver, first by oxidation and then conjunction by the CYP3A subgroup of the hepatic cytochrome P450 system. The metabolites have no significant antiepileptic action. About 10–20% of the drug is excreted unchanged in the urine. Ethosuximide is cleared slowly, with a mean half-life in adults of 50–60 hours and 30–40 hours in children and neonates. Steady state is reached in 12 days in adults and 6 days in children. There is considerable inter-individual variability, but the elimination half-life is unaffected by drug dosage. The total body clearance is 0.010–0.015 l/kg/h and may be slightly lower in women. Ethosuximide does not induce hepatic microsomal enzymes, nor is there auto-induction.

Renal disease, unless very severe, does not affect ethosuximide concentrations. 50% of the drug is removed by 6 hours of dialysis. The effect of hepatic disease has not been formally studied, but as ethosuximide is heavily metabolized, one would expect severe hepatic disease to alter its pharmacokinetics.

## Drug interactions

Ethosuximide does not generally affect serum levels of other antiepileptic or non-antiepileptic drugs. However, co-medication can effect ethosuximide levels. Sodium valproate has variable and complex effects, but can result in an increase of up to 50% in ethosuximide levels owing to valproate-induced inhibition of ethosuximide metabolism. Co-medication with carbamazepine can result in a significant decrease (up to 50%) in ethosuximide plasma concentrations, owing to the hepatic enzyme inducing properties of carbamazepine. Rifampicin, a classic inducer of CYP3A, has been shown to increase the clearance of ethosuximide by 90%. Other drugs acting on this enzyme system would also be expected to have a similar effect.

## Adverse effects
### Idiosyncratic reactions

Ethosuximide has the potential to cause severe idiosyncratic reactions. The skin is most commonly affected followed by the formed elements of the blood and the liver, and to a lesser extent the nervous system and kidneys. These reactions range from non-specific symptoms such as lymphadenopathy, arthralgias, eosinophilia and fever to more severe allergic dermatitis, rash, erythema multiforme, Stevens–Johnson syndrome, auto-immune thyroiditis, myocarditis, pericarditis and systemic lupus erythematosus. Blood dyscrasias have occurred but are rare, and include aplastic anaemia and agranulocytosis. In the early years of therapy, severe haematological effects were thought to be relatively common. However, only eight cases of ethosuximide-associated aplastic anaemia were reported between 1958 and 1994, all with onset 6 weeks to 8 months after initiation of ethosuximide therapy. Most patients were on polypharmacy, and five of the eight patients died.

### Other side-effects

The side-effects in 12 clinical trials published between 1958 and 1966 are summarized in Table 3.6. The overall incidence of adverse effects ranged from 26 to 46%. The most common adverse effects involve the gastrointestinal system, and include nausea, abdominal discomfort, anorexia, vomiting and diarrhoea. These are dose dependent but occasionally are severe enough to preclude therapy. Ethosuximide can also cause a wide range of dose-dependent CNS effects. The most common are insomnia, nervousness, dizziness, hiccups, lethargy, fatigue, ataxia, and behavioural changes such as aggression, euphoria, irritability and hyperactivity. Headache is a particular problem, occurring in one in eight treated children and is often not dose-dependent. The effect of ethosuximide on cognition is

**Table 3.6** Summary of the adverse effects due to ethosuximide; data from 12 early studies, published between 1958 and 1966, each involving 50 or more subjects receiving ethosuximide.

| Adverse effect | Range (median), % |
|---|---|
| Any adverse effect | 26–46 (37) |
| Gastrointestinal disturbances (nausea, abdominal discomfort, anorexia, vomiting and diarrhoea) | 4–29 (13) |
| Drowsiness | 0–16 (7) |
| Rash | 0–6 (0) |
| Ataxia | 0–1 (0) |
| Dizziness | 0–4 (1) |
| Hiccups | 0–5 (0) |

unclear. There are some reports of memory, speech and emotional disturbances, and ethosuximide can certainly occasionally cause severe behavioural changes, particularly irritability, depression and anxiety, and occasionally a psychotic reaction. The psychotic reaction has been attributed to 'forced normalization', and seems to occur with a higher frequency with ethosuximide than with other antiabsence drugs. For this reason, the drug should be used with caution in patients with a history of psychiatric disturbance. However, other reports show striking cognitive improvement on ethosuximide therapy, possibly related to the better control of spike-wave discharges. Other rarer neurological side-effects include bradykinesia and Parkinsonism. Sedation can be a problem and is not uncommon following the increase in plasma level of ethosuximide in patients in whom valproate has been added. Occasionally, a severe encephalopathy can be induced by ethosuximide, as it can by other succinimide drugs.

The incidence of ethosuximide-related granulocytopenia ranged from 0 to 7% in early studies, and is dose dependent. This is of no concern, but must be distinguished from the severe marrow depression in ethosuximide hypersensitivity. Some teratogenic effects have been reported, but the incidence of these is quite unknown.

### Overdose

Cases of ethosuximide overdose have been reported. Coma and respiratory depression occur and treatment is by supportive measures. Additional recommended measures include the use of activated charcoal, gastric lavage and haemodialysis. Exchange transfusion and forced diuresis have no value.

### Antiepileptic effect

Ethosuximide, like valproate, is highly effective in controlling generalized absence seizures. Although it was introduced before the current vogue for randomized controlled trials, well-conducted open studies in the 1970s demonstrated a clear and powerful effect in often previously resistant patients. In one study of 37 patients, 19% were rendered free from seizures, and 49% had a greater than 90% reduction and 95% a greater than 50% reduction in seizures. In another study complete control of seizures was obtained in 47% of patients, an effect closely correlated to plasma level.

The effectiveness of the drug has been shown to be equal to that of valproate in five controlled trials, and furthermore the drugs in combination can have a synergistic effect in patients who have not responded adequately to either drug alone. Tolerance does not develop with ethosuximide. Although ethosuximide does not generally control tonic–clonic seizures, a gratifying effect is occasionally encountered in resistant idiopathic generalized epilepsy. The usual lack of effect in tonic–clonic seizures is

a disadvantage compared with valproate, which has a much broader spectrum of action.

Ethosuximide has a moderate effect in atypical absence seizures (in the Lennox–Gastaut syndrome), and is reported to be helpful in absence status epilepticus, severe myoclonic epilepsy in infancy, juvenile myoclonic epilepsy, epilepsy with myoclonic absences, eyelid myoclonia with absences, epilepsy with continuous spike and wave during slow-wave sleep, photosensitive seizures and gelastic seizures. It probably has little or no effect in simple partial, complex partial or partial secondarily generalized tonic–clonic seizures.

Plasma level measurements of ethosuximide are useful in defining dosage, and there is a clear relationship between plasma level and clinical effectiveness. The target range of drug levels is between 300 and 700 $\mu$mol/l.

### Clinical use in epilepsy

Ethosuximide remains a useful drug in the treatment of childhood absence seizures, although its first-line use has been largely supplanted, particularly in older children or young adults, by valproate because of the latter drug's superior action in tonic–clonic seizures. It still has a place in the treatment of young children where there is a risk of valproate-induced hepatotoxicity. It may be usefully added to valproate in patients whose absence seizures are not controlled on valproic acid monotherapy. It also has a limited role in other seizure types where more conventional therapy has failed.

A common starting dose for children is 10–15 mg/kg/day, with subsequent titration according to the patient's clinical response. Older children and adults often initiate ethosuximide at 250 mg/day and increase by 250 mg increments until the desired clinical response is reached. Ethosuximide can be administered either as once, twice or even thrice daily dosing, with meals to maximize seizure control while minimizing adverse effects. In younger children, maintenance dosages are usually between 15 and 40 mg/kg/day. In older children and adults, common maintenance doses are 750–2000 mg/day. Ethosuximide withdrawal should be carried out at a decremental rate not exceeding 250 mg every 2 weeks.

Serum level monitoring of ethosuximide is more useful than for any other antiepileptic drug with the exception of phenytoin, and effectiveness is closely correlated to serum levels. Nevertheless, the dose should be escalated according to clinical response rather than serum level. The therapeutic range is generally between 40 and 100 $\mu$g/ml, although patients with refractory seizures may need serum concentrations up to 150 $\mu$g/ml. Routine laboratory monitoring of blood count is not useful in preventing idiosyncratic haematological reactions. However, if the total white blood-cell count falls below 3500 or the proportion of granulocytes below 25% of the total white blood-cell count, the dose should be reduced or the drug withdrawn.

# GABAPENTIN

NH$_2$   COOH

| | |
|---|---|
| **Primary indications** | Partial or secondarily generalized epilepsy. Adults and children (over age of 6 years) |
| **Licensed for monotherapy/add-on therapy** | Add-on therapy only |
| **Usual preparations** | Capsules: 100, 300, 400 mg |
| **Usual dosage—adults** | Initial: 300 mg/day<br>Maintenance: 900–2400 mg/day |
| **Usual dosage—children** | Initial: 50–100 mg/kg |
| **Dosing intervals** | 2–3 times/day |
| **Dose commonly affected by co-medication** | No |
| **Dose affected by renal/hepatic disease** | Severe renal disease |
| **Common drug interactions** | None |
| **Serum level monitoring** | Not useful |
| **Common/important adverse events** | Drowsiness, dizziness, seizure exacerbation, ataxia, headache, tremor, diplopia, nausea, vomiting, rhinitis |
| **Major mechanism of action** | Not known |
| **Main advantages** | Lack of side-effects, especially at low doses; good pharmacokinetic profile |
| **Main disadvantages** | Lack of therapeutic effect in severe cases; absorption variable, especially at high doses; seizure exacerbation in some cases |
| **COMMENT** | Effective second-choice antiepileptic drug for partial epilepsy, particularly in mild cases. Easy to use and few side-effects at low doses |

Gabapentin is one of the newer antiepileptic drugs and was designed as a GABA agonist, with a close structural relationship to GABA, although subsequent clinical and experimental evidence has shown little or no action at the GABA receptor. It was first studied as an antispastic drug and an analgesic, but early clinical trials of its antispastic action proved disappointing. Attention then turned to its antiepileptic action, and on the basis of a series of clinical trials, it became licensed widely in the USA, Britain, Europe, and other countries for this indication. Initial clinical experience in routine practice in epilepsy, however, was rather disappointing, although its off-label effects on neurogenic pain were generally considered stronger. This indication was pursued and licensing achieved in many countries, and now the majority of prescriptions for Gabapentin worldwide are for the alleviation of neuropathic pain. In epilepsy it was then realized that greater effectiveness was possible with higher doses than those used in the clinical trials, and this has revived interest in the drug. Gabapentin has now achieved a solid place as second-line treatment in partial epilepsy, with moderate effect and certain advantages over other, possibly stronger, therapy.

It is currently approved for adjunctive therapy in partial epilepsy in many countries and for monotherapy for epilepsy in 30 countries (but not the USA).

## Physical and chemical characteristics

Gabapentin is a highly soluble crystalline substance (molecular weight 172.24), with pKa values of 3.7 and 10.7. It has a chemical structure which is very similar to that of GABA, with the same 4-carbon chain but with an additional cyclohexyl ring incorporated.

## Mode of action

Like pregabalin, gabapentin binds to the alpha-2-delta protein associated with the voltage-gated calcium channel. This, however, does not affect inward calcium flux to a marked extent (for example, in comparison with pregabalin). Whether this is its mode of antiepileptic action is unknown. It does not act at the GABA-A receptor, in spite of its close structural similarity. It may, however, increase GABA synthesis and it possibly reduces GABA reuptake. It has no major action on glutamate receptor systems, although it may reduce brain concentrations of glutamate

**Gabapentin**
Pharmacokinetics—average adult values

| | |
|---|---|
| Oral bioavailability | < 65% (dose dependent) |
| Time to peak levels | 2–3 h |
| Volume of distribution | 0.65–1.04 l/kg |
| Biotransformation | Not metabolized |
| Elimination half-life | 5–7 h |
| Plasma clearance | 0.120–0.130 l/kg/h |
| Protein binding | None |
| Active metabolite | None |

and glutamine, nor on sodium or calcium channel conductance. In experimental models it has a profile that differentiates it from other antiepileptics used for these indications.

## Pharmacokinetics
### Absorption and distribution
The bioavailability of gabapentin is only about 60% at doses of 1800 mg/day or less and 35% or less for doses over 3600 mg/day, even when given in a thrice daily regimen. This is because gabapentin is actively transported across the gut wall by an L-amino acid transporter that is saturable. What few data there are suggest that age has little effect on absorption nor does food, although food rich in neutral amino acids or monosaccharides may enhance absorption. Because absorption is incomplete and relies on an active transport system, caution should be exercised when gabapentin is used in those clinical circumstances in which absorption might be expected to be compromised. Peak serum levels are achieved within 2–4 hours of oral dosing. The volume of distribution of the drug is 0.65–1.04 l/kg at steady state.

Gabapentin is not bound to plasma proteins at all. The drug readily crosses the blood–brain barrier, utilizing the L-amino acid transport system, which is saturable, and plasma to brain concentrations fall at higher plasma concentrations. Two clearance mechanisms, active transport and passive diffusion, limit its accumulation

### Biotransformation and elimination
The drug is not metabolized at all and is completely excreted in an unchanged form. This lack of hepatic metabolism is of course a great advantage, and there are no pharmacokinetic drug interactions.

Gabapentin is eliminated unchanged entirely by renal excretion with an elimination half-life of 5–7 hours. The renal clearance is 0.120–0.13 l/kg/h and is linearly correlated with creatinine clearance. Gabapentin clearance varies with age-related changes in creatinine clearance and glomerular filtration rate. Clearance is highest in young children, and children between the ages of 1 month and 5 years of age require approximately 30% higher doses to achieve a given plasma concentration than children aged 5–12 years. Age- and disease-related decreases in renal function significantly reduce gabapentin clearance, and the dose needs to be reduced progressively in patients with creatinine clearance levels below 60 ml/min. In haemodialysis, the dosing should be related to creatinine clearance with small supplemental doses given immediately after each 4 hours of dialysis. Steady-state levels are achieved within a few days, however, and the half-life does not change on chronic administration nor is it influenced by co-medication. Serum levels of gabapentin are not routinely measured and there are few data on the correlation between serum level and effectiveness.

### Drug interactions
Gabapentin has no known pharmacokinetic drug interactions owing to its lack of protein binding and hepatic metabolism. There is potential for interaction at the renal level, but no specific effects have been reported.

### Adverse effects
Gabapentin has a remarkably good side-effect profile, with only sedation, dizziness and ataxia being at all prominent (Table 3.7). In the early double-blind studies, 44% of patients reported adverse effects on gabapentin 900 mg. Similar levels of side-effects were recorded in later studies on 1200 mg. In the US study, at 1200 and 1800 mg/day, the following adverse effects were most commonly reported: somnolence 20–36%, dizziness 18–24%, ataxia 18–26%, headache 9–20%, tremor 13–15% and fatigue 11–13%. In the UK study, at 1200 mg/day, somnolence occurred in 15% of gabapentin-treated patients, fatigue in 13%, dizziness in 7%, and weight increase in 5%. Most of the adverse effects were mild and only seven of the 61 and five of the 208 treated patients in the UK and US studies, respectively, withdrew medication because of adverse events. In Table 3.7 the side-effects reported by 485 patients treated with gabapentin and 307 given placebo in controlled studies are shown. Overall, only 7.4% of 1748 patients who received gabapentin in any clinical study have been withdrawn from the study owing to adverse events.

The effect of gabapentin on mood is unpredictable. It has been variously reported to improve, have no effect upon, and adversely affect mood, and there are reports of aggressive behaviour, hyperactivity and irritability in patients with learning disability. In formal studies of cognition, no adverse effects have been reported on attention, psychomotor speed, language and speech in healthy volunteers or in patients with complex partial seizure.

**Table 3.7** The 10 most common adverse effects of gabapentin reported in clinical trials; number (percent) of patients with adverse effects.

| | Controlled studies | | All studies |
|---|---|---|---|
| | Placebo (*n* = 307) | Gabapentin (*n* = 485) | Gabapentin (*n* = 1160) |
| | 174 (56.7) | 369 (76.1) | 944 (81.4) |
| *Adverse events* | | | |
| Somnolence | 30 (9.8) | 98 (20.2) | 283 (24.4) |
| Dizziness | 24 (7.8) | 87 (17.9) | 235 (20.3) |
| Ataxia | 16 (5.2) | 64 (13.2) | 202 (17.4) |
| Fatigue | 15 (4.9) | 54 (11.1) | 171 (14.7) |
| Nystagmus | 15 (4.9) | 45 (9.3) | 174 (15.0) |
| Headache | 28 (9.1) | 42 (8.7) | 176 (15.2) |
| Tremor | 12 (3.9) | 35 (7.2) | 174 (15.0) |
| Diplopia | 6 (2.0) | 31 (6.4) | 124 (10.7) |
| Nausea and/or vomiting | 23 (7.5) | 29 (6.0) | 108 (9.3) |
| Rhinitis | 12 (3.9) | 22 (4.5) | 101 (8.7) |

Worsening of seizures is a particularly marked phenomenon in some patients treated with gabapentin. In the US study, 19% of patients treated with 1800 mg/day gabapentin and in the UK study 20% treated with 1200 mg/day experienced a worsening of seizure frequency. Gabapentin can also worsen myoclonus.

Gabapentin has been given to over 10 million patients, and remarkably few potentially serious side-effects have been reported. The incidence of rash is 0.5% and that of neutropenia 0.2%. ECG changes and/or angina were found in 0.05%. No cases of hepatotoxicity have been recorded. There are no consistent changes in any other clinical or laboratory measure, and no serious idiosyncratic or hypersensitivity reactions. Pancreatic carcinoma was reported in the animal toxicology studies, but there have been no clinical reports of pancreatic disease. Three cases of massive gabapentin overdose have been reported without serious effects.

The abrupt withdrawal of gabapentin has been associated with a range of symptoms, many related to sympathetic overactivity, and as with all other antiepileptics in routine practice the drug should be withdrawn gradually.

### Antiepileptic effects

Gabapentin has been studied in a series of open and double-blind randomized controlled investigations in partial epilepsy, and a consistent picture has emerged. The large multicentre study carried out in the UK randomized patients to add-on therapy with either gabapentin 1200 mg or placebo. Twenty-five percent of the gabapentin patients showed a reduction in partial seizures of at least 50% compared with 9.8% of those taking placebo. In a similar study from the USA, patients were randomized to 600, 1200 or 1800 mg/day of gabapentin or placebo. The percentage of patients with a reduction in seizures of at least 50% ranged from 18 to 26% with gabapentin and 8% with placebo. These trials showed that the drug has antiepileptic action in partial epilepsy, however, the number of responders is disappointingly low, and at the doses tried, the drug seems rather weak. Since licensing, it has become customary to prescribe much higher doses, and although these doses have not been studied in double-blind controlled trials, there is a universal clinical impression that higher doses are markedly more effective, at least in some patients. The side-effects at higher doses are also more prominent. Gabapentin has a narrow spectrum of activity and is not effective in primary generalized seizures, absence seizures and myoclonus (and indeed absence seizures and myoclonus are frequently worsened by the drug).

In newly diagnosed patients with partial epilepsy, double-blind studies have shown that gabapentin, lamotrigine and carbamazepine have similar efficacy in monotherapy. In addition a large number of open and retrospective studies have been reported, showing similar results. Long-term follow-up studies have demonstrated sustained benefit without the emergence of longer-term toxicity or new toxicity. However, in long-term retention studies, fewer than 40% of patients taking gabapentin remained on the drug for 6 years and fewer than 4% became free from seizures. A double-blind trial of gabapentin for benign rolandic epilepsy (with centrotemporal spikes) demonstrated statistically significant superiority of gabapentin over placebo.

### Clinical use in epilepsy

Gabapentin is a useful drug in the treatment of partial and secondarily generalized tonic–clonic seizures. It has an excellent pharmacological profile, and its lack of protein binding, its lack of metabolism, and its lack of drug interactions are attractive properties. It has particular value in renal or hepatic disease and in patients on complicated drug regimens. Also, it is relatively well tolerated although it does have some side-effects, particularly at higher doses, but apart from drowsiness these are usually relatively minor. Certainly, the severe behavioural or psychiatric disturbances found with other drugs do not occur with gabapentin nor do idiosyncratic or serious systemic side-effects. There are, however, disadvantages. The drug appears to have only a rather modest efficacy, and most patients with severe epilepsy derive little benefit. Furthermore, a substantial minority of patients treated with gabapentin suffer a worsening of seizure frequency and occasionally this deterioration can be marked. Also the drug is ineffective in most generalized seizure types including tonic–clonic and absence seizures and in myoclonus. Although its pharmacokinetic profile is generally good, its absorption is erratic, particularly at higher doses, and this can be problematic.

Gabapentin is available in 100, 300 and 400 mg capsules, and in 600 and 800 mg tablets. It is common practice to titrate this dose up at weekly intervals to a maximum of 3600 mg/day. The usual initial maintenance doses are between 900 and 2400 mg/day. Although all the trials used three times a day dosing, a twice a day regimen seems equally effective. However, at high doses, three or four times daily dosing may avoid saturation of the processes of absorption. In routine practice withdrawal can be carried out at weekly decremental rates of 400 mg. Serum antiepileptic drug levels can be helpful to assess absorption, particularly where higher doses are contemplated, but serum level is not closely related to effectiveness. The dose should be halved in patients with creatinine clearance values between 30 and 59 ml/min, reduced by a further half where creatinine clearance is between 15 and 29 ml/min, and reduced further at lower levels.

# LAMOTRIGINE

| | |
|---|---|
| **Primary indications** | Partial and generalized epilepsy. Also in Lennox–Gastaut syndrome and other generalized epilepsy syndromes. Adults and children over 2 years of age |
| **Licensed for monotherapy/add-on therapy** | Both (monotherapy in patients ≥ 12 years) |
| **Usual preparations** | Tablets: 25, 50, 100, 200 mg; chewtabs: 5, 25, 100 mg |
| **Usual dosage—adults** | Initial: 12.5–25 mg/day<br>Maintenance: 200–600 mg/day<br>But depends on co-medication; see Tables 3.11 and 3.12 |
| **Usual dosage—children** | Depends on co-medication; see Tables 3.11 and 3.12 |
| **Dosing intervals** | 2 times/day |
| **Dose commonly affected by co-medication** | Yes |
| **Dose affected by renal/hepatic disease** | Avoid in hepatic disease |
| **Common drug interactions** | Extensive drug interactions; see p. 138 |
| **Serum level monitoring** | Useful in some cases |
| **Target range** | 10–60 µmol/l |
| **Common/important adverse events** | Rash (sometimes severe), headache, blood dyscrasia, ataxia, asthenia, diplopia, nausea, vomiting, dizziness, somnolence, insomnia, depression, psychosis, tremor, hypersensitivity reactions |
| **Major mechanism of action** | Inhibition of voltage-dependent sodium conductance |
| **Main advantages** | Moderate effectiveness, and generally well-tolerated |
| **Main disadvantages** | High instance of rash (occasionally severe) and other side-effects; complicated pharmacokinetics |
| **COMMENT** | A useful antiepileptic, especially in generalized epilepsies |

The history of medicine has seen many drugs developed on incorrect premises, and lamotrigine is a recent example. In the 1960s it was postulated—wrongly—that the antiepileptic effects of phenytoin and phenobarbital could be mediated through their antifolate properties. Lamotrigine was then developed as an anti-folate drug. However, as it turns out, lamotrigine does not have a marked antifolate action and there is no correlation between antifolate action and antiepileptic effects. Such is fortune, however, that lamotrigine was then found to have a pronounced antiepileptic effect.

## Physical and chemical characteristics
Lamotrigine (3,5-diamino-6-[2,3-dichorophenyl]-1,2,4-triazine; molecular weight 256.1) is a triazine compound unrelated chemically to any other antiepileptic. It is a weak base, pKa 5.5, and is poorly soluble in water or in ethanol.

## Mode of action
In its short life, a whole range of mechanisms of action have been postulated, only later to be discounted. It seems now that the antiepileptic action is largely due to its effect in blocking voltage-dependent sodium channel conductance, an action similar to that of carbamazepine or phenytoin. Indeed, the drug binds to the same amino-acid residues as phenytoin, although it has different binding kinetics. Whether or not the drug has any more direct neurotransmitter action is uncertain, although antiglutamate and antiaspartate actions have been suggested, and lamotrigine also modulates voltage-dependent calcium conductance at N-type calcium channels. In experimental seizure models lamotrigine has a rather similar profile of action to that of phenytoin.

# Pharmacokinetics

---

### Lamotrigine
Pharmacokinetics—average adult values

| | |
|---|---|
| Oral bioavailability | < 100% |
| Time to peak levels | 1–3 h |
| Volume of distribution | 0.9–1.31 l/kg |
| Biotransformation | Hepatic glucuronidation without phase 1 reaction (UDPGT family enzymes) |
| Elimination half-life | 12–60 h (varies considerably with co-medication) |
| Plasma clearance | 0.044–0.084 l/kg/h (but variable) |
| Protein binding | 55% |
| Active metabolite | None |

---

### Absorption and distribution

The drug is well absorbed orally with a bioavailability approaching 100%. Peak concentrations occur within 1–3 hours after dosing in adults (1–6 hours in children), and a linear relationship exists between dose and concentration in the normal clinical dosing ranges. There is a second smaller lamotrigine peak after oral administration attributed to intestinal re-absorption of the drug sequestered in the stomach. Absorption is not affected by food. Lamotrigine is 55% bound to plasma proteins and has a volume of distribution of between 0.9 and 1.3 l/kg in adults and 1.5 l/kg in children. Brain concentrations are 1.5–2.5 times plasma concentrations.

### Metabolism and elimination

The drug undergoes extensive metabolism in the liver largely to the inert glucuronide conjugate, most of which is renally excreted, and its metabolism results in complex pharmacokinetics. In chronic therapy, less than 10% of the drug is excreted unchanged in the urine.

Plasma clearance shows marked intra-individual variation and is affected by age and co-medication. In monotherapy, plasma clearance values are higher in children (0.038 l/kg/h) than in adults (0.044–0.084 l/kg/h). Elimination half-lives are broadly similar in children and in adults (32 hours in children vs 23–37 hours in adults). Younger children have higher clearance values than older children, and older children and adults higher levels than the elderly. These differences may be due to a relative reduction in liver size and hepatic blood flow in adolescents compared with young children, and diminished glucuronidation at older ages. A comparison of single 150 mg oral doses in healthy young and elderly volunteers revealed a 37% lower clearance in the elderly and a 27% higher maximum plasma concentration ($C_{max}$) and 55% higher values of AUC (area under the plasma concentration–time curve). Some but not all investigators have shown autoinduction. Peculiarly, the plasma clearance of lamotrigine can greatly increase towards the end of pregnancy, and as a result doses of lamotrigine may need to be doubled during pregnancy to maintain constant serum levels. Clearance is not significantly affected by renal impairment. Gilbert syndrome, a disorder of conjugation characterized by altered uridine diphosphate glucuronyl transferase (UDGT) activity, results in decreased clearance and prolongation (by appro-ximately 35%) of half-life. Lamotrigine is excreted in considerable amounts in breast milk, which in combination with slow elimination in the infant may result in similar plasma concentrations in the infant and mother.

### Drug interactions

The hepatic glucuronidation of lamotrigine is not via P450 enzymes, and thus lamotrigine does not induce P450 activity and hence has little effect on the metabolism of other lipid-soluble drugs, including the enzyme-inducing antiepileptic drugs or warfarin.

Unfortunately, the concomitant administration of other antiepileptic drugs does have a profound effect on the metabolism of lamotrigine. Enzyme inducers reduce the half-life from a mean of 29 hours to 15 hours in adults, and this effect is even greater in young children. Sodium valproate lengthens the half-life, by mechanisms that are unclear, to 60 hours or more. In children, the half-life falls to less than 10 hours in those co-medicated with enzyme-inducing antiepileptics and is between 15 and 27 hours when valproate is given with inducers, and 44 and 94 hours with valproate alone. As a result of these major interactions, lamotrigine dosage needs to be modified according to concomitant therapy, and conversely, when the dose of co-medication is altered, lamotrigine levels will also change. In young children, pronounced peak–trough fluctuations may occur in co-medication with enzyme-inducing drugs, and more frequent dosing intervals may be required.

Ethosuximide, vigabatrin, gabapentin, zonisamide and tiagabine have no significant effect on hepatic metabolism and are therefore not expected to have an effect on lamo-trigine pharmacokinetics. No clear differences have been observed in combination with felbamate, and co-medication with topiramate results in either slightly decreased or un-changed plasma concentrations. The clearance of lamotrigine can be affected by non-antiepileptic enzyme-inducing drugs. A common example is the increased clearance of lamotrigine when the oral contraceptive is added as co-medication, and this can require dosage change.

**Table 3.8** Adverse events reported by newly diagnosed patients on lamotrigine, carbamazepine and phenytoin monotherapy; pooled data from comparative trials of lamotrigine and carbamazepine or phenytoin.

| | Lamotrigine (n = 443) | Carbamazepine (n = 246) | Phenytoin (n = 95) |
|---|---|---|---|
| *Median-modal dose* | *100–200 mg/day* | *600 mg/day* | *300 mg/day* |
| Headache | 89 (20) | 43 (17) | 18 (19) |
| Asthenia | 70 (16) | 60 (24) | 28 (29) |
| Rash | 52 (12) | 35 (14) | 9 (9) |
| Nausea | 44 (10) | 25 (10) | 4 (4) |
| Sleepiness | 36 (8) | 49 (20) | 27 (28) |
| Dizziness | 36 (8) | 34 (14) | 11 (12) |

## Adverse effects

### Neurotoxic effects

The most common side-effects of lamotrigine—noted both in adjunctive and monotherapy—are headache, nausea and vomiting, diplopia, dizziness, ataxia, and tremor (Tables 3.8 and 3.9). Sedation can occur but is usually not prominent and the lack of sedation is an advantage of this drug over others. There have been reports of behavioural change, aggression, irritability, agitation, confusion, hallucinations and psychoses, but these side-effects are uncommon. In isolated individual cases, however, severe reactions do occur. Diplopia and unsteadiness seem particularly common when the drug is used in combination with carbamazepine, but whether this is a pharmacodynamic or pharmacokinetic interaction is not known. Certainly, lowering either the carbamazepine or the lamotrigine dose in this situation will usually reverse the visual disturbance.

**Table 3.9** Adverse events reported by 10% or more of patients receiving lamotrigine in a double-blind study of lamotrigine tolerability; n (%).

| | Lamotrigine (n = 334) | Placebo (n = 112) |
|---|---|---|
| Dizziness | 166 (50)* | 20 (18) |
| Headache | 125 (37) | 40 (36) |
| Diplopia | 109 (33)* | 12 (11) |
| Ataxia | 80 (24)* | 5 (5) |
| Blurred vision | 77 (23)* | 10 (9) |
| Nausea | 73 (22) | 17 (15) |
| Rhinitis | 58 (17) | 21 (19) |
| Somnolence | 46 (14)* | 8 (7) |
| Pharyngitis | 42 (13) | 13 (12) |
| Co-ordination abnormality | 39 (12) | 7 (6) |
| Flu syndrome | 38 (11) | 10 (9) |
| Cough | 35 (10) | 9 (8) |
| Rash | 34 (10) | 6 (5) |
| Dyspepsia | 32 (10) | 6 (5) |
| Vomiting | 32 (10) | 10 (9) |

*, Statistically significant against placebo.

### Hypersensitivity

Idiosyncratic hypersensitivity has been a major concern particularly in children, and predominantly affects the skin (Table 3.10). Many antiepileptic drugs cause allergic skin rash, but the incidence of rash and its severity separate lamotrigine from other antiepileptic drugs in this regard. The lamotrigine-associated skin rash is typically maculopapular or erythematous, associated with pruritus, and usually appears within the first 4 weeks of initiating treatment. Occasionally, the rash may be more severe (erythema multiforme) or progress to desquamation with involvement of the mucous membrane (Stevens–Johnson syndrome) and to toxic epidermal necrolysis. The frequency of skin rash is higher in children than in adults, and early reports suggested that as many as 1 in 50 to 1 in 100 children developed a potentially life-threatening rash. This high frequency was probably due to the effects of valproate co-medication on lamotrigine levels, and the frequency of rash is greatly reduced with slow escalation of lamotrigine doses or its use in low doses or as monotherapy. Hypersensitivity can be accompanied by a systemic illness with fever, malaise, arthralgia, lymphadenopathy and eosinophilia. Sporadic cases of multiorgan failure associated with disseminated intravascular coagulation have also been reported as part of a hypersensitivity reaction, sometimes associated with acute renal

| AED therapy | Total no. of patients | All rash (%) | DC rash (%)* | Hosp/SJSrash (%)** |
|---|---|---|---|---|
| *Paediatric (younger than 16 years)* | | | | |
| LTG + EIAED | 394 | 9.6 | 4.1 | 0.8 |
| LTG + VPA only | 145 | 20.0 | 9.0 | 1.4 |
| LTG + VPA + NEIAED | 145 | 21.4 | 10.3 | 1.4 |
| *Adult (older than 16 years)* | | | | |
| LTG + EIAED | 2240 | 6.7 | 2.0 | 0.1 |
| LTG + VPA only | 205 | 19.5 | 12.2 | 2.0 |
| LTG + VPA + NEIAED | 10 | 20.0 | 10.0 | 0 |

**Table 3.10** The rates of rash due to lamotrigine in children and adults in relation to co-medication with other antiepileptic drugs.

EIAED, enzyme-inducing antiepileptic drugs; NEIAED, non-enzyme-inducing antiepileptic drugs; LTG, lamotrigine; VPA, valproic acid. *, rash leading to discontinuation of treatment; **, rash leading to hospitalization or Stevens–Johnson syndrome (SJS).

failure. Isolated cases of pseudolymphoma, agranulocytosis and hepatotoxicity have also been recorded.

### Other adverse effects

Other side-effects reported with lamotrigine include diarrhoea, abdominal pain, dyspepsia, rhinitis, tremor, infection, fever, bronchitis and flu-like symptoms. The drug can increase the requirement for therapy in diabetes insipidus and precipitate a flare-up of ulcerative colitis. A paradoxical increase in seizures occasionally occurs.

### Overdose

Cases of overdose up to 15 g have been reported, and can be fatal. Ingestion of up to 4500 mg are not associated with respiratory depression, although stupor and other cerebral and metabolic disturbances occur. Supportive therapy can be supplemented by gastric lavage and the use of activated charcoal, midazolam and fluid loads.

### Antiepileptic effect

#### Partial-onset seizures

There have been 10 placebo-controlled trials exploring the use of lamotrigine as add-on therapy in refractory epilepsy. Nine of the 10 showed lamotrigine to be significantly better than placebo, with a total decrease in seizures on lamotrigine of between 17 and 59%. Most trials showed a reduction in seizures of approximately 25–30%, and a 20–30% responder rate. In the largest of the trials lamotrigine at a dose of 500 mg/day proved more effective than lamotrigine 300 mg/day or placebo as add-on therapy, reducing the total frequency of seizures by 36% and producing a reduction in seizure frequency of more than 50% in 34% of patients. Lamotrigine has also been studied in a large double-blind trial in 199 children, and a reduction in partial seizures of more than 50%, compared with the baseline frequency, was seen in 42% of lamotrigine-treated and 16% of placebo-treated children.

#### Newly diagnosed epilepsy

In monotherapy in newly diagnosed partial and generalized tonic–clonic seizures, lamotrigine has been shown to be as effective as carbamazepine or phenytoin in newly diagnosed patients. For instance, in one study of adults with newly diagnosed epilepsy randomized to lamotrigine 100–300 mg/day or CBZ 300–1400 mg/day for 48 weeks, the percentages of patients who remained free from seizures over the final 24 weeks of treatment were similar, in terms of overall seizures (39 vs 38%), partial seizures (35 vs 37%), and idiopathic generalized seizures (both 47%). In a study of 150 elderly patients, lamotrigine was shown to be as effective as carbamazepine and better tolerated.

#### Generalized seizures

There is also now good evidence that lamotrigine is effective in generalized tonic–clonic seizures, typical and atypical absence, and atonic seizures. This is a significant advantage over other newer anticonvulsants, and is indeed in this author's opinion the drug's main merit. Lamotrigine can have a marked effect on seizures in the Lennox–Gastaut syndrome, and in one pivotal randomized, controlled, double-blind study, for instance, in a total of 169 patients, the median frequency of all major seizures decreased in the lamotrigine group from 16.4 to 9.9 vs 13.5 to 14.2 compared with placebo. Seizure reduction of greater than 50% was seen significantly more often in the lamotrigine-treated patients (33% vs 16%).

The influence of lamotrigine on myoclonus is however variable. Some cases are improved, but in some the myoclonus is aggravated. Exacerbation of myoclonus has been reported, particularly in the progressive myoclonic epilepsies. In myoclonus in the idiopathic generalized epilepsies, lamotrigine is not as effective as valproate, but it is a useful second-line therapy. Lamotrigine has a useful action in newly diagnosed absence epilepsy. In one placebo-controlled trial, 30 of 42 patients (71%) aged 2–16 years became free from seizures at a median dose of 5 mg/kg/day, and 60% of 15 patients remained free from seizures with lamotrigine treatment compared with 21% of the 14 patients receiving placebo.

Lamotrigine has also been shown to be effective in neonatal seizures and in infantile spasms, although it is not currently considered a drug of first choice in either clinical situation.

## Clinical use in epilepsy

The drug is available in tablets containing 25, 50, 100 and 200 mg. Formulations of 5, 25 and 100 mg tablets are also available. There is no parenteral preparation. The drug is usually prescribed on a twice daily basis, although a single daily dose can be used if it is taken with valproate alone. The drug is currently licensed as first- or second-line treatment for primary generalized epilepsy or partial and secondarily generalized seizures, in polytherapy or as monotherapy. It is generally well tolerated but the risk of rash remains a clinical problem in children. If a rash develops, the drug should be immediately stopped, and it seems sensible to avoid using the drug in patients with severe hepatic impairment.

There is a general clinical consensus that the effectiveness of the drug in chronic partial epilepsy is only moderate, comparable to that of gabapentin, but less effective than other first-line drugs. Its lack of sedative side-effects is a positive feature. It has a wide spectrum of activity, and is particular useful in generalized epilepsies, for instance the Lennox–Gastaut syndrome, and in patients with learning disability. This is considered by many to be its most valuable contribution to current epilepsy practice. However, it can exacerbate myoclonus. It has some use in the idiopathic generalized epilepsies, although it is not as effective as valproate against myoclonus in this condition.

Dosing regimens depend on age and co-medication. In monotherapy, 25 mg at night should be given for 2 weeks, then 50 mg at night for 2 weeks followed by target maintenance doses of 100–400 mg/day in two divided doses. The maintenance dose can be increased to 600 mg/day if required, with 50 or 100 mg increments every 2 weeks. Suggested dosing regimens for co-medicated patients are shown in Tables 3.11 and 3.12.

Although plasma levels can be measured, and a therapeutic range has been postulated, there is only a loose relationship between serum concentration and clinical effectiveness (or indeed with side-effects). The routine measurement of blood levels is therefore unnecessary. However, because of the com-plex effects of co-medication, monitoring of plasma levels when concomitant medication is changed can be helpful. This applies to the addition of both antiepileptic and non-antiepileptic drugs including the oral contraceptive. In later pregnancy, lamotrigine levels can fall precipitously (often to less than half the pre-conception levels), and plasma levels should be frequently measured; a rapid escalation of dose is sometime required to maintain consistent levels.

**Table 3.11** Lamotrigine (LTG) dose regimens, when co-medicated with valproate.

*Patients over 12 years of age*
- Weeks 1 and 2: 25 mg every other day: Weeks 3 and 4: 25 mg every day
- Usual maintenance dose: 100–400 mg/day (1or 2 divided doses)
- To achieve maintenance, doses may be increased by 25–50 mg/day every 1–2 weeks
- Usual maintenance dose, when adding LTG to valproate alone, ranges from 100 to 200 mg/day

*Patients 2–12 years of age*
- Weeks 1 and 2: 0.15 mg/kg/day in 1 or 2 divided doses
- Weeks 3 and 4: 0.3 mg/kg/day in 1 or 2 divided doses
- Usual maintenance dose: 1–5 mg/kg/day in 1 or 2 divided doses (maximum 200 mg/day)
- To achieve the usual maintenance dose, subsequent doses should be increased every 1–2 weeks (calculate 0.3 mg/kg/day)

**Table 3.12** Lamotrigine dose regimens when co-medicated with enzyme-inducing antiepileptic drugs.

*Patients over 12 years of age*
- Weeks 1 and 2: 50 mg/day: Weeks 3 and 4: 100 mg/day in 2 divided doses
- Usual maintenance dose: 300–500 mg/day in 2 divided doses
- To achieve maintenance, doses may be increased by 100 mg/day every 1–2 weeks

*Patients 2–12 years of age*
- Weeks 1 and 2: 0.6 mg/kg/day in 2 divided doses
- Weeks 3 and 4: 1.2 mg/kg/day in 2 divided doses
- Usual maintenance dose: 5–15 mg/kg/day in 2 divided doses (maximum 400 mg/day)
- To achieve the usual maintenance dose, subsequent doses should be increased every 1–2 weeks (calculate 1.2 mg/kg/day)

# LEVETIRACETAM

| | |
|---|---|
| **Primary indications** | Partial seizures with or without secondarily generalized seizures. Adults only |
| **Licensed for monotherapy/add-on therapy** | Add-on therapy in patients aged ≥ 16 years |
| **Usual preparations** | Tablets: 250, 500, 1000 mg |
| **Usual dosage—adults** | Initial: 125–250 mg/day<br>Maintenance: 750–4000 mg/day |
| **Dosing intervals** | 2 times/day |
| **Dose commonly affected by co-medication** | Yes |
| **Dose affected by renal/hepatic disease** | Renal disease |
| **Common drug interactions** | None |
| **Serum level monitoring** | Not useful |
| **Common/important adverse events** | Somnolence, asthenia, infection, dizziness, headache, irritability, aggression, behavioural and mood changes |
| **Major mechanism of action** | Action via binding to SV2A synaptic vesicle protein |
| **Main disadvantages** | Mood and behavioural changes |
| **Main advantages** | Highly effective and generally well tolerated; mode of action not shared by other drugs |
| **COMMENT** | Well-tolerated and powerful antiepileptic drug. Preliminary trial evidence suggests also a broad spectrum of activity |

Levetiracetam (ucb L059) was first investigated in the early 1980s as a drug with cognitive enhancing and anxiolytic effects. More than 2000 patients were included in these early studies, the majority receiving doses ranging from 250 to 1000 mg/day, but the findings were disappointing. Pivotal clinical studies were then initiated in epilepsy, with excellent results, and clinical trials of the drug as adjunctive therapy in the treatment of partial onset seizures began in 1991. The drug was licensed in 1999 in the USA and in 2000 in Europe. It is a powerful antiepileptic compound which has gained an important place in clinical practice. It is currently available only in an oral form, although an IV formulation is under development.

## Physical and chemical characteristics

Levetiracetam bears a close structural similarity to piracetam, and is one of a large family of pyrrolidine drugs. Early studies in other indications used the racemic mixture, etiracetam. Levetiracetam is the L-enantiomer of etiracetam (the R-enantiomer, ucb L060, is inactive). It is a white powder (molecular weight 170.21) and is freely soluble in water, soluble in ethanol but not in other organic solvents.

## Mode of action

Levetiracetam binds selectively, and with high affinity, to a synaptic vesicle protein known as SV2A, which is involved in synaptic vesicle exocytosis and presynaptic neurotransmitter release. This is a novel bindings site, not shared by other conventional antiepileptic drugs, and exactly how binding confers antiepileptic action is unclear. It has an antikindling action and carries neuroprotective potential. Levetiracetam has no action against the maximal electroshock and pentylenetetrazol seizure models, unlike many conventional antiepileptics, but does provide protection in a broad range of other models, especially those of chronic epilepsy. A systematic search for other drugs with a related pyrrolidone acetamide scaffold has been recently undertaken. This has resulted in the identification of a new drug (ucb 34714), chemically closely related to levetiracetam, which is 10 times as potent in animal models, and is currently undergoing clinical trials. This is an exciting prospect.

## Pharmacokinetics

### Levetiracetam
Pharmacokinetics—average adult values

| | |
|---|---|
| Oral bioavailability | < 100% |
| Time to peak levels | 1–2 h |
| Volume of distribution | 0.5–0.7 l/kg |
| Biotransformation | Hydrolysis in many body tissues. Not metabolized by hepatic enzymes |
| Elimination half-life | 12–60 h (depending on co-medication) |
| Plasma clearance | 0.036 l/kg/h |
| Protein binding | None |
| Active metabolite | None |

### Absorption

Levetiracetam is rapidly absorbed following oral administration. The peak concentration is reached at about 1–2 hours after ingestion and oral bioavailability approaches 100%. The speed of absorption—but not its extent—is slowed by food. There is no protein binding.

### Distribution

The drug is widely distributed, with a volume of distribution of approximately 0.5–0.7 l/kg. Despite its water solubility, it freely crosses the blood–brain barrier and it also crosses the placenta, and fetal and maternal plasma levels are similar. It is less than 10% bound to plasma proteins.

### Metabolism and elimination

The major metabolic pathway is to a carboxylic acidic metabolite (ucb L057) by hydrolysis of the acetamide group. Metabolism occurs in various body tissues, including red blood cells, and does not involve the enzymes of the cytochrome P450 system. The half-life of levetiracetam in young healthy people ranges between 7 and 8 hours and does not vary either with dose within the usual dose ranges, or with the frequency of dosing. The principal metabolite (ucb L057) is inactive. There is no auto-induction and the kinetics of the drug are linear in clinical dose ranges. Levetiracetam and its metabolites are excreted renally, with cumulative urinary excretion of unchanged levetiracetam and of L057 of 66% and 24%, respectively, after 48 hours. In persons with normal renal function, the renal clearance of levetiracetam is about 0.6 ml/min/kg. However, elimination is proportional to renal clearance, and the half-life increases in renal impairment. In a comparison of healthy controls and patients with severe renal impairment, the half-life of levetiracetam was 7.6 hours in controls and 24.1 hours in those with renal disease. Both the drug and its principal metabolite are removed from the plasma during haemodialysis.

In severe hepatic impairment, the half-life and the exposure to both levetiracetam and ucb L057 were increased, but this is probably owing to co-existent renal disease, and hepatic impairment *per se* does not seem to affect the kinetics of the drug. The half-life in children (6–12 years of age) is about 6 hours, the clearance 1.43 ml/min/kg and the $C_{max}$ about 30% lower than in adults. In elderly persons the half-life increases to 10–11 hours, possibly owing largely to a decrease in renal function. Serum level monitoring is possible, but wide ranges of serum levels are observed with marked individual variation and little correlation with clinical effect.

### Drug interactions

No significant drug interactions have been identified with other antiepileptic drugs with the exception of inconsistent changes in phenytoin level in some cases where the phenytoin level is close to saturation levels. No clinically significant drug interactions have been observed in interaction studies with the oral contraceptive, warfarin or digoxin. The drug has no inhibitory effect on drug-metabolizing enzymes including CYP3A4, CYP1A2, CYP2C19, CYP2C9, CYP2E1, CYP2D6, epoxide hydrolase and various uridine glucuronyltransferases even at high concentrations. Other antiepileptic drugs have no effect on the metabolism of levetiracetam.

### Adverse effects

Levetiracetam is generally well tolerated, and has a good safety profile (Table 3.13). The most commonly reported side-effects in the adult population are somnolence and asthenia. In a pooled analysis, somnolence was seen in 14.8% of epilepsy patients treated with levetiracetam compared with 8.4% with placebo. The effect was not clearly dose related, and in one study somnolence was seen in 20.4% of patients on 1000 mg of levetiracetam and 18.8% on 3000 mg, as compared with 13.7% of patients on placebo. The second most common side-effect in clinical trials was asthenia, with an overall incidence of 14.7% compared with 9.1% with placebo, and again it was not clearly dose related. Other adverse effects include nausea, dizziness and headache. The incidence of side-effects is greatest during titration, and slow titration improves tolerability significantly. Infections, including those of the upper respiratory tract (rhinitis and pharyngitis) and those of the urinary tract, were increased in some of the controlled trials, but the clinical relevance of this finding is still unclear.

In open label studies in paediatric patients, the adverse events reported are shown in Tables 3.14.

**Table 3.13** Adverse effects in adults patients in the placebo-controlled studies of levetiracetam; NB Only adverse effects occurring in > 5% of patients listed.

| Adverse event | Placebo (n = 351) % affected | Levetiracetam (n = 672) % affected |
|---|---|---|
| Dizziness | 4.3 | 9.2 |
| Asthenia | 9.7 | 14.1 |
| Infection | 7.4 | 13.2 |
| Somnolence | 9.7 | 14.9 |

**Table 3.14** Summary of adverse effects due to levetiracetam in paediatric patients in four open-label studies; NB Only adverse effects occurring in > 3% of patients listed.

| Adverse event | % of patients afected |
|---|---|
| Behavioural | 15–22 |
| Lethargy | 6–7 |
| Ataxia | 7 |
| Dizziness | 7 |
| Decreased appetite | 4 |
| Tremor | 4 |
| Hypotonia | 4 |

Since licensing, the most troublesome side-effects of levetiracetam, not appreciated in the clinical trials, are behavioural symptoms, notably agitation, hostility, and anxiety. Levetiracetam therapy can also precipitate acute psychosis, and this may persist in some cases in spite of drug withdrawal. Other neurological side-effects have included apathy, emotional lability, depersonalization and depression, and a small number of patients have psychotic symptoms and suicidal behaviour. A marked increase in the frequency of seizures is noted in some patients in routine practice, and there is a suggestion that a paradoxical increase in seizures can occur at high doses, especially in those with generalized abnormalities on the EEG. A similar adverse event profile is seen in children, with behavioural disturbances the most prominent problem, and these occur especially in those with a history of pre-existing behavioural disorder.

Hypersensitivity and skin rash are very uncommon, and there are no reports of serious idiosyncratic adverse effects. There are no definitive studies of levetiracetam in pregnancy, and currently levetiracetam is categorized as a pregnancy category C drug (demonstrated teratogenicity in animals, human risk not known) in the USA. One side-effect recently reported is enterocolitis, and this should be suspected in patients developing persistent diarrhoea.

Overdose of levetiracteam is probably safe although no case series have been reported. In animal studies, doses of up to 5000 mg/kg/day produced only mild and transient signs. Haemodialysis would be expected to be effective therapy.

## Antiepileptic effect
### Partial-onset seizures
In the clinical development programme of levetiracetam, four placebo-controlled studies of 1023 persons were carried out in refractory partial epilepsy. Three had a 'similar parallel group randomized to placebo-controlled design' and studied 904 patients, and it was on the basis of these that the drug was licensed. Efficacy was measured over a 12–14 week evaluation period at a daily dose of between 1 and 3 g of levetiracetam or placebo. The three studies showed a consistent, statistically significant, reduction in the weekly frequency of seizures compared with baseline of 18–33% on 1 g, 27% on 2 g, and 37–40% on 3 g (compared with a placebo rate of 6–7%). In all three studies the trend towards a larger improvement was seen in the highest dosage group. The responder rate, defined as the proportion of patients who had a reduction in frequency of partial seizures of at least 50%, was 23–33% on 1 g, 32% on 2 g and 40–42% on 3 g (compared with placebo rates of 10–17%). In one study 3% of the treated patients were rendered seizure-free on 1 g and 9% on 3 g, compared with 0% of the placebo group, during the 14-week evaluation period. The proportion of patients entering the long-term extension studies and the retention rates in these studies were high (> 90% and > 70%, respectively) indicating the favourable effects of the drug without loss of efficacy. A dose–response relationship is demonstrated only in some studies of levetiracetam, and in routine clinical practice many patients respond to lower doses than were used in the clinical trials. In most patients, raising the dose to levels above 4000 mg/day will have no beneficial effect. In the long-term extension studies concomitant antiepileptic drugs were withdrawn in some patients and the favourable effect maintained on monotherapy with levetiracetam.

### Photosensitivity
Levetiracetam also has a marked effect on the photoparoxysmal response in patients with photosensitive epilepsy, and a single 750 or 1000 mg dose will diminish or abolish the photosensitivity in over 50% of photosensitive patients studied (Figure 3.4). The duration of suppression of photosensitivity greatly exceeds the plasma half-life of the drug in all patients, and an effect was noted for more than 24 hours in one-third of patients.

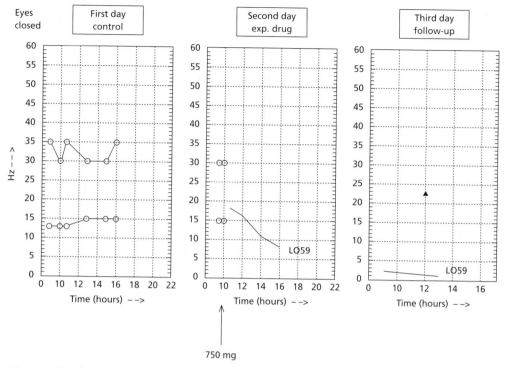

**Figure 3.4** The effect of oral intake of 750 mg levetiracetam (ucb LO59) on the photosensitivity range (upper minus lower limit, in Hz) in patient no. 8 is shown. The limits are graphically expressed as small circles. An abolishment of the reaction to intermittent photic stimulation (IPS) is seen 1 hour after intake of the experimental drug on day 2. On the third day at 12 hours an epileptogenic reaction to IPS has returned, although not yet complete (▲) and only at one frequency (23/Hz). A correlation can be seen between the serum levels of LO59 and the suppressive effect of the drug.

### Generalized seizures

A large number of open studies have been carried out in other types of epilepsy. These have shown undoubted efficacy, particularly in generalized seizure disorders, and a similar experience is noted in routine clinical practice. Striking effects occur especially in absence, myoclonus and tonic–clonic seizures in idiopathic generalized epilepsy. In one open study of 36 patients with primary generalized epilepsy which was not controlled on other antiepileptic drugs, 42% became free from seizures and 75% were considered seizure responders on levetiracetam. Similarly, in patients with intractable myoclonic seizures in juvenile myoclonic epilepsy or absence seizures in childhood or juvenile absence epilepsy (JME), the drug can be strikingly effective. Levetiracetam is also very effective in treating myoclonus in the progressive myoclonic epilepsies and in postanoxic myoclonus. It is also probably useful in atypical absence epilepsy and in the Lennox–Gastaut syndrome and other generalized childhood epilepsy syndromes, but studies in these areas are limited. Dose-related improvements in several domains of quality of life have been noted in a series of formal studies.

## Clinical use in epilepsy

Levetiracetam is a highly effective new antiepileptic drug, with a good safety and tolerability profile. It has a novel mode of action, and the drug is effective in cases resistant to other antiepileptics. The pharmacokinetics of the drug are generally felicitous, and there are few if any drug interactions.

It is highly effective in a wide range of seizure types. The clinical trials, and its current licensing, demonstrate efficacy and safety as add-on therapy for refractory partial onset seizures with or without secondary generalization. However, there is evidence of its value in monotherapy, and many patients in routine practice are well controlled on single drug therapy, often at low doses. It is also clearly apparent from routine clinical practice that the drug is effective in generalized epilepsies, including absence and myoclonus in a wide variety of syndromes, although definitive controlled data have not been obtained. The effects of the drug seem to be maintained during long-term follow-up. Indeed, on the basis of this early experience and provided that no serious adverse effects are encountered, levetiracetam seems likely eventually to become a first-line drug in both partial and generalized epilepsies, rivalling carbamazepine and valproate in this role.

In the clinical trials, there were few serious adverse effects and few withdrawals due to adverse effects. The most common were asthenia, dizziness and somnolence. In clinical practice, somnolence is a problem and can be minimized by slow titration and the use of low doses. Changes in behaviour —notably hostility, aggressive tendencies and agitation- —and also the induction of acute psychosis are the effects in routine practice that cause most difficulty, and patients should be warned about these. Whether the drug increases the risk of infection is unclear, and cases of enterocolitis have also been reported.

Levetiracetam is available in 250, 500 and 1000 mg tablets. In the clinical trials antiepileptic effect was noted at 2–4 g/day, but many patients respond to lower doses, and it is the author's current practice to aim initially for lower doses (750–1500 mg/day) in many patients. The starting dose in routine practice can be 125–250 mg/day in adults, and the dose incremented fortnightly by 250 mg steps in a twice daily regimen. Doses above 4000 mg seem not usually to increase efficacy, and there is indeed a tendency for seizures to be exacerbated at higher doses. Children metabolize levetiracetam faster, and therefore might be expected to require higher doses per unit of body weight than adults. Clinical trials in children aged 6–12 years used mean doses of 40 mg/kg/day, but initial doses used in children are typically 10–20 mg/kg/day. In patients with severe renal impairment and in the elderly, clearance is lowered and the dose should be reduced (Table 3.15). Serum level monitoring seems not to be of any great clinical utility.

**Table 3.15** Levetiracetam dosing in patients with renal impairment.

| Renal function | Creatinine clearance (ml/min/1.73 m$^2$) | Dose administered b.i.d. |
|---|---|---|
| Normal | > 80 | 500–1500 |
| Mild | 50–80 | 500–1000 |
| Moderate | 30–50 | 250–750 |
| Severe | < 30 | 250–500 |

# OXCARBAZEPINE

| | |
|---|---|
| **Primary indications** | Partial and secondarily generalized seizures. Adults and children |
| **Licensed for monotherapy/add-on therapy** | Both for patients ≥ 1 month |
| **Usual preparations** | Tablets: 150, 300, 600 mg<br>Oral suspension: 300 mg/5 ml |
| **Usual dosage—adults** | Initial: 600 mg/day<br>Maintenance: 900–2400 mg/day |
| **Usual dosage—children** | Initial: 8–10 mg/kg per day<br>Maintenance: 30–60 mg/kg/day (maximum 60 mg/kg/day) |
| **Dosing intervals** | 2 times/day |
| **Dose commonly affected by co-medication** | Yes |
| **Dose affected by renal/hepatic disease** | Severe renal disease |
| **Common drug interactions** | Some drug interactions; see p. 149 |
| **Serum level monitoring** | Useful in some cases |
| **Target range** | 50–140 µmol/l (MHD derivative) |
| **Common/important adverse events** | Somnolence, headache, dizziness, diplopia, ataxia, rash, hyponatraemia, weight gain, alopecia, nausea, gastrointestinal disturbance |
| **Major mechanism of action** | Inhibition of voltage-dependent sodium conductance. Also effects on potassium conductance, N-type calcium channels, NMDA receptors |
| **Main advantages** | Similar to carbamazepine, but adverse event profile is different and fewer drug interactions |
| **Main disadvantages** | Higher incidence of hyponatraemia than with carbamazepine |
| **COMMENT** | Powerful antiepileptic for use in partial-onset epilepsy. Clinical indications and effects similar to those of carbamazepine |

Oxcarbazepine is the 10-keto analogue of carbamazepine. Although it was synthesized in 1963, clinical trials did not begin until 1977 and its clinical development was initially slow and irregular, reflecting, perhaps, a lack of clarity within the company about its role vis-à-vis carbamazepine. It was introduced into clinical practice early in Denmark and it was widely accepted, but by the time more general licensing was considered, a second set of modern clinical trials was required for regulatory purposes. These were completed in the 1990s and the drug was introduced into EU countries in 1999 and into the USA in 2000. The drug was trialled in monotherapy initially, which is unusual for an antiepileptic drug, and is available for single and combination drug therapy. Oxcarbazepine is metabolized first by reduction, and thus avoids the oxidative step that carbamazepine undergoes, an important difference as the oxidative metabolite of carbamazepine (CBZ-epoxide) is responsible for some of the side-effects of carbamazepine.

Although oxcarbazepine has a different range of side-effects and drug interactions when compared with carbamazepine, its antiepilepsy effects are very similar.

## Physical and chemical characteristics

Oxcarbazepine (molecular weight 252.3) is, chemically speaking, very similar to carbamazepine. It is a neutral lipophylic compound, and like carbamazepine it is very insoluble in water. It is not clear whether it is as unstable in humid conditions as carbamazepine. Its monohydroxylated derivative (MHD) is more soluble. An aqueous solution of MHD, which may allow parenteral administration, is under development, but at present only an oral preparation is available.

## Mode of action

The pharmacological action of oxcarbazepine is exerted almost exclusively through its 10-monohydroxy metabolite.

| Oxcarbazepine Pharmacokinetics—average adult values | |
| --- | --- |
| Oral bioavailability | < 100% |
| Time to peak levels | 4–6 h |
| Volume of distribution | 0.3–0.8 l/kg |
| Biotransformation | Reduction then conjugation (cytochrome P450 system; UDPGT family enzymes) |
| Elimination half-life | 8–10 h (MHD) |
| Protein binding | 38% (MHD) |
| Active metabolite | MHD |

The mechanism of action in experimental models is very similar to that of carbamazepine. The primary action is blockade of voltage-sensitive sodium channels resulting in stabilization of hyperexcited neural membranes, inhibition of repetitive neuronal firing, and inhibition of the spread of discharges. Unlike carbamazepine, MHD also increases potassium conductance and modulates high-voltage N-type calcium channel activity. Like carbamazepine, it has actions on NMDA receptors, but it has no action on serotonin, GABA or acetylcholine (ACh) receptors.

## Pharmacokinetics

### Absorption and distribution
Oxcarbazepine is absorbed almost completely after oral ingestion, and this is an advantage over carbamazepine. Absorption is not affected by food. Oxcarbazepine is rapidly reduced to the biologically active 10-monohydroxy metabolite MHD (10,11 dihydro-10-hydroxy-5H-dibenzol[b,f]azepine-5-carboxamide), and its pharmacological action is due to this metabolite. MHD reaches peak levels 4–6 hours after oxcarbazepine ingestion and it is widely distributed to brain and other lipid tissues. The volume of distribution is 0.3–0.8 l/kg, suggesting distribution in body water, and is 38% bound to plasma proteins. Fetal and maternal plasma concentrations of oxcarbazepine and MHD are similar, and the plasma to breast milk ratio of both compounds is approximately 0.5.

### Biotransformation and excretion
Oxcarbazepine is rapidly and extensively metabolized in the liver, and less than 1% of the drug is excreted unchanged in the urine. After conversion to MHD, which is responsible for the antiepileptic action of the drug, this is then conjugated to a glucuronide compound (Figure 3.5). The half-life of conversion is 1–2.5 hours and the elimination half-life of MHD is 8–10 hours. In contrast to carbamazepine, there

is no auto-induction. This metabolic pathway avoids the oxidation step (to the epoxide) which is exhibited by carbamazepine and which is mediated via CYP3A4 and CYP2C8, both of which make the metabolism of carbamazepine prone to enzyme induction and drug interaction. The clearance of the drug in children over 8 years of age is similar to that of adults. In younger children, clearance is 30–40% higher. In the elderly clearance may be reduced, but usually in proportion to changes in renal function. The disposition of oxcarbazepine or MHD is not greatly influenced by hepatic disease nor by mild renal disease. However, in patients with creatinine clearance below 30 ml/min, doses should be reduced by 50% or more. MHD levels can be measured, and levels of 20–200 μmols/l are associated with antiepileptic effect. The place of monitoring in routine practice has not been established.

### Drug interactions
Oxcarbazepine has the advantage of not inhibiting or inducing hepatic microsomal enzymes to the same extent as carbamazepine. It does not affect cytochrome P450 enzymes, including CYP1A2, CYP2A6, CYP2C19, CYP2D6, CYP2E1, CYP4A9 and CYP4A11. However, the important isoforms CYP2C19, CYP3A4 and CYP3A5 can be inhibited. Thus, interactions with phenobarbital, carbamazepine and phenytoin may occur (via CYP2C19) resulting in elevation of phenytoin, carbamazepine epoxide and phenobarbital levels. Lamotrigine levels can fall on co-medication by about one-third. Co-medication with the same three drugs reduces MHD concentrations by 30–40%, but there is usually no interaction between oxcarbazepine and valproate. As is the case with carbamazepine, oral contraceptive levels may be lower on co-medication with oxcarbazepine (via CYP3A family enzymes) and this may render low oestrogen contraceptives in effective. No interactions have been noted with warfarin, cimetidine, viloxazine or erythromycin.

## Adverse effects
The side-effect profile of oxcarbazepine is generally similar in nature to that of carbamazepine. Although oxcarbazepine is probably generally better tolerated than standard formulations of carbamazepine, the tolerability of oxcarbazepine has not been compared with slow-release carbamazepine. This would be of interest, as carbamazepine tolerability is itself significantly improved by the use of the slow-release formulation.

### Neurotoxic and gastrointestinal side-effects
The most common are effects on the central nervous system (Table 3.16). The most common dose-related side-effects are fatigue, headache, dizziness and ataxia, and the side-effect profile in this regard is very similar to that of carbamazepine. Nausea and vomiting can also be prominent, especially in children. Other side-effects include weight

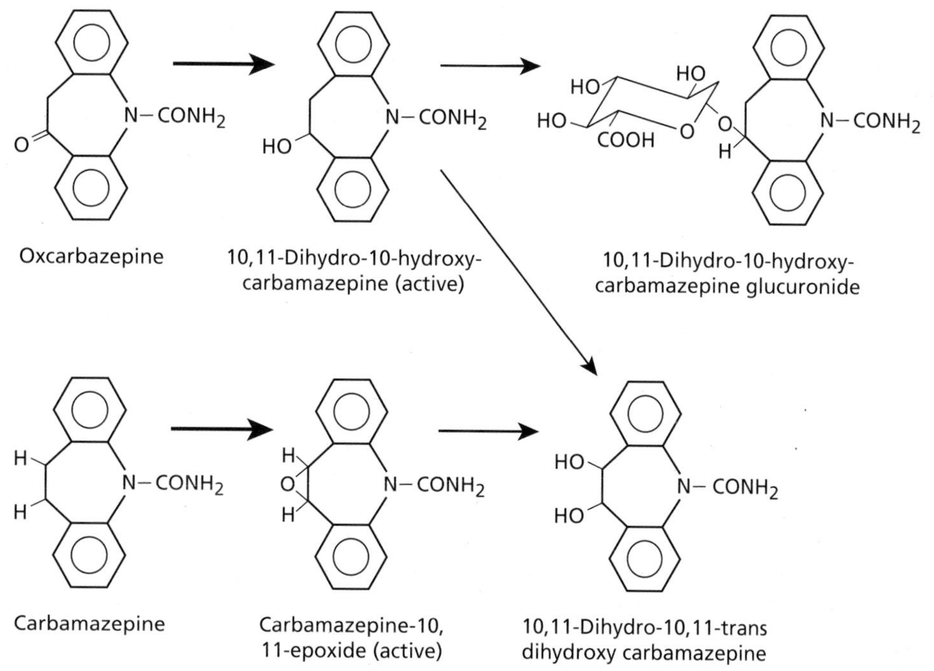

**Figure 3.5** Comparison of metabolism of carbamazepine and oxcarbazepine. Note that the latter drug does not have an active epoxide metabolite.

| | Initial monotherapy trials | | Adjunctive trials* | |
|---|---|---|---|---|
| Side-effect | OXC ($n = 440$) | Placebo ($n = 66$) | OXC ($n = 705$) | Placebo ($n = 302$) |
| Headache | 37 | 12 | 26 | 21 |
| Somnolnce | 22 | 6 | 26 | 12 |
| Dizziness | 20 | 4 | 30 | 11 |
| Ataxia | 2 | 0 | 17 | 5 |
| Diplopia | 0.5 | 0 | 24 | 3 |

*, Combined data from randomized placebo-controlled studies of oxcarbazepine add-on therapy in refractory partial epilepsy in adults and children.

**Table 3.16** The five most common CNS side-effects on oxcarbazepine (OXC) therapy. Comparison of initial monotherapy with adjunctive therapy studies.

increase, tremor, vertigo, alopecia, nervousness, oculogyric crises and gastrointestinal disturbance. Two formal controlled studies have shown no impairment of cognitive function after 4–12 months of therapy with oxcarbazepine.

### Hyponatraemia

Oxcarbazepine, like carbamazepine, results in hyponatraemia owing to an alteration of the regulation of antidiuretic hormone. The effect is, however, more common and more severe with oxcarbazepine and is a particular problem in the elderly patient. In one study comparing sodium levels in patients switched from carbamazepine to oxcarbazepine, a mean drop in sodium levels of 9 mmol/l was observed.

Between 25 and 50% of patients on chronic therapy have serum sodium levels below 135 mmol/l, but this is usually asymptomatic. If the serum sodium level falls below 125 mmol/l (as is reported in < 5% of patients) careful monitoring is advised, and dose reductions should be made if symptoms of hyponatraemia are present. It also seems sensible to advise dose reduction or drug withdrawal if the level falls below 120 mmol/l even in the absence of symptoms.

### Hypersensitivity

The risk of serious life-threatening idiosyncratic side-effects is low, and lower than that of carbamazepine. However, skin rash is relatively common (about 5–10% of all patients) and was the main reason for discontinuation of the drug in the comparative monotherapy studies (10% vs 16% on carbamazepine in one study). Although the rate of occurrence of rash is somewhat lower with carbamazepine, there is significant cross-reactivity, with oxcarbazepine-induced rash occurring in 25–30% of those experiencing rash on carbamazepine. No cases of Stevens–Johnson syndrome or toxic epidermal necrolysis have been reported.

### Overdose

Six cases are reported with a maximum dose of 24 g and all recovered. Potential risks include cardiac arrhythmia, respiratory depression, anticholinergic effects and gastro-intestinal effects. By analogy with experience with carbamazepine, in addition to supportive therapy, gastric lavage, activated charcoal and dialysis are likely to be helpful.

### Antiepileptic effect

Oxcarbazepine has been subjected to twelve randomized double-blind trials, including eight in monotherapy. Comparisons were made with placebo or between high and low doses of oxcarbazepine. All these studies demonstrated effectiveness.

Monotherapy studies preceded add-on studies, uniquely in modern antiepileptic drug development programmes, largely because safety had been established in older open studies. There are, in fact, more monotherapy data on this drug than on any other new antiepileptic.

In newly diagnosed epilepsy, oxcarbazepine monotherapy has been shown to have similar efficacy to valproate, carbamazepine and phenytoin, in studies including nearly 1000 patients. Overall, about 50–60% of newly diagnosed patients become free of seizures on initiation of oxcarbazepine therapy.

Two randomized double-blind add-on studies have also been carried out in refractory adult patients with partial seizures, and the superiority of oxcarbazepine over placebo was demonstrated in both. In the add-on trials, the median reduction in the frequency of partial seizures was between 26.4% at 600 mg/day and 50% at 2400 mg/day. Twenty-two per cent of patients on 2400 mg/day were free of seizures, which is an impressive number for adjunctive therapy in refractory patients. This figure may be high partly because the duration of treatment with 2400 mg was relatively short for patients who dropped out early because of adverse effects.

In a randomized, double-blind placebo-controlled study in children, 41% of patients treated with oxcarbazepine had a reduction in the frequency of seizures of at least 50%, and a 34.8% reduction in the median frequency of seizures. Recent trials in children have shown excellent results with higher doses than previously used (up to 60 mg/kg/day) extending the dose range and potential of oxcarbazepine in paediatric practice. Three controlled studies have compared the efficacy of oxcarbazepine with carbamazepine, and no overall differences were found.

### Clinical use in epilepsy

The indications for oxcarbazepine are similar to those of carbamazepine. Its efficacy is similar to that of other first-line drugs, including carbamazepine, and it is reasonably well tolerated. It has fewer enzyme-inducing effects than some other antiepileptic drugs, including carbamazepine, and thus fewer interactions. If the drug is being substituted for carbamazepine, care is needed, as the removal of the carbamazepine enzyme-inducing effects could alter levels of the concomitant medication. Oxcarbazepine, however, interacts with the contraceptive pill, and low-dose oestrogen contraceptives should not be used. There are few human data concerning pregnancy, but fetal abnormalities have been recorded in animal experimentation and the drug should be avoided where possible in pregnancy. Oxcarbazepine is currently clased as a category C teratogen.

The most common chronic effect is hyponatraemia, but this is usually mild and of no clinical significance. The hyponatraemia is due to a marked antidiuretic effect, and the consumption of large volumes of fluid (including large quantities of beer) should be discouraged.

Oxcarbazepine is only available as an oral preparation. It can be introduced more quickly than carbamazepine. In adults a starting dose of 600 mg/day can be increased weekly in 600 mg increments to a usual maintenance dose of 900–2400 mg/day, in two or three daily doses, although infrequently doses up to 3000 mg/day are used. It has been claimed that carbamazepine can be abruptly substituted with oxcarbazepine (in a dosing ratio of 200 : 300 mg), although there is widespread anecdotal evidence that a rapid switch carries a real risk of severe seizure exacerbations, and should not be routinely carried out. It has also been suggested that oxcarbazepine and carbamazepine can be combined to obtain high combined doses without the side-effects that would be expected at equivalent doses in monotherapy, but again in routine practice this seems not to be the case, and high-dose combinations of the two drugs are frequently poorly tolerated. In children the usual initial dosage is 8–10 mg/kg/day, given in divided doses, and increasing in steps of 10 mg/kg. For example, a 30 kg child would start treatment with one 150 mg tablet twice a day. The usual maintenance dose for a child is 30 mg/kg/day and the maximum dose for a child is 60 mg/kg/day. In severe renal disease (creatinine clearance below 30 ml/min) oxcarbazepine should be started at half the usual dose, and the dose incremented at a slower than usual rate until the desired clinical response is attained.

In routine practice, serum level monitoring of MHD has some role, but experience is not as favourable as for carbamazepine. Serum sodium should be measured as a baseline and then after 1–2 months of establishing therapy in all patients, and then at regular intervals depending on clinical circumstances.

# PHENOBARBITAL

| | |
|---|---|
| Primary indications | Partial or generalized seizures (including absence and myoclonus). Status epilepticus. Lennox–Gastaut syndrome. Other childhood epilepsy syndromes. Febrile convulsions. Neonatal seizures |
| Licensed for monotherapy/add-on therapy | Both |
| Usual preparations | Tablets: 15, 30, 50, 60, 100 mg; elixir: 15 mg/5ml; injection: 200 mg/ml |
| Usual dosage—adults | Initial: 30 mg/day<br>Maintenance: 30–180 mg/day |
| Usual dosage—children | Neonates: 3–4 mg/day<br>Children: 3–4 mg/kg/day |
| Dosing intervals | 1–2 times/day |
| Dose commonly affected by co-medication | Yes |
| Dose affected by renal/hepatic disease | Severe hepatic and renal disease |
| Common drug interactions | Extensive; see p. 154 |
| Serum level monitoring | Useful |
| Target range | 50–130 µmol/l |
| Common/important adverse events | Sedation, ataxia, dizziness, insomnia, hyperkinesis (children), mood changes (especially depression), aggressiveness, cognitive dysfunction, impotence, reduced libido, folate deficiency, vitamin K and vitamin D deficiency, osteomalacia, Dupuytren contracture, frozen shoulder, connective tissue abnormalities, rash. Risk of dependency. Potential for abuse |
| Major mechanism of action | Enhances activity of GABA-A receptor; also depresses glutamate excitability, and affects sodium, potassium and calcium conductance |
| Main advantages | Highly effective and low-cost antiepileptic drug |
| Main disadvantages | CNS side-effects, especially in children; a controlled drug in many countries |
| COMMENT | Highly effective well-tried antiepileptic. Often reserved for second-choice therapy because of potential for side-effects |

Phenobarbital (PB) is a remarkable drug. It was introduced into practice in 1912, and is still, in volume terms, the most commonly prescribed antiepileptic drug in the world. It is highly effective, and its introduction opened a new chapter in the history of epilepsy treatment. Its efficacy has not generally been bettered by any subsequent drug, it is well tolerated by many persons, and it is by far the cheapest of the antiepileptic drugs commonly available.

## Physical and chemical characteristics

Phenobarbital (molecular weight 232.23) is a crystalline substance which is a free acid, soluble in non-polar solvents but relatively insoluble in water. The pKa of phenobarbital is 7.2. Changes in pH, common in active epilepsy, can result in substantial shifts of phenobarbital between compartments. The sodium salt is soluble in water, but can be unstable in solution.

## Mode of action

Phenobarbital seems to act in a relatively non-selective manner both limiting the spread of epileptic activity and elevating the seizure threshold. It binds strongly to the GABA-A receptor, and its major action is at this receptor, post-synaptically, where it increases the duration of channel opening without affecting the frequency of opening (and differs from the benzodiazepine drugs, which bind to

**Phenobarbital**
Pharmacokinetics—average adult values

| | |
|---|---|
| Oral bioavailability | 80–100% |
| Time to peak levels | 1–3 h |
| Volume of distribution | 0.42–0.75 l/kg |
| Biotransformation | Hepatic oxidation, glucosidation and hydroxylation, then conjugation (cytochrome P450 enzymes CYP2C9, CYP2C19, CYP 2E1; UDPGT family enzymes) |
| Elimination half-life | 75–120 h |
| Plasma clearance | 0.006–0.009 l/kg/h |
| Protein binding | 45–60% |
| Active metabolite | None |

adjacent sites). At higher concentrations it also directly reduces sodium and potassium conductance. It also reduces presynaptic calcium influx and depresses glutamate excitability. It has profound effects in a wide variety of experimental models.

## Pharmacokinetics
### Absorption
Phenobarbital has a bioavailability of 80–100% in adults after oral or intramuscular administration. Peak plasma concentrations occur 1–3 hours after oral administration, but can be significantly delayed in patients with poor circulation or reduced gastrointestinal motility. After intramuscular administration, peak serum concentrations occur within 4 hours, and peak plasma concentrations are similar to those after oral administration (Figure 3.6). Absorption is slowed by the presence of food, but ethanol, in the stomach or blood, can increase the rate of phenobarbital absorption. Absorption occurs mostly in the small intestine because of its larger surface area and longer intra-luminal dwell time, and disease at this site can markedly reduce absorption. In the newborn and young infants, bioavailability is reduced and oral absorption is incomplete compared to that after IM injection.

### Distribution
Phenobarbital distributes rapidly to all body tissues. In adults, the relative volume of distribution ranges from 0.36 to 0.67 l/kg after IM administration and from 0.42 to 0.73 l/kg after oral dosing. The volume of distribution is larger in newborns, where it ranges from 0.39 to 2.25 l/kg after IV or IM injection. The distribution of phenobarbital is very sensitive to variations in the plasma pH and acidosis results in an increase of the transfer of phenobarbital from plasma into tissue. This is of potential importance in the treatment of, for instance, status epilepticus. After IV administration the distribution of phenobarbital into body organs is diphasic. In the first phase there is rapid distribution to high-blood-flow organs including the liver, kidney and heart, but not into the brain. During the second phase there is a fairly uniform distribution throughout the body except for the fat tissue. This pattern of relatively slow entry into the brain (12–60 minutes) and late exclusion from fat is related to the drug's low lipid solubility; however, in status epilepticus, because of focal acidosis and increased blood flow, the transfer of phenobarbital into the brain is much faster. Phenobarbital is 40–60% bound to plasma protein. Binding in newborns is lower (35–45%). The concentration of phenobarbital in CSF in adults is about 50% of that in plasma, and correlates well with the unbound phenobarbital plasma concentrations. The drug rapidly crosses the placenta, so that maternally-derived phenobarbital serum concentrations in neonates are similar to those in the mother. Concentrations in breast milk are about 40% of those in the mother's serum.

### Metabolism and elimination
Phenobarbital has a median half-life of 75–120 hours, the longest among any of the commonly used antiepileptic drugs. This is age-dependent. Premature and full-term newborns have the longest PB half-lives (ranging from 59 to 400 hours), infants (aged 6 weeks to 12 months) have the shortest, and the half-life diminishes from an average of 115 to 67 hours between birth and the first month of life. By the time the child is 6 months old, however, the half-life has fallen to 21–75 hours. The elimination of phenobarbital is reduced when the urine has acidified, and by age, genetic

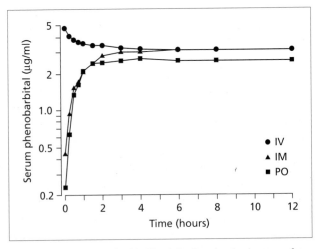

**Figure 3.6** Mean phenobarbital levels in six normal volunteers after single IV or IM injections of 130 mg or a single oral dose of 100 mg. This demonstrates the complete absorption of the drug after IM and oral ingestion and their comparable rates of absorption.

factors, nutritional status and drug interactions. Phenobarbital is subject to extensive biotransformation in the liver. The major metabolite of phenobarbital is p-hydroxyphenobarbital, and approximately 8–34% of the daily dose is converted to this metabolite, which is then largely excreted as the glucuronide conjugate. N-glucosidation is another important metabolic pathway, inactive at birth and becoming effective only after about 2 weeks of life. Other metabolites include an epoxide, a dihydrodiol catechol and methylcatechol derivatives, but these are of less clinical significance. The amount of drug excreted unchanged is very variable between individuals, with mean values of 20–25% of the total dose (range 7–55%). Although phenobarbital is a powerful inducer of hepatic microsomal enzymes, it does not exhibit auto-induction in humans.

The total renal clearance of phenobarbital ranges from 0.006 to 0.009 l/kg/h in adults, and is considerably less than the glomerular filtration rate, indicating extensive resorption. Acidification of the urine increases resorption, and a combination of sodium bicarbonate administration to alkalinize the urine and forced diuresis can increase clearance by up to fivefold. There is no enterohepatic recirculation and faecal excretion of phenobarbital is of little consequence. Elimination is linear at normal dose-rate ranges. Oral administration of activated charcoal can assist elimination, by increasing intestinal absorption.

### Drug interactions

Phenobarbital is involved in a number of pharmacokinetic drug interactions, the magnitude of which varies greatly from person to person depending on genetic factors and concomitant medication. Phenytoin, valproate, felbamate and dextropropoxephene inhibit phenobarbital metabolism leading to elevation of phenobarbital levels. The interaction with valproate is clinically the most significant and is complex. Severe somnolence or even stupor can be induced by this combination, a side-effect not entirely explained by high serum levels. Rifampicin is a powerful enzyme inducer and may lower phenobarbital levels.

Phenobarbital is itself a potent inducer of hepatic enzyme activity and increases the metabolism of other drugs including a number of analgesics and antipyretics (antipyrine, amidopyrine, acetaminophen, meperidine, methadone), antiasthma agents (theophylline), antibiotics (chloramphenicol, doxicycline, griseofulvin), anticoagulants (bishydroxycoumarin, warfarin), antiulcer agents (cimetidine), immunosuppressants (ciclosporin), psychotropic drugs (chlorpromazine, haloperidol, desipramine, nortriptyline, benzodiazepines), oral steroid contraceptives, and antiepileptic agents. Among the antiepileptic drugs, phenobarbital particularly induces the metabolism of valproate. It has also been suggested that induction of valproate metabolism by phenobarbital may contribute to valproate hepatotoxicity, by stimulating the production of several valproate metabolites. Phenobarbital may cause a decline in plasma carbamazepine levels in some patients, but the effect is often negligible. The effect on phenytoin is complex, involving induction and competitive inhibition, and is difficult to predict in any individual. The conversion of carbamazepine, diazepam and clobazam to active metabolites is also accelerated by phenobarbital.

## Adverse effects
### Neurotoxic side-effects

The most important side-effects are alterations of behaviour, sedation and cognitive impairment. Sedation and cognitive impairment occur in adults and children. Impairments include motor slowness, memory disturbance, loss of concentration and mental slowness. To what extent these problems are common is uncertain but it is a clinical impression that in adults these deficiencies are usually of minor importance. The frequency of sedation was no greater on phenobarbital than on phenytoin or carbamazepine in the large Veterans' Administration (VA) co-operative study, possibly owing to the slow rate of incrementation. Changes in cognitive function have been measured by various standardized neuropsychological tests. A decrease in verbal and performance IQ scores has been observed in children treated with PB compared with normal controls or patients receiving valproate or carbamazepine. Memory and concentration scores, visuomotor performance and spatial memory, and short-term memory can also be significantly impaired, especially in children.

Behavioural changes, primarily hyperactivity, irritability and aggressiveness are most prominent in children, but also occur in the elderly and in those with organic brain damage. In one study 42% of children developed these paradoxical behavioural changes after febrile seizures. The disturbances were not correlated with plasma PB concentrations, and improved in all children when PB was discontinued. In another study comparing phenobarbital with other first-line agents in newly diagnosed epileptic children, phenobarbital was associated with the highest chance of withdrawal because of behavioural problems. Problems with memory or compromised work and school performance can develop even in the absence of sedation or hyperkinetic activity. Because of these behavioural disturbances, great caution should be exercised in using phenobarbital in children, especially those with learning disabilities or organic brain syndromes.

Alteration of affect, particularly depression, also occurs. A complex picture including depression, apathy, impotence, decreased libido and sluggishness is sometimes observed in adults. In the VA co-operative study, decreased libido and/or potency was found to be more common in patients treated with phenobarbital than in those taking phenytoin or carbamazepine. During chronic therapy other side-effects include nystagmus and ataxia, and more rarely peripheral neuropathy and dyskinesia. Elderly patients with organic cerebral disease may also become confused and irritable rather than sedated.

### Effects on blood, bone, connective tissue and skin

Phenobarbital commonly lowers the serum folate level but frank megaloblastic anaemia is rare. A severe coagulation defect has been reported in neonates born to epileptic mothers taking phenobarbital due to drug-induced vitamin K deficiency, and supplementation of vitamin K at birth will prevent this complication. Phenobarbital can affect calcium and vitamin D metabolism, by inducing hydroxylation of vitamin D, resulting in frequent reductions in calcium levels but only occasionally in overt rickets or osteomalacia. The extent to which phenobarbital induces osteoporosis is unclear, but it is likely to be clinically relevant only in post-menopausal women or in the infirm. The drug has marked effects on connective tissue, resulting in an increased tendency to fibrosis, with increased rates of Dupuytren contractures with palmar nodules, frozen shoulder, plantar fibromatosis, Peyronie disease, heel and knuckle pads, and generalized joint pain. The incidence of these disorders ranges from 5 to 38%, depending on the population studied. In one study, for instance, a shoulder–hand syndrome was observed in 28% of 126 neurosurgical patients treated with barbiturates but in none of 108 control patients receiving carbamazepine or phenytoin. Mild skin reactions, usually maculopapular, morbilliform or scarlatiniform rashes, occur in 1–3% of all patients receiving phenobarbital.

### Hypersensitivity and immunological reactions

Serious skin reactions, such as exfoliative dermatitis, erythema multiforme, Stevens–Johnson syndrome or toxic epidermal necrolysis are remarkably rare. A barbiturate hypersensitivity syndrome, characterized by rash, eosinophilia and fever, is also rare. An immunologically mediated hepatitis has also been reported. Systemic lupus erythematosus and acute intermittent porphyria may be unmasked or precipitated by phenobarbital.

### Teratogenicity

In spite of its use for over 90 years, the teratogenic potential of phenobarbital is quite unclear. Although a barbiturate fetal syndrome has been identified, there are few reports of major malformations. However, current use is inadequate in developed countries to make definitive recommendations. The drug is widely used in developing countries, but until their pregnancy registry data are published, no reliable estimates of risk are available.

### Dependency and withdrawal symptoms

Phenobarbital, like other barbiturates, when used chronically can cause physical dependence, and abrupt cessation can lead to withdrawal seizures. Withdrawal seizures can also be a problem in neonates of a mother receiving phenobarbital, and the neonatal withdrawal syndrome includes hyperexcitability, tremor, irritability and gastrointestinal upset. This can last for days or even months. An increase in the frequency of seizures or a relapse in controlled patients has often been noted during or after withdrawal of phenobarbital, and the drug should be tapered very slowly to avoid convulsive withdrawal seizures.

### Overdose

Levels of phenobarbital above 350 μmol/l are potentially fatal, and many deaths from overdose are reported. Characteristic cerebral and EEG changes are seen as levels increase (Figure 3.7). Drug-naïve patients are much more sensitive to the effects, and coma occurs in most cases with levels over 300 μmol/l. Coma, respiratory depression and hypothermia are leading symptoms. Supportive treatment is, however, usually successful, and additional effective measures include forced diuresis, the alkalinization of urine and the use of activated charcoal and ion-exchange resins.

### Antiepileptic effect

Phenobarbital has been extensively used in a wide variety of epileptic seizure types for many years. Because of its venerable age, the drug has not been subjected to the usual panoply of pre-licensing controlled trials, and indeed there are very few controlled data to document the extent of its self-evident effectiveness.

In the VA co-operative double-blind study, the efficacy and tolerability of four drugs (phenobarbital, primidone, carbamazepine and phenytoin) were assessed in 622 adults with previously untreated or under-treated partial and secondarily generalized tonic–clonic seizures. Similar rates of overall seizure control were obtained with each drug (36%, 35%, 47% and 38%, respectively). Carbamazepine, however, provided better total control of partial seizures (43%) than phenobarbital (16%) or primidone (15%). Interestingly, phenobarbital was associated with the lowest incidence of motor, gastrointestinal or idiosyncratic side-effects. In another large long-term prospective randomized pragmatic trial the comparative efficacy and toxicity of phenobarbital, phenytoin, carbamazepine and valproate were assessed in both adults and children newly diagnosed with epilepsy. In 243 adults, the overall control of seizures on all four drugs was similar, with 27% of patients being free from seizures throughout the follow-up, and 75% entering 1 year of remission by 3 years of follow-up. Similar results were reported in 167 children (aged 3–16 years) who entered the study. Twenty per cent remained free from seizures and 73% achieved 1-year remission by 3 years of follow-up. Again there was no difference in efficacy between the drugs for either measure of efficacy at 1, 2 or 3 years of follow-up. In drug-resistant patients, there are small trials showing

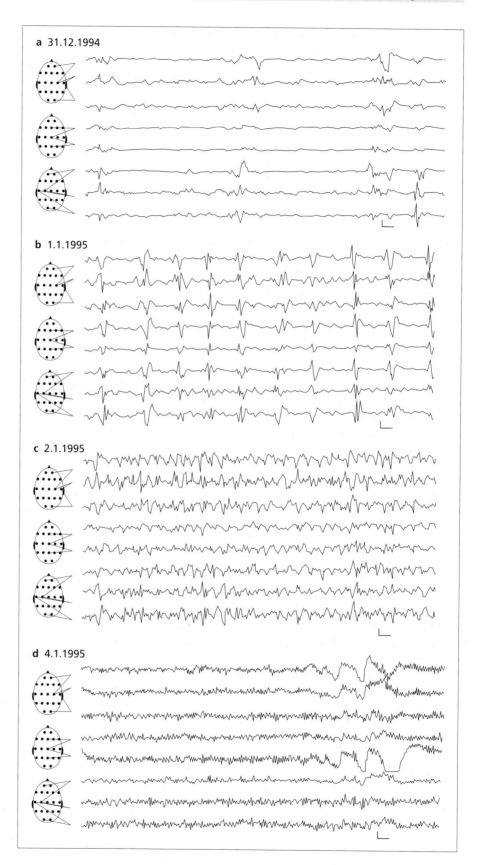

**a** 31.12.1994

**b** 1.1.1995

**c** 2.1.1995

**d** 4.1.1995

**Figure 3.7** PB overdose in a 47-year-old woman with a 34-year history of focal motor and secondarily generalized seizures, on chronic treatment with PB 100 mg daily. There was no apparent aetiology for epilepsy. The patient was found comatose in her bed; on admission to the hospital, the patient was in deep coma and required assisted ventilation; the EEG showed a burst-suppression pattern (a). The plasma levels of PB were 82 μg/ml. On the subsequent day, there was some improvement of the EEG, with shortening of the 'inter-bursts' flattenings (b). The corresponding plasma levels were 60 μg/ml. Progressive improvement of the EEG continued (c), with a normal tracing on the fifth day (d) after overdose. When awake, the patient admitted to have taken 'many' pills to attempt suicide (R. Michelucci, personal observation).

that phenobarbital is equal in efficacy to established drugs, but there are no large randomized controlled studies.

### Idiopathic generalized epilepsy

Phenobarbital has also been shown to be effective in the treatment of seizures (generalized tonic–clonic, myoclonic, and absence) in the syndrome of idiopathic generalized epi-lepsy, and is a useful alternative if valproate is ineffective or not well tolerated. The drug is also effective against myo-clonic, atonic, and tonic seizures, although evidence from clinical trials of its value in these attacks is largely lacking.

### Neonatal seizures

Phenobarbital is also a drug of choice for the treatment of neonatal seizures. There is familiarity and long experience, but controlled evidence of its efficacy or superiority above other drugs.

### Febrile convulsions

Phenobarbital has also been extensively used as an anticonvulsant for the prophylaxis of febrile seizures. In one study, 59 patients were compared with 72 untreated children, and the recurrence rate of febrile convulsions was 13% in the treated group compared with 20% in the control group. In cerebral malaria, phenobarbital has been traditionally used to control seizures, but a recent study showed that although the frequency of seizures was significantly lower in a phenobarbital group than in a placebo group (11% vs 27%), mortality was doubled (18% vs 8% deaths), leading to the recommendation that, in this special population, phenobarbital should not be used.

## Clinical use in epilepsy

There is no large pharmaceutical company promoting or marketing phenobarbital, and as a result its value is underestimated. It has a strikingly low cost and ease of use, which renders phenobarbital an important antiepileptic drug, especially in the developing world. It can be given once a day, and has a low risk of idiosyncratic reactions and probably also of teratogenicity. Its efficacy is not in question, but its general use as a first-line drug is limited by its potential to cause sedation and mental slowness in adults and the risk of paradoxical reactions in children. To what extent the sedative potential of small doses of phenobarbital is actually greater or less than that of other antiepileptics has not really been very clearly established. Individuals can experience severe sedation, but many patients take the drug without any noticeable side-effects. Nevertheless, its use is now largely confined to second-line therapy in patients with

focal or generalized seizures intractable to other more modern first-line alternatives. Other indications are in primary generalized epilepsy (where valproate has failed), first-line therapy for neonatal seizures, and as second-line therapy for severe secondarily generalized seizure disorders. The drug is valuable in status epilepticus (see pp. 228–9).

The drug is available in a large number of formulations and preparations. Tablet sizes include 30, 50, 60 and 100 mg sizes, and elixirs (15 mg per 5 ml) and injections (200 mg in 1 ml) or propylene glycol and water (90/10%) are also in common use. In adults the starting dose is 30–60 mg, given at night. The dose can be increased in 15 or 30 mg increments for a maintenance dose of between 60 and 180 mg/day, the most common dose for adults being between 60 and 120 mg/day. Too rapid an initiation of therapy can produce drowsiness, which may persist for several weeks, and it is usually better to introduce the drug slowly.

Many patients are well controlled on low serum levels and low doses. Indeed, it seems likely that low-dose phenobarbital therapy is as effective as any other first-line therapy, with few side-effects, at least in adults, and the low cost of the drug ($2–5 per year) confers remarkable value. There is a need for randomized head-to-head comparisons against the newer drugs, but none have been carried out. In adults, the side-effects develop mainly at the higher doses, which are anyway largely redundant in contemporary practice. In children the usual starting dose is 3 mg/kg/day with maintenance doses in the range 3–6 mg/kg/day. Twice daily dosing may be necessary in younger children because of the shorter half-life. The drug is widely used in neonatal seizures, where rapid seizure control is needed, and intravenous administration is used. Loading doses of 15–20 mg/kg intravenously followed by maintenance doses of 3–4 mg/kg/day are usually used. Side-effects (particularly behavioural changes and hyperkinetic behaviour) are more severe in children than in adults, and these effects need to be particularly monitored. In the elderly, paroxysmal agitation and irritability can also occur, as they can in patients with learning difficulty or cerebral damage. The use of the drug in these patients should, therefore, be circumspect.

Serum level measurement of phenobarbital has been widely used, and for most patients concentrations of 40–170 μmol/l are associated with optimal seizure control. Some patients, however, will experience good seizure control above or below this limit, and although side-effects are usually not too troublesome when levels are maintained in this range, there is a relatively inconsistent relationship between side-effect and level even on a statistical basis. This is possibly because of the tendency for tolerance of the side-effects of phenobarbital to develop over time.

# PHENYTOIN

| | |
|---|---|
| **Primary indications** | Partial and primary and secondarily generalized seizures (excluding myoclonus and absence). Status epilepticus. Childhood epilepsy syndromes |
| **Licensed for monotherapy/add-on therapy** | Both |
| **Usual preparations** | Capsules: 25, 30, 50, 100, 200 mg; chewtabs: 50 mg; liquid suspension: 30 mg/5ml, 125 mg/50 ml; injection: 250 mg/5 ml |
| **Usual dosage—adults** | Initial: 200 mg at night<br>Maintenance: 200–450 mg/day<br>(higher doses can be used; guided by serum level monitoring) |
| **Usual dosage—children** | 10 mg/kg/day<br>(higher doses can be used; guided by serum level monitoring) |
| **Dosing intervals** | 1–2 times/day |
| **Dose commonly affected by co-medication** | Yes |
| **Dose affected by renal/hepatic disease** | Severe hepatic disease |
| **Common drug interactions** | Extensive; see Table 3.17, p. 162 |
| **Serum level monitoring** | Useful |
| **Target range** | 40–80 µmol/l |
| **Common/important adverse events** | Ataxia, dizziness, lethargy, sedation, headaches, dyskinesia, acute encephalopathy (phenytoin intoxication), hypersensitivity, rash, fever, blood dyscrasia, gingival hyperplasia, folate deficiency, megaloblastic anaemia, vitamin K deficiency, thyroid dysfunction, decreased immunoglobulins, mood changes, depression, coarsened facies, hirsutism, peripheral neuropathy, osteomalacia, hypocalcaemia, hormonal dysfunction, loss of libido, connective tissue alterations, pseudolymphoma, hepatitis, vasculitis, myopathy, coagulation defects, bone marrow hypoplasia |
| **Major mechanism of action** | Inhibition of voltage-dependent sodium channels |
| **Main advantages** | Highly effective and low-cost antiepileptic drug |
| **Main disadvantages** | CNS and systemic side-effects; non-linear elimination kinetics; drug interaction profile |
| **COMMENT** | Powerful antiepileptic drug. Use reserved increasingly for second-choice therapy because of side-effects and pharmacokinetic properties |

Phenytoin was introduced into clinical practice in 1938, as Lennox put it 'a year of jubilee' for epileptics. Since then phenytoin has been a major first-line antiepileptic drug in the treatment of partial and secondarily generalized seizures. When it was introduced, only potassium bromide and phenobarbital showed equal effectiveness, but phenytoin was found to cause less sedation. Although phenobarbital continues to be used, the introduction of phenytoin meant that bromides were finally, after nearly 100 years of prescription, redundant. Now many alternative drugs are available, and the use of phenytoin has diminished. Nevertheless, it has both low cost and strong antiepileptic effects, and is still considered a drug of first choice in many parts of the world. It has had a huge effect on the treatment of epilepsy during the last 50 years, and has been a paradigm for epilepsy clinical and experimental therapeutics and drug development. Phenytoin has also been used as second-line treatment in trigeminal neuralgia, neuropathic pain, certain cardiac arrhythmias, as a prophylactic in occasional varieties of migraine, and in paroxysmal choreoathetosis and myotonia.

### Physical and chemical characteristics

Phenytoin (5,5'-diphenylhydantoin) is usually available as the free acid (molecular weight 252.3), or, more commonly, as the sodium salt (molecular weight 274.3). It is a white crystalline solid, a weak acid with a pKa of 8.3−9.2, and is relatively insoluble in water. A parenteral formulation is available with a pH of about 12. The storage of phenytoin capsules under conditions of high temperature and humidity may reduce the oral bioavailability of the drug.

### Mode of action

Phenytoin exerts its antiepileptic effect largely by binding to and thus prolonging the inactivation of voltage-dependent sodium ion channels in neuronal cell membranes. This effect is greater when the cell membrane is depolarized than when it is hyperpolarized. With repeated depolarization the ion channel block becomes use-dependent. Phenytoin binds to the same site on the outer surface of the cell membrane sodium ion channel as carbamazepine and lamotrigine; however, the drugs have different binding affinities. Phenytoin at high concentration may also inhibit axonal and nerve terminal calcium ion channels, an action that stabilizes axonal cell membranes and diminishes neurotransmitter release at axon terminals in response to action potentials. The drug has no effect on the function of the T-type calcium ion channels in the thalamus. At high concentrations, phenytoin inhibits calcium ion calmodulin-mediated protein phosphorylation. The drug also binds to the peripheral type of benzodiazepine receptor in brain membranes, but it is not clear whether this action leads to any antiepileptic effect. Phenytoin also has mild dopamine antagonist effects.

## Pharmacokinetics

**Phenytoin**
Pharmacokinetics—average adult values

| | |
|---|---|
| Oral bioavailability | 95% |
| Time to peak levels | 4−12 h |
| Volume of distribution | 0.5−0.8 l/kg |
| Biotransformation | Oxidation, glucosidation, hydroxylation, conjugation (cytochrome P450 enzymes CYP2C9, CYP2C19, CYP3A4; UDPGT family enzymes) |
| Elimination half-life | 7−42 h (dependent on plasma level and co-medication) |
| Plasma clearance | 0.003−0.02 l/kg/h (dependent on plasma level) |
| Protein binding | 85−95% |
| Active metabolite | None |

### Absorption and distribution

Phenytoin is usually given to patients as the sodium salt, a crystalline preparation which is absorbed rather slowly from the gastrointestinal tract. Absorption through the stomach is relatively poor because phenytoin is very insoluble at the pH of gastrointestinal juice. The high pH of the small intestine, however, enhances phenytoin solubility and absorption. The presence of food alters phenytoin absorption as do diseases of the small bowel. In an average healthy person, the oral bioavailability is about 95%, and the time to peak levels following oral administration is 4−12 hours. Any factor that interferes with the dissolution of phenytoin in the gastrointestinal tract will retard or prevent absorption. There is a wide intra- and inter-individual variability in absorption, and occasional patients have very unusual patterns for no obvious reason. Pregnancy reduces absorption, occasionally to extreme levels. Neonates absorb the drug poorly and erratically. The difference in formulation of some generic preparations of phenytoin can result in altered absorption, and so it is usually recommended that the same formulation of phenytoin is dispensed—this is particularly important in patients where metabolism is close to saturation levels. Phenytoin can also be given intravenously (see p. 29). Intramuscular phenytoin must not be given, as the drug precipitates in muscle resulting in a profound delay in absorption and sometimes in muscle necrosis. The rectal bioavailability of phenytoin is low, around 24 ± 3%.

Phenytoin is distributed throughout total body water with relatively little selective regional concentration. The apparent volume of distribution is about 0.5–0.8 l/kg. The drug achieves a slightly higher concentration in the brain than in plasma, and is at higher concentration in white than in grey matter. Phenytoin is transported out of the brain by P-glycoprotein activity. Phenytoin is 70–95% bound to plasma proteins. The concentration of free phenytoin is higher in the neonate than the adult, in the elderly, in later pregnancy, in the presence of hypoalbuminaemia as occurs in malnutrition, liver disease, nephrotic or uraemic states, AIDS, and with high levels of glycated albumin as in diabetics. The cerebrospinal fluid levels of phenytoin are equal to the free plasma fraction, as are the salivary and tear levels. Bioavailability is not significantly altered during pregnancy, and the phenytoin breast milk to plasma ratio is about 0.2. A number of acidic drugs, e.g. salicylates and valproate, and certain endogenous substances (fatty acids, bilirubin) displace phenytoin from its plasma protein binding sites, but these effects are rarely of importance clinically.

## Metabolism and excretion

Phenytoin is extensively metabolized by the hepatic P450 mixed oxidase system (Figure 3.8), and at normal doses 90% of the metabolism is by the isoform CYP2C9 activity. The first step involves zero-order kinetics, accounting for the non-linear dose to serum level relationship (see below). The para-hydroxylation step is mainly followed by glucuronidation, although there is a range of other minor metabolites. None of the phenytoin metabolites have anticonvulsant activity, and all are excreted via the kidney. The major metabolite of phenytoin found in urine, p-hydroxyphenytoin (HPPH), accounts for the elimination of some 60–80% of usual doses of the drug. This particular oxidative metabolite

is formed via a postulated short-lived arene oxide intermediate in a reaction catalysed by the CYP450 isoforms 2C9 and 2C19. The glucuronide conjugate [S]-isomer of p-hydroxyphenytoin is the predominant one in human urine, accounting for 75–95% of the total phenytoin metabolite present. None of these metabolites has any known biological activity. There is some evidence that the postulated arene oxide intermediate and also epoxide products can interact with tissue proteins, and that the reaction products formed are responsible for some unwanted effects of the drug. About 1 in 500 of the Japanese population is a slow hydroxylator of phenytoin, and hereditary poor metabolizers of the drug have more rarely been encountered in other populations. Mutations of the *CYP2C9* gene appear to be responsible for the slow metabolism. Minor degrees of auto-induction occur in phenytoin metabolism.

Because the first step in the enzymic degradation of phenytoin is rate limited, the dose to serum level ratio is not linear. As the dose is increased, plasma levels initially rise linearly until the point of enzymic saturation is reached, and then in a much steeper fashion. There is marked inter-individual variability (Figure 3.9). The clearance and half-life of phenytoin therefore both vary considerably within populations, and also depend on the plasma level. At higher plasma concentrations, the half-life is much longer and the clearance much reduced owing to saturation of the enzyme systems. The time to steady state will also vary non-linearly with dose (but linearly with plasma level) and as many as 28 days may need to elapse before steady state is reached after certain dose changes. The Michaelis constant of phenytoin is around 6 mg/l (24 μmol/l), lower than the usual plasma concentration in clinical practice.

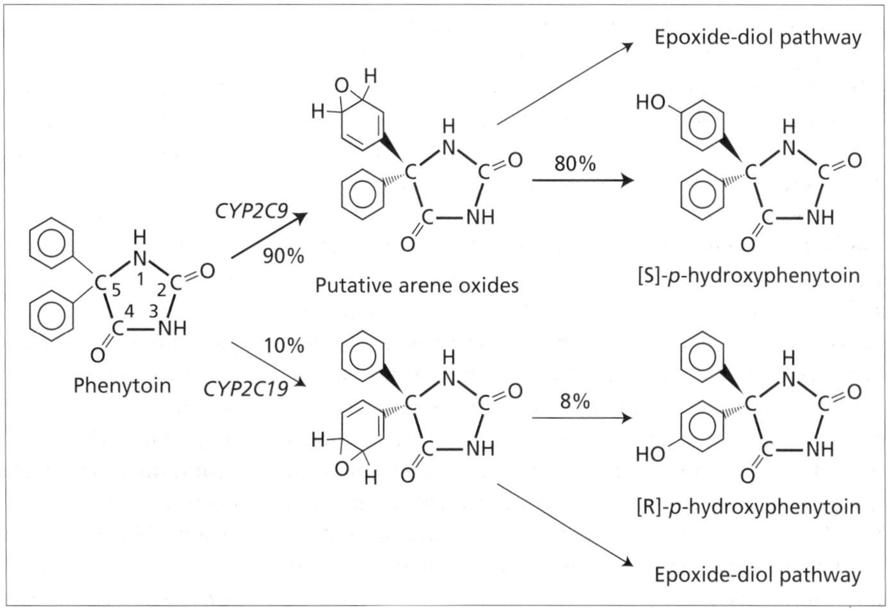

**Figure 3.8** The principal pathways of metabolism of phenytoin, and the involvement of CYP2C9 and CYP2C19.

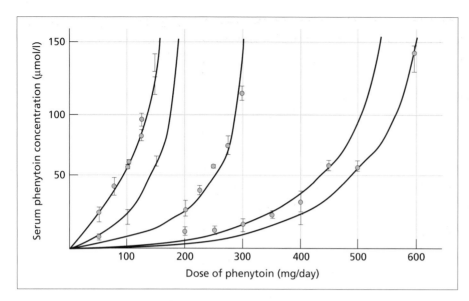

**Figure 3.9** Relationship between serum phenytoin concentration and daily dose in five patients. Each point represents the mean (± SD) of three to eight measurements of serum phenytoin concentration at steady state. The curves were fitted by computer using the Michaelis–Menten equation.

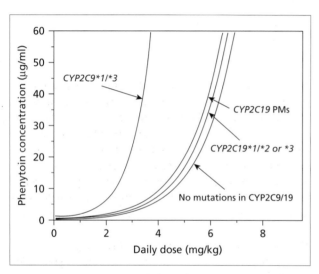

**Figure 3.10** Estimated phenytoin dose–concentration relationships in groups of patients with differing CYP2C9 and CYP2C19 genotypes—showing the importance of CYP genotype in determining rates of phenytoin metabolism.

Neonates eliminate phenytoin more slowly and young children more rapidly than adults. In the elderly, metabolism is less rapid than in younger adults. Phenytoin doses need to be reduced in severe hepatic failure. In renal failure phenytoin levels fall, although those of its major metabolite rise. Haemodialysis has little effect on phenytoin plasma concentrations. In pregnancy, phenytoin metabolism is increased, the elimination half-life of phenytoin shortens, and total plasma levels fall, especially in the last trimester, although free levels may be maintained, and doses may need to be increased to maintain therapeutic effects. Pre-pregnancy values are regained within a few weeks of childbirth.

## Drug interactions

Phenytoin is probably the antiepileptic drug with the most problematic drug interaction profile (Table 3.17). This is partly because of the saturable kinetics of phenytoin itself, which results in different interaction behaviour at different doses/serum levels. Phenytoin also is a strong enzyme inducer, prone to induction and inhibition, and is also highly protein bound.

### The effect of other antiepileptic drugs on phenytoin levels

*Carbamazepine and phenobarbital*: There is a complex pattern of interactions between phenytoin and these two drugs. Phenytoin levels can be raised or lowered by carbamazepine or phenobarbital co-medication, as both induce and compete for hepatic enzyme metabolism. The overall effect on phenytoin levels is highly variable.

*Valproate*: Valproate displaces phenytoin from its protein binding sites and also inhibits its metabolism. There is a transient rise in free levels, but within weeks, owing to redistribution, the free levels return to their previous values, although total levels may be somewhat lower (and dosage should not be increased). Near saturation levels, however, the combination of protein binding displacement and metabolic inhibition can result in marked rises in phenytoin levels and toxicity. Care therefore needs to be taken, particularly when high phenytoin doses are used or when pre-interaction serum levels are near the top of the therapeutic range.

*Vigabatrin*: Vigabatrin leads to an approximately 25% fall in phenytoin levels in most patients when introduced as co-medication. The mechanism of this interaction is not known.

*Other antiepileptics*: Felbamate, oxcarbazepine and stiripentol act as competitive inhibitors of CYP2C9 and CYP2C19 and thus often elevate phenytoin levels.

| | Effect of phenytoin on the drug | Effect of the drug on phenytoin |
|---|---|---|
| Carbamazepine (CBZ) | ↑CBZ epoxide and ↓ CBZ concentration | Variable ↓↑ |
| Ethosuximide (ESM) | ↓ ESM concentration | No effect |
| Felbamate (FLM) | ↓ FLM concentrations | ↑ PHT concentrations |
| Lamotrigine (LTG) | ↓ LTG concentration | No effect |
| Oxcarbazepine (OXC) | ↓ OXC concentrations | ↑ PHT concentrations |
| Phenobarbital (PB) | Variable ↓↑ in PB concentration | Variable ↓↑ in PHT concentration |
| Primidone (PRM) | ↓ PRM concentration | Variable ↓↑ PHT concentrations |
| Tiagabine (TGB) | ↓ TGB concentrations | No effect |
| Topiramate (TPM) | ↓ TPM concentration | No effect |
| Valproate (VPA) | ↓ VPA concentration | ↑ PHT concentration at high levels |
| Vigabatrin (VGB) | No effect | ↓ PHT concentrations |
| Zonisamide (ZNS) | ↓ ZNS concentration | No effect |

**Table 3.17** Pharmacokinetic interactions between phenytoin (PHT) and other antiepileptic drugs.

Gabapentin, levetiracetam and pregabalin have no interactions with phenytoin.

Sulthiame comedication markedly increases plasma phenytoin levels.

### The effect of non-antiepileptic drugs on phenytoin levels

Phenytoin levels are affected by a wide range of other drugs. These are all more marked when phenytoin is close to the top of its therapeutic level. Amiodorone increases serum phenytoin concentrations by as much as 100–200% and its signs of toxicity are similar to those of phenytoin. Antacids and protein hydrolysates and theophylline can reduce the bioavailability of phenytoin, although the effect is variable, reflecting the complex effects on phenytoin dissolution, chelation and gastrointestinal motility. Dosing should be separated by at least 2 hours. Some nutritional formulas can reduce phenytoin absorption by up to 75%; Isocal® and Osmolite® are the main culprits, while Ensure® apparently does not have a marked effect. Other drugs that, in co-medication, can reduce phenytoin concentrations include: aciclovir, aspirin, cisplatin, dexamethazone, doxycycline, diazoxide, methotrexate, nitrofurantoin and vinblastine.

Drugs that inhibit CYP2C9 and CYP2C19 will elevate phenytoin concentrations, by impairing oxidation to *p*-hydroxyphenytoin. Such drugs include: sulfaphenazole, phenylbutazole, fluconazole, azapropazone, co-trimoxazole, dextropropoxyphene, disulfiram, fluoxamine, fluoxetine, ketoconazole, losartan, metronidazole, miconazole, paroxetine, proguanyl, propranolol, sertraline, trimethoprim, omeprazole, cimetidine, imipramine and diazepam. Cimetidine is a potent inhibitor of phenytoin metabolism and can rapidly cause phenytoin toxicity if phenytoin metabolism is close to saturation. Isoniazid markedly inhibits phenytoin metabolism, and symptoms of phenytoin intoxication are common within days of the introduction of isoniazid as co-medication. The effects are greatest in those individuals who are slow acetylators of isoniazid, and who therefore have higher isoniazid levels. Azapropazone, diazoxide, phenylbutazone, salicylate, sulfafurazone, sulfamethoxypyrine, and tolbutamide displace phenytoin from its protein binding sites (in the same way as valproate) and will affect phenytoin dosage only when levels are close to saturation.

### The effect of phenytoin on levels of other drugs

Phenytoin is a potent enzyme-inducing agent. Co-medication with phenytoin results in falling concentrations of carbamazepine, clobazam, clonazepam, felbamate, lamotrigine, midazolam, primidone, tiagabine, topiramate, valproate and zonisamide. The effect of phenytoin on phenobarbital concentrations is variable, and levels may rise or fall.

The most clinically common interactions with non-antiepileptic drugs include the inhibition of warfarin metabolism, and clotting times need to be monitored frequently if phenytoin dosage changes are made. Corticosteroid metabolism (including dexamethazone) is induced, and doses may need to be twice normal to obtain the desired therapeutic effects. The levels, and thus effectiveness, of busulfan and possibly other anti-mitotic agents can also be significantly affected by phenytoin co-medication. Theophylline levels can be lowered by as much as 35–75% by phenytoin co-medication. Furosemide clearance can be increased by as much as 50% and ciclosporin clearance is increased by 75%. Serum folate levels are reduced in about 50%

of patients receiving phenytoin. Praziquantel levels are reduced by a mean of 75% by phenytoin co-medication; this compares to a 10% reduction by carbamazepine, which may therefore be the drug of first choice in treating active cysticercosis. Enhanced metabolism of the combined oral contraceptives renders low-oestrogen contraceptives potentially inactive, and patients on phenytoin frequently need contraception with higher oestrogen content (see p. 102). Other drugs affected include: atorvastatin, chloramphenicol, dicoumarol, digoxin, disopyramide, doxycycline, haloperidol, methadone, mexilitine, isoniazide, nortryptyline, pethidine, phenazone, quinidine, simvastatin and the tricyclic antidepressants.

## Adverse effects

Phenytoin is one of the oldest drugs in the pharmacopoeia (although outflanked by phenobarbital in venerability) and the most studied. There is therefore a large body of information about adverse effects. It is salutary to contemplate how long some, even common, side-effects took to be recognized. Many patients, however, taking phenytoin suffer no or only minimal side-effects even after decades of therapy; an important point to emphasize when discussing the pros and cons of therapy.

### Phenytoin intoxication and encephalopathy

Acute dose-related effects of phenytoin are usually seen at serum levels above 80 μmol/l, although there is individual variation, and some patients have no side-effects at much higher levels. These effects, known as 'phenytoin intoxication', include ataxia, dysarthria, motor slowing, lethargy and sedative mental changes. A reversible encephalopathy can occur at high doses (levels usually over 160 μmol/l) with mental changes, confusion progressing to stupor or even coma (at levels above 200 μmol/l) and a paradoxical exacerbation of seizures.

### Chronic neurological side-effects

The most common neurological side-effects are the acute dose-related side-effects listed above, and these reverse when the blood levels of phenytoin are lowered. Phenytoin also has more chronic side-effects which occur at normal levels, usually after years of chronic therapy. A phenytoin-induced cerebellar syndrome has been postulated, although its existence has been disputed, and occasionally asterixis, dystonia, orofacial dyskinesia and ophthalmoplegia have occurred. Phenytoin can also induce a peripheral neuropathy, and two patterns are described: a reversible neuropathy associated with phenytoin intoxication, and a mild usually asymptomatic sensori-motor neuropathy on chronic therapy. Phenytoin has been reported clinically to cause chronic motor slowing or mental dulling, although rigorous studies have failed to detect any clear-cut effects.

**Table 3.18** Signs and symptoms in 38 cases of phenytoin hypersensitivity reaction.

| Sign or symptom | Percentage of patients |
| --- | --- |
| *Rash* | |
| Morbilliform or licheniform | 66 |
| Erythema multiforme | 18 |
| Stevens–Johnson syndrome | 13 |
| Total | 74 |
| Fever | 13 |
| Abnormal liver function tests | 29 |
| Lymphoid hyperplasia | 24 |
| Eosinophilia | 21 |
| *Blood dyscrasias* | |
| Leucopenia | 16 |
| Thrombocytopenia | 5 |
| Anaemia | 16 |
| Increased atypical lymphocytes | 3 |
| Total | 31 |
| Serum sickness | 5 |
| Albuminuria | 5 |
| Renal failure | 3 |

### Hypersensitivity and immunologically related side-effects

Phenytoin hypersensitivity is idiosyncratic and immunologically mediated (Table 3.18). Skin rash occurs in up to 5% of patients started on phenytoin, and is most common in the first 4 weeks of treatment. The rash is usually minor and recedes when the drug is discontinued. It is occasionally associated with fever, leucopenia and lymphadenopathy, and very occasionally evolves into exfoliative dermatitis, toxic epidermal necrolysis or Stevens–Johnson syndrome. The incidence of phenytoin-related rashes is higher in post-operative patients or those receiving radiotherapy. Serious agranulocytosis, thrombocytopenia or red cell aplasia have been recorded but are fortunately rare.

Phenytoin can suppress both humoral and cellular mechanisms. However, there is no clear evidence that patients taking phenytoin are more prone to infection, and the immunological effects are largely subclinical. Very rarely, pulmonary fibrosis has occurred in patients taking phenytoin and may be due to an immune complex disorder. Lymph-node enlargement is not uncommon on phenytoin therapy, and this has led to a controversy about the relationship of phenytoin therapy and malignant lymphoma. Most cases take the form of 'pseudolymphomas', which resolve when phenytoin therapy is withdrawn, but a small number of persisting lymphomas have also been recorded in patients on phenytoin therapy. This may be a chance association. An illness similar to systemic lupus erythematosus has also been reported but the immunological markers of drug-induced cases differ from those of the idiopathic form. Phenytoin exacerbates myasthenia gravis, and has been recorded to precipitate the condition. Acute hepatitis and hepatic necrosis have been rarely caused by phenytoin, usually in the context of an acute hypersensitivity reaction. A 'serum sickness'-like syndrome of rash, fever, arthralgia and atypical lymphocytes has also been recorded, as have cases of auto-immune nephritis and thyroiditis.

### Connective tissue effects

Gum hypertrophy occurs in up to 10–40% of adult patients on phenytoin and there is possibly a higher incidence in children. In the past, before the widespread availability of plasma level monitoring, gum hypertrophy was often severe, but the effects nowadays are usually mild. The reduction in frequency is due to the introduction of serum level monitoring, and thus the avoidance of high phenytoin levels, and also an emphasis on better dental hygiene. Gum hypertrophy usually develops within 3 months of commencing phenytoin therapy and will regress within 6 months of discontinuing the drug, and can be reduced by good dental hygiene and periodic gingivectomy. The cause of the gum hypertrophy is unclear. It has been suggested that because phenytoin is metabolized in gum tissue to p-hydroxyphenytoin, the resulting arene-oxide metabolic intermediate forms adducts with various tissue proteins in the gums leading to gum overgrowth. An alternative hypothesis is that gum hypertrophy is due to increased serum concentrations of basic fibroblast growth factor, which is elevated by phenytoin. Facial changes including coarsening, enlargement of the lips and nose, hirsuitism, acne, and pigmentation can result from chronic phenytoin therapy. The overgrowth of body hair can be marked and of cosmetic importance, especially in dark-haired females. These effects too have become much less prominent since the introduction of drug level monitoring.

### Haematological effects

Mild leucopenia is very common in patients taking phenytoin, and does not require attention unless the neutrophil count falls below 1500/mm$^3$. Macrocytosis occurs in up to one-third of patients on chronic therapy, a subnormal folate level in at least half the patients, and low CSF folate levels in up to 45%. Despite this, less than 1% develop a frank megaloblastic anaemia. The mechanism of the folate deficiency is uncertain, but may reflect impaired absorption. Folate supplementation is not usually required unless the patient develops a megaloblastic anaemia, or in pregnancy. In up to 10% of patients, low serum vitamin $B_{12}$ levels are also noted. Evidence that the folate deficiency results in depression or mental side-effects is weak.

Neonatal blood coagulation defects due to a relative deficiency of vitamin K-catalysed clotting factors can occur in neonates exposed to phenytoin during pregnancy, carrying the risk of neonatal haemorrhage. This is prevented by prophylactic vitamin K administration immediately after birth.

### Endocrine and biochemical effects

Phenytoin affects a range of endocrine values, but these changes are, in the majority of cases, of no clinical significance. The drug impairs the absorption of vitamin D and calcium, and increases the hepatic metabolism of vitamin D. Biochemical abnormalities include an elevated plasma alkaline phosphatase and reduced plasma calcium and plasma 2-hydroxycholecalciferol. This can result in loss of bone density, and occasionally in frank osteomalacia, especially in institutionalized patients and in Asian immigrants to northern climates—reflecting the contribution of dietary factors and sunlight exposure. There may also be secondary hyperparathyroidism. The osteomalacia may lead to repeated fractures, and sometimes presents with a painful proximal myopathy. Asymptomatic biochemical changes require no specific treatment, but long-term therapy with vitamin B can be given. Osteomalacia or rickets reverses with appropriate therapy. Whether phenytoin causes osteoporosis is also unclear, but there has been a recent suggestion that all patients over 60 years of age, and also symptomatic patients of any age, on chronic phenytoin therapy should have regular dual X-ray absorptiometry (DEXA) bone density scans to monitor osteopenia and osteoporosis. Phenytoin can displace thyroxin from its plasma globulin binding. This may result in a decrease in total thyroxin levels, but triiodothyronine ($T_3$) and thyroid-stimulating hormone (TSH) levels are usually normal and the patients are clinically euthyroid. The acute administration of phenytoin can increase adrenocorticotropic hormone (ACTH) and cortisol levels but this reverses on chronic administration. Phenytoin can affect the result of the dexamethasone suppression test. Free testosterone levels are lowered by chronic phenytoin therapy, and follicle-stimulating hormone (FSH), leutinizing hormone, and prolactin levels are raised. Phenytoin treatment in experimental models does not affect fertility, but there is a higher incidence of hyposexuality and sperm abnormalities recorded in patients taking phenytoin.

Other biochemical effects, which are usually asymptomatic, include: raised serum or plasma levels of high-density lipoprotein (HDL) cholesterol, caeruloplasmin, copper, prolactin and sex hormone binding globulin. It has also been associated with reduced concentrations of IgA, IgG, IgE, IgM, fibrinogen, vitamin K, vitamin E, oestrogens, progesterone, free testosterone, pyridoxal phosphate, tryptophan and thiamine. Phenytoin intake can precipitate attacks of porphyria in those who suffer from the disorder, and it can diminish insulin secretion from the pancreas, resulting in a tendency to hyperglycaemia.

### Teratogenicity

Phenytoin is a category D teratogen according to the FDA (i.e. a drug in which studies have shown a fetal risk in humans). Fetal abnormalities due to phenytoin were first recorded in 1970, but much still remains to be discovered about the extent of the risk and its mechanisms. The individual role of phenytoin has been difficult to interpret, partly because of the tendency to treat the teratogenicity of antiepileptic drugs as a class effect, and the large number of women on multiple drug therapy. Although these initial reports attributed to phenytoin a marked teratogenic potential, more recent studies have not shown this. In an analysis of five prospective European studies of malformation rates following fetal exposure to antiepileptic drugs during pregnancy, the malformation rate for phenytoin monotherapy was 6%, and the relative risk for phenytoin being associated with malformations, compared with the background risk, was 2.2 (95% CI, 0.7–6.7). In that study, phenytoin in monotherapy seemed safer than other established major antiepileptic drugs. It seems therefore that, in monotherapy and particularly at low doses, the teratogenic risk is not high and may be less than that of alternative drugs.

A range of different malformations have been reported. The most severe include facial clefts, diaphragmatic hernias, hip dysplasias and congenital heart abnormalities. That these can be due to phenytoin therapy seems well established, and animal experimentation has confirmed this. Phenytoin is less likely to cause serious spinal malformations than carbamazepine or valproate. A 'fetal hydantoin syndrome' has been described, comprising characteristic facies with wide-spaced eyes, deformities of the fingernails, slender and shortened terminal phalanges, mild mental retardation, and poor infantile growth and development. Many of these minor abnormalities become unrecognizable within the first few years of life. Partial rather than full syndromes are more commonly encountered, and the extent to which there are really teratogenic effects or simply variations in healthy development, unrelated to phenytoin exposure, is unclear. The mechanism of teratogenicity may relate to the production of reactive metabolic intermediates, notably arene-oxide derivatives, which form adducts with fetal tissue proteins. Free radical intermediates produced by the activity of tissue peroxidases may also play

a part. The arene-oxide adducts would be more likely to be present at higher concentrations if the activity of the enzyme epoxide hydrolase (which catalyses the further metabolism of arene oxides and epoxides) is deficient, and there is evidence that low levels of the enzyme epoxide hydrolase in amniocytes and fetal fibroblasts are associated with the fetal hydantoin syndrome.

### Antiepileptic effect

Phenytoin was introduced for the treatment of partial and tonic–clonic seizures on the basis of a small number of open uncontrolled investigations. In the first study in the late 1930s, phenytoin was added for 2–11 months to 142 patients with active seizures on phenobarbital and bromides. Bromides were withdrawn but the phenobarbital was continued, and 'complete relief' was obtained in 58% of the 118 patients with frequent 'grand mal' seizures, and there was a 'marked decrease' in seizures in another 32%. The corresponding figures for the 74 patients with 'petit mal' (probably some cases would now be classified as having complex partial seizures) were 35% and 49%, respectively, and for the six with 'psychomotor seizures' 67% and 33%. Similar excellent findings were reproduced in many other open studies. In the past decade, blinded controlled comparisons of new drugs with phenytoin, phenobarbital and carbamazepine have been carried out (notably the VA study and studies from King's College Hospital in London). None of these demonstrated any significant differences in antiepileptic effect between phenytoin and either phenobarbital or carbamazepine in the control of either partial or generalized tonic–clonic seizures. In a series of similar studies of partial and generalized tonic–clonic seizures, phenytoin has also been compared in a controlled fashion with valproate, carbamazepine, clobazam and lamotrigine, without significant differences in efficacy or withdrawal rates due to toxicity. In one study only, of newly diagnosed patients, was phenytoin found to control tonic–clonic seizures better than carbamazepine (but not valproate). There is consensus, therefore, that phenytoin is as effective as any other first-line drug in partial and tonic–clonic seizures (especially when secondarily generalized). Dispute exists about its relative tolerability.

The effectiveness of phenytoin in partial and secondarily generalized seizures is clearly dependent on serum level. In any individual, better control is consistently obtained at higher serum levels. The concept of a therapeutic range was established on the basis of experience with phenytoin, and applies more to phenytoin than to any other antiepileptic drug. The upper limit of the target range is 80 $\mu$mol/l, although there are patients who respond better to higher levels without serious side-effects. Equally, there are large numbers of patients with low serum levels that are quite adequate for seizure control. At least 70% of patients with newly diagnosed epilepsy (partial or tonic–clonic seizures) will be controlled by phenytoin monotherapy. A recent study showed that functional polymorphisms in *CYP2C9* and an intronic polymorphism in the *SCNIA* gene were related to the dosage of phenytoin (and, in the latter case, carbamazepine) needed in clinical practice. This is the first example in epilepsy of how a individual genetic variation influences drug effectiveness and this study is a paradigm for future investigation into tailoring individual drug treatment.

There is also general agreement that phenytoin is ineffective for treating myoclonic seizures (irrespective of their age of onset or epilepsy syndrome), typical absence seizures (petit mal), atonic seizures, or atypical absence seizures of the Lennox–Gastaut syndrome. In some of these seizure types phenytoin can cause an exacerbation of seizures, although this is unusual. The drug can worsen myoclonus in patients with progressive myoclonic epilepsy. The drug has also proved ineffective in treating two reasonably common varieties of situation-related human epilepsy, namely febrile convulsions of infancy, and the eclamptic seizures of pregnancy toxaemia.

Intravenous phenytoin has been used successfully in treating neonatal seizures and status epilepticus .

## Clinical use in epilepsy

Phenytoin is one of the most commonly used antiepileptics in the world. In North America, for instance, until recently phenytoin accounted for nearly 50% of all new prescriptions and 45% of the total antiepileptic drug market, eclipsing carbamazepine and valproate for instance. In Britain and Scandinavia, phenytoin is used less commonly than carbamazepine or valproate, but in other countries it remains a drug of first choice. As the efficacy of the major antiepileptic drugs in partial and secondarily generalized epilepsy has not been shown to differ, the rational choice of a drug will depend on other factors such as cost, ease of use, and the side-effect profile. Phenytoin is extremely cheap. However, its use requires serum level monitoring, and the list of side-effects is long. In most patients on chronic therapy, no serious side-effects are experienced, and evidence of any general difference in tolerability between phenytoin and other old (or new) drugs is weak. The marketing budget of newer antiepileptic drugs has profoundly eclipsed that of phenytoin (or other older antiepileptics), and marketing pressures exert an additional influence on prescribing choice beyond scientific evidence.

In the author's practice, phenytoin is a drug of second choice in partial and secondarily generalized seizures, and also in primary generalized tonic–clonic seizures. The difficult pharmacokinetics of the drug, rather than its side-effect profile, weigh against its first-line use. Because of the non-linear kinetics of phenytoin, blood level monitoring is essential. The therapeutic range of plasma phenytoin concentrations is usually considered to be 40–80 μmol/l (10–20 mg/100 ml). However, many patients achieve total control of seizures at lower levels, and others require higher levels (100–120 μmol/l). It is often claimed that lower levels are required to control tonic–clonic seizures than partial seizures. Drug interactions are common, complex and troublesome, and where possible phenytoin should be used as monotherapy. Once a satisfactory phenytoin dosage regimen has been achieved in a particular patient, it will rarely be necessary to alter that regimen over many years.

Phenytoin is also often recommended after head trauma or neurosurgical procedures, although the frequency of rash and immunologically mediated side-effects seems greater in these acute situations than in routine therapy. Phenytoin is, after phenobarbital, a drug of choice in neonatal seizures when administered parenterally. The drug also has a major role in the treatment of status epilepticus (see p. 228).

Phenytoin is available in tablets and capsules of 25, 50, 100 and 200 mg sizes. It is also available as a solution for intravenous injection and as a suspension and chewable tablet. In most patients it is given on a once, or more commonly twice, daily basis. A typical starting dose in an adult is 200 mg/day and this can be increased up to 450 mg as initial maintenance therapy, although the dose will depend to some extent on the serum level and some patients require higher doses. Serum concentrations usually take about a week to reach steady state after a change in dose, but occasionally steady state may not be reached for up to 4 weeks. In children the usual starting dose is 5 mg/kg/day and the drug given twice per day. Phenytoin can also be loaded intravenously or orally in emergency situations, the oral loading dose being 15 mg/kg in three doses at 1 hourly intervals. A serum level in the low therapeutic range is usually achieved 12 hours following such a loading dose.

# PREGABALIN

$H_2N$ —— $CO_2H$
       |
       H
      |
   (isobutyl)

| | |
|---|---|
| Primary indications | Partial seizures with or without secondary generalization. Adults only |
| Licensed for monotherapy/add-on therapy | Add-on therapy only |
| Usual preparations | Capsules: 25, 50, 75, 150, 300 mg |
| Usual dosage—adults | Initial: 150 mg/day<br>Maintenance: 150–600 mg/day |
| Dosing intervals | 2 or 3 times/day |
| Dose commonly affected by co-medication | No |
| Dose affected by renal/hepatic disease | No definitive clinical data |
| Common drug interactions | None |
| Serum level monitoring | Not useful |
| Common/important adverse events | Somnolence, dizziness, ataxia, asthenia, weight gain, blurred vision, diplopia, tremor |
| Major mechanism of action | Binds to alpha-2-delta subunit of the voltage-gated calcium channel. Also reduces release of glutamate and other excitatory neurotransmitters |
| Main advantages | Effective and well tolerated |
| Main disadvantages | Limited routine clinical experience to date |
| COMMENT | Recently licensed drug for adjunctive therapy in partial-onset epilepsy in adults |

Pregabalin was licensed as an antiepileptic drug in July 2004 in Europe and has received approval in 40 countries as of May 2005. In addition to its epilepsy indications, it is licensed as an analgesic for neuropathic pain and is undergoing clinical studies as an anxiolytic.

## Physical and chemical properties

Pregabalin (S-(+)-3-isobutyl GABA) is a structural analogue of GABA. It is a white solid and is stable in storage at 25 °C. Although pregabalin has structural similarities to gabapentin, the potency in animal models of epilepsy, pain and anxiety is significantly greater. The R-isomer, R-isobutyl GABA, appears to be 10-fold less potent in animal models of epilepsy and pain.

## Mode of action

Pregabalin binds in a very potent fashion to the alpha-2-delta protein subunit of the voltage-gated calcium channel, binding much more strongly, for instance, than gaba-pentin. Its binding reduces calcium influx in response to depolarization, and this in turn reduces nerve terminal release of neurotransmitters including glutamate. This is likely to be responsible for the antiepileptic effect, although it is possible that other additional mechanisms of action exist. It has strong analgesic and anxiolytic actions, probably due to the same binding properties. The S-isomer binds 10 times more strongly than the R-isomer, and only the S-isomer has antiepileptic action. In spite of its close structural similarity to GABA, pregabalin is inactive at GABA-A and GABA-B receptors and it is not converted metabolically into GABA or a GABA antagonist, nor does it, like gabapentin, alter GABA uptake or degradation. It has no effect on GABA in the retina or optic nerve, in contrast to vigabatrin. In animal experimentation, pregabalin has a similar profile to gabapentin in all animal models tested, but pregabalin was consistently three- to sixfold more potent on a milligram per kilogram dose basis. It is effective in a wide range of animal models of epilepsy.

## Pharmacokinetics

---

**Pregabalin**
Pharmacokinetics—average adult values

---

| | |
|---|---|
| Oral bioavailability | ≥ 90% |
| Time to peak levels | 1 h |
| Volume of distribution | 0.56 l/kg |
| Biotransformation | None |
| Elimination half-life | 6 h |
| Plasma clearance | 0.083 l/kg/h |
| Protein binding | None |
| Active metabolite | None |

---

### Absorption and distribution

Pregabalin is rapidly absorbed with a bioavailability of over 90%, and peak levels are reached within 1 hour. The serum level concentration rises linearly with dose and there is little intra-individual variation. Steady state is reached within 24–48 hours after repeated administration. It is transported into the brain by the system L active transport system.

### Metabolism and elimination

Pregabalin is not metabolized to any extent in humans. Pregabalin has linear pharmacokinetics in the normal dosing ranges. Its plasma half-life is approximately 6 hours, independent of dose and repeated administration. Food has no clinically significant effect on absorption, in contrast for instance to tiagabine. Plasma pregabalin concentration–time profiles are similar following twice or three times daily dosing. It does not bind to plasma proteins.

Approximately 98% of the drug can be recovered unchanged in the urine. The amount excreted is independent of dose and is not significantly different whether given as single or repeated administrations, but it is affected by severe renal disease. Dose reductions are needed if the creatinine clearance falls below 60 ml/min.

No differences in pharmacokinetic parameters have been noted in different ethnic groups or by gender and, although limited data only are available, the pharmacokinetics seem to be unchanged in the elderly.

### Drug interactions

Pregabalin has no effect or action on the cytochrome P450 system in humans at therapeutic doses, nor is it protein bound. There have been no reports of drug interactions and, on the basis of its pharmacology, none would be expected. There is no interaction with the combined contraceptive pill.

### Adverse effects

Although there has been little experience of the drug in routine epilepsy practice, a large number of subjects (more than 10,000 by mid-2003) had received oral pregabalin in studies of epilepsy, anxiety and pain, as well as healthy volunteers, and a consistent picture of the side-effect profile, at least in early therapy, has been obtained.

In healthy volunteers given doses up to 900 mg/day with little or no titration, the main side-effects were headache, dizziness and somnolence, which were mild or moderate in intensity. No major serious adverse events due to pregabalin treatment were reported. Mild transient increases in hepatic enzymes in the multiple-dose study at 900 mg/day were noted in healthy volunteers, and for this reason the highest recommended dose in clinical trials is 600 mg/day.

In the clinical trials adverse events resulted in discontinuation of pregabalin in between 10 and 14% of patients at 300 mg/day and in 19–26% of patients at 600 mg/day, with no difference between twice and three times daily regimens. Common adverse events were dizziness, somnolence, ataxia and asthenia and these appear to be dose related. Other side-effects include increased appetite, blurred vision, diplopia, dry mouth, constipation, peripheral oedema and weight gain. Most adverse events were transient and mild to moderate in intensity. Overall, pregabalin seems reasonably well tolerated, and 83% of pregabalin-treated patients in the clinical trials enrolled in the open-label extension phases. Only 0.3% of all PGB patients developed myoclonus vs. 1.5% for all epilepsy controlled trials. Only 0.37% of patients discontinued due to myoclonus. No life-threatening adverse events have been recorded. Table 3.19 gives the most common adverse events and withdrawal rates reported in the clinical trials of pregabalin and placebo.

No information is yet available on the effect of pregabalin on pregnancy. However, pregabalin is not teratogenic in mice or rabbits, but teratogenicity was observed in rats at very high doses of 1250–2500 mg/kg.

### Antiepileptic effect

Due to pregabalin's recent approval, there is little open experience or routine clinical experience of the drug at present, and data on its efficacy are drawn largely from three multicentre, double-blind, placebo-controlled, parallel-group, randomized trials of pregabalin as add-on therapy in patients with refractory partial epilepsy.

The first trial enrolled 453 patients in the USA and Canada, and reported percentage reductions in the frequency of seizures between baseline and treatment periods were 7, 12, 34, 44 and 54 for the placebo and pregabalin 50, 150, 300 and 600 mg/day without titration, respectively.

| | Frequency of side-effects (%) | | Frequency of withdrawals due to side-effects (%) | |
|---|---|---|---|---|
| | Pregabalin ($n = 758$) | Placebo ($n = 294$) | Pregabalin ($n = 758$) | Placebo ($n = 294$) |
| Dizziness | 28.9 | 10.5 | 5.3 | 0.3 |
| Somnolence | 20.8 | 10.9 | 3.3 | 0.0 |
| Ataxia | 13.2 | 4.1 | 3.0 | 0.3 |
| Asthenia | 11.2 | 8.2 | 1.8 | 0.3 |
| Weight gain | 10.4 | 1.4 | 0.4 | 0.0 |
| Accidental injury | 9.9 | 5.4 | 0.9 | 0.0 |
| Headache | 9.1 | 11.6 | 1.2 | 0.0 |
| Amblyopia (blurred vision) | 9.0 | 4.4 | 1.6 | 0.0 |
| Diplopia | 8.4 | 3.7 | 1.6 | 0.7 |
| Tremor | 7.5 | 3.7 | 1.5 | 0.0 |
| Abnormal thinking (difficulty concentrating) | 7.0 | 2.0 | 1.3 | 0.0 |

**Table 3.19** Most common adverse events and reason for withdrawals from study in the regulatory clinical trials of pregabalin as adjunctive therapy in refractory partial epilepsy.

**Table 3.20** Mean seizure reductions on placebo and pregabalin in three clinical trials as adjunctive therapy in refractory partial epilepsy (expressed as RRatio).

| | | Pregabalin dose | | | |
|---|---|---|---|---|---|
| | Placebo | 50 mg | 150 mg | 300 mg | 600 mg |
| Simple and complex partial seizures | 1.2 | −5.1 | −10.6/−28.3***/* | −28.3*** | −29.1/−32.5*** |
| Secondarily generalized seizures | −3.7 | 18.5 | 1.5/6.8 | −24.7 | −30.6/−35.3*/** |
| All partial-onset seizures | −0.8 | −6.2 | −20.5/−11.6***/** | −27.8*** | −32.5/−34.0*** |

The table shows the RRatio which was the primary end-point of the study (see text). The two values in the 150 and 600 mg dose columns refer to different trials.

*, Significant difference compared with placebo, $P \leq 0.05$; **, significant difference compared with placebo, $P \leq 0.001$; ***, significant difference compared with placebo, $P \leq 0.0001$.

Seizure reduction for all partial seizures was statistically significantly lower in the pregabalin 150, 300 and 600 mg/day groups compared with the placebo group. Responder rates were 14, 15, 31, 40 and 51% across all treatment gruops, respectively, and the rate was significantly greater than for placebo in the pregabalin 150, 300 and 600 mg-treated groups. Seizure-free rates for the intent-to-treat population (ITT) were 8, 5, 6, 11 and 17, respectively.

The second study enrolled 287 patients in Europe and South Africa and studied placebo and pregabalin at two doses (150 and 600 mg/day). Seizure reduction for all partial seizures was found to be statistically significantly lower in both the pregabalin groups. Responder rates were 6, 14

and 44, for placebo, pregabalin 150 mg and 600 mg/day respectively. Seizure-free rates were 1, 7 and 12, respectively for the ITT population.

The third study enrolled 312 patients at 43 centres in the USA and Canada, and compared twice and three times daily dosing at 600 mg with placebo. There was a percentage reduction in the frequency of seizures between baseline and treatment periods of −1%, 48% and 36% for the placebo, pregabalin 600 mg/day three times daily and pregabalin 600 mg/day twice daily groups, respectively. The percentage reduction in seizure rate for the pregabalin two and three times daily groups were similar and not statistically significantly different. Responder rates were 9, 49 and 43%, respectively; the responder rates for the pregabalin two and three times daily groups were similar. Seizure-free rates were 3, 14 and 3%, respectively for the ITT population.

The mean reduction in seizures in all three studies combined is shown in Table 3.20, which uses the RRatio (defined as the difference between treatment and placebo rates divided by the sum of the two rates) to compare treatment with placebo rates. This ratio was accepted as a primary end-point of the study, and is a transformed symmetrized ratio which allows statistical comparisons to be made. As the figures in Table 3.20 show, there were highly significant reductions in the frequencies of seizures at doses between 150 and 600 mg/day for partial seizures and at 600 mg/day for secondarily generalized seizures. It was notable too that significant reductions in seizure frequency were recorded from day 2 onward of the titration phase (with a dosage of 150 mg/day). These are impressive results.

The results from four long-term open studies of adjunctive therapy in adults have also been analysed. Of 1480 patients enrolled (512 started *de novo* and 968 from the randomized placebo-controlled studies of adjunctive therapy), 77.2% and 59.4% took pregabalin (up to a dose of 600 mg/day) for more than 6 or 12 months (maximum 4.8 years), and at the time of analysis, 8.8% of the patients were seizure free over the previous 6 months of observation and 5.8% over the previous 12 months. Although these results are to some extent due to the self-selected nature of the cohort, they do suggest that pregabalin has persisting effectiveness over long time periods in a significant number of cases. Other anecdotal experience with pregabalin confirm this, and has shown that some patients with severe epilepsy experience impressive and long-lasting seizure control where other therapies have been totally ineffective.

## Clinical use in epilepsy

Pregabalin has recently been licensed in Europe, the USA and 40 additional countries, as adjunctive therapy in partial-onset epilepsy in adults, and its place in routine therapy has not yet been fully ascertained. However, the results from the clinical trials are encouraging, and pregabalin appears to be effective. The lack of interactions and its excellent pharmacokinetic properties make pregabalin an easy drug to use. It has no drug interactions and no interactions with the combined oral contraceptive pill. There is not enough experience to recommend use in preganancy, but in animal experimentation, no teratogenic effects were observed. Pregabalin has a reasonable side-effect profile, and the frequency of adverse effects may be reduced by slow titration. No life-threatening or serious idiosyncratic effects have been recorded. In addition to its effects in epilepsy, pregabalin shows a marked analgesic effect, especially against neuropathic pain and the drug is now widely licensed for this indication. Preliminary results also suggest that pregabalin has marked anxiolytic properties also. The usual starting dose in routine clinical practice is 150 mg/day given in two or three divided doses, and dose escalation up to 600 mg/day will depend on individual tolerability and response to the drug. The drug can be given either in a twice or three times daily regimen.

# PRIMIDONE

| | |
|---|---|
| **Primary indications** | Partial and primary and secondarily generalized seizures. Adults and children |
| **Licensed for monotherapy/add-on therapy** | Both |
| **Usual preparations** | Tablet: 250 mg |
| **Usual dosage—adults** | Initial: 62.5–125 mg/day<br>Maintenance 250–1000 mg/day |
| **Usual dosage—children** | Initial 1–2 mg/kg/day<br>Maintenance 10–20 mg/kg/day |
| **Dosing intervals** | 1–2 times/day |
| **Dose commonly affected by co-medication** | Yes |
| **Dose affected by renal/hepatic disease** | Severe hepatic and renal disease |
| **Common drug interactions** | Extensive; see p. 172 |
| **Serum level monitoring** | Useful to measure the levels of derived phenobarbital |
| **Target range** | 25–50 µmol/l (and derived phenobarbital 50–130 µmol/l) |
| **Common/important adverse events** | As for phenobarbital. Also dizziness and nausea on initiation of therapy |
| **Major mechanism of action** | — |
| **Main advantages** | Not a controlled drug; less risk of abuse than phenobarbital |
| **Main disadvantages** | Adverse event profile, as for phenobarbital |
| **COMMENT** | A prodrug of phenobarbital with probably some minor additional efficacy |

Primidone was introduced into clinical practice in 1952. Although it has strong advocates, most clinicians feel that it functions simply as a prodrug of phenobarbital, with little clinical advantage (and significant disadvantages) compared with the parent drug. In most countries it is not, like phenobarbital, a drug of abuse and therefore it is not subject to special controls—a practical (and rather illogical!) benefit enjoyed by the drug.

## Physical and chemical characteristics and mode of action

Primidone (molecular weight 218.25) is a crystalline powder with low solubility in water. The main action of primidone is due to the derived phenobarbital, and whether either primidone itself or a second active metabolite, phenylethylmalonamide, adds anything to its antiepileptic properties in controversial.

## Pharmacokinetics

**Primidone**
Pharmacokinetics—average adult values

| | |
|---|---|
| Oral bioavailability | < 100% |
| Time to peak levels | 3 h |
| Biotransformation | Metabolized to phenobarbital, and then further oxidation, glucosidation and hydroxylation, then conjugation as per phenobarbital (P450 system and oxidation in liver) |
| Elimination half-life | 5–18 h |
| Protein binding | 25% |
| Active metabolite | Phenobarbital |

### Absorption and distribution

Primidone is well absorbed orally, with a bioavailability approaching 100%, although there does seem to be quite significant intra-individual variation (and possibly differences in different formulations). Peak levels are obtained after about 3 hours. The drug is 25% bound to proteins and concentrations in fluids, including CSF, saliva and breast milk approach those in plasma. The distribution of the drug through tissues is similar to that of phenobarbital.

### Metabolism, elimination and drug interactions

Primidone is rapidly metabolized into phenobarbital, which is its primary metabolite, and phenylethylmalonamide. The elimination half-life of primidone is very variable (range 3–22 hours) and of the derived phenobarbital it is 40–60 hours. As it is metabolized by the cytochrome oxidase system, there is a potential for drug interactions, not only between primidone and other drugs but also between primidone and the derived phenobarbital. Phenytoin and carbamazepine increase the rate of conversion of primidone to phenobarbital, and primidone lowers carbamazepine levels. There is a complex interaction with valproate, which usually elevates the ratio of phenobarbital to primidone. The ratio of primidone to phenobarbital in the plasma also seems variable, depending on co-medication, age, duration of therapy, and factors such as pregnancy and disease. Valproate can have variable and unpredictable effects on the rate of conversion of primidone to phenobarbital. In contrast to other antiepileptics, clonazepam seems to increase primidone levels.

## Adverse and antiepileptic effects

The side-effects are largely those of phenobarbital. The drug, however, is often considered to be less well tolerated, and this is because of intense dizziness, nausea and sedation which occur commonly at the onset of therapy (sometimes after only one tablet). These reactions are probably due to the initially high concentration of the parent drug. These side-effects disappear over a week or so, but it is always advisable to start primidone at a low dose. The effects of primidone overdose are largely related to the levels of derived phenobarbital, and management of overdose of both drugs is similar.

There is an unresolved debate as to whether primidone itself (or its other metabolite phenylethylmalonamide) exerts any greater antiepileptic action than its derived phenobarbital. A number of studies appear to demonstrate independent action, but although this evidence is reasonably strong, it is not conclusive. Perhaps the best clinical study is the VA co-operative study, in which primidone, phenobarbital, carbamazepine and phenytoin were compared. The efficacy of primidone and phenobarbital was similar but primidone showed fewer behavioural side-effects than either phenobarbital or phenytoin. There is also an interesting report of a patient in whom primidone generic formulations were substituted on two occasions for the proprietary formulation (mysoline), with loss of seizure control on both occasions. The phenobarbital level was virtually unaltered but the primidone level was reduced by 53%. These and other studies suggest that primidone does have independent actions, but these are probably relatively slight.

## Clinical use in epilepsy

Primidone is available as 250 mg tablets, which have sim-ilar efficacy to 60 mg phenobarbital. Measurement of the derived phenobarbital (and not primidone) levels is usually carried out if plasma concentration monitoring is required. An average starting dose for an adult would be 62.5–125 mg at night, with increments every 2–4 weeks to an average maintenance dose of 250–1000 mg/day in one or two divided doses. A low starting dose is essential to avoid the risk of intense side-effects on drug initiation. In routine therapy, the efficacy of primidone can be assumed to be close to that of phenobarbital. However, it is doubtful whether there is any advantage in prescribing primidone rather than phenobarbital, other than in exceptional circumstances.

# TIAGABINE

| | |
|---|---|
| **Primary indications** | Partial and secondarily generalized seizures. Patients ≥ 12 years of age only |
| **Licensed for monotherapy/add-on therapy** | Add-on therapy only |
| **Usual preparations** | Tablets: 2, 4, 12, 16 (USA); 5, 10, 15 (Europe) |
| **Usual dosage—adults** | Initial: 15 mg/day<br>Maintenance: 30–45 mg/day |
| **Dosing intervals** | 2–3 times/day |
| **Dose commonly affected by co-medication** | Yes |
| **Dose affected by renal/hepatic disease** | Hepatic disease |
| **Common drug interactions** | Yes |
| **Serum level monitoring** | Usefulness not established |
| **Common/important adverse events** | Dizziness, tiredness, nervousness, tremor, diarrhoea, nausea, headache, confusion, psychosis, flu-like symptoms, ataxia, depression, word-finding difficulties, encephalopathy, non-convulsive status epilepticus |
| **Major mechanism of action** | Inhibits GABA reuptake |
| **Main advantages** | Effective antiepileptic drug, with possible particular effect in lesional epilepsy |
| **Main disadvantages** | CNS and gastrointestinal side-effects |
| **COMMENT** | Recently licensed drug for adjunctive therapy in partial-onset epilepsy in adults |

Tiagabine was introduced into clinical practice in 1998, first in the UK. It has been the subject of a well-conducted programme of clinical trials, but post-licensing experience is rather limited and the relative role of the drug in routine therapy is not yet established.

## Chemical and physical characteristics

Tiagabine is a derivative of the GABA uptake inhibitor nipecotic acid, rendering the parent compound lipid-soluble by the attachment of a lipophylic side chain. Tiagabine is thus able freely to cross the blood–brain barrier, unlike the parent compound.

## Mode of action

Tiagabine greatly increases cerebral GABA concentrations, via the inhibition of the GABA transporter-1 (GAT-1), which is one of at least four specific GABA transporting compounds that carry GABA from the synaptic space into neurones and glial cells. Measurements in human and experimental models have confirmed that extracellular GABA concentrations are indeed raised after administration of tiagabine. The action of tiagabine on GAT-1 is reversible (unlike the action of vigabatrin on GABA-T), and its affinity is greater for glial than for neuronal uptake. Although its primary effect is similar to that of vigabatrin, the range of pharmacological changes differs, and tiagabine does not result in the widespread increase in brain GABA levels which accompany vigabatrin therapy, and nor does it increase retinal GABA levels. Its effect seems remarkably specific, and studies have shown little or no effect at other receptor systems, including the glutamate, benzodiazepine, 5-HT, dopamine 1 or 2, adenosine, serotonin, glycine, adrenergic or muscarinic receptors. Tiagabine also appears not to affect the sodium or calcium channels. It has antiepileptic effects in a wide range of animal models, and an experimental profile which differs from that of vigabatrin.

## Pharmacokinetics

**Tiagabine**
Pharmacokinetics—average adult values

| | |
|---|---|
| Oral bioavailability | < 100% |
| Time to peak levels | 1–2 h |
| Volume of distribution | 1.0 l/kg |
| Biotransformation | Hepatic oxidation then conjugation (cytochrome P450 enzymes CYP3A4; UDPGT family enzymes) |
| Elimination half-life | 5–9 h (in monotherapy) |
| Plasma clearance | 0.109 l/kg/h |
| Protein binding | 96% |
| Active metabolite | None |

### Absorption and distribution

The oral bioavailability of the drug approaches 100% and absorption is almost complete at all ages. Drug concentrations are linear over the range of usual clinical dosages, and peak concentrations occur about 30–90 minutes after intake. A second peak of the plasma concentration of tiagabine is seen 12 hours after ingestion, and is presumably due to enterohepatic recycling. Food slows down absorption by two or three times; however, the total amount absorbed is unchanged by food. The peak concentration ($C_{max}$) is also reduced by food. In view of its rapid absorption and short half-life, taking the drug with food avoids excessive peaking of blood level, and it is recommended that the drug is always taken with food, preferably at the end of a meal; this greatly improves tolerability. The volume of distribution is about 1 l/kg, and the drug is extensively bound (96%) to human plasma proteins.

### Metabolism and excretion

Tiagabine is extensively metabolized in the liver. This is a relative disadvantage of the drug, although one shared by many other antiepileptics. *In vitro* studies suggest that the main enzymatic degradation is by the isoform CYP3A of the cytochrome P450 family. At least five major metabolites are found both in plasma and in urine two additional metabolites in faeces. None of these known metabolites has any antiepileptic action. After oral ingestion of a single dose, less than 3% of the drug appears in the urine unchanged.

The plasma half-life of tiagabine is about 5–9 hours in healthy volunteers, and 2–3 hours in patients with epilepsy co-medicated with enzyme-inducing drugs. The shorter half-life in patients is presumably due largely to the hepatic-inducing effects of other antiepileptics. The plasma clearance of tiagabine has been found to be 12.8 l/kg/h in patients with epilepsy without concomitant therapy and is faster in patients receiving adjunctive therapy with enzyme-inducing antiepileptic drugs. There are no differences in metabolism in the elderly. The kinetics in young children seem to be more variable and are less well studied, but generally speaking the clearance of tiagabine is greater in children. Co-medication with enzyme-inducing drugs greatly increases metabolism in children as in adults, and the tiagabine half-life can fall to 2–3 hours. The elimination of the drug is reduced in patients with mild to moderate liver impairment. In a study of four subjects with mild hepatic impairment, three with moderate impairment, and six matched normal controls, tiagabine half-life was found to be 7, 12 and 16 hours, respectively, and similar affects on $C_{max}$ and AUC were found. The patients with hepatic impairment also have more neurological side-effects, and the drug should be used only with caution in those with hepatic disease. The pharmacokinetics of tiagabine are unaffected in patients with renal impairment or in subjects with renal failure requiring haemodialysis. The pharmacokinetics of tiagabine in elderly patients are similar to those observed in younger patients, hence there should be no need for dosage modification.

### Drug interactions

Tiagabine does not itself induce or inhibit hepatic metabolic enzymatic activity, and therefore should not alter the concentration of other adjunctive antiepileptic drugs. A small decrease in valproate concentrations has, however, been reported in patients taking concomitant tiagabine, but the mechanism of this effect is uncertain and the extent of the change is unlikely to be clinically significant. Interaction studies with carbamazepine, phenytoin, theophylline, warfarin, digoxin, cimetidine, alcohol and triazolam have not demonstrated any change in kinetics caused by tiagabine co-medication. No significant change in plasma concentrations of progesterone, oestradiol, follicle-stimulating hormone or luteinizing hormone were found in one small short-term study of co-medication with the contraceptive pill.

Although tiagabine co-medication does not affect the kinetics of other drugs, the metabolism of tiagabine itself is markedly changed by co-administration of hepatic inducing drugs such as carbamazepine, phenytoin and primidone. In one large-population kinetic analysis, the clearance of tiagabine was increased by two-thirds, and the AUC and $C_{max}$ are similarly reduced in patients taking concomitant anticonvulsants. Higher tiagabine doses are therefore necessary for those receiving concomitant enzyme-inducing antiepileptic drug therapy. Valproate, cimetidine and erythromycin havd been found not to affect tiagabine plasma concentrations.

**Table 3.21** Adverse effects of tiagabine in the randomized placebo-controlled studies as add-on therapy in refractory partial epilepsy in adults (%).

|  | Tiagabine, (n = 675) | Placebo, (n = 276) |
|---|---|---|
| Dizziness | 30 | 13 |
| Tiredness | 24 | 12 |
| Nervousness | 12 | 3 |
| Tremor | 9 | 3 |
| Diarrhoea | 7 | 2 |
| Depressed mood | 5 | 1 |

This table lists the adverse events that occurred significantly more frequently on tiagabine than placebo, from combined data from the placebo-controlled randomized clinical trials.

## Adverse effects
### Neurotoxic and other side-effects
In the randomized placebo-controlled trials, 91% of the 675 patients taking tiagabine reported at least one side-effect compared with 79% of those taking placebo. The most common adverse events are listed in Table 3.21. Other side-effects—which included somnolence, headaches, abnormal thinking, abdominal pain, pharyngitis, ataxia, confusion, psychosis and skin rash—occurred at a similar frequency in treated and placebo groups. Most of these side-effects were categorized as mild or moderate in severity, and only 15% of patients on tiagabine withdrew therapy because of side-effects. In the clinical trials, these CNS-related adverse events occurred at greater frequency in patients on tiagabine than in those on placebo only in the titration period, and there is now also recognition that the dizziness, light-headedness and unsteadiness occurring within 1–2 hours of taking a tiagabine dose are due to peaking of the drug concentration. This has led to the practice of titrating tiagabine slowly, and taking the drug after food, which has greatly improved tolerability.

Because of its action on GABAergic mechanisms, the question has been raised as to whether tiagabine, like vigabatrin, can result in visual field abnormalities. To date, however, there is no evidence of an increased risk of concentric visual field defects, in spite of careful testing. Both prospective and cross-sectional studies have been carried out, without a single tiagabine-treated patient showing abnormalities.

Again, on the basis of the experience with vigabatrin, the potential of tiagabine to cause psychosis, depression or severe behavioural disturbance has been carefully studied. In the three main clinical trials the incidence of psychosis was 0.8% in the tiagabine-treated patients and 0.4% in the placebo-treated patients, which was a non-significant

difference. However, depression occurred more often on tiagabine than on placebo (5 vs 2%). Because of this, tiagabine should be carefully monitored in patients with a history of behavioural problems or depression.

No adverse effect on cognitive abilities has been demonstrated in extensive neuropsychological studies of tiagabine add-on therapy and monotherapy. Indeed, there is evidence that monotherapy with tiagabine results in modest improvements in cognitive abilities and adjustment and also causes less fatigue when compared with standard antiepileptic drugs.

### Non-convulsive status epilepticus and encephalopathy
Several cases of non-convulsive status epilepticus have been reported, usually in patients with spike-wave epilepsy. The extent of this risk is unclear, and some of the cases reported were probably not cases of status epilepticus but rather drug-induced encephalopathy. However, in view of this risk, tiagabine should not be used routinely in patients with generalized epilepsy, especially those with a history of absence or myoclonic seizures, with a history of spike-and-wave discharges on EEG, or non-convulsive status epilepticus.

### Idiosyncratic side-effects and changes in laboratory parameters
No idiosyncratic reactions have as yet been linked to the use of tiagabine. There are no systematic abnormalities in haematology values or common biochemical parameters, and routine monitoring of laboratory values is not required. The relationship of adverse events has correlated more strongly with dose than with the plasma concentration of tiagabine, and there is therefore no need to check plasma concentrations routinely.

### Teratogenicity
There is no definitive information on the teratogenic risk of tiagabine in humans and the drug cannot therefore be recommended for treatment during pregnancy. Effects were seen in the offspring of rats exposed to maternally toxic doses of tiagabine, but not in animals receiving non-toxic doses.

### Overdose
Forty-seven cases are reported and all survived. One patient took 400 mg and developed convulsive status epilepticus. In addition to respiratory and cerebral depression, other symptoms included agitation and myoclonus. Treatment with simple supportive measures is effective.

## Antiepileptic effect
### Partial-onset seizures
Tiagabine has been the subject of a series of clinical trials designed to demonstrate efficacy, including five double-blind placebo-controlled studies of the drug as adjunctive

therapy, three trials (one open and two double-blinded) in monotherapy and six long-term open studies. The randomized double-bind placebo-controlled studies in refractory partial epilepsy in adults form the core of the definitive efficacy studies. Pooling the results, 661 of the 951 enrolled patients entered into a double-blind phase, and 23% of patients showed a reduction of more than 50%, versus 9% of patients on placebo. The overall frequency of seizures was also reduced, by 25% on tiagabine versus 0.1% on placebo. Tiagabine was effective at doses of 32 and 56 mg/day. A meta-analysis across all three trials for 50% responders showed an odds ratio of 3.03 (95% CI, 2.01–4.58) in favour of tiagabine, with no significant differences in efficacy between tiagabine, gabapentin, lamotrigine, topiramate, vigabatrin or zonisamide. The summary odds ratios for each dose indicated increasing efficacy with increasing dose, with no suggestion that the effect of the drug had reached a plateau at the doses examined in these studies. A 16-mg dose has a fairly small effect of 2.40 (95% CI, 0.65–8.87), and this was substantially increased with doses of 30 or 32 mg to an odds ratio of 3.17 (95% CI, 2.03–4.96).

Randomized studies have also been performed to compare twice and three times daily dosing, and greater numbers of patients completed the study in the three times daily group, suggesting that this regimen is better tolerated. The proportion of responders is similar whatever regimen is chosen. Studies of combination therapy with carbamazepine and phenytoin have been carried out. These did not show that any particular drug combination was more efficacious, although tiagabine combinations were better tolerated than the combination of phenytoin and carbamazepine. In the long-term extension studies (i.e. of responders in the short-term clinical trials), a total of 772 patients were treated with tiagabine (at less than 80 mg/day), with a reduction in the frequency of seizures of at least 50% in about 30–40% of patients treated for between 3 and 6 months. For partial seizures this effect was maintained during 12 months, but not for secondarily generalized seizures.

In open studies in 2248 patients, of whom more than half were treated with tiagabine for more than 1 year, 30–40% of the patients obtained considerable treatment effect, which was maintained after 12 months of treatment. Daily doses in the long-term studies were between 24 and 60 mg in the majority of patients and mean and median doses were 45 mg/day for most studies. However, up to 15% of patients received a dose of between 80 and 120 mg/day after their first year of treatment.

### Monotherapy

Tiagabine has also been studied in monotherapy. The efficacy of tiagabine monotherapy in patients with chronic partial epilepsy has been studied in a double-blind parallel-group study in 198 patients with refractory epilepsy, comparing 6 mg/day tiagabine with 36 mg/day after gradual withdrawal of other antiepileptic drugs over 29 weeks. Thirty-three per cent of the patients on the low dose completed the study compared with 47% taking the higher dose, and in both groups the median complex partial seizure rates decreased significantly during treatment compared with baseline. However, a higher proportion of patients in the 36 mg/day group experienced a reduction in complex partial seizures of at least 50% compared with the 6 mg/day group (31 vs 18%). The conclusions of this study were that although higher doses were more effective, as low a dose as 6 mg/day of tiagabine may be effective when used as monotherapy or with non-inducing antipileptics. Another double-blind, randomized comparison of a slow and fast switch to tiagabine monotherapy from another monotherapy has been carried out. Thirty-four (85%) out of the 40 patients were successfully switched to tiagabine monotherapy. The retention rate in the study for 12 weeks on tiagabine monotherapy was 63% (25/40) and 48% for 48 weeks (19/40). The median dose in the open phase was 20 mg/day and the range was from 7.5 to 42.5 mg/day during the first 48 weeks.

### Children

Tiagabine has also been studied as adjunctive therapy in children in several studies. Effectiveness is reported in partial seizures, to a similar extent as in adults, but tiagabine was also shown to be effective in absence and atonic seizures. The mean maximum daily tiagabine dose level tolerated was 0.65 mg/kg. In another long-term open-label extension study in 140 children aged 2–11 years, 10 patients were rendered free from seizures with tiagabine add-on therapy and 13 patients achieved seizure freedom with tiagabine monotherapy for periods ranging from 9 to 109 weeks. The dose range in this study was from 4 to 66 mg/day, and the average dose was 23.5 mg/day.

### Clinical use in epilepsy

Tiagabine is available for use as add-on therapy in refractory patients with partial or secondarily generalized seizures, in adults and in children over the age of 12 years. It has been claimed that the drug has a particular place in patients with lesional epilepsy (e.g. tumoural epilepsy) and in patients who are prone to agitation or anxiety.

It is an effective drug, but its use is complicated by the need to titrate slowly, the potential for drug interactions, and the frequent need for three times daily dosing. In adults tiagabine should be initiated at a dose of 4–5 mg/day and incremented by weekly increments of 4–5 mg until a maintenance dose is reached. This titration rate is slower than that used in the labelling or in the clinical trials, but minimizes CNS-related side-effects. Initial doses can be given twice a day, but a change to thrice-daily dosing is recommended with doses above 30–32 mg/day. Tiagabine should always be taken with food, and preferably at the end of meals, to avoid rapid rises in plasma concentrations, and taking it with food will greatly improve tolerability. Individual dosing four times daily may also be helpful, at least with higher doses.

The recommended initial target maintenance dose is between 30 and 32 mg/day in patients co-medicated with enzyme-inducing drugs, and 15–16 mg/day for those who are not. The usual maximum recommended dose is 50–56 mg/day in patients taking enzyme-inducing drugs, and 30–32 mg/day for those not taking enzyme-inducing drugs. However, high daily doses of at least 70–80 mg have been used in occasional patients and seem to be well tolerated. An an anecdotal level, there is a general view that the higher doses of tiagabine particularly can be strikingly effective; and certainly, there are series of patients reported, by different authorities, who had been resistant to all previous antiepileptic therapies and who gained total seizure control with tiagabine. Patients taking a combination of inducing and non-inducing drugs (e.g. carbamazepine and valproate) should be considered to be enzyme-induced.

Routine tiagabine withdrawal should be carried out at rates of no greater than 5 mg per week.

Although minor dose-related side-effects are common, the frequency of idiosyncratic drug-related reactions, including cutaneous reactions, is very low, and an advantage of tiagabine over other conventional drugs is its favourable cognitive profile. It does not suffer the major side-effects encountered with vigabatrin, namely psychosis and depression, or the induction of visual-field defects.

If there is a history of depression, treatment with tiagabine should be initiated at a low initial dose under close supervision as there may be an increased risk of recurrence. In view of the risk of inducing an encephalopathic state (with stupor and confusion) or non-convulsive status epilepticus, tiagabine should not be used in patients with generalized epilepsy, especially those with a history of absence or myoclonic seizures, with a history of spike-and-wave discharges or non-convulsive status epilepticus. Tiagabine is contraindicated in severe hepatic impairment. Dosage recommendations in children are not yet available. The drug should not be used in pregnant or lactating women.

# TOPIRAMATE

| | |
|---|---|
| **Primary indications** | Partial and secondarily generalized seizures. Also for Lennox–Gastaut syndrome. Idiopathic generalized epilepsy. Adults and children over 2 years of age |
| **Licensed for monotherapy/add-on therapy** | Both (monotherapy ≥ 6 years of age) |
| **Usual preparations** | Tablets: 25, 50, 100, 200 mg; sprinkle: 15, 25, 50 mg |
| **Usual dosage—adults** | Initial: 25–50 mg/day<br>Maintenance: 100–500 mg/day |
| **Usual dosage—children** | Initial: 0.5–1 mg/kg/day<br>Maintenance: 5–9 mg/kg/day |
| **Dosing intervals** | 2 times/day |
| **Dose commonly affected by co-medication** | Yes |
| **Dose affected by renal/hepatic disease** | Renal disease |
| **Common drug interactions** | Some drug interactions; see p. 179 |
| **Serum level monitoring** | Utility not established |
| **Target range** | 10–60 µmol/L |
| **Common/important adverse events** | Dizziness, ataxia, headache, paraesthesia, tremor, somnolence, cognitive dysfunction, confusion, agitation, amnesia, depression, emotional lability, nausea, diarrhoea, diplopia, weight loss |
| **Major mechanism of action** | Inhibition of voltage-gated sodium channels; potentiation of GABA-mediated inhibition at the GABA-A receptor; reduction of AMPA receptor activity; inhibition of high-voltage calcium channels; carbonic anhydrase activity |
| **Main advantages** | Powerful antiepilepitc action; weight loss a common effect |
| **Main disadvantages** | Potential for CNS and other side-effects |
| **COMMENT** | Powerful antiepileptic drug. Its use has been limited by side-effects, although slow titration and lower doses reduce the incidence of adverse effects |

Topiramate was initially developed as an antidiabetic drug. It was found to have striking antiepileptic action in animal models on routine screening, and then underwent a series of controlled trials in North America and Europe. It was licensed, first in the UK, in 1994 and subsequently in the USA and Europe and many countries worldwide. Its strong antiepileptic action has differentiated topiramate from some other newer antiepileptics, and it has gained a reputation as a powerful antiepileptic drug, effective in some patients in whom all other medications have failed.

## Physical and chemical properties

Topiramate (2,3:4,5-bis-O-(1-methylethylidene)-α-D-fructo-pyranose sulphamate; molecular weight 339.36) is a sulphamate substituted monosaccharide, derived from D fructose, a naturally occurring sugar. It is mildly acidic, moderately soluble in water, and its solubility is increased in alkaline solutions. It is freely soluble in ethanol and other organic solvents.

## Mode of action

Topiramate appears to have multiple actions which potentially contribute to its antiepileptic potential. The relative contribution of each mechanism is not known, and probably varies in different individuals and types of epilepsy. The drug exerts an inhibitory effect on sodium conductance in neuronal membranes. This action is similar to that of phenytoin and carbamazepine although its action is not as rapid or as complete as that of phenytoin or lamotrigine. It also enhances GABA-A receptor activity, and, like phenobarbital and the benzodiazepine drugs, increases GABA-mediated chloride influx into neurones. However,

**Topiramate**
Pharmacokinetics—average adult values

| | |
|---|---|
| Oral bioavailability | < 100% |
| Time to peak levels | 2–4 h |
| Volume of distribution | 0.6–1.0 l/kg |
| Biotransformation | When hepatic enzymes are not induced, most of the drug is excreted without metabolism. In the presence of enzyme-inducing drugs, some of the drug is hydoxylated or hydrolysed and then conjugated (cytochrome P450 system; UDPGT family enzymes) |
| Elimination half-life | 19–25 h (varies considerably with co-medication) |
| Plasma clearance | 0.022–0.036 l/kg/h; higher in children than in adults |
| Protein binding | 13–17% |
| Active metabolite | None |

topiramate does not bind at the benzodiazepine binding site, and the exact mechanism of action at the GABA site is not known. Topiramate also inhibits glutamate receptors, particularly of the aminohydroxymethylisozole propionic acid (AMPA) subtype, but has no action on NMDA receptor activity. It is unique among the antiepileptic drugs in this regard. It also reduces l-type high-voltage activated calcium channel activity. Finally, topiramate is a weak inhibitor of carbonic anhydrase, 10–100 times less potent than acetazolamide in this regard. Topiramate exerts a powerful antiepileptic action in a wide range of experimental models of epilepsy. There is also a body of experimental work suggesting a promising potential for neuroprotection, but no human studies have yet been carried out to explore this.

## Pharmacokinetics
### Absorption and distribution
Topiramate is rapidly absorbed after oral dosing with a bioavailability approaching 100%. The time to peak blood levels is about 2 hours. Food delays absorption by several hours, but does not affect its extent and the drug need not be given at any fixed time in relation to food. Topiramate is widely distributed in tissues, including brain. The volume of distribution is between 0.6 and 1.0 l/kg, although this falls at higher doses. Approximately 13–17% of topiramate is bound to plasma protein. Plasma concentrations increase linearly with dose within the normal dosing range.

### Metabolism and elimination
Topiramate is metabolized in the liver by the P450 microsomal enzymes. At least eight metabolites have been identified, formed by hydroxylation, hydrolysis or cleavage of the sulphamate group. None of the metabolites have antiepileptic action. The plasma elimination half-life of topiramate is between 19 and 25 hours, and is independent of dose over the normal clinical range. In monotherapy metabolism is slight, plasma concentrations show little intra-individual variability, and the majority of the drug (85%) is excreted unchanged in the urine. In polytherapy, however, metabolism is much more extensive, presumably due to enzyme induction. The elimination of topiramate and its metabolites is via renal mechanisms.

In children, topiramate clearance is higher than in adults. In older children, clearance values are about 50% higher than in adults. In children between the ages of 4 and 7 years, renal clearance is 40% higher than in children over 8 years old. In infants, topiramate clearance is further increased, and the dose requirement in infants (mg/kg/day) necessary to maintain a similar plasma concentration is twice that of adults. No change in clearance or elimination half-life of topiramate has been seen among elderly adults with healthy renal function. Topiramate clearance is reduced by 42% in patients with moderate renal impairment and 54% in patients with severe renal impairment, and topiramate doses should be reduced in such patients. However, topiramate is cleared rapidly by haemodialysis, and supplemental dosing may be required during haemodialysis. Severe hepatic disease results in about a 30% decrease in clearance, and about a 30% increase in plasma concentrations.

### Drug interactions
Topiramate is a mild inhibitor of P450 isoenzyme CYP2C19 and, although it thus has the potential to interact with other drugs, in most patients in practice topiramate does not affect the steady-state concentrations of other antiepileptic drugs. However, where phenytoin metabolism is close to saturation, the inhibitory action of topiramate may cause phenytoin levels to increase. It has been shown to have no effect on carbamazepine or CBZ-epoxide levels and no consistent effect on valproate concentrations. In children, co-medication has been shown to result in a slight decrease in lamotrigine levels. Topiramate also increases the clearance of warfarin and the oestrogen component of the oral contraceptive.

Enzyme-inducing antiepileptic drugs such as phenytoin, phenobarbital and carbamazepine decrease topiramate serum concentrations by approximately 50%, and because of this interaction, topiramate dosage in combination therapy with these drugs needs to be increased. Valproate administration has no effect on topiramate concentrations. A similar effect is noted in children, and studies have shown a reduction in average half-life from 15.4 to 7.5 hours in the

| Adverse event | Percentage of patients in each target mg/kg dosage group | | | | | |
|---|---|---|---|---|---|---|
| | Placebo (*n* = 174) | 200 (*n* = 45) | 400 (*n* = 68) | 600 (*n* = 124) | 800 (*n* = 76) | 1000 (*n* = 47) |
| Ataxia | 7 | 20 | 22 | 17 | 16 | 21 |
| Concentration impaired | 1 | 11 | 9 | 12 | 15 | 21 |
| Confusion | 5 | 9 | 15 | 18 | 14 | 28 |
| Dizziness | 13 | 36 | 22 | 31 | 32 | 40 |
| Fatigue | 16 | 13 | 18 | 31 | 49 | 32 |
| Somnolence | 10 | 27 | 26 | 17 | 20 | 28 |
| Abnormal thinking | 2 | 20 | 12 | 29 | 28 | 26 |
| Anorexia | 3 | 4 | 4 | 8 | 9 | 21 |
| Paraesthesia | 3 | 18 | 20 | 13 | 18 | 13 |

**Table 3.22** Percentage of patients in placebo-controlled trials of topiramate experiencing adverse effects in different dosage groups.

| Adverse event | Adjunctive therapy | | Monotherapy (*n* = 114) |
|---|---|---|---|
| | Placebo + AEDs (*n* = 101) | TPM + AEDs (*n* = 98) | |
| Somnolence | 16 | 26 | 10 |
| Anorexia | 15 | 24 | 13 |
| Fatigue | 5 | 16 | 19 |
| Nervousness | 7 | 14 | 4 |
| Concentration/attention difficulty | 2 | 10 | 8 |
| Aggressiveness | 4 | 9 | 4 |
| Weight loss | 1 | 9 | 5 |
| Memory difficulty | 0 | 5 | 5 |

AED, antiepileptic drug.

**Table 3.23** Adverse effects of topiramate (TPM) experienced by children in add-on and monotherapy trials; figures are percentages. The first two columns refer to events with a difference in incidence of ≥ 5% vs placebo on TPM 6 mg/kg/day, the last column gives the data for 25–50 mg/day TPM.

presence of enzyme-inducing drugs. In infants, treatment with enzyme inducers has been shown to reduce the half-life of topiramate to 6.4 hours.

## Adverse effects

Topiramate side-effects have been extensively studied in the controlled trials, and also during the extensive open experience of the drug. The adverse effects noted as adjunctive therapy and as monotherapy in the randomized clinical trials are shown in Tables 3.22 and 3.23. In the early trials, 14% of those randomized to topiramate withdrew prematurely because of adverse events, but this rate is less in subsequent studies, which have used lower doses and slower rates of titration. Adverse events seen in trials in children have been similar to those seen in adults (see Table 3.23),

and as in adults, these effects were more prevalent in polytherapy than monotherapy, and with a more rapid titration of the dose.

## Neurotoxic effects

The most prominent side-effects noted in clinical practice are somnolence, mental slowing (with a particular effect on word finding and language), and impairment of concentration. Cognitive testing has shown significant effects, particularly on word fluency, list learning and verbal IQ. These are very much dose-related and their frequency increases markedly at higher doses. Other side-effects are not uncommon and include dizziness, ataxia, fatigue, paresthesiae in the extremities, ataxia, disturbance of memory, depression and agitation. These adverse events are prominent in about 15% of patients, and topiramate is badly tolerated by a higher proportion of patients than other less effective medication. However, tolerance to many of the side-effects does develop within a few weeks if the drug is continued, and it is worth emphasizing this point in clinical practice. Furthermore, the adverse events can be greatly reduced by slow titration of the drug, and the high frequency of side-effects noted in the clinical trials largely occurred as the dose was being rapidly titrated upwards, often to high doses. The importance of slow titration was emphasized in a randomized parallel double-blind study evaluating two rates of titration, in which incremental steps of 100/200 mg/day resulted in twice the withdrawal rate of 50 mg/day increments.

The effect on cognition has been formally studied, and these investigations demonstrate the importance of slow titration. In healthy young adults, the cognitive profile at baseline was compared, after rapid titration, with that at 2 and 4 weeks of treatment with either topiramate 5.7 mg/kg/day, lamotrigine 7.1 mg/kg or gabapentin 35 mg/kg. The verbal fluency rate of the topiramate group dropped an average of 50% per subject compared with a negligible change for the other two groups, and a threefold error occurred for the visual attention task. At the 2- and 4-week test periods only the topiramate subjects continued to display adverse cognitive effects from drug administration. In a second study, the cognitive effects of topiramate were compared with those of valproate with slow titration to a dose of 200–400 mg/day for topiramate (weekly increments of 25 mg) and 1800 mg/day for valproate. Of 10 baseline to end-point comparisons, only one test (measuring short-term verbal memory) showed a statistically significant worsening for topiramate and improvement for valproate. None of the tests of mood or of subjective complaints showed significant differences between the treatments.

## Weight loss

Topiramate also causes weight loss in many patients. This effect is dose related and also greatest in those who are overweight. In the early clinical trials, mean decreases were 1.1 kg at 200 mg/day and 5.9 kg at doses over 800 mg/day, and the mean loss in patients over 60 kg was 8%, compared with 3% in those under 60 kg. The weight loss can be marked—a loss of over 10 kg has been reported in one case—and patients need to be warned about this to prevent misinterpretation. The effect is probably due to a suppressive effect on appetite, although this has not been unequivocally shown. To some patients, weight loss is welcome, and counters the tendency of other antiepileptic drugs (notably valproate, gabapentin and vigabatrin) to promote weight gain. However, the possible long-term implications of weight loss in children are uncertain, and further studies are required.

## Other side-effects

As the drug is a carbonic anhydrase inhibitor, topiramate also has a propensity to cause paraesthesia, and this is not an infrequent minor complaint. The formation of renal calculi has also been reported, and is presumably related to the carbonic anhydrase activity. Symptomatic calculi are reported to occur in one patient per thousand per year, and topiramate should be used cautiously in those with a history of renal calculi or a family history. Patients should be encouraged to drink plenty of fluids because of this risk. A decrease in serum bicarbonate may occur, particularly in children, although clinical acidosis is rare. Hypohyolosis can result in significant hyperpyrexia especially in children; mothers should be cautioned about this. Acute rises in intra-ocular pressure can occur, which resolve on discontinuation of therapy. There are no reports of significant cardiotoxicity or gastrointestinal toxicity. Allergic rash is extremely rare. One case of fulminant hepatic failure has been reported. There have been no reports of haematological toxicity with topiramate.

There are no definitive data on the teratogenic effects of topiramate in humans, although teratogenicity has been reported in animals. The drug is not recommended for use in pregnancy.

## Antiepileptic effect
### Partial-onset seizures

Topiramate has been intensively studied in various types of epilepsy and in various syndromes over the past 10 years. The initial studies were, as with all antiepileptic drugs, in adults with refractory partial epilepsy. These include five double-blind parallel-group placebo-controlled add-on trials (Table 3.24), which aimed initially at high maintenance doses (600–1000 mg) and then, based on subsequent experience, at substantially lower doses. The pivotal clinical trials demonstrated a reduction in the frequency of seizures of at least 50% (treatment responders) in 35–50% of subjects. A meta-analysis of these placebo-controlled studies showed a greater effect on topiramate than any of the other drugs, although the power of these studies was insufficient to demonstrate significant differences. In an intention to treat meta-analysis, significantly smaller numbers of patients were required to find a responder to topiramate treatment than to gabapentin or lamotrigine.

A pooled analysis of initial studies in 527 patients randomized to topiramate and 216 patients to placebo found a median per cent reduction in topiramate-treated patients of 44% compared with 2% in placebo-treated patients. The first pivotal studies included patients randomized to high doses (600–1000 mg/day), and it was quickly realized that the gains in efficacy were outweighed by poor tolerability at these high levels. Thus, subsequent double-blind, placebo-controlled studies were carried out at 300 and 200 mg/day. In these studies, 48% and 45% of patients showed a reduc-

| Placebo topiramate (mg/day) | No. of subjects | Median percent reduction in monthly seizure rate | Percentage of patients with 50% decrease in seizures | Percentage of patients with 75–100% decrease in seizures |
|---|---|---|---|---|
| Placebo | 24 | 1 | 8 | 4 |
| Topiramate 400 | 23 | 41* | 35† | 22 |
| Placebo | 30 | −12†† | 10 | 3 |
| Topiramate 600 | 30 | 46‡ | 47§ | 23 |
| Placebo | 28 | −18†† | 0 | 0 |
| Topiramate 800 | 28 | 36§ | 43§ | 36 |
| Placebo | 45 | 13 | 18 | 9 |
| Topiramate 200 | 45 | 30§ | 27 | 9 |
| Topiramate 400 | 45 | 48** | 47† | 22 |
| Topiramate 600 | 46 | 45§ | 46† | 22 |
| Placebo | 47 | 1 | 9 | 0 |
| Topiramate 600 | 48 | 41§ | 44§ | 23 |
| Topiramate 800 | 48 | 41§ | 40§ | 13 |
| Topiramate 1000 | 47 | 38§ | 38§ | 13 |

**Table 3.24** The results of five double-blind, placebo-controlled clinical trials of topiramate in adults with partial epilepsy.

*, $P = 0.065$; †, $P \leq 0.05$; ‡, $P \leq 0.005$; §, $P \leq 0.001$; **, $P \leq 0.01$; ††, negative number indicates an increase in seizure rate.

tion in seizures of at least 50% compared with 13% and 24% of placebo-treated patients. In these low-dose studies, only 8% of topiramate-treated patients and 2% of patients receiving placebo discontinued the trial owing to adverse events. Most of these patients were receiving other enzyme-inducing antiepileptics, and even in these cases, 100–200 mg/day appears to be an appropriate target dosage. Data from open studies have confirmed the effectiveness of topiramate in partial seizures, and one pragmatic study of 901 adults, for instance, showed a median reduction in seizures of 73%, with 68% of patients achieving a 50% or more reduction. In a retrospective review the 1-year retention rates in the open extension phases of clinical trials were 52% for topiramate compared with 46% for lamotrigine and 23% for gabapentin. At 5 years, retention rates were 28% (topiramate), 12% (lamotrigine) and 2% (gabapentin).

### Partial-onset seizures in children

In children with partial-onset seizures, similar results have been obtained in formal regulatory studies. The pivotal randomized double-blind controlled trial found a median reduction in seizures of 33% in topiramate-treated compared with 11% in placebo-treated children. The proportion of topiramate-treated children achieving a 50% or more seizure reduction was 39%, compared with 20% in

the placebo group. Five per cent of children receiving topiramate were free from seizures during the 16-week study and none in the placebo-treated group. No children discontinued topiramate treatment because of adverse events.

### Monotherapy

Topiramate has been evaluated as monotherapy in a series of double-blind comparative studies. The first study was of 252 patients with recent-onset epilepsy (less than 3 years) not responding to initial therapy. Two dose regimens were compared. Fifty-four per cent of patients receiving 200/500 mg/day topiramate were free from seizures compared with 39% of patients receiving 25/50 mg/day topiramate (in each case, the lower dose—200 or 25 mg—was given to patients who weighed ≤ 50 kg). In another study, the seizure-free rates were 35–48% at 6 months and 54–61% at 1 year with 400 mg/day topiramate. In a randomized controlled trial comparing topiramate monotherapy (100 and 200 mg/day) with carbamazepine (600 mg/day) and valproate (1250 mg/day), in a broad spectrum of patients, the 6-month seizure-free rates with 100 and 200 mg/day were 49% and 44%, compared with 44% on carbamazepine and valproate. The discontinuation rates owing to adverse events for 100 mg/day topiramate, 200 mg/day topiramate, carbamazepine, and valproate were 19%, 28%, 25% and

23%, respectively. In recent open flexible-dose studies of monotherapy in recently diagnosed epilepsy, topiramate therapy was shown to be highly effective at low doses. At doses of 100–125 mg/day, 80% of patients exhibited a >50% reduction in seizures and at month 7 and 13 of therapy, 44% and 35% respectively of patients had remained seizure free.

### Primarily generalized seizures

There have also been two double-blind placebo-controlled add-on trials of topiramate in primarily generalized tonic–clonic seizures. There was a statistically significant reduction of seizures in one study but not the other. When data from both studies were pooled, the median per cent reduction was 57% in topiramate-treated patients and 27% in the placebo group. Fifty-five per cent of topiramate-treated patients had a reduction of seizures of at least 50% compared with 28% in the placebo group. The effects were similar in children and adults. Adverse events led o discontinuation of therapy in 10% of the topiramate-treated patients and 8% in the placebo group. These good results are con-firmed at an anecdotal level in routine clinical practice. Topiramate has also been shown to reduce myoclonus and absence seizures (petit mal) in patients with juvenile myo-clonic epilepsy (JME) and idiopathic generalized epilepsy.

### Other epilepsy syndromes

A controlled study of patients with the Lennox–Gastaut syndrome has also been carried out. The median per cent reduction in drop attacks was 15% (compared with a 5% increase in those on placebo), and in major motor seizures (drop attacks and tonic–clonic seizures combined) the reduction was 26% (compared with a 5% increase in those on placebo). The effectiveness of topiramate against major motor seizures was comparable to that reported with lam-otrigine. Topiramate also shows effectiveness in atypical absence and tonic seizures. In the long-term extension of this study, drop attacks were reduced by 50% or more in 55% of patients receiving topiramate, and despite an average baseline frequency of 90 drop attacks per day, 15% of patients had no drop attacks for at least 6 months. Sub-stantial reductions were also observed in atypical absence, myoclonic, and tonic–clonic seizures.

Open studies have also shown effectiveness in various childhood epilepsy syndromes. In a study of 11 patients with West syndrome, infantile spasms were reduced in nine patients (82%), and five patients (45%) became spasm free. In an open study of 18 patients with severe myoclonic epilepsy of infancy (SMEI), after a mean period of 10 months of treatment 72% of the patients had achieved a reduction in seizure rate of at least 50%, and 16.6% were seizure free. In five children with Angelman syndrome after a mean 8.8 months on topiramate, two were seizure free. Finally, pilot and experimental work suggests topiramate is highly effective in controlling tonic–clonic status epilepticus.

## Clinical use in epilepsy

Topiramate is a powerful antiepileptic drug. It is effective in a broad spectrum of epilepsies and epilepsies syndromes, but has a particular place in the treatment of resistant focal seizures, and symptomatic generalized epilepsies. It is useful in children and in adults, and in those with learning disability and epilepsy. The drug is available in 50, 100 and 200 mg tablets, and as a sprinkle and syrup. There are no parenteral preparations. It is now licensed for use as initial single drug therapy in newly diagnosed patients as well as adjunctive therapy in patients with refractory epilepsy.

The early clinical trials were carried out at higher doses than are now currently recommended, and although these studies showed marked efficacy, the rate of neurological and cognitive side-effects was also high. The drug gained a reputation for being strikingly effective, but also poorly tolerated. However, subsequent experience has shown that lower doses are also effective and confer much better tolerability. In routine practice, the rate of side-effects is thus lower than initially feared. The risk of side-effects can also be greatly reduced by starting the drug at a very low dose and titrating upwards slowly.

In adults on adjunctive therapy, my own practice is to initiate therapy at 25 mg/day and increase this fortnightly to 50 mg, then 100 mg, and then increase in 50 mg increments to an initial mainten-ance dose of between 100 and 300 mg/day (the higher dose ranges are needed usually for patients co-medicated with enzyme-inducing antiepileptics). The drug is given in two divided doses. The usual maximum maintenance dose is 600 mg/day, but occasionally up to 1000 mg/day has been given without side-effects. Much lower doses are needed in newly diagnosed patients, and in monotherapy, and it is my practice to aim for maintenance doses of 75–150 mg/day initially, building the dose up slowly at 25 mg increments every 2–4 weeks. On this regimen, good efficacy is usually obtained with very few side-effects.

In children on adjunctive therapy, the usual recommended dose is 0.5–1 mg/kg/day for the first week, with weekly increments of 0.5–1 mg/kg/day until an initial maintenance dose of 4–6 mg/kg/day is reached. Higher doses, up to 20–30 mg/kg/day, have been used and are sometimes necessary, especially in those co-medicated with enzyme-inducing drugs.

Blood levels can be measured, but are not routinely useful. The most common side-effects are on cognitive function (notably effects on language and word finding), paraesthesia and weight loss. These are reversible when doses are reduced. There is also a risk of renal calculi and acute rises in intra-ocular pressure.

# VALPROATE

COOH

| | |
|---|---|
| **Primary indications** | Primary and secondarily generalized seizures (including myoclonus and absence) and partial seizures. Lennox–Gastaut syndrome. Idiopathic generalized epilepsy. Childhood epilepsy syndromes. Febrile convulsions |
| **Licensed for monotherapy/add-on therapy** | Both |
| **Usual preparations** | Enteric-coated tablets: 200, 500 mg; crushable tablets: 100 mg; capsules: 150, 300, 500 mg; syrup: 200 mg/5 ml; liquid: 200 mg/5 ml; slow-release tablets; 200, 300, 500 mg; divalproex tablets: 125, 300, 500 mg; sprinkle |
| **Usual dosage—adults** | Initial: 200–500 mg/day<br>Maintenance: 500–3000 mg/day |
| **Usual dosage—children** | Initial: 20 mg/kg/day (children under 20 kg); 40 mg/kg/day (children over 20 kg)<br>Maintenance:<br>Children under 20 kg: 20–30 mg/kg/day<br>Children over 20 kg: 20–40 mg/kg/day |
| **Dosing intervals** | 2–3 times/day |
| **Dose commonly affected by co-medication** | Yes |
| **Dose affected by renal/hepatic disease** | Avoid in hepatic disease |
| **Common drug interactions** | Extensive; see Table 3.25 and p. 186 |
| **Serum level monitoring** | Useful in occasional patients |
| **Target range** | 300–700 μmol/l |
| **Common/important adverse events** | Nausea, vomiting, hyperammonaemia and other metabolic effects, endocrine effects, severe hepatic toxicity, pancreatitis, drowsiness, cognitive disturbance, aggressiveness, tremor, weakness, encephalopathy, thrombocytopenia, neutropenia, aplastic anemia, hair thinning and hair loss, weight gain, polycystic ovarian syndrome |
| **Major mechanism of action** | Effects on GABA and glutaminergic activity, calcium (T) conductance and potassium conductance |
| **Main advantages** | A wide spectrum of activity; drug of choice in most patients with idiopathic generalized epilepsy |
| **Main disadvantages** | Weight gain, CNS and other side-effects; risk of severe hepatic disturbance in children; teratogenicity |
| **COMMENT** | Effective, well-tried and broad spectrum antiepileptic drug. Use limited by side-effects |

Valproate (VPA) was first sythesized in 1882 as an organic solvent. Its antiepileptic properties were recognized in the 1960s, entirely by accident, while being used as a solvent for the screening of new antiepileptic compounds. It was licensed in Europe in the early 1960s, where it became very widely used, and then in the USA in 1978. It has been marketed as a magnesium or calcium salt, an acid, and also as sodium hydrogen divalproate (Depakote®). Sodium valproate is the usual form in the UK and Depakote in Europe.

Valpromide (dipropylacetamide), a prodrug of valproate, is also marketed, as is a delayed-release formulation of sodium valproate. The term valproate is usually adopted to refer to all these forms, and although properties vary to some extent, none of these formulations has been shown to confer any real superiority over the others. Valproate is widely available throughout the world, and has become a drug of choice in primary generalized epilepsy and for treating a wide spectrum of seizure types.

**Valproate**
Pharmacokinetics—average adult values

| | |
|---|---|
| Oral bioavailability | < 100% |
| Time to peak levels | 0.5–8 h |
| Volume of distribution | 0.1–0.4 l/kg |
| Biotransformation | Oxidation, epoxydation, reduction and glucuronidation. (Some metabolism via cytochrome P450 enzymes CYP4B1, CYP2C9, CYP2A6, CYP2B6, CYP2C19; UDPGT family enzymes, but other non-cytochrome enzymes involved) |
| Elimination half-life | 12–17 h |
| Plasma clearance | 0.010–0.115 l/kg/h |
| Protein binding | 85–95% |
| Active metabolite | None |

## Physical and chemical properties

Valproic acid is a simple molecule, a branched chain carboxylic acid, similar in clinical structure to endogenous fatty acids. It is slightly soluble in water and very soluble in organic solvents. Its pKa is 4.8. The sodium salt is extremely soluble in water, whereas the calcium and magnesium salts are insoluble.

## Mode of action

The mechanism of action is not entirely clear. Valproate has a number of actions at the GABA-A receptor, and this is postulated to be the main antiepileptic effect. It increases synaptosomal GABA concentrations through the activation of the GABA-synthesizing enzyme glutamic acid decarboxylase and also inhibits GABA catabolism through inhibition of GABA transaminase and succinic semialdehyde dehydrogenase. However, valproate also inhibits excitatory neurotransmission mediated by aspartic acid, glutamic acid and γ-hydroxybutyric acid, and reduces cellular excitability through modulation of voltage-dependent sodium currents. In hippocampal slices, valproate also reduces the threshold for calcium and potassium conductance. The relative importance of these mechanisms in human epilepsy is unclear. In animal models valproate is highly effective against a range of seizures.

## Pharmacokinetics

### Absorption and distribution

Valproate is rapidly and nearly completely absorbed, with bioavailability approaching 100%. The peak plasma concentration of sodium valproate, after oral administration, is usually reached within 30 minutes to 2 hours. Other formulations have slightly different absorption properties, and administration with food slightly delays the absorption of most forms, but not their extent. Sodium valproate is available in an enteric-coated formulation which results in peak plasma concentrations within 3–8 hours, and this is the commonly used form in the UK. Rectal administration also results in complete absorption.

Valproate has a restricted distribution, probably mainly in the vascular compartment and extracellular fluid, and has an apparent volume of distribution of 0.1–0.4 l/kg. High concentrations, however, are found in the liver, intestinal tract, gall bladder, kidney and urinary bladder. Valproate also enters the CSF compartment and brain rapidly, via an active transport mechanism which is saturable, and absorption at high doses is much less efficient. Peak concentrations can be achieved in the brain within minutes and the CSF concentration is lower than the free plasma concentration, and there is great variation. The mean total CSF to plasma ratio is about 0.15. Valproate is removed from the brain by a probenecid-sensitive monoamine transport system. This has implications for its use in acute seizures or status epilepticus.

Valproate is 85–95% bound to plasma proteins. The free faction is concentration dependent and at higher plasma concentrations (above 700 µmol/l) protein binding decreases. Protein binding is reduced in renal and hepatic disease and during pregnancy, and other drugs may displace valproate from its protein binding sites (e.g. aspirin, phenylbutazone). The other antiepileptics do not influence binding, however.

## Metabolism and elimination

Valproate is rapidly eliminated from the body by hepatic metabolism. Uniquely amongst antiepileptics, the enzymes involved are mainly not those of the P450 system. There are a variety of pathways, the main one being beta-oxidation followed by glucuronidation. At least 30 metabolites have been identified, some of which may be responsible for adverse side-effects (notably the 4-ene metabolite and hepatic toxicity). Less than 4% of the drug is excreted unchanged. The elimination half-life is between 12 and 15 hours in young adults and between 14 and 17 hours in the elderly. In children, the half-life is somewhat lower. However, in neonates the drug is slowly metabolized and the half-life is 40–60 hours. The clearance of valproate and its metabolites follows linear kinetics at most dosage ranges, although at higher plasma concentrations reduced protein binding results in an increased clearance.

Because of the relatively short half-life of the drug, there are marked diurnal variations in plasma levels (100% differences between peak and trough levels) on twice-daily dosing. Also there is marked intra-individual variation.

Valproate is relatively contraindicated in hepatic disease, because of concern about its toxicity. Its pharmacokinetic properties are not altered by renal impairment. The protein binding of valproate decreases during pregnancy and total concentration is also reduced owing to an increased volume of distribution. The free drug fraction concentration increases, sometimes by 100%, from the first to the third trimester. Concentrations of valproate in breast milk range from 1 to 3% of those in maternal plasma.

### Drug interactions

Valproate is involved in a number of interactions with other antiepileptic drugs, the mechanism of which is often obscure. Valproate is extensively protein bound; it is metabolized in the liver but does not induce the metabolism of other drugs. However, its own metabolism is greatly affected by co-medication with enzyme-inducing antiepileptic drugs which can increase valproate clearance, often by 100%. The clinical consequences of the complex interactions are not clear, and in most patients these interactions do not pose much of a clinical problem. This may be partly because the clinical effectiveness of the drug is not closely correlated to serum level.

The interactions with other antiepileptic drugs are shown in Table 3.25. Phenytoin, phenobarbital and carbamazepine can induce the hepatic metabolism of valproate, and levels can be reduced by co-medication by as much as 50%. Valproate is also a potent inhibitor of both oxidation and glucuronidation, and via this mechanism elevates diazepam, phenobarbital, phenytoin, ethosuximide, carbamazepine and lamotrigine levels. Among non-antiepileptic drugs, the antacids, Adriamycin and cisplatin have been shown to impair the absorption of valproate. Naproxen, phenylbutazone and salicylate displace valproate from its albumin binding sites and occasionally result in significant toxicity. The metabolism of some drugs is inhibited, notably of nimodipine, levels of which can be almost doubled.

## Adverse effects

As valproate was introduced before the wide use of large controlled and blinded studies, the frequency of side-effects has not been fully established. However, clinical experience has led to the view that the drug is well tolerated, and at least as well tolerated as carbamazepine, phenytoin or another of the newer antiepileptic drugs.

### Neurotoxic side-effects

The sedative side-effects typical of antiepileptic drugs also occur with valproate, severely so in about 2% of patients, and sometimes associated with other neurological symptoms such as confusion and irritability. Tremor occurs in about 10% of patients on valproate, and is dose-related but usually mild. Parkinsonism seems to be another uncommon but unusual side-effect of vaproate therapy, usually developing on long-term treatment and reversible on drug withdrawal. The mechanism is unclear.

### Encephalopathy

Rarely, severe sedation amounting to stupor or even coma has been reported (valproate encephalopathy). Encephalopathy usually occurs in the first weeks of treatment but may appear months after the initiation of therapy. In many cases, serum concentrations and serum ammonia levels are within healthy limits. The encephalopathy worsens if treated with benzodiazepines and, in fact, an improvement with flumazenil (a benzodiazepine receptor antagonist) has been reported. Occult carbamyl phosphate synthetase-1

**Table 3.25** Pharmacokinetic interactions between valproate (VPA) and other antiepileptic drugs.

| Drug | Effect of VPA on the drug | Effect of the drug on VPA |
| --- | --- | --- |
| Benzodiazepines | ↑ Benzodiazepine concentration | No significant effect* |
| Carbamazepine (CBZ) | ↑ CBZ-epoxide (25–100%) | ↓ VPA (30–40%) |
| Ethosuximide (ESM) | ↑ ESM concentration (50%) | No effect |
| Felbamate (FLM) | ↑ FLM concentration | ↑ VPA concentration |
| Lamotrigine (LTG) | ↑ LTG concentration (up to 164%) | No effect |
| Phenytoin (PHT) | ↑ PHT unbound fraction | ↓ VPA (30–40%) |
| Phenobarbital (PB) | ↑ PB concentration (30–40%) | ↓ VPA (30–40%) |
| Primidone (PRM) | ↑ PB concentration (30–40%) | ↓ VPA (30–40%) |
| Vigabatrin (VGB) | No effect | No effect |
| Zonisamide | ↓ ZNS (15%) | No effect |

Gabapentin, levetiracetam, oxcarbazepine, tiagabine and zonisamide have no interactions with VPA;
*, clobazam co-medication can result in an increase in VPA levels.

deficiency may be responsible for some cases at least. Co-medication with phenobarbital also seems to induce severe sedation or even stupor, and this seems to be a pharmacodynamic reaction, usually unrelated to plasma ammonia levels. The EEG usually shows high-voltage slow activity and the stupor or coma rapidly reverses when valproate is withdrawn. The encephalopathy should be differentiated from valproate-induced hyperammonaemia (see below).

### Weight gain and gastrointestinal side-effects

The common dose-related side-effects include nausea, vomiting and gastrointestinal effects, common on initiation of therapy and avoided by the administration of enteric-coated formulations.

Weight gain is a frequent problem (seen in 30% of all patients), often troublesome and occasionally profound, especially in females. This is dose-related and a problem mainly only at higher doses. A recent study showed a mean gain of 5.8 kg after 8 months of treatment at a mean dose of 1800 mg/day. The cause of weight gain is not completely known, but is likely to be due to an increase in appetite due to impaired β-oxidation of fatty acids with hyperinsulinaemia.

### Metabolic and endocrine effects

Valproate has various metabolic effects resulting from interference in mitochondrial-based intermediate metabolism. The common results are hypocarnitinaemia, hyperglycinaemia and hyperammonaemia. The metabolic effects may be exacerbated by genetically determined enzymic defects or by enzymic pathways already stressed owing to acute illness or co-medication. Ammonia levels are often slightly raised on valproate therapy and are asymptomatic. When hyperammonaemia is severe, stupor, coma or even death can result, and hyperammonaemia should be suspected whenever drowsiness occurs on valproate therapy. Patients with existing urea cycle enzymic defects or those with hepatic disease are at particular risk. The most common enzymic defect is partial deficiency (heterozygosity) of ornithine transcarbamylase (OTC deficiency) which may be asymptomatic until valproate is prescribed or until valproate and metabolic stress combine to precipitate acute hyperammonaemia. The hyperammonaemic encephalopathy can be severe and is occasionally fatal.

### Endocrine effects

Valproate also has endocrine effects. The importance of these is uncertain, and data are somewhat conflicting. Polycystic ovarian syndrome (PCOS)—a syndrome with polycystic ovaries, hyperandrogenism, obesity, hirsutism, anovulatory cycles and menstrual disorders—occurs more frequently in women with epilepsy than in the general population (prevalence rate of 13–25% vs 4–6%, respectively).

It has been particularly, but not exclusively, associated with valproate therapy, and with insulin resistance and changes in levels of sex hormones. Serum androgen concentrations increase in valproate-treated patients but with a different profile of hormonal changes in women than in men. Polycystic ovaries are a common finding in young women and do not necessarily imply PCOS. Assessment is further complicated by the confounding effects of weight gain and other medications. However, the presence of a menstrual disorder, hirsutism or weight gain should trigger a thorough evaluation, and favours discontinuation of valproate.

### Other effects: on hair, pancreatic function, HIV replication

Another unusual side-effect of valproate is its propensity, rarely, to cause hair loss, or change in colour or more usually curling of hair. Some degree of hair loss occurs in up to 12% of patients. The mechanism is unclear, but it may be due to the formation of abnormal metabolites. The hair curling can sometimes be profound, and striking changes of appearance (not always unwelcome) may result. It is said that the hair changes reverse if therapy is continued, but in the author's experience this is certainly not true in all cases.

Treatment with VPA may increase serum amylase concentration in up to 24% of the asymptomatic patients. This requires no particular action, provided that other hepatic and pancreatic enzymes (lipase, trypsin) are within healthy limits. However, valproate can also induce acute pancreatitis. This is a rare but serious complication, due possibly to a drug-induced reduction in free radical scavenging enzyme activity. Pancreatitis usually presents with progressive epigastric pain, nausea and vomiting, three-quarters of reported patients are under the age of 20 years, and one-third are under the age of 10 years. One-quarter occurred during valproate monotherapy, half within 3 months of initiating therapy and two-thirds within 12 months of the initiation of treatment. The pancreatitis appears not to be related to dose or serum concentration. In most cases the illness is relatively mild, although occasional fatalities have been reported. It is not appropriate to rechallenge patients after pancreatitis because there is a high risk of relapse.

Valproate appears to increase the viral burden in patients infected with HIV by potentiating viral replication. The clinical consequences of this effect for HIV-positive patients are unknown. Recently, a 14% reduction in bone mineral density during long-term treatment with VPA was reported in both men and women.

### Hypersensitivity, hepatic and haematological side-effects

Acute allergic rashes have been only rarely reported, as have severe bone marrow depression and neutropenia. The most common haematological effects of valproate are effects on clotting; these include thrombocytopenia, inhibition of platelet aggregation, reduction of factor VII complex and fibrinogen depletion. These can result in bruising and haematoma. Usually mild, these are of little clinical significance except during surgical intervention, and it is advised that valproate is withdrawn, especially in children, prior to intracranial surgery (including epilepsy surgery).

The serious idiosyncratic side-effect that has caused most concern is acute hepatic failure. This has been most frequently observed in children under the age of 2 years on polytherapy and with neurological handicaps. Initially, a rate of 1 case of hepatic failure per 500 children on polytherapy under the age of 2 years was found. Some of these initial cases were in fact multi-factorial, with valproate precipitating an already existing diathesis, and with more careful prescribing to avoid high-risk cases, the rate of valproate-induced hepatic failure has now fallen considerably (to 0.2 cases per 10,000). The risk factors for hepatotoxicity seem to be: young age (less than 2 years), use in polytherapy, presence of psychomotor retardation, and the presence of certain underlying metabolic disorders (organic acidaemias, mitochondrial disorders, Alper disease).

Hepatotoxicity usually appears during the first 3 months of therapy. The pathology is microvesicular steatosis with necrosis, and may be caused by an unsaturated metabolite of the drug (2-*n*-propyl-4-pentenoic acid) that is a potent inducer of microvesicular steatosis. However, routine measurement of this and other metabolites has not been useful in predicting hepatic disease, nor have routine measurements of bilirubin or liver function tests. In addition to the usual general and supportive measures, it has been suggested that an infusion of intravenous L-carnitine (100 mg/kg/day, up to a maximum of 2 g/day) should be given. Oral L-carnitine has also been advocated for patients with symptomatic valproate-associated hyperammonaemia. Hepatic failure has occasionally occurred in older children and adults, but no fatalities associated with valproate monotherapy have occurred in patients over the age of 10 years.

Hepatic hypersensitivity should be differentiated from dose-related elevations of liver enzymes, which are present in up to 44% of VPA-treated patients. However, those elevations are usually not associated with clinical symptoms and resolve with drug reduction or withdrawal.

### Teratogenicity

Overall risks of major malformations in the offspring of women treated with valproate monotherapy are between 4 and 9%. This includes a 1–2% increased risk of spina bifida and other congenital anomalies such as cardiovascular malformations and craniofacial defects. The rate of major malformation is thus somewhat worse than that on carbamazepine or lamotrigine (risks of 2–4%). Many of these abnormalities can be detected prenatally, however, and termination of pregnancy reduces the risk to live offspring to almost baseline rates. In addition to these risks, valproate is also said to cause 'fetal valproate syndrome', which comprises minor changes in facial appearance and

skeletal effects such as a high forehead, long digits, long philtrum and small flat nose. To what extent these are simply healthy population variations, or if 'unhealthy' are related to genetic influences or are drug-related, is quite unknown, as is the frequency of these effects. Another issue is the possibility that maternal valproate therapy can result in learning disability and behavioural problems in the offspring, often manifest only in the school years. Evidence on these points is rather weak, and is based on retrospective series with potential for bias and with data that exhibit internal inconsistencies. Nevertheless, these effects may be common and the possibility (even if unproven) will preclude the use of valproate during pregnancy unless there are pressing reasons.

If valproate is to be given during pregnancy, the dose should be reduced (to less than 1000 mg/day), and monotherapy used, wherever possible. A recent study shows that the teratogenic risk of valproate at dose < 100 mg is approximately the same as that of lamotrigine at doses > 200 mg. The daily dose should be divided into three or more administrations per day to avoid high peak plasma levels of VPA (as these may be a mechanism for teratogenic effects) and the controlled-release formulation should be used. It is also possible that administration of folic acid during pregnancy will reduce the risk of spina bifida, and although not formally studied in valproate-treated women, folic acid supplements (1 mg/day) should be given from the onset of pregnancy.

Counselling on all these points is essential in all fertile women contemplating pregnancy; not to do so, is now negligent practice.

### Overdose

Overdose causes coma, convulsions and respiratory depression; cardiac conduction defects, hypotension, and gastrointestinal and multiple metabolic effects can also occur. Profound coma occurs at doses above 200 mg/kg. Death is rare but has been reported. Supportive treatment should be supplemented by gastric lavage and the use of activated charcoal. Haemodialysis and haemoperfusion may be helpful. Naloxone has been reported to reverse coma, and L-carnitine infusions may prevent hepatic damage.

## Antiepileptic effect

Valproate has been the subject of many open and uncontrolled studies, in many types of epilepsy, since its introduction in the 1960s. The standards of monitoring and documentation do not match modern regulatory studies, yet these investigations showed indubitable effectiveness.

### *Partial-onset seizures*

Existing evidence suggests that the drug has similar efficacy to other main-line therapies, although most clinicians use carbamazepine as a first choice, a decision based, mainly, on a large and influential study that compared valproate and carbamazepine in 480 previously untreated adults with partial-onset epilepsy. Both drugs were similarly effective in controlling secondarily generalized seizures, but a greater percentage of patients with partial seizures remained free from seizures on carbamazepine. However, other controlled studies have not found differences between valproate and other drugs. In randomized double-blind monotherapy studies in newly diagnosed patients, for instance, similar efficacy was found when comparing valproate and oxcarbazepine (seizure-free rates of 54% and 57%, respectively, over 1 year in 249 adults) and valproate and lamotrigine (26% on valproate and 29% on lamotrigine free from seizures at 8 months).

The absolute effect of valproate can be estimated from two randomized controlled studies that compared valproate and placebo in uncontrolled partial epilepsy, in one of which a 38% responder rate (at a dose of 1200 mg/day) was found (and in both valproate was significantly more efficacious than placebo), a rate which compares favourably with that of many more modern drugs. Also, a controlled comparison of the effect of low-dose and high-dose valproate (defined by plasma concentrations of 25–50 and 80–150 µg/ml) found 30% and 70% median reductions of complex partial seizures and of tonic–clonic seizures, respectively, in the high-dose group, compared with 19% and 22% in the low-dose (active control) group.

In children, three large open-label studies (with 837 children included) have compared valproate with carbamazepine, phenytoin and phenobarbital, finding no differences in efficacy between the drugs.

### Generalized epilepsy and epilepsy syndromes

Valproate is often considered the drug of first choice for generalized epilepsies, and indeed it shows striking efficacy in a wide range of generalized epileptic disorders: childhood and juvenile absence epilepsy, juvenile myoclonic epilepsy, photosensitive epilepsies, Lennox–Gastaut syndrome, West syndrome and myoclonic epilepsies. However, most data in these indications are based on open-label or retrospective studies. Two randomized double-blind controlled studies have compared valproate with ethosuximide in children with absence epilepsy in a cross-over design. Both drugs had similar effects on absence seizures, but valproate was more effective in controlling convulsive seizures. The effectiveness of the drug in Lennox–Gastaut syndrome has been shown in numerous open studies, and one small controlled investigation. It is said to control seizures in about 10% of cases and reduce attacks by 50% or more in one-third, but this seems optimistic and experience suggests more modest outcomes. In West syndrome, high-dose valproate is sometimes used if steroids and vigabatrin are ineffective or contra-indicated. One series reported a 90% rate of seizure control, but this seems high, and most studies report less good results. In open studies

of juvenile myoclonic epilepsy, around 85% of patients are rendered free from seizures. In one open study of 142 young patients with generalized epilepsy, 50% of whom were having daily seizures prior to therapy, valproate controlled the epilepsy in 63% of all cases overall, and a further 18% showed improvement greater than 50%. Of the 69 patients with 3 Hz spike-wave discharges, 81% became free from seizures, as did 77% of those with myoclonic jerks. VPA also controlled the seizures in 8/32 patients with myoclonic-astatic epilepsy, and 8/32 were improved by more than 50%. VPA is effective in controlling photosensitivity and abolishes it in more than half of the patients. In patients with photosensitive seizures, total seizure control is attained in 84%. Valproate is also a drug of first choice in the progressive myoclonic epilepsies, although it seldom fully controls the myoclonus in these cases. Valproate has been used in neonatal seizures and to prevent febrile seizures, although other drugs are preferable in children under 2 years of age in view of the potential hepatotoxic effects. The use of valproate in status epilepticus is discussed on p. 230.

### Clinical use in epilepsy

Valproate is still one of the most commonly used antiepileptics throughout the world. It is a drug of first choice in all seizure types (absence, myoclonus, tonic–clonic) in idiopathic generalized epilepsy (including juvenile myoclonic epilepsy). It is strikingly more effective than lamotrigine and topiramate in this indication, and probably more useful than the benzodiazepine or barbiturate drugs. Whether levetiracetam can compete with its effectiveness is not yet clear. It is a drug of first choice in the Lennox–Gastaut syndrome, where it controls atypical absence and atonic seizures better than most other first-line drugs. It is also a drug of first choice in the syndromes of myoclonic epilepsy and the progressive myoclonic epilepsies, and for epilepsies with photosensitivity and/or generalized spike wave electrographically. In partial and secondarily generalized epilepsy, carbamazepine is usually tried before valproate, although there is no real evidence that valproate is less effective in new or mild cases.

Valproate is presented in different formulations in different countries, and this can be very confusing. It exists as the sodium, calcium and magnesium salts, as the acid, as sodium hydrogen divalproate or as valpromide. Enteric-coated, immediate and slow-release formulations also exist, as well as syrup, sprinkle, IV forms and a rectal suppository. There are no convincing therapeutic differences between any of these forms, although the enteric-coated form reduces gastrointestinal side-effects, and rates of absorption differ in different formulations. The pharmacokinetics of individual patients vary much more than any difference in formulation, and there is little logic in having so many different manufactured products. In the UK the most popular form of sodium valproate is as 200 and 500 mg enteric-coated tablets, although evidence that this is better tolerated than the conventional sodium valproate is very weak.

The usual starting dose for an adult is 200 mg at night increasing in fortnightly steps by 200 or 500 mg increments to a usual maintenance dose of between 600 and 1500 mg. Doses as high as 3000 mg/day are occasionally given. Twice daily dosing is usual. Valproate has complex interactions, and general rules are difficult to make. However, generally, patients on co-medication require higher doses than those on monotherapy. In children, the usual starting dose is 20 mg/kg/day and the maintenance dose is 40 mg/kg/day, and on combination therapy doses may need to be higher. Although a target serum level range has been suggested by clinical studies, the levels fluctuate widely during a 24-hour period even on three times daily doses, although the antiepileptic effectiveness is not influenced by these fluctuations. The controlled-release formulation lessens this fluctuation, but does not improve seizure control.

Serum level estimations can be made, but there is a poor relationship between level and effect. Moreover, the marked diurnal swings in blood levels on twice or three times daily dosing often render measurements rather meaningless. There is little point in a rigid adherence to the so-called therapeutic range (300–700 μmol/l).

Side-effects remain a problem, and it is because of these that enthusiasm for valproate has waned in recent years. Weight gain is common and often problematic. Other side-effects, such as the neurotoxic effects and effects on hair growth, are also common, but often are only slight and usually are not a reason for drug withdrawal. In female patients, the hints that valproate increases the frequency of polycystic ovaries, causes menstrual irregularities, and reduces fertility are enough for many to avoid its use. Scientific evidence on these points, however, is generally slight, and has tended to come from one (potentially unreliable) source; nevertheless, this and a marketing onslaught from valproate's competitors have reduced its usage, particularly in partial epilepsy. Valproate teratogenicity is a major concern and is a further reason for avoiding valproate in female patients where pregnancy is an issue. Its use in young children, especially those under 2 years of age, carries a small but definite risk of hepatic failure, and where other drugs are available, these tend now to be used. It is contra-indicated in the presence of hepatic or pancreatic disease.

# VIGABATRIN

| | |
|---|---|
| **Primary indications** | Partial and secondarily generalized epilepsy. West syndrome |
| **Licensed for monotherapy/add-on therapy** | Add-on therapy only |
| **Usual preparations** | Tablets: 500 mg; powder sachet: 500 mg |
| **Usual dosage—adults** | 1000–3000 mg/day |
| **Usual dosage—children** | Body weight 10–15 kg: 40 mg/kg/day or 500–1000 mg/day<br>Body weight 15–30 kg: 1000–1500 mg/day<br>Body weight > 30 kg: 1500–3000 mg/day |
| **Dosing intervals** | 2 times/day |
| **Dose commonly affected by co-medication** | No |
| **Dose affected by renal/hepatic disease** | Renal disease |
| **Common drug interactions** | No |
| **Serum level monitoring** | Not useful |
| **Common/important adverse events** | Mood change, depression, psychosis, aggression, confusion, weight gain, insomnia, changes in muscle tone in children, tremor, diplopia, severe visual field constriction |
| **Major mechanism of action** | Inhibition of GABA transaminase activity |
| **Main advantages** | Highly effective antiepileptic drug. Excellent effect in West syndrome |
| **Main disadvantages** | Adverse effect on visual fields and potential for cognitive side-effects |
| **COMMENT** | Because of effects on visual fields, prescribing now restricted to last-resort use in partial epilepsy. However, remains a drug of choice in infantile spasm, especially when due to tuberous sclerosis |

Recognition in the 1970s that γ-aminobutyric acid (GABA) was an important inhibitory neurotransmitter in the central nervous system raised the possibility that boosting GABA action might suppress seizures. This led the worldwide pharmaceutical industry to turn their attention to GABA analogues. The first developed and the most successful was vigabatrin. This was synthesized in 1974 and then trialled in epilepsy, and licensed in Britain in 1989 and subsequently in 65 other European countries and worldwide, but not in the USA. It was the first of a new wave of antiepileptic drugs introduced in the last 15 years. It was marketed as the prime example of a 'designer drug' engineered to produce a specific and rational mechanism of action. It had gained an important role in the treatment of epilepsy, but the recognition of its effects on retinal function have resulted in a dramatic decline in its usage, and it is now considered a drug of last resort.

## Physical and chemical characteristics

Vigabatrin (γ-vinyl-GABA; 4-amino-hex-5-enoic acid; molecular weight 129.16) is a close structural analogue of GABA. The drug is a racemic mixture, but only the S-(+)-enantiomer is biologically active. It is a crystalline substance, highly soluble in water but only slightly soluble in ethanol.

## Mode of action

Vigabatrin is a close structural analogue of GABA and acts on GABA transaminase, the enzyme that metabolizes GABA in the synaptic cleft. Vigabatrin binds irreversibly to the enzyme, and binding results in non-competitive inhibition of the enzyme. Extra-cellular GABA concentrations in brain are thereby greatly elevated. This elevation has been demonstrated in vitro, in animal experimentation, and in human CSF and magnetic resonance spectroscopy studies,

| **Vigabatrin** Pharmacokinetics—average adult values | |
| --- | --- |
| Oral bioavailability | < 100% |
| Time to peak levels | 0.5–2 h |
| Volume of distribution | 0.8 l/kg |
| Biotransformation | None |
| Elimination half-life | 4–7 h |
| Plasma clearance | 0.102–0.114 l/kg/h |
| Protein binding | None |
| Active metabolite | None |

and the extent of GABA elevation is similar in humans and animal models. Enzyme activity only recovers when new enzyme is synthesized, and this occurs over 4–6 days. Vigabatrin is effective in some but not all animal models of epilepsy. The time scale of the effect of local brain injections of vigabatrin mirrors that of the recovery of GABA-transaminase concentrations. Vigabatrin has no other known action.

Vigabatrin has simple pharmacokinetics, which pose few problems. As the drug acts by irreversibly inhibiting the cerebral enzyme GABA transaminase, its effect is dependent on the rate of production of new enzyme rather than on any pharmacokinetic parameters. The biological half-life of the drug—i.e. the time taken for the enzyme concentrations to recover to half their previous level—is several days, even after a single dose.

## Pharmacokinetics
### Absorption and distribution
Absorption is rapid following oral ingestion, with a peak concentration at about 2 hours. The oral bioavailability is at least 60–70%. Food has little effect on the rate or extent of absorption. There is no appreciable protein binding in plasma, and the volume of distribution of the drug is 0.8 l/kg. The drug is distributed widely. The CSF concentration of vigabatrin is about 10% that of the plasma. In neonates and young children, bioavailability and $C_{max}$ of the active (S+) enantiomer are somewhat lower than in adults. Only a small amount of the drug crosses the placenta. The concentration in breast milk compared with plasma is less than 0.5.

### Metabolism and excretion
Vigabatrin is only minimally metabolized by humans (< 5%), and is eliminated primarily by renal excretion. Vigabatrin does not induce the activity of hepatic enzymes.

Elimination is not dose dependent, and the elimination half-life in subjects with healthy renal function is between 4 and 7 hours. The plasma clearance is 0.102–0.114 l/kg/h. Elimination is slower in the elderly. A steady state is attained after stable dosing regimes within 2 days. Sixty per cent of the drug is removed by haemodialysis and so dosage supplementations in these circumstances are needed.

### Drug interactions
Vigabatrin has virtually no pharmacokinetic or pharmaco-dynamic interactions with any other antiepileptic drug, except phenytoin. The addition of vigabatrin can result in a fall on plasma concentration of phenytoin by a mean of 25%, usually within a few weeks of polytherapy. The mechanism of this effect is uncertain, but presumably it is due to impairment of phenytoin absorption as phenytoin protein binding, metabolism and excretion are unchanged. Serum levels of phenobarbital can also be slightly reduced. Vigabatrin has no effect on the metabolism of the oral contraceptive, nor known effects on other non-antiepileptic drugs.

## Adverse effects
During the initial development of the drug, neuropathological studies in rats and dogs showed that vigabatrin caused widespread intramyelinic vacuolization throughout the brain. This could also be demonstrated *in vivo* by magnetic resonance spectroscopy (MRS). Primate studies, human surgical and postmortem pathology, human MRS and human evoked potential studies, however, failed to demonstrate any similar changes. On the basis of the generally reassuring data the drug was licensed, but vigilance still needs to be maintained to assess the possible development of neuropathological changes over more prolonged treatment periods, and there is one report of focal changes on imaging in the splenium of the corpus callosum which reversed on therapy. The drug also affects the retina in some rodent species, but until recently problems in the human retina were not recognized clinically.

### Neurotoxic side-effects
Minor neurotoxic side-effects were noted in about 40% of all patients taking vigabatrin in the clinical trials, and these are listed in Table 3.26. The most troublesome common effects are the tendency of vigabatrin to cause occasionally severe neuropsychiatric adverse events, notably depression, agitation or confusion, and in a few cases psychosis. The psychosis caused by vigabatrin usually has paranoid features and visual hallucinations. In the reported series these psychotic reactions often occured when seizure control had been improved, and some cases at least can be attributed to the process of forced normalization rather than to a direct toxic effect of the drug. Depression can be severe, and

**Table 3.26** Adverse effects due to vigabatrin (% of patients affected); pooled data from 2692 patients from the clinical trials of vigabatrin.

| Adverse event | Frequency |
| --- | --- |
| Drowsiness | 18.6 |
| Fatigue | 15.1 |
| Headache | 12.7 |
| Dizziness | 10.3 |
| Weight gain | 7.9 |
| Agitation | 6.9 |
| Abnormal vision | 5.3 |
| Diplopia | 5.1 |
| Tremor | 5.1 |
| Depression | 5.1 |

occasionally is a threat to life. An increase in body weight of more than 10% is seen in about 10–15% of adults taking long-term vigabatrin therapy, an effect which seems particularly to develop in the first 6 months of therapy, but the mechanism is unknown. Vigabatrin has little if any effect on cognitive function.

### Peripheral visual failure

In 1997—eight years after the licensing of the drug, and 15 years after its introduction into clinical trials—three cases of constriction of the peripheral visual fields were reported. In the following year, other cases were noted, and it has now been established that between 30 and 40% of persons treated with vigabatrin therapy develop this side-effect. Typically, the visual field loss is asymptomatic, although there are a growing number of patients (perhaps 10% of all those taking vigabatrin) who notice deterioration in peripheral vision and on occasion this deterioration has been severe. Visual fields show the pattern of bilateral nasal then concentric constriction (tunnel vision), with central vision preserved (Figure 3.11). Field testing to confrontation in the clinic is usually healthy, and the visual field disturbances are picked up by careful testing by experienced personnel using techniques such as Goldman perimetry and the computerized Humphries testing battery. The mechanism of this effect is likely to be due to GABA inhibition in the retina, which is a structure rich in GABA-C receptors, and GABA levels in the retina have been shown to be greatly raised on treatment with vigabatrin. It is unclear whether this effect is dose related or when is the period of greatest risk, although most people developing field defects do so within 2 years of the initiation of therapy. The field defects are irreversible, and if chronic therapy with

vigabatrin is to be contemplated, baseline field testing should be carried out and repeated initially at 6 monthly and then annually. The patients should be fully counselled about this risk.

### Hypersensitivity and other effects

Acute idiosyncratic immunological adverse events (e.g. rash, hepatic disturbance, marrow dysplasia) are extremely rare, and vigabatrin has proved a safe drug in this regard. One case of fatal hepatotoxicity has been reported, but was probably due to an undetected metabolic disorder rather than vigabatrin. One unusual effect of vigabatrin is to increase levels of α-aminoadipic acid in plasma and urine, and this can mimic α-aminoadipic aciduria, causing diagnostic confusion. Similar confusion can be caused by abnormal urinary amino-acid measurements due to inhibition of β-alanine metabolism.

### Antiepileptic effect
#### Partial-onset seizures

Adults with refractory partial epilepsy were the first target group in clinical trials in the clinical evaluation of vigabatrin. The pivotal European studies were of 479 such patients, in an add-on parallel group design. These demonstrated a 50% or greater response rate in 40–50% of adult patients with refractory partial seizures. Up to 10% of patients in these clinical trials became free from seizures. Essentially similar figures were then shown in similar studies from the USA, with 40–50% response rates at doses of 2–4 g/day. These are evidence of good efficacy, and of the newer drugs only topiramate showed better response rates. In paediatric studies, too, vigabatrin had a good effect against complex partial seizures, with seizure-free rates of between 10 and 40% in some studies.

#### Generalized seizures

However, secondarily generalized seizures are notably less well controlled than partial seizures, and less well than with other first-line antiepileptic drugs, even where the two seizure types co-exist. Vigabatrin has no effect either in primary generalized tonic–clonic seizures, or against absence or myoclonus; indeed these seizure types are frequently worsened by vigabatrin therapy. In placebo-controlled trials in refractory epilepsy, 20% of children and 5% of adults showed an increase in seizures. Absence status can be precipitated by vigabatrin therapy. Anecdotal experience suggests that vigabatrin has little utility in patients with Lennox–Gastaut syndrome, although studies have shown conflicting results.

#### Newly diagnosed epilepsy

A comparative study of monotherapy with vigabatrin or carbamazepine in newly diagnosed patients showed significantly fewer patients becoming seizure free on vigabatrin

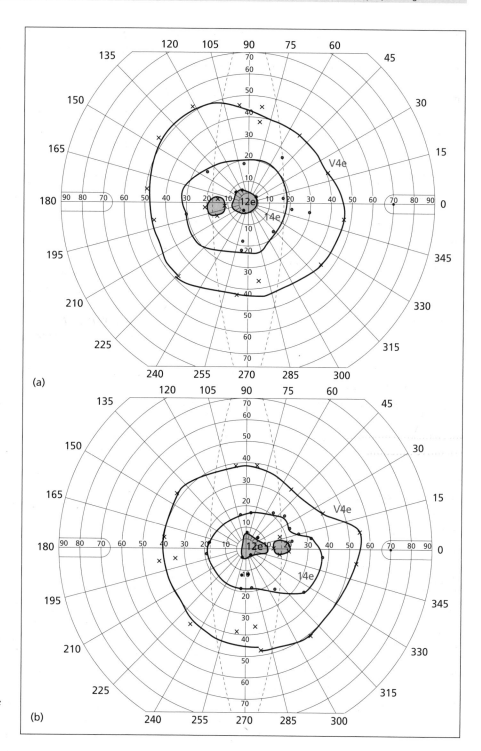

**Figure 3.11** Perimetry showing severe bilateral visual field constriction caused by vigabatrin therapy.

(32%) than with carbamazepine (52%), and this poor result was perhaps partly due to the heterogeneous patient population, which included generalized epilepsies. This evidence suggests that vigabatrin cannot be considered as first-line therapy in newly diagnosed epilepsy.

### Infantile spasm

Vigabatrin is particularly effective in controlling infantile spasms, with the majority of patients experiencing a great reduction in spasms and many becoming free from seizures. Vigabatrin seems to be superior to corticosteroids or ACTH in this indication, and does not have the problematic steroid side-effects. It has become a drug of choice especially for children whose infantile spasm is due to tuberous sclerosis. One study at a dose of 150 mg/kg/day showed complete control of patients randomized to vigabatrin, and complete control in all those who were initially uncontrolled when randomized to hydrocortisone and were then switched to vigabatrin. In a retrospective review of all studies of vigabatrin (at doses between 20 and 400 mg/kg/ day), complete control of spasms was noted in 68%, and 97% of the 28 cases with underlying tuberous sclerosis.

Seizures show a tendency to flare up during too rapid vigabatrin withdrawal, and withdrawal should be slow.

### Clinical use in epilepsy

The usual starting dose for an adult is 250–500 mg once or twice per day, increasing by 250–500 mg incremental steps every 1–2 weeks. The average maintenance dose is between 1 and 2 g/day, although 25% of patients have better control on 3 g than on 2 g. The maximum dose is 4 g. In children, 40 mg/kg/day is the usual starting dose, with maintenance doses of 80–100 mg/kg/day. Lower doses should be used in patients with renal impairment, especially when the creatinine clearance is less than 60 ml/min. When the drug is being withdrawn it is recommended that this be done slowly, with 250 or 500 mg decrements every 2–4 weeks.

As the drug irreversibly inhibits a cerebral enzyme, therapeutic drug monitoring of the serum concentrations is unhelpful. It is possible to measure the activity of the same enzyme in platelets, and to use this as a guide to dosing, but these measurements have not proved useful in clinical practice.

The use of vigabatrin has been severely curtailed by the discovery of its effects on vision (and to some extent its other side-effects). What seemed, only a few years ago, to be a promising drug is now reserved for use in exceptional cases only. Indeed, in view of the ready availability of other drugs for partial epilepsy, the whole future of the drug is in jeopardy. There are several lessons here. The side-effects should have been picked up earlier, 'rational design' of antiepileptic drugs still seems an elusive quest, predictable effects should be actively sought, and licensing procedures are not foolproof.

The drug, however, is effective in partial seizures, and indeed has efficacy unmatched by many other drugs, but is not useful in the generalized seizures, even if of partial onset (in this respect it is similar to gabapentin, but not to lamotrigine, topiramate or levetiracetam). It has a niche position as a drug of first choice for infantile spasm, and it appears (on circumstantial evidence) to be particularly useful where the spasms are due to tuberous sclerosis.

# ZONISAMIDE

| | |
|---|---|
| **Primary indications** | Refractory partial epilepsy and generalized epilepsy (all types). Lennox–Gastaut syndrome. West syndrome. Progressive myoclonic epilepsy. |
| **Licensed for monotherapy/add-on therapy** | Monotherapy and adjunctive therapy in children and adults for a broad range of epilepsy (Japan and Asia); adjunctive therapy for partial epilepsy (+/− 2° generalisation) USA, UK and Europe. |
| **Usual preparations** | Capsules: 25, 50, 1200 mg (USA); Tablets: 100 mg (Japan, Korea); Powder: 20% (Japan, Korea) |
| **Usual dosage—adults** | 200–600 mg/day |
| **Usual dosage—children** | Initial: 2–4 mg/kg/day<br>Maintenance: 4–8 mg/kg/day |
| **Dosing intervals** | 1–2 times/day |
| **Dose commonly affected by co-medication** | Yes |
| **Dose affected by renal/hepatic disease** | Avoid in severe renal disease |
| **Common drug interactions** | Extensive |
| **Serum level monitoring** | Potentially useful |
| **Target range** | 30–140 µmol/l |
| **Common/important adverse events** | Somnolence, ataxia, dizziness, fatigue, nausea, vomiting, irritability, anorexia, impaired concentration, mental slowing, itching, diplopia, insomnia, abdominal pain, depression, skin rashes, hypersensitivity. Significant risk of renal calculi. Weight loss, oligohidrosis and risk of heat stroke |
| **Major mechanism of action** | Inhibition of voltage-gated sodium channel, T-type calcium currents, benzodiazepine GABA-A receptor excitatory glutaminergic transmission, carbonic anhydrase |
| **Main advantages** | Shown to be effective in broad spectrum of epilepsies; also a particular place in Lennox–Gastaut syndrome, infantile spasm and progressive myoclonic epilepsies |
| **Main disadvantages** | Side-effect profile. |
| **COMMENT** | Recently introduced drug in Western countries for adjunctive therapy in partial-onset epilepsy. Experience in Japan suggests a broader spectrum of epilepsy indications |

Zonisamide (ZNS) is a sulphonamide derivative chemically distinct from any of the previously established antiepileptic drugs. Its antiepileptic action was discovered by chance in 1974, and it was approved for use in Japan in 1989 and in the USA in 2003, and is expected to be licensed in Europe in 2005. It was subjected to intensive study in Japan in the 1980s and then a further three pivotal clinical studies were carried out in the USA and Europe, and it is now licensed for monotherapy and adjunctive therapy in a wide spectrum of epilepsies in Japan, but as adjunctive therapy in refractory partial epilepsy only in USA, UK and Europe.

## Chemical and physical properties

Zonisamide (1,2-benzisoxazole-3-methanesulphonamide; molecular weight 212) is a white crystalline powder, slightly soluble in acidic and neutral aqueous solutions, with a $pK_a$ of 10.2. Solubility markedly increases as pH increases.

**Zonisamide**
Pharmacokinetics—average adult values

| | |
|---|---|
| Oral bioavailability | < 100% |
| Time to peak levels | 2–4 h |
| Volume of distribution | 0.9–1.2 l/kg |
| Biotransformation | Acetylation, reduction, glucuronidation (cytochrome P450 enzyme CYP3A4; UDPGT family enzymes) |
| Elimination half-life | 49–69 h |
| Plasma clearance | 0.0089–0.001 l/kg/h |
| Protein binding | 30–60% |
| Active metabolite | None |

## Mode of action

Zonisamide has a number of different properties that contribute to its antiepileptic effect. It reduces conductance at the voltage-gated sodium channel by affecting the kinetics of sodium-channel inactivation, an action similar to that of phenytoin but with different kinetics. It also affects T-type calcium currents, increasing the proportion of channels in the inactivated state. It binds to the benzodiazepine GABA-A, receptor where it has valproate-like actions. It also has effects on excitatory glutaminergic transmission and acetylcholine metabolism, and it inhibits dopamine turnover and carbonic anhydrase activity, but the relevance of these actions to its anticonvulsant action is unclear. It is effective in a wide variety of animal models of epilepsy. In addition to its antiepileptic action, it has marked neuroprotective properties in some experimental models, by its ability to scavenge free radicals and its antioxidant properties.

## Pharmacokinetics
### Absorption and distribution

Zonisamide is rapidly and completely absorbed, and peak concentrations are achieved in 2–6 hours. Bioavailability is close to 100% and not affected by food. The mean volume of distribution is betwen 0.9–1.2 l/kg. The drug is widely distributed in the body, involving active transport systems, and is particularly highly concentrated in erythrocytes. Concentrations in the cerebral cortex are higher than in the midbrain. Protein binding is 30–60%. There is a linear dose to serum level relationship at doses up to 800 mg, but the $C_{max}$ and AUC increase disproportionately at higher doses, perhaps owing to saturation of the binding to red blood cells. It is not known to what extent the drug is excreted in breast milk.

## Metabolism and excretion

Zonisamide is metabolized by acetylation and cleavage of the isoxazole ring followed by conjugation with glucuronic acid by the CYP3A species of the P450 system. The plasma half-life is between 50 and 70 hours. The drug exhibits first-order kinetics at normal doses. Steady state is reached within 7 days, and diurnal variations in the levels are small, with peak–trough differences of only 14–27% at steady-state concentrations. The metabolites are not active and are excreted in the urine. In chronic therapy about 35% of the drug is excreted unchanged. Zonisamide does not induce its own metabolism. Plasma clearance is low, in various studies between 0.0089 and 0.001 l/kg/h in patients who are not receiving enzyme-inducing co-medication. It increases to about 0.015 in co-medicated patients. In renal disease clearance is markedly reduced.

## Drug interactions

Zonisamide does have drug interactions that might be expected to alter dosing requirements in some situations. Adjunctive administration of enzyme-inducing antiepileptic drugs reduced the half-life of zonisamide, in one study, from 52–66 hours to less than 27 hours with phenytoin, 38 hours with carbamazepine, 38 hours with phenobarbital, and 46 hours with valproate. Lamotrigine may inhibit the metabolism of zonisamide.

Conversely, co-medication with zonisamide generally has no effect on concentrations of phenytoin, carbamazepine or valproate. There is no autoinduction.

## Adverse effects
### Neurotoxic and other side-effects

In the pooled data of three double-blind placebo-controlled studies in the USA and Europe, the incidence of adverse drug reactions was 78.1%, compared with 61.3% on placebo. Side-effects which occurred at an incidence greater than 5% in the placebo-controlled studies are listed in Table 3.27. 11.5% of the treated patients and 6.5% of the placebo group discontinued treatment because of side-effects, mainly sedation and effects on behaviour and cognition. Speech and language problems were also recorded, especially after 6–10 weeks of therapy and at doses above 300 mg/day. In the placebo-controlled studies, 2.2% of patients were hospitalized for depression and 2.2% were hospitalized for psychosis. Weight loss is a common side-effect, often welcomed by patients. Pancreatitis has been reported.

### Renal stones and oligohydrosis

A striking difference that has been noted between Japanese studies and the US and European studies is the occurrence of renal stones. In pre-approval studies in Japan, only two patients (0.2%) developed urinary stones, compared with a rate of 2.6% in the early studies in the USA and Europe.

**Table 3.27** Adverse events of zonisamide (%) in double-blind placebo-controlled studies; pooled data: events occurred in more than 5% of patients.

| Adverse event | Placebo ($n = 230$) | Zonisamide ($n = 269$) |
|---|---|---|
| Somnolence | 12.2 | 19.3 |
| Ataxia | 5.7 | 16.7 |
| Anorexia | 6.1 | 15.6 |
| Dizziness | 10.9 | 15.6 |
| Fatigue | 10.4 | 14.1 |
| Nausea and/or vomiting | 11.7 | 11.5 |
| Irritability | 5.2 | 11.5 |
| Diplopia | 4.3 | 8.9 |
| Headache | 8.3 | 8.6 |
| Decreased concentration | 0.9 | 8.2 |
| Insomnia | 3.5 | 7.8 |
| Abdominal pain/discomfort | 1.7 | 7.4 |
| Depression | 3.0 | 7.4 |
| Forgetfulness | 2.2 | 7.1 |
| Rhinitis | 6.1 | 6.7 |
| Confusion | 1.3 | 5.6 |
| Anxiety | 2.6 | 5.6 |
| *All events* | *61.3* | *78.1* |

In another US study, the occurrence of renal stones was assessed by means of renal ultrasound, repeated annually during the study, in 501 patients treated with zonisamide and 85 patients with placebo. Calculi were demonstrated in two out of 85 patients (2.4%) during placebo treatment, and in 17 out of 501 patients (3.4%) treated with ZNS. The reason for the difference is not known. Overall, during the developmental studies of zonisamide, the rate of occurrence of kidney stones was 28.7 per 1000 patient-years of exposure in the first 6 months, 62.6 per 1000 patient-years of exposure between 6 and 12 months, and 24.3 per 1000 patient-years of exposure after 12 months.

Zonisamide had a mild effect on renal function in some clinical studies. A mean 8% elevation of serum creatinine occurred in some studies during the first 4 weeks of therapy, and this returned to baseline values on discontinuation of the drug. It is advised that zonisamide is not used in patients with severe renal failure (gromerular filtration rate below 50 ml/min).

Oligohydrosis (impairment of sweating) is another unusual side-effect of zonisamide. This was identified in 17–25% of cases in two studies in children, but less than 1% in post-marketing surveillance. Zonisamde can be shown to suppress the sweating response to acetylcholine loading in humans. This adverse effect is a particular problem in infants and young children and may predispose to heat stroke.

### Hypersensitivity
Of patients in the controlled trials 2.2% withdrew the drug because of the occurrence of rash, and across all trials the rate of rash is 12 events per 1000 patient-years of treatment. Eighty-five per cent of the rashes occurred within 16 weeks of the initiation of therapy in the US studies.

Two cases of aplastic anaemia and one case of agranulocytosis were reported during the first 11 years post-marketing of zonisamide in Japan. Forty-nine cases of Stevens–Johnson syndrome and toxic epidermal necrolysis were reported in the same period (with seven deaths)—a rate of 46 cases per million patient-years of exposure. All patients were taking other drugs. No cases have been reported in the European or US development programmes.

### Teratogenicity
Zonisamide has demonstrated teratogenic potential in animal studies. Of 25 known human pregnancies in which zonisamide was taken in combination with other anti-epileptics, one infant had anencephaly (with co-medication with phenytoin) and one an atrial septal defect (with co-medication with valproate and phenobarbital). It is classified as a category C teratogen by the FDA.

### Overdose
One patient is reported who took 7400 mg zonisamide. It is thought that her peak levels may have reached 200 µg/ml. She developed coma and respiratory depression. She was treated with supportive measures, fluids and gastric lavage, and recovered.

## Antiepileptic effect
### Double-blind placebo-controlled trials in partial-onset epilepsy
In the three definitive placebo-controlled studies in the USA and Europe, zonisamide (400, 200 or 100 mg/day) was used in 499 patients with refractory partial or generalized epileptic seizures. In these three studies, responder rates (i.e. those showing a reduction in seizures of at least 50%) were 41.8% at 400 mg/day, 29.0% at 200 mg/day, and 28.0% at 100 mg/day (compared with 22.2%, 15.0% and 12.0% on placebo). The median reduction in seizures was 40.5% at 400 mg/day, 27.2% at 200 mg/day, and 29.5% at 100 mg/day (compared with 9.0%, −3.2% and −1.1%

on placebo). In one of the trials, dose effects could be studied; in this trial the median reduction in seizures at 100 mg/day was 24.7% (8.3% on placebo); at 200 mg/day it was 20.4% (4.0% on placebo); and at 400 mg/day it was 40.5% (9% on placebo). All (bar one) of these findings showed significant improvements compared with placebo (at $P < 0.05$).

## Comparative controlled studies with carbamazepine and valproate

A randomized comparison of zonisamide and carbamazepine in 123 patients with refractory partial epilepsy showed mean reductions in seizures of 68.4% on zonisamide compared with 46.6% on carbamazepine (69.7 and 70.2% for tonic–clonic seizures), and responder rates were 81.8 and 70.7%, respectively. These were not significant differences. Zonisamide (mean daily dose of 7.3 mg/kg/day) was compared with valproate (mean daily dose 27.6 mg/kg/day) in 34 children with refractory generalized seizures, with overall improvement rates of 50.0% on zonisamide and 43.8% on valproate.

## Other studies

The responder rates in the 1008 adults and children who had been enrolled in the controlled studies and non-comparative multicentre studies are shown in Table 3.28. Among the partial seizures, responder rates were similar in temporal lobe epilepsy (54%; $n = 428$) and those with extratemporal lobe epilepsy (51%; $n = 224$). Sixty-six per cent (of 41 patients) with idiopathic epilepsy responded, as did 32% of 132 patients with Lennox–Gastaut syndrome and 22% of 9 patients with West syndrome.

## Monotherapy

In the 1008 epileptic patients recruited in studies in Japan, 55 patients were treated with zonisamide monotherapy and there was a responder rate (a reduction in seizures of at least 50%) of 72%. In two later Japanese studies of 38 and 72 children, rates of freedom from seizures of 78% and 79% were recorded, with follow-up in the second study of between 6 and 43 months. The dosages used were 2–8 mg/kg/day.

## Progressive myoclonic epilepsy (PME)

Zonisamide seems to have a specific effect in patients with progressive myoclonic epilepsy. Dramatic improvements in all seizure types (tonic–clonic and myoclonic) were first reported in 1988 and have been repeatedly confirmed. The improvement occurs in patients with Unverricht–Lundborg type and in mitochondrial disease.

## Clinical use in epilepsy

Zonisamide has a chemically distinctive drug with striking effectiveness in a broad range of seizure types and epilepsies

**Table 3.28** Clinical efficacy of zonisamide in 1008 patients from the clinical trials of the drug.

| Seizure type | No. of patients | Responder rate (%) |
|---|---|---|
| *Partial* | | |
| Simple partial | 63 | 57 |
| Simple partial followed by complex partial | 82 | 50 |
| Complex partial | 362 | 50 |
| Partial-onset generalized tonic–clonic | 168 | 60 |
| *Generalized* | | |
| Generalized tonic–clonic | 46 | 59 |
| Generalized tonic | 74 | 26 |
| Atypical absences | 9 | 67 |
| Typical absences | 4 | 50 |
| Atonic | 10 | 50 |
| Myoclonic | 7 | 43 |
| Clonic | 1 | 100 |
| Combination | 129 | 41 |

and notably also in epilepsy syndromes that are otherwise often reisistant to therapy. The effects are maintained and there is no evidence of tachyphylaxis. It may have a particular role in the progressive myoclonic epilepsies, and also has intriguing possibilities as a neuroprotective agent. Because of its long usage, there are now over 2 million patient-years of experience and its side effect profile is well understood. The CNS side-effects can be prominent but can be lessened by starting at a low dose and incrementing the dose at 50–100 mg/week in adults.

Other side-effects are less common, but can be troublesome and include renal stones and oligohydrosis and a risk of hypersensitivity. It is licensed currently in USA, UK and Europe currently only for adjunctive therapy in adults with partial epilepsy (+/– 2° generalisation), but has much wider indications in Asia.

The initial recommended dose is 25 mg bd in adults and 2–4 mg/kg/day in children.

Usual mainten-ance doses are 200–400 mg/day in adults (maximum dose 600 mg/day) and 4–8 mg/kg/day in children (maximum dose 12 mg/kg/day). The drug can be given once or twice a day. The half life is long in monotherapy, but considerably reduced in adjunctive therapy. Serum level monitoring is not usually needed, but it has been suggested that the usual range of therapeutic levels is 30–140 μmol/l.

Because of the risk of hypersensitivity, patients should report to their physicians immediately if a skin rash, fever, sore throat or bruising occurs. Renal function should be monitored, and the drug avoided in severe renal failure.

## OTHER DRUGS USED IN THE TREATMENT OF EPILEPSY

In 1861 Sir Edward Sieveking closed the treatment chapter in his book on epilepsy with the words 'there is scarcely a substance in the world capable of passing through the gullet of man that has not at one time or other enjoyed the reputation of being an antiepileptic'. Things have changed, but still unsubstantiated claims are made about numerous medicinal and non-medicinal products, with varying degrees of hope or cynicism. Among prescribed medicines there are a number whose claims are based on highly unsatisfactory open studies, often in small numbers of patients and for short periods of time. Some of these are listed in Table 3.29, and some are still occasionally encountered in clinical practice. Some carry significant risks of severe side-effects and in others the evidence of any antiepileptic efficacy is extremely slight; this is therapeutic nihilism familiar to Sieveking. There are also many different herbal remedies for epilepsy, at least 30 of which have some evidence of antiepileptic effect in animal models, but most of which have not led to pharmaceutical development.

There are, however, other drugs for which utility has been proven, and these are considered further here.

### Acetazolamide

Acetazolamide, 2-acetylamido-1,3,4-thiadiazole-5 sulphonamide, is a sulphonamide derivative ($C_4H_6N_4O_3S_2$) (Table 3.30). It is a carbonic anhydrase inhibitor and this is probably the mechanism of its antiepileptic action. It has a clear effect in animal models of epilepsy, and its antiepileptic action was first reported in humans in the 1950s. The drug has had a place in therapy ever since.

**Table 3.29** Prescription drugs licensed for other indications that have also been reported to have been used as antiepileptics.

| |
| --- |
| Allopurinol |
| Calcium channel blockers (diltiazem, nimodipine, nifedipine, verapamil) |
| Carbenoxolone |
| Furosemide (and other diuretics) |
| Mannitol |
| Propranolol and other beta-blockers |
| Quinidine |
| Vitamin E |

### Pharmacokinetics

Acetazolamide is a weak acid with a pKa of 7.4. The drug is absorbed largely in the duodenum and upper jejunum. The oral bioavailablity is more than 90% in the dose range used in epilepsy. The peak plasma concentrations (10–18 µg/ml) are reached 1–3 hours after oral ingestion of a single 250-mg dose. It is concentrated in erythrocytes (like zonisamide). Acetazolamide is 90–95% bound to plasma proteins. The drug diffuses into tissue water and binds strongly in an enzyme complex to carbonic anhydrase. The plasma half-life of freely available acetazolamide is about 2 hours, although most of the drug is in the form of an enzyme complex which has a half-life of 10–12 hours. The volume of distribution of acetazolamide is 1.8 l/kg, and the drug is preferentially concentrated in erythrocytes and other tissues where carbonic anhydrase concentrations are high— in the brain, for instance, to glia. The concentration in brain is rather lower than in other tissues owing to an active transport system of the drug out of brain. The drug is not metabolized. Twenty per cent of the elimination is by glomerular filtration and 80% by renal tubular excretion. The whole of a single oral dose of acetazolamide is recovered in the urine in 24 hours. Less than 0.7% of the dose per kilogram of body weight of the mother is transferred in breast milk, and breast-feeding therefore is likely to be harmless. There are no significant drug interactions, except at the level of protein binding.

### Side-effects

#### Idiosyncratic reaction

Like any sulphonamide drug, acetazolamide can cause acute hypersensitivity. Stevens–Johnson syndrome, aplastic anaemia, agranulocytosis, acute thrombocytopenia, and acute renal failure can occur. These are rare, but patients should be warned about the risk.

#### Common side-effects

Mild side-effects are common (recorded in 10–30% of most series). In one study, 11% of 277 patients reported the following side-effects in descending order of frequency: drow-siness, anorexia, irritability, nausea, vomiting, enuresis, headache, thirst, dizziness and hyperventilation. Other effects that are commonly recorded include paraesthesia of the hands and feet, diarrhoea, loss of libido, diuresis and transient distortion of healthy taste sensations. A metabolic acidosis can be induced by acetazolamide, owing to inhibition of carbonic anhydrase activity in the proximal renal tubules. In 44 of 92 (48%) patients treated with acetazolamide for chronic glaucoma, malaise, fatigue, weight loss, depression, anorexia and loss of libido were common and attributed to acidosis. Treatment with sodium bicarbonate 56–70 mmol/day orally may alleviate some of these effects.

**Table 3.30** Acetazolamide—summary table.

| | |
|---|---|
| **Primary indications** | All seizure types. Catamenial epilepsy |
| **Licensed for monotherapy/add-on therapy** | Both |
| **Usual preparations** | Tablets: 250 mg |
| **Usual dosage—adults** | Initial: 250 mg/day<br>Maintenance: 250–750 mg/day |
| **Usual dosage—children** | Initial: 10 mg/kg/day<br>Maintenance: 30 mg/kg/day |
| **Dosing intervals** | Once or twice daily |
| **Dose commonly affected by co-medication** | No |
| **Dose affected by renal/hepatic disease** | Contra-indicated in renal and hepatic disease |
| **Common drug interactions** | None |
| **Common/important adverse events** | Severe hypersensitivity reactions, renal stones, acidosis, drowsiness, anorexia, irritability, nausea and vomiting, enuresis, headache, thirst, dizziness, hyperventilation |
| **Major mechanism of action** | Carbonic anhydrase inhibition |
| **Main advantages** | Powerful broad-spectrum action |
| **Main disadvantages** | Tolerance to the antiepileptic effects very common; hypersensitivity reactions; renal stones; acidosis; other side-effects |
| **Pharmacokinetics** (average adult values) | |
|    Oral bioavailability | > 90% |
|    Time to peak levels | 1–3 h |
|    Volume of distribution | 1.8 l/kg |
|    Biotransformation | None |
|    Elimination half-life | 10–12 h |
|    Protein binding | 90–95% |
|    Active metabolite | None |
| **COMMENT** | Useful adjunctive therapy in severe epilepsy. Also used in catamenial epilepsy |

### Renal calculi

Renal calculi can be caused by acetazolamide, owing to renal tubular acidosis with resultant hypercalciuria and hypocitraturia. The frequency of stone formation has varied between studies from 0 to 43%. Citrate supplementation and hydration may be effective in reducing stone formation.

### Teratogenicity

There are no adequate studies in pregnancy and the risk of malformations has not been established. However, animal experimentation has demonstrated a teratogenic potential, and there are at least two human case reports of major malformations.

### Antiepleptic effect

Acetazolamide has a very broad spectrum of activity. It is effective in most forms of generalized seizures and also partial and secondarily generalized seizures, and this has been confirmed in a variety of open case series. There is one double-blind placebo-controlled study of 14 children with refractory post-traumatic seizures, and this showed initial therapy with acetazolamide to be superior to placebo, and comparable to phenytoin. Eight of the 14 patients (57%) had a seizure reduction of at least 75%.

The drug will have an initial effect in almost all patients. However, there is an almost universal tendency for the effects of therapy to diminish over time, and this has been demonstrated in all seizures types. In idiopathic generalized epilepsy, for instance, on initial therapy, tonic–clonic seizures are controlled in about 50–70% of cases, myoclonic seizures in about 20–40% of cases, and absence seizures in nearly all cases. However, in one study the control of absence seizures fell from over 90% of cases initially to only 7% at 3 years of therapy. Similarly, about 30% of patients with complex partial seizures became seizure free within the first 3 months of therapy, but the proportion fell to about 10% at 1 and 2 years.

Because of this tendency for tolerance to develop, the drug is often given intermittently, notably in catamenial epilepsy. It is usually given at dosages of 250–750 mg/day for 5–7 days prior to the onset of the menstrual period and for its duration. There are a variety of case reports recommending its use in this way, although my own clinical experience is less positive, and most women with catamenial exacerbations of seizures seem to derive little benefit from the drug. Clobazam used in this way is probably more efficacious.

In one retrospective study, the drug was given as adjunctive therapy continuously in 55% and intermittently in 45% of subjects. A 59% decrease in the frequency of seizures was reported by 40% (both of focal and generalized seizures), and there was no difference in effectiveness between continuous and intermittent regimens. Loss of efficacy was reported by 15% of patients over 6–24 months.

### Clinical use in epilepsy

Acetazolamide is an interesting broad-spectrum antiepileptic drug. It has a place in modern therapy, and is probably generally under-employed. Indeed, it can have a spectacular effect (although more often it is ineffective) and is worth a trial in any patient with severe epilepsy in whom other more conventional therapies have failed. It is usually given as adjunctive therapy, and has the advantage of not interacting with other antiepileptic drugs. The recommended dose in children is between 10 and 30 mg/kg, and in adults 250–750 mg/day, given twice daily. The usually quoted plasma levels are 10–14 µg/ml. The antiepileptic effect is immediate, and so it can be quickly evaluated.

The major drawback of the drug is the frequent development of tolerance, which can occur weeks or months after initiating therapy, and this limits its usefulness. Once tolerance has developed the drug should be withdrawn. Its restitution after a period of 'drug holiday' sometimes restores its effect, and cyclical regimens may also reduce the development of tolerance. Acetazolamide is often used as adjunctive therapy in catamenial epilepsy for this reason.

The drug is generally simple and easy to use and well tolerated. However, because of the risk of acute and severe hypersensitivity (a risk shared with all sulphonamide drugs), a blood count should be obtained before initiating treatment and patients should be warned of this risk. The

drug should be avoided in renal failure, and also in hepatic failure, because alkalinization of the urine diverts ammonia of renal origin from urine into the systemic circulation, causing hepatic encephalopathy. It increases potassium loss and should not be used in Addison disease or adrenal insufficiency. It should be used cautiously in combination with carbamazepine and oxcarbazepine because of its tendency to cause hyponatraemia, and should not be given with topiramate or zonisamide because of the risk of renal calculi.

## Benzodiazepines

The benzodiazepines are widely used as antiepileptic drugs, as well as for anxiolytic, hypnotic and antispastic indications. The main role in epilepsy for diazepam, lorazepam and midazolam is as acute therapy for status epilepticus, acute seizures and in febrile convulsions, and this is covered on pp. 211–13, 218–21. In chronic epilepsy, in addition to clobazam (pp. 123–6) and clonazepam (pp. 127–9), three other benzodiazepines—diazepam, clorazepate and nitrazepam—still have a minor role.

The benzodiazepines all bind to the GABA-A receptors and exert their antiepileptic action by enhancing inhibitory neurotransmission. Differences between the drugs relate to their differential binding at the receptor and their pharmacokinetic properties. The similarities between the drugs are greater than the differences (Figure 3.12).

### Diazepam

Diazepam was the first benzodiazepine to be used in epilepsy. It is highly lipophilic, allowing rapid entry into the brain, but this high lipid solubility also results in rapid subsequent redistribution into peripheral tissues. It is 90–99% bound to plasma proteins. The volume of distribution for the free component of diazepam (i.e. the active, unbound fraction) is 1.1 l/kg. The initial half-life is 1 hour. Enterohepatic circulation result in a second peak in blood levels 6–8 hours after ingestion. Diazepam undergoes demethylation to desmethyldiazepam (DMD; nordiazepam), a metabolite with anticonvulsant activity and a long half-life (> 20 hours), and then slow hydroxylation to oxazepam, which is also active. Both metabolites are conjugated with glucuronic acid in the liver, with an elimination half-life of 24–48 hours. Diazepam induces cytochrome P450 CYP2B, and enhances the metabolism of phenobarbital and phenytoin. Valproate displaces diazepam bound to plasma proteins, leading to increased free diazepam levels.

Drowsiness, fatigue, amnesia, mental slowing, depression, sleep disturbances and ataxia are common side-effects in chronic therapy. Less common are dizziness, weakness, headache, agitation or restlessness, aggression, and mood and personality changes. Occasionally hallucinations and delirium occur. Hypersensitivity includes neutropenia or thrombocytopenia, nephritis, skin reactions and anaphy-

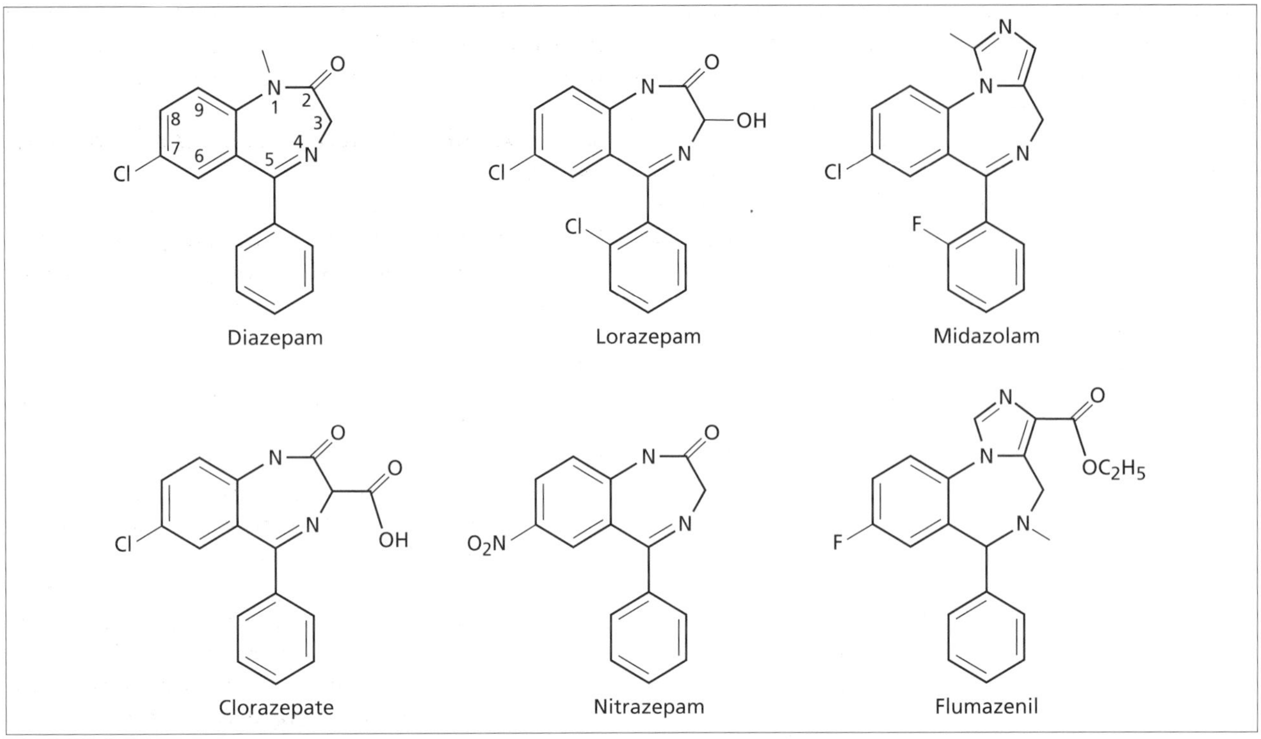

**Figure 3.12** Chemical structures of some benzodiazepine drugs used in epilepsy.

laxis. There is significant potential for abuse and dependency. The teratogenicity of diazepam has not been clearly quantified, but a 'fetal syndrome' and major malformations have been described.

Diazepam is given occasionally as a long-term antiepileptic, especially in the presence of anxiety. It is used largely as adjunctive therapy in severe partial and generalized epilepsy, and also in the Lennox–Gastaut syndrome. The dose is between 5 and 20 mg/day, and its use is limited by the sedative side-effects, the risk of dependency, and the marked potential for tolerance.

### Clorazepate

Clorazepate is a benzodiazepine used in adjunctive treatment of seizure disorders, anxiety and alcohol withdrawal. It is a prodrug which is rapidly converted to nordiazepam, the major active metabolite produced by diazepam. Ninety per cent of clorazepate is converted in the stomach to nordiazepam in less than 10 minutes. Clorazepate is 100% bioavailable by the intramuscular route, and conversion to nordiazepam occurs more slowly in the blood. Clorazepate and nordiazepam are 97–98% protein bound. The time to peak concentration is 0.7–1.5 hours. The volume of distribution ranges from 0.9 to 1.5 l/kg, and is greater in the elderly and in obese subjects. The elimination half-life of clorazepate is 2.3 hours, but the half-life of nordiazepam is about 46 hours, longer in the elderly and neonates. Nordiazepam is excreted predominantly by the kidneys (62–67%) with

renal clearance of 0.15–0.27 ml/min/kg. Plasma DMD levels of 0.5–1.9 μg/ml may represent the therapeutic range.

The side-effects of clorazepate are similar to those of diazepam. Hepatotoxicity and transient skin rashes have also been reported. Clorazepate has teratogenic potential (and FDA category D status) and has been associated with major and minor malformations.

Open and blinded studies have been performed, and one double-blind, add-on study found no difference in control of seizures between clorazepate and phenobarbital or phenytoin.

Its use is restricted to add-on therapy in refractory partial and generalized epilepsy. The recommended initial dose of clorazepate for the adjunctive treatment of epilepsy is 7.5 mg three times daily, with slow increases as required, to a maximal daily dose of 90 mg in twice or three times a day regimens.

### Nitrazepam

Nitrazepam is a benzodiazepine derivative with a nitro group at the 7 position of the benzodiazepine ring.

Oral bioavailability is about 78%. Peak concentrations are reached in about 1.5 hours. Nitrazepam is 85–88% protein bound. The volume of distribution is 2.4 l/kg, and is higher in the elderly. The plasma half-life is about 27 hours, but the drug is rapidly taken up into the CSF and brain tissue and the CSF elimination half-life is 68 hours. Nitrazepam is metabolized in the liver by nitro-reduction to the inactive aromatic amine (7-aminonitrazepam), followed by acetylation to 7-acetoamidonitrazepam. Excretion occurs in both urine (45–65%) and faeces (14–20%), with the remainder bound in tissues for prolonged periods.

Like most benzodiazepines, nitrazepam can produce sedation, disorientation, sleep disturbance, nightmares, confusion, drowsiness and ataxia. Hypotonia, weakness, hypersalivation, drooling, and impaired swallowing and aspiration seem to particularly common with nitrazepam, particularly in young children. Confusion and pseudo-dementia can occur in the elderly. Withdrawal symptoms include delirium, mood and behavioural change, insomnia, involuntary movements, paraesthesia and confusion. The tolerability profile of many other AEDs differs in children compared with adults. There is a risk of sudden death in young children due to nitrazepam therapy, probably because of pharyngeal hypotonia in children given nitrazepam doses over 0.7 mg/kg. In a retrospective analysis of 302 patients treated for periods ranging from 3 days to 10 years, 21 patients died, 14 of whom were taking nitrazepam at the time of death. In patients younger than 3.4 years, the death rate was 3.98 per 100 patient-years, compared with 0.26 deaths per 100 patient-years in patients not taking nitrazepam. Conversely, nitrazepam had a slight protective effect (death rate of 0.50 vs 0.86) in children older than 3.4 years. Nitrazepam is in FDA pregnancy category C (teratogenic effects demonstrated in animals but no studies in humans).

Nitrazepam has been used mainly in West syndrome, febrile seizures, Lennox–Gastaut syndrome and myoclonic epilepsy, and as adjunctive therapy for refractory epilepsy, particularly in children. Its main residual use is in refractory childhood epilepsy. One study showed a reduction in average daily seizure number from 17.7 to 7.2 in 36 infants and children (aged 3 months to 12 years) when nitrazepam was added to existing therapy. Myoclonic seizures particularly improved. In another study, of 31 children with learning disability aged between 2 months and 15 years, complete control of seizures was obtained in seven patients and moderate control in 10. In West syndrome, a study of 52 patients (aged 1–24 months) demonstrated similar efficacy when nitrazepam (0.2–0.4 mg/kg/day in two divided doses) and adrenocorticotropic hormone (ACTH, 40 IU intramuscularly daily) were compared. Both regimens resulted in a reduction in seizure frequency of 75–100% in 50–60% of patients.

The usual initial dose is 1–6 mg/day, and the maintenance dose is usually 0.25–10 mg/day in children. Optimal seizure control has been related to a mean plasma concentration of 114 ng/ml. Occasionally, very high maintenance doses have been used (up to 60 mg/day). There was also a common practice among paediatricians of using very small doses (1.25–5 mg a day), sometimes on alternate days—a practice which seems to have no published evidential support. In view of the alarming suggestion of increased mortality rates, nitrazepam should be used with extreme caution, if at all, in children younger than 4 years.

## Corticosteroids and adrenocorticotropic hormone (ACTH)

Since the 1950s ACTH and corticosteroids have been used to treat a variety of seizure types and epileptic syndromes. Although these compounds have clear antiepileptic action, the mechanisms of the effects are quite unclear.

### Adverse effects

Steroids (including ACTH) produce important and serious side-effects that severely limit their usefulness, particularly as long-term therapy. Most children will develop cushingoid features and behavioural changes, especially irritability. Hypertension develops in 4–33% of children with infantile spasms, and infections—including pneumonia, septicaemia, urinary tract infections, gastroenteritis, ear infections, candidiasis and encephalitis—are commoner. Hypokalaemia may sometimes occur in patients receiving higher doses and longer durations of hormonal therapy. Myocardial hypertrophy develops in 72–90%, but this reverses within months after discontinuation of ACTH therapy.

### Clinical use in epilepsy

Steroids are used mainly for the treatment of West syndrome. Where formal comparisons have been made, ACTH and corticosteroids seem to be of equal efficacy, although many paediatricians still opt for ACTH. ACTH has an-all-or-nothing effect in infantile spasms, and monitoring is therefore relatively straightforward. In about 70–75% of children the spasms are controlled. The following regimen is recommended: $150\ IU/m^2/day$ in two divided doses for 1 week, followed by $75\ IU/m^2/day$ in a single dose for another week, and then this same dose only on alternate days for 2 weeks. Four weeks after starting treatment the alternate-day dose of ACTH is gradually reduced over 8 or 9 weeks, until discontinued.

ACTH has also been reported to be effective in patients with intractable seizures and particularly convulsive status epilepticus and epilepsia partialis continua (EPC). The drug is also used to control seizures in Rasmussen encephalitis, although evidence of benefit is slight.

## Felbamate

Felbamate (2-phenyl-1,3-propanediol dicarbamate), was synthesized by in 1954, investigated in the Antiepileptic Drug Development Program of the National Institutes of Health, and licensed for use in the USA in 1993 (Table 3.31). Within a year, reports of aplastic anaemia and hepatic failure emerged and the drug was withdrawn. However, because of its effectiveness, it remains available, with special

**Table 3.31** Felbamate—summary table.

| | |
|---|---|
| **Primary indications** | Refractory partial and secondarily generalized epilepsy. Lennox–Gastaut syndrome |
| **Licensed for monotherapy/add-on therapy** | Both |
| **Usual preparations** | Tablets: 400, 600 mg; syrup: 600 mg/5 ml |
| **Usual dosage—adults** | Initial: 1200 mg/day<br>Maintenance: 1200–3600 mg/day |
| **Usual dosage—children** | Initial: 15 mg/kg/day<br>Maintenance: 45–80 mg/kg/day |
| **Dosing intervals** | 3–4 times/day |
| **Dose commonly affected by co-medication** | Yes |
| **Dose affected by renal/hepatic disease** | Dose reductions in renal disease. Avoid in hepatic disease |
| **Common drug interactions** | Extensive |
| **Serum level monitoring** | Potentially useful |
| **Target range** | 30–100 mg/l |
| **Common/important adverse events** | Severe hepatic disturbance and aplastic anaemia, insomnia, weight loss, gastrointestinal symptoms, fatigue, dizziness, lethargy, behavioural change, ataxia, visual disturbance, mood change, psychotic reaction, rash, neurological symptoms |
| **Major mechanism of action** | Inhibition of NMDA receptor (glycine recognition site) and sodium-channel conductance |
| **Main advantages** | Powerful broad-spectrum action |
| **Main disadvantages** | Severe hepatic and aplastic anaemia in occasional patients |
| **Pharmacokinetics** (average adult values) | |
|    Oral bioavailability | < 100% |
|    Time to peak levels | 1–4 h |
|    Volume of distribution | 0.75 l/kg |
|    Biotransformation | Hepatic hydroxylation and conjunction (cytochrome P450 system; UDPGT family enzymes) |
|    Elimination half-life | 20 h |
|    Plasma clearance | 0.027–0.032 l/kg/h |
|    Protein binding | 20–25% |
|    Active metabolite | None |
| **COMMENT** | Used only by specialists as last-resort therapy |

precautions for specialist use, in the USA, Britain and many other countries.

## Mode of action

Felbamate blocks the N-methyl-D-aspartate (NMDA) receptor, and also modulates sodium channel conductance. It has no major effect on the GABA-A receptor. It is active in a wide variety of seizure models, and in addition to its antiepileptic action, felbamate seems to possess neuro-protective action.

## Absorption and distribution

Felbamate is rapidly and almost completely absorbed after oral administration, the time to peak plasma concentration being 1–4 hours. It is distributed rapidly and widely to many tissues, including the brain. Twenty to 25% of the total concentration is bound, primarily to serum albumin.

## Biotransformation and excretion

Felbamate is extensively metabolized in the liver via hydroxylation and conjugation. A number of potentially pharmacoactive and toxic metabolites may be formed, including 2-phenylpropenal, an $\alpha,\beta$-unsaturated aldehyde (atropaldehyde). The latter compound is suspected to be largely responsible for hepatic failure and bone marrow suppression. Forty to 49% of the drug is excreted unchanged in the urine. The half-life of felbamate is approximately 20 hours (range, 13–23 hours) in monotherapy and shortened to 13–14 hours (range, 11–20 hours) in co-medication with enzyme-inducing drugs. In renal failure lower doses are required. In children, clearance is faster, and higher doses are needed.

## Drug interactions

Felbamate is both an inhibitor of some drugs and an inducer of others. Phenytoin metabolism is inhibited by felbamate, and phenytoin dose decreases of about 20% were needed in the add-on felbamate study to maintain stable phenytoin concentrations. Conversely, carbamazepine concentrations are lowered by felbamate, and CBZ-epoxide concentrations elevated by up to 30%. Valproate levels are increased by felbamate by 20–30%. Felbamate metabolism is also affected by co-medication; the half-life of felbamate is shortened by about 30% on co-medication with phenytoin or carbamazepine, and can be doubled on co-medication with valproate. There are few other formal studies, but any substance metabolized via the cytochrome P450 system is likely to be affected.

## Adverse effects

### Neurotoxic and other effects

In the clinical trials felbamate was found to be well tolerated, a fact that figured prominently in its advertisements, ironically in view of subsequent developments. The most common side-effects of felbamate as monotherapy were anorexia, vomiting, insomnia, nausea and headache. One case of

urolithiasis has been reported and one case of crystalluria and renal failure. Toxic epidermal necrolysis after initiation of felbamate has also been reported.

### Marrow aplasia

Scattered case reports of marrow aplasia began to occur within 12 months of the launch of the drug. The incidence has subsequently been calculated to be approximately 127 per million patients (in a range lying between 27 and 209) compared with a general population risk of about 2 per million. In the cases studied, a prior history of antiepileptic drug allergy or toxicity, especially rash, was observed in 52%, a history of prior cytopenia in 42%, and evidence of immune disease, especially lupus erythematosus, in 33%. If two of the above three factors were present, the patient's relative risk for aplastic anaemia quadrupled. Aplastic anaemia developed after 23 to 339 days (mean 173 days), and no cases have occurred in persons treated for more than 1 year.

### Hepatic failure

Hepatic failure was also recorded within a year of the drug being licensed, and in total 18 cases have been reported, with a clear relationship to felbamate therapy in seven. The overall risk has been estimated to be 1 per 18,500–25,000 drug exposures, using seven cases as the numerator, or one case per 9,000–12,000 if one assumes all 18 cases were related to felbamate therapy. This compares to hepatic-related fatality estimates of one case in 10,000–49,000 in patients treated with valproate. Although the overall risk is similar to that of valproate, felbamate cases occurred largely in adults.

## Antiepileptic effect

Various randomized controlled blinded and open studies have been undertaken, in adults and in children, and in polytherapy and monotherapy. In all, felbamate was shown to be highly efficacious. It has demonstrated effectiveness in partial and secondarily generalized epilepsy, in primary generalized tonic–clonic and absence seizures, and in the various seizure types in the Lennox–Gastaut syndrome. In a double-blind study in the Lennox–Gastaut syndrome, a 34% decrease in the frequency of atonic seizures ($P = 0.01$) and a 19% decrease in the frequency of all seizures were observed.

## Clinical use in epilepsy

Following the catastrophe of cases exhibiting hypersensitivity, 1 year after licensing, felbamate was close to being withdrawn. However, it is now recognized that the drug still has a place in therapy, in view of its outstanding efficacy. It should be used only by experienced specialists, and after full counselling. Its use is confined to therapy in patients with severe epilepsy, unresponsive to other more conventional antiepileptics. A full haematological evaluation is needed before initiation of felbamate therapy, and blood counts should be monitored frequently during therapy. Liver function tests are recommended every 4 weeks. Patients should be warned to report any symptom such as lethargy, nausea and vomiting, flu-like symptoms, easy bruising and unusual bleeding, and haematological and biochemical parameters should immediately be checked. There is no definite 'therapeutic range', but concentrations between 40 and 100 µg/ml are commonly found in persons responding favourably.

In adults therapy should be initiated at 1200 mg/day in three divided doses, with increases to 2400 or 3600 mg/day in weekly or bi-weekly increments of 600 or 1200 mg steps, as tolerated, as outpatients. Some patients have tolerated doses as high as 7200 mg/day as monotherapy. In children, recommended starting doses have been 15 mg/kg/day with weekly incremental increases to 45–80 mg/kg/day. Blood levels of concomitant therapy need to be monitored, and doses of felbamate and concomitant therapy may need modification in polytherapy. Monotherapy should be a goal. Felbamate is available as 600 mg tablets and a suspension containing 600 mg/5 ml.

## Mesuximide

Mesuximide is an *N*,2-dimethyl-2-phenyl-succinimide, chemically related to ethosuximide, but with a phenyl substituent similar to that of phenytoin.

Mesuximide is indicated for the treatment of absence seizures when conventional treatment has failed, and is, unlike ethosuximide, also indicated as adjunctive therapy for complex partial seizures. The mechanism of action of mesuximide is unknown. It has been shown to be effective against pentylenetetrazol-induced seizures and against maximal electroshock seizures, but less so than ethosuximide.

### Pharmacokinetics

Mesuximide is rapidly absorbed after oral administration and thereafter undergoes rapid and complete demethylation to *N*-desmethylmesuximide (NDMSM). This compound is pharmacologically active and is assumed to be primarily responsible for the anticonvulsant effect of mesuximide. During chronic treatment, NDMSM plasma levels are about 700 times that of mesuximide. *N*-desmethylmesuximide is slowly metabolized, with an apparent half-life of 34–80 hours. The therapeutic plasma level of mesuximide has been proposed to be between 10 and 40 µg/ml. In one clinical trial the optimal effect was obtained with plasma levels of 20–24 µg/ml.

The recommended starting dose of mesuximide is 150 mg/day with a gradual increase of the dose up to a maximal daily dose of 1200 mg. Studies have reported that the addition of mesuximide as concomitant therapy significantly increases the plasma level of phenytoin by 43.4%, and of phenobarbital derived from primidone by 17%, whereas carbamazepine levels are decreased by a mean of 23.2%. In one study, plasma phenobarbital levels increased by 40% and those of phenytoin by 78%.

### Adverse effects

The incidence of side-effects is similar to that of ethosuximide, but the side-effects are more severe and persistent. The most commonly reported side-effects are drowsiness, lethargy, gastrointestinal disturbances, hiccups, irritability and headache. In one study two of 26 patients experienced psychic changes including depression, weepiness and impulsive behaviour.

### Indications and efficacy

The efficacy of mesuximide in the treatment of absence seizures has not been systematically studied and no studies seem to have compared the drug with ethosuximide. Ten of 16 patients with absences in one study became free from seizures and there was a reduction of 75% in seizures in another five. Of four patients with juvenile myoclonic epilepsy, two became free from seizures and in two there was a reduction in seizures of more than 75%. Only 20% of patients with absence seizures had a 50% or greater reduction in seizure frequency when mesuximide was used in previously untreated patients, and no patients achieved complete seizure control.

Unlike ethosuximide, mesuximide is also effective against complex partial and secondarily generalized seizures. In a study of previously untreated complex partial seizures, 27% of patients achieved a 50% or greater reduction and 18% became completely seizure-free. When mesuximide was used as an adjunctive drug for refractory complex partial seizures, 71% of the patients had 90–100% seizure control. More than 50% of the patients complained of adverse effects, particularly somnolence and lethargy. Only 30% of patients with refractory complex partial seizures had a 50% seizure reduction following addition of mesuximide, and only five of eight patients continued a 50% seizure reduction after 3–34 months of follow-up. This study controlled for alterations of plasma levels of concomitant drugs, which were reduced when plasma concentrations increased by more than 10%. Mesuximide is rarely used today, as less toxic drugs are available. Nevertheless, it is a powerful antiepileptic with a wide spectrum of action, and still has a place as adjunctive therapy in the occasional patient.

## Piracetam

Piracetam is a drug with an unusual clinical history (Table 3.32). It was developed in 1967 by the research laboratory of UCB-Pharma in Belgium and deployed in clinical practice as a 'memory enhancing drug'. Its efficacy in this role has been highly contentious and the drug has not been licensed for this indication, either in the USA or the UK, although it is widely used in other, particularly developing countries (the manufacturers report over a million prescriptions). Recent controlled trials do show a small but definite effect in improving memory. In 1978 its anti-

**Table 3.32** Piracetam—summary table.

| | |
|---|---|
| **Primary indications** | Myoclonus, especially in progressive myoclonic epilepsies |
| **Licensed for monotherapy/add-on therapy** | Both |
| **Usual preparations** | Tablets or capsules: 400, 800, 1200 mg; solution: 20, 33% |
| **Usual dosage—adults** | Initial: 7.2 g/day<br>Maintenance: up to 32 g/day |
| **Dosing intervals** | 2–3 times/day |
| **Dose commonly affected by co-medication** | No |
| **Dose affected by renal/hepatic disease** | Severe renal disease |
| **Common drug interactions** | None |
| **Serum level monitoring** | Not useful |
| **Common/important adverse events** | Dizziness, insomnia, nausea, gastrointestinal discomfort, hyperkinesis, weight gain, tremulousness, agitation, drowsiness, rash |
| **Major mechanism of action** | Not known |
| **Main advantages** | Well-tolerated and highly effective in some resistant cases |
| **Main disadvantages** | Not effective in many cases |
| **Pharmacokinetics** (average adult values) | |
| Oral bioavailability | < 100% |
| Time to peak levels | 30–40 min |
| Volume of distribution | 0.6 l/kg |
| Biotransformation | None |
| Elimination half-life | 5–6 h |
| Protein binding | None |
| Active metabolite | None |

myoclonic effect was first noted in a case of post-anoxic myoclonus after cardiac arrest, where it was being given as a neuroprotective agent. In the last 10 years or so the remarkable effectiveness of this drug in cortical myoclonus of various aetiologies has been confirmed by controlled trial. It has received a licence in the UK and elsewhere for its use in this indication. Interestingly, levetiracetam (see p. 142), which is closely related to the laevo-isomer of piracetam, has a more marked and broad-spectrum antiepileptic action and antimyoclonic effects.

### Physical and chemical properties and mode of action

Piracetam is a white crystalline powder. Its mechanism of action is unexplained. It has effects on brain vasculature, but these are probably not related to its antimyoclonic effects. Piracetam appears to have no effect on brain GABAergic function, nor to affect cerebral serotonin or dopamine levels.

### Pharmacokinetics

The drug has an oral bioavailability of 100%. The time to peak levels is between 30 and 40 minutes. Absorption of the drug is not affected by food. Piracetam is not bound to plasma proteins. The drug does not undergo metabolism and is completely excreted by the kidneys, with an elimination half-life of 5–6 hours and almost complete elimination from the body after 30 hours. There are no drug interactions. The elimination from cerebrospinal fluid occurs with a half-life of about 7 hours.

### Adverse effects

The drug is very well tolerated and there is a low incidence of reported side-effects. Those that do occur (at a frequency of less than 10%) include dizziness, insomnia, nausea, gastrointestinal discomfort, hyperkinesis, weight gain, tremulousness and agitation. Rash occurs at a frequency of less than 1% and there have been no serious idiosyncratic reactions. In a placebo-controlled double-blind crossover study, the only adverse effects were a sore throat and headache in one patient and single seizures in two, and these side-effects may well not have been treatment related. At the very high doses used in the treatment of myoclonus, most patients report a few side-effects, although there are no formal studies of side-effects at these very high doses.

### Use in myoclonus

Piracetam is useful in cortical myoclonus of various types and causes. The drug has been shown to be effective in post-anoxic action myoclonus, some cases of progressive myoclonic epilepsy, myoclonus due to carbon monoxide poisoning, some cases of primary generalized epilepsy with myoclonus, post-electrocution myoclonus, myoclonus in Huntington disease, and in other symptomatic metabolic disorders (e.g. sialidosis). Initial case reports and then case series were followed by a well-conducted double-blind placebo-controlled study in 21 patients with severe myoclonus. A medium 22% improvement was noted on piracetam on global rating scales of disability, and some patients became free from seizures. The results were impressive in this severe condition, and on this basis the drug was licensed for myoclonus in the UK and elsewhere. There are now numerous reported cases of complete 'cure' of severe myoclonus by the drug, often in cases where all other therapy had failed, and indeed it may be the only drug that improves myoclonus in some patients.

Cortical myoclonus may produce profound disabilities. The jerks are often exacerbated by actions and patients may be bed-bound and immobile, unable to move without severe jerking disrupting all motor activity. In some cases (but not all), piracetam can have a truly remarkable effect in suppressing the myoclonus and reversing completely even severe disability. There does not seem to be a loss of the antimyoclonic effect over time. It has been said that the drug works best in combination, say with clonazepam, although there is no doubt that monotherapy with piracetam can be highly efficacious.

### Clinical use in epilepsy

Piracetam is only indicated in myoclonus, and is used usually as a second line for patients resistant to treatment with valproate or benzodiazepine drugs. Its remarkable effectiveness in some patients, even with severe and disabling myoclonus, combined with its almost complete lack of side-effects, gives the drug a special place in the therapy of myoclonus. Whether this place will be superseded by the use of levetiracetam remains to be seen.

It is available as 800 and 1200 mg tablets and as a solution. The initial dose is 4.8–8 g/day and this may be rapidly increased (in 1600 mg incremental steps weekly) to 18–24 g/day. Some patients require up to 32 g/day. The drug can be given in two or three divided doses, and is usually given in combination with other antimyoclonic drugs. The major drawback at these higher doses is the number of tablets taken (sometimes 30 or 40 a day) and their bulk. Serum level monitoring is not available. Dosage reductions in patients with moderate or severe renal disease are recommended and the drug is contra-indicated in patients with creatinine clearances below 20 ml/min. There is no published experience of the drug in children. Withdrawal needs to be gradual (2 weekly decrements of 800 or 1600 mg), and abrupt cessation has been associated with a severe exacerbation of seizures.

## Rufinamide

Rufinamide, 1-(2,6-difluoro-benzyl)-$^1$H-1,2,3-triazole-4-carboxide ($C_{10}H_8F_2N_4O$, molecular weight 238.20), is a triazole drug, insoluble in water. Its chemical structure is dissimilar to any other currently marketed antiepileptic drug and its mode of action is uncertain. The licensing rights were recently acquired by Eisai from Novartis, and it is expected to be launched in the latter part of 2005 in Europe and then later in the USA, both for the usual indication of refractory partial-onset seizures in adults, and gratifyingly also for use in the Lennox–Gastaut syndrome under the scheme for orphan indications in the European regulatory framework. In experimental studies, it was found to be both effective and also to have an extremely wide therapeutic index, suggesting promise as an efficacious drug with low potential for dose-related side-effects. The experimental studies also suggest a broad-spectrum profile. Preclinical studies showed excellent clinical pharmacological characteristics, good pharmacokinetic properties and no evidence of either mutagenicity or teratogenicity.

### Pharmacokinetics

The drug is moderately well absorbed with a bioavailability is about 85%. Absorption is influenced by food, and the rate and the extent of absorption are lowered if the drug is taken with a meal. Rufinamide is extensively metabolized (4% only recovered), predominately by hydrolysis. The P450 system is not involved and therefore rufinamide would not be expected to alter levels of hepatically-metabolized antiepileptic drugs. The dose : blood level ratio is linear in the normal dose range and with antiepileptic drug co-medication. There is no evidence of auto-induction and rufinamide is 34% bound to plasma proteins. The half-life lies between 8.5–12 hours, and excretion is largely renal and complete with 7 days. Studies in elderly populations show no marked pharmacokinetic differences.

**Table 3.33** Rufinamide

| | |
|---|---|
| **Primary indications** | Adjunctive therapy in refractory partial-onset seizures in adults; Lennox–Gastaut syndrome |
| **Usual preparations** | Tablets: 100, 200, 400 mg |
| **Usual dosage—adults** | Up to 3200 mg/day |
| **Dosing intervals** | 2 times/day |
| **Common drug interactions** | The levels of rufinamide may be elevated by valproate and reduced by drugs metabolised by the P450 enzyme system; rufinamide does not affect levels of commonly used antiepileptics |
| **Common/important adverse events** | Dizziness, headache, nausea, somnolence, double vision, fatigue, ataxia, vomiting, abnormal vision |
| **Major mechanism of action** | Not known |
| **Pharmacokinetics** (average adult values) | |
| Oral bioavailability | 60–85% (affected by food) |
| Time to peak levels | 5–6 h |
| Volume of distribution | 0.6 l/kg |
| Biotransformation | Extensive hydrolysis but not involving P450 enzyme system |
| Elimination half-life | 8.5–12 h |
| Protein binding | 34% |
| Active metabolite | None |

*Drug interactions*

One study has shown that valproate reduces the plasma clearance of rufinamide by approximately 22%, that phenobarbital, phenytoin and primidone increase rufinamide clearance by approximately 25%, and that clearance is unaffected by co-medication with carbamazepine, vigabatrin, oxcarbazepine or clobazam. Rufinamide had no effect on the trough concentrations of any of these drugs. The mechanism of these interactions is not clear, and *in vitro* studies confirm that rufinamide does not inhibit P450 isoenzyme activity (CYP1A2, CYP2A6, CYP2C9, CYP2C19, CYP2D6, CYP2E1, CYP3A4/5 and CYP4A9/11). Rufinamide significantly increases the metabolism of oestrogen, and so the use of the low-oestrogen dose combined oral contraceptive pill should be avoided in patients co-medicated with rufinamide.

**Adverse effects**

In the first double blind study of rufinamide, the most commonly reported side-effects were: headache (20% vs 12% on placebo: tiredness/fatigue/lethargy (20% rufinamide, 4% placebo), tremor (12% rufinamide, 0% placebo) and gait disturbance/balance difficulty (8% rufinamide, 4% placebo). In the two definitive blinded studies, reports of

adverse events were more common on rufinamide (~53%) than placebo (46%), but the proportion of patients discontinuing therapy because of side-effects was similar on rufinamide and placebo (10% rufinamide, ~7% placebo). No changes in haematological, hepatic or other laboratory parameters and no life-threatening side-effects have been reported.

Amongst the 1054 patients in all clinical studies, the adverse events reported by at least 10% of the patients included: dizziness, headaches, nausea, somnolence, diplopia, fatigue, ataxia, vomiting, abnormal vision and infection (this was more common on placebo).

**Antiepileptic effectiveness**

Rufinamide has been evaluated in two adjunctive therapy, double-blind, placebo-controlled studies in patients with refractory partial-onset epilepsy. In the first, the median seizure frequency was reduced by 42% in the rufinamide group compared with an increase of 52% in the placebo-treated patients ($P = 0.00397$). The 25% responder rate was significantly higher in the patients treated with rufinamide, but the 50% responder rate showed a trend only. In the second study, seizure frequency improved significantly, and there was also a significant difference in 50% responder rates when analysed using a linear dose–response trend. In an open label extension in nine children, four (45%) had a 50% reduction in their complex partial seizure frequency compared with baseline. Studies are ongoing in monotherapy, in children with partial epilepsy, and in the Lennox–Gastaut syndrome where rufinamide seems particularly effective in preventing falls and drop attacks.

### Clinical use in epilepsy

It is too early to say what place rufinamide will have in clinical practice, but its excellent tolerability and lack of side-effects (to date) are promising features. In preclinical studies, it has a broad-spectrum antiepileptic action, and it will be interesting to see its effects in a wider range of types of epilepsy. The drug was used in doses up to 3200 mg/day in the clinical trials in adults. Its first license will be for refractory partial (and secondarily generalized) seizures in adults – as is almost always the case for newly licensed antiepileptic drugs. However, under the scheme for orphan indications, the drugs is also to be licensed for add-on use in Lennox–Gastaut syndrome in children and adults, and has the potential to be of great utility in this currently intractable form of epilepsy.

# 4 The emergency treatment of epilepsy

## THE IMMEDIATE MANAGEMENT OF A SEIZURE

### General measures

Short-lived tonic–clonic seizures do not require emergency drug treatment, and nothing anyway can be done to influence the course of the seizure. The patient should be made as comfortable as possible, preferably lying down (or eased to the floor if seated), the head should be protected, and tight clothing or neckwear released. During the attack measures should be taken to avoid injury (e.g. from hot radiators, top of stairs, hot water, road traffic). No attempt should be made to open the mouth or force anything between the teeth. After the convulsive movements have subsided, roll the person into the recovery position, and check that the airway is not obstructed and that there are no injuries. Ensure that there is no apnoea and that the pulse is maintained. When fully recovered, the patient should be comforted and reassured. An ambulance or emergency treatment is required only if:

• injury has occurred
• convulsive movements continue for longer than 10 minutes, or longer than is customary for the individual patient
• the patient does not recover consciousness rapidly
• seizures rapidly recur
• the cardio-respiratory system is impaired.

Non-convulsive seizures are less dramatic but can still be disturbing to onlookers and embarrassing to the victim. Again, drug treatment is not indicated in short attacks. If consciousness is not lost, the patient should be treated sympathetically and with the minimum of fuss. If consciousness is impaired or in the presence of confusion, it is necessary to prevent injury or danger (for instance from wandering about), at the same time minimizing restraint as attempts at restraint will often increase confusion and cause agitation or occasionally violence.

If a person with epilepsy is likely to have a seizure in any particular situation (for instance at school or at work) it is usually best to inform those who might be present (e.g. fellow students, workmates, supervisors), and to provide simple advice about first-aid measures. This lessens the impact of a sudden epileptic seizure, which can be particularly frightening and disturbing if unexpected.

### Emergency antiepileptic drug therapy

This is needed in convulsive attacks if the convulsions persist for more than 10 minutes, recur rapidly or last longer than is customary for the individual patient. It is usual to give a fast-acting benzodiazepine. The traditional choice is diazepam, administered either intravenously or rectally. Intravenous diazepam is given in its undiluted form at a rate not exceeding 2–5 mg/min, using the Diazemuls© formulation. Because of the high lipid solubility of diazepam, injections given at a faster rate carry the risk of high first-pass concentrations causing respiratory arrest or cardiovascular collapse. Rectal administration is either as the intravenous preparation infused from a syringe via a plastic catheter, or as the ready-made proprietary rectal tube preparation Stesolid©, which is convenient and easy. Diazepam suppositories should not be used, as absorption is too slow. The adult bolus intravenous or rectal dose is 10–20 mg, and in children the equivalent bolus dose is 0.2–0.3 mg/kg.

Intravenous lorazepam is an alternative with some advantages over IV diazepam. It is longer lasting and—because it is less lipid-soluble—the intravenous injection can be given faster without the need to limit the rate of injection. The potentially dangerous first-pass effects possible with diazepam are not a risk with lorazepam. The dose is 4 mg in adults or 0.1 mg/kg in children.

Midazolam has the advantage that it can be given by IM injection or buccal or intra-nasal instillation. A published randomized trial has shown that buccal midazolam has equal efficacy and as rapid an action as rectal diazepam, and is more convenient, potentially faster to administer, and less stigmatizing. The dose used is 10 mg drawn up into a syringe and instilled into the mouth or between the cheeks and gums.

### Precautions needed with parenteral benzodiazepines

Although benzodiazepines are the drugs of first choice for

emergency therapy, they do carry a risk of respiratory depression, hypotension and cardio-respiratory collapse. In a well-controlled study in anaesthetic practice, for example, diazepam 10 mg was given intravenously to 15 patients and resulted in a drop in blood pressure of 10 mmHg or more in eight patients, a mean 28% decrease in ventilation, and a 23% decrease in tidal volume. The effects on cardio-respiratory function are as great (or even greater) with midazolam or lorazepam. In the occasional patient, the cardio-respiratory effects can be extremely severe, and for this reason it is essential that no patient given parenteral benzodiazepine should be left unattended. After parenteral benzodiazepine administration (buccally, intra-nasally, rectally, IM or IV) pulse, respiration, blood pressure, and (where possible) oxygen saturation should be frequently monitored, until the patient has recovered full consciousness. Resuscitation is occasionally needed, and deaths have occurred owing to lax post-administration care.

### Serial seizures

Serial seizures are defined as seizures recurring at frequent short intervals, with full recovery between attacks, and in the latter sense differ from status epilepticus. The premonitory stage of status, however, often takes the form of serial seizures, and drug therapy is advisable even if the individual seizures are short. The emergency antiepileptic drug treatment is as outlined above for acute seizures.

### Seizures occurring in clusters

In some patients clusters of seizures regularly occur, often at certain times (for instance around menstruation). In a cluster, seizures typically recur over periods of hours or days. Acute therapy after the first seizure can be given in an attempt to prevent subsequent attacks. Clobazam (10–20 mg) is a common choice. An oral dose of clobazam will take effect within 1–2 hours and last for 12–24 hours. Clobazam has the advantage that it causes much less sedation than either diazepam or lorazepam.

A cluster of seizures is sometimes the result of the withdrawal or dose reduction of an antiepileptic drug. The reintroduction of the drug will usually terminate the seizure cluster.

## STATUS EPILEPTICUS

### Classification of status epilepticus

Status epilepticus is defined as a condition in which epileptic activity persists for 30 minutes or more. The seizures can take the form of prolonged seizures or repetitive attacks without recovery in between. There are a variety of types with clinical features that are dependent on age, seizure type, syndrome and aetiology. A simplified classification of the types of status epilepticus is shown in Table 4.1.

**Table 4.1** Classification of status epilepticus (SE).

*Status epilepticus confined to early childhood*
Neonatal status epilepticus
Status epilepticus in specific infantile epilepsy syndromes

*Status epilepticus confined to later childhood*
Febrile status epilepticus
Non-convulsive SE in benign partial epilepsy syndromes
Non-convulsive SE in severe childhood epileptic encephalopathies

*Status epilepticus occurring in childhood and adult life*
Tonic–clonic status epilepticus
Absence SE (in childhood absence epilepsy)
Atypical absence SE (in severe epileptic encephalopathies)
Absence SE (in other categories of idiopathic generalized epilepsy)
Non-convulsive status epilepticus in specific epilepsy syndromes (other forms)
Myoclonic SE in coma
Myoclonic SE (other forms)
Tonic SE (in severe epileptic encephalopathies)
Epilepsia partialis continua
Simple partial status epilepticus
Complex partial status epilepticus

*Status epilepticus confined to adult life*
*De novo* absence status of late onset

## Pharmacokinetics and pharmacodynamics in status epilepticus

The pharmacokinetic properties of antiepileptic drugs in status epilepticus are noteworthy for a number of reasons:
• Rapid action is needed.
• The pharmacokinetics of a drug administered parenterally in large doses can differ greatly from those of the drug administered chronically.
• Drug distribution can be affected by seizures.
• Drug effectiveness can lessen the longer the seizures continue.

### Rapid action and parenteral pharmacokinetics

Fast drug absorption is essential in the treatment of status epilepticus, and thus almost all drugs need to be administered intravenously. Midazolam is the only drug that is absorbed fast enough by the intra-muscular, intra-nasal or buccal routes. Diazepam and other drugs can be given rectally in out-of-hospital situations, but in hospital the intra-venous route is favoured.

In order to act rapidly, the drugs need to cross the blood–brain barrier readily, and thus the drugs that are effective in status epilepticus usually have a high lipid solubility. The intravenous infusion of lipid-soluble drugs, however, carries the particular problem of drug accumulation, especially if the elimination half-life is long and the volume of distribution large. During parenteral administration, the drug first enters the central compartment (blood and the extracellular spaces of highly perfused organs) and then is rapidly redistributed to peripheral compartments such as fat and muscle, which act as 'sumps'. Thus, large doses are needed, as this redistribution leads to rapid falls in plasma levels. The initial drug half-life depends on redistribution and elimination, the former being more important. The half-life of redistribution—the distribution half-life—is usually very short. As these 'sumps' become saturated, redistribution begins to fail, and the half-life of the drug then depends on elimination via hepatic and renal mechanisms (as in chronic therapy). The elimination half-life is much longer than the distribution half-life. Thus, the dose—serum level relationship changes as the duration of therapy lengthens, sometimes dangerously. This is a problem with drugs given by repeated bolus injections or by continuous infusions. The doses needed initially become dangerous as time passes, and unless this is recognized, sudden rises in blood level can result in respiratory or cardiovascular collapse. This is a problem with the benzodiazepine drugs, barbiturates and clomethiazole particularly. Midazolam infusion, because of its rapid elimination, is much safer than diazepam in this regard.

### Kinetics of drugs during seizures

Seizures (especially convulsive seizures) can affect both the peripheral and central pharmacokinetics of drugs. During convulsive seizures there is a fall in the pH of the blood resulting in a change in the degree of ionization (and thus lipid solubility) of drugs in plasma. This will affect the distribution half-lives, the ability to cross the blood–brain barrier, and the protein binding. Blood pH decreases to a greater degree than brain pH, and this pH gradient facilitates the movement of a weakly acidic drug from blood to brain. This effect is prominent, for instance, with phenobarbital. Other peripheral pharmacokinetic changes occur during status epilepticus, resulting from increased blood flow to muscle, and hepatic and renal compromise. The permeability of the blood–brain barrier increases during convulsive seizures, especially at the seizure foci where blood flow increases. As a result of these changes, cortical blood flow can largely determine the rate at which some drugs, notably phenobarbital, cross the blood–brain barrier. The concentration of these drugs at the seizure foci enhances their effectiveness.

### *Drug responsiveness*

As status epilepticus progresses it becomes more difficult to treat, probably largely because of brain receptor changes triggered by continued seizure activity. Many treatments effective in the initial stages are ineffective later. The potency of benzodiazepines decreases as status epilepticus progresses, although their efficacy remains, probably because of acute down-regulation of their GABA-A receptor target (Figure 4.1). Non-GABAergic drugs lose their effects even

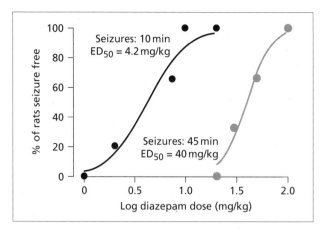

**Figure 4.1** Diazepam was more effective in controlling seizures when given early (before 10 mins) than when given later (45 mins) in the lithium-pilocarpine rat model of status epilepticus.

more, and phenytoin, for example, is generally largely ineffective in the later stages of status.

### Clinical features of tonic–clonic status epilepticus

Tonic–clonic status epilepticus is the classic form of status epilepticus, first described in the early 19th century. It is a common and important form, not least because urgent therapy is required to prevent consequent permanent cerebral damage.

Tonic–clonic status epilepticus is defined as a condition in which prolonged or recurrent tonic–clonic seizures persist for 30 minutes or more. The annual incidence has been estimated to be approximately 18–28 cases per 100,000 persons, with the highest rates in children, the learning-disabled, and in those with structural cerebral pathology, especially in the frontal lobes. About two-thirds of cases develop *de novo*, without a prior history of epilepsy, and such cases are almost always due to acute cerebral disturbances; common causes are cerebral infection, trauma, cerebrovascular disease, cerebral tumour, acute toxic or metabolic disturbances, or childhood febrile illness. In patients with pre-existing epilepsy tonic–clonic status can be precipitated by drug withdrawal, intercurrent illness, metabolic disturbance or the progression of the underlying disease, and is more common in symptomatic than in idiopathic epilepsy (Table 4.2). About 5% of all adult patients attending an epilepsy clinic will have at least one episode of status in the course of their epilepsy, and in children the proportion is higher (10–25%).

The mortality of tonic–clonic status is about 5–10%, most patients dying of the underlying condition rather than the status itself or its treatment. Permanent neurological and mental deterioration may result from status, particularly in young children. The risks of morbidity are greatly increased the longer the duration of the status episode.

| Underlying aetiology | No previous history of epilepsy (%) | Previous history of epilepsy (%) | All patients (%) |
|---|---|---|---|
| Cerebral trauma | 12 | 17 | 14 |
| Cerebral tumour | 16 | 10 | 13 |
| Cerebrovascular disease | 20 | 19 | 20 |
| Intracranial infection | 15 | 6 | 11 |
| Acute metabolic disturbance | 12 | 5 | 9 |
| Other acute event | 14 | 3 | 10 |
| No cause found | 11 | 41 | 23 |

**Table 4.2** Aetiology of status epilepticus in 554 patients from five case series.

## Physiological and clinical changes during tonic–clonic status epilepticus

At the onset of status, the attacks typically take the form of discrete tonic–clonic seizures. The motor activity then becomes continuous and the seizures become very prolonged. As neuronal function becomes progressively impaired, the jerking begins to fade, and if the status is allowed to progress may cease altogether or take the form of irregular myoclonus. This is the stage of subtle status epilepticus, by which time the patient will be deeply unconscious. This stage develops in some patients within a few hours of the onset of status and indicates severe cerebral compromise, and is reflected also in progressive change in the EEG. Once this state has developed there is a risk of permanent cerebral damage.

There is also often a premonitory stage of several hours, during which epileptic activity increases in frequency or severity from its habitual level. This clinical deterioration is a warning of impending status, and urgent therapy at this stage can prevent full-blown status.

The physiological changes in status can be divided into two phases, the transition from phase 1 to phase 2 occurring after about 30–60 minutes of continuous seizures (Table 4.3 and Figure 4.2).

### Phase 1 (phase of compensation)

The initial consequence of a prolonged convulsion is a massive release of plasma catecholamines, with resulting increases in heart rate, blood pressure and plasma glucose. During this stage cardiac arrhythmias frequently occur and can be fatal. As the seizure continues, there is a steady rise in the core body temperature, and prolonged hyperthermia (above 40 °C) can itself cause cerebral damage, and carries a poor prognosis. Acidosis also commonly occurs, and in one series 25% of the patients had an arterial pH below 7.0. This acidosis is mainly the result of lactic acid production, but there is also a rise in carbon dioxide tension that can, in itself, result in life-threatening narcosis. The acidosis increases the risk of cardiac arrhythmias and hypotension,

and in conjunction with the cardiovascular compromise may result in severe pulmonary oedema. The autonomic activity also results in sweating, bronchial secretion, salivation, and hypersecretion and vomiting.

However, within the brain, homoeostatic physiological mechanisms (autoregulation) are initially sufficient to compensate for these changes. There is a massive increase in cerebral blood flow, and the delivery of glucose to the active cerebral tissue is maintained. At this stage neuronal integrity is maintained, the blood–brain barrier is not impaired, and there is little risk of cerebral damage.

### Phase 2 (phase of decompensation)

The status epilepticus may then enter a second late phase in which cerebral protective measures progressively fail. The main systemic characteristics of this phase are a fall in systemic blood pressure and progressive hypoxia. Hypotension is due to seizure-related autonomic and cardio-respiratory changes and drug treatment, and in the later stages can be severe and intractable. At a critical stage cerebral autoregulation begins to fail and the control of blood flow then becomes dependent on systemic blood pressure. This is potentially hazardous, as falling blood pressure leads to a failure of cerebral perfusion. The high metabolic demands of the epileptic cerebral tissue cannot be met and this results in ischaemic or metabolic damage. The hypotension can be greatly exacerbated by intravenous antiepileptic drug therapy, especially if infusion rates are too fast. Intracranial pressure can rise dramatically in late status, and the combined effects of systemic hypotension and intracranial hypertension cause cerebral oedema, particularly in children.

Physiological changes are not confined to the brain metabolism. Pulmonary hypertension and pulmonary oedema occur, and pulmonary artery pressures can exceed the osmotic pressure of blood, causing oedema and stretch injuries to lung capillaries. Cardiac output can fall owing to decreasing left ventricular contractility and stroke volume, and cardiac failure can ensue. Profound hyperpyrexia

**Table 4.3** Physiological changes in tonic–clonic status epilepticus.

### Phase I: compensation

During this phase, cerebral metabolism is greatly increased because of seizure activity, but physiological mechanisms are sufficient to meet the metabolic demands, and cerebral tissue is protected from hypoxia or metabolic damage. The major physiological changes are related to the greatly increased cerebral blood flow and metabolism, massive autonomic activity and cardio-vascular changes.

| Cerebral changes | Systemic and metabolic changes | Autonomic and cardiovascular changes |
|---|---|---|
| Increased blood flow | Hyperglycaemia | Hypertension (initial) |
| Increased metabolism | Lactic acidosis | Increased cardiac output |
| Energy requirements matched by supply of oxygen and glucose (increased glucose and oxygen utilization) | | Increased central venous pressure |
| | | Massive catecholamine release |
| Increased lactate concentration | | Tachycardia |
| Increased glucose concentration | | Cardiac dysrhythmia |
| | | Salivation |
| | | Hyperpyrexia |
| | | Vomiting |
| | | Incontinence |

### Phase II: decompensation

During this phase, the greatly increased cerebral metabolic demands cannot be fully met, resulting in hypoxia and altered cerebral and systemic metabolic patterns. Autonomic changes persist and cardio-respiratory functions may progressively fail to maintain homoeostasis.

| Cerebral changes | Systemic and metabolic changes | Autonomic and cardiovascular changes |
|---|---|---|
| Failure of cerebral autoregulation; thus cerebral blood flow becomes dependent on systemic blood pressure | Hypoglycaemia | Systemic hypoxia |
| | Hyponatraemia | Falling blood pressure |
| | Hypokalaemia/hyperkalaemia | Falling cardiac output |
| Hypoxia | Metabolic and respiratory acidosis | Respiratory and cardiac impairment (pulmonary oedema, pulmonary embolism, respiratory collapse, cardiac failure, dysrhythmia) |
| Hypoglycaemia | Hepatic and renal dysfunction | |
| Falling lactate concentrations | Consumptive coagulopathy, DIC, multi-organ failure | |
| Falling energy state | | |
| Rise in intracranial pressure and cerebral oedema | Rhabdomyolysis, myoglobulinuria | Hyperpyrexia |
| | Leucocytosis | |

DIC, disseminated intravascular coagulopathy.

*Note*: the physiological changes listed above do not necessarily occur in all cases. The type and extent of the changes depend on aetiology, clinical circumstances and the methods of therapy employed.

is a common consequence. There are many metabolic and endocrine disturbances in status, the most common and most important being acidosis (including lactic acidosis), hypoglycaemia, hypo/hyperkalaemia and hyponatraemia. Other potentially fatal metabolic complications include acute tubular necrosis, renal failure, hepatic failure and disseminated intravascular coagulation (DIC). Rhabdo-myolysis, resulting from persistent convulsive movements, can precipitate renal failure if severe.

### Risk of cerebral damage

The major reason for treating tonic–clonic status epilepticus as a medical emergency is the risk of permanent cerebral damage, a consequence amply demonstrated in animal and

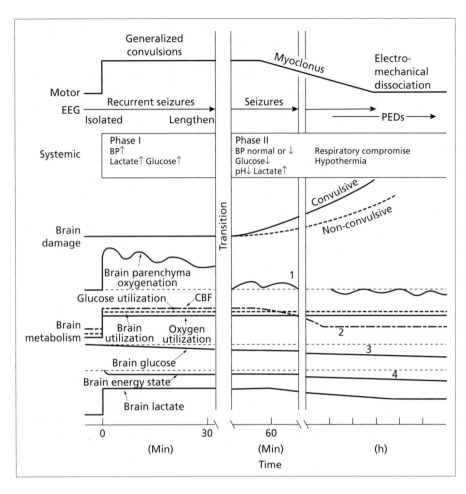

**Figure 4.2** Temporal changes which occur as tonic–clonic status epilepticus progresses. Motor activity lessens, the electroencephalogram (EEG) evolves and profound physiological changes occur, both systemically and cerebrally. In the first 30 min or so, physiological changes are largely compensatory, but as the seizures continue these compensatory mechanisms break down. The biphasic evolution is emphasized. PED, periodic epileptic discharge; 1, loss of reactivity of brain oxygen tension; 2, mismatch between the sustained increase in oxygen and glucose utilization and a fall in cerebral blood flow; 3, a depletion of cerebral glucose and glycogen concentrations; 4, a decline in cerebral energy state.

human studies. Brain damage has a number of mechanisms. Hypoxia, ischaemia or metabolic disturbances can certainly be a cause, but the predominant risk is of excitotoxic brain damage. This is damage due to the continuous electrographic activity itself, and the repeated depolarization of neurones which occurs during continuous seizures. The electrographic activity results in progressively increasing calcium influx into the affected neurones, and the calcium influx triggers processes of cell death and apoptosis. The result is neuronal loss, particularly in the hippocampus, but also in other areas of the cerebral cortex. The process of excitotoxic cell death is exacerbated by the energy failures inherent in the stage 2 physiological changes, and vulnerability to cellular damage is usually felt to begin after 1–2 hours of continuous seizure activity. The longer the status continues the greater is the risk of damage. For this reason it is important to abolish electrographic changes and not just the motor changes of status. If antiepileptic drug therapy has not controlled both the clinical and electrical manifestations of seizures within 2 hours, general anaesthesia should be applied as a method of abolishing all neuronal activity.

## General measures in the management of tonic–clonic status epilepticus
### Cardio-respiratory function

In all patients presenting in status, the protection of cardio-respiratory function takes first priority. It should be assessed, the airway secured, and resuscitation carried out if necessary. Hypoxia is usually much worse than appreciated, not least because of the higher metabolic demands of convulsing muscles and increased cerebral activity, and oxygen should always be administered.

### Respiratory compromise

This can arise from cardiovascular collapse, pulmonary oedema, and from the respiratory depressant properties of the drugs used to treat status epilepticus. There should be a low threshold for instituting ventilatory support, and it should be borne in mind that hypoxia is often much greater than initially suspected. The use of subanaesthetic doses of anaesthetic agents without ventilatory support is not recommended. Even 10 mg of intravenous diazepam has been shown to depress respiration in anaesthetic practice by a mean of about 30%. Aspiration pneumonia is common and broad-spectrum antibiotics should be started in any patients requiring assisted ventilation.

## Monitoring

Regular neurological observations and measurements of pulse, blood pressure, ECG and temperature should be initiated. Metabolic abnormalities may cause status epilepticus, or develop during its course, and biochemical, blood gas, pH, clotting and haematological measures should be regularly monitored.

## Intravenous lines

These should be set up for fluid replacement and drug administration. The drugs should not be mixed and, if two antiepileptic drugs are needed (for example, phenytoin and diazepam), two intravenous lines should be sited. The lines should be in large veins, as many antiepileptic drugs cause phlebitis and thrombosis at the site of infusion. Arterial lines must never be used for drug administration, as potentially fatal arterial necrosis and spasm can occur.

## Emergency investigations

Blood should be drawn for the emergency measurement of blood gases, sugar, renal and liver function, calcium and magnesium levels, full haematological screen (including platelets), blood clotting measures, and antiepileptic drug levels. Fifty millilitres of serum should also be saved for future analysis, especially if the cause of the status epilepticus is uncertain. Other investigations depend on the clinical circumstances.

## Intravenous glucose and thiamine

Glucose—50 ml of a 50% solution—should be given immediately by intravenous injection if hypoglycaemia is suspected. Routine glucose administration in non-hypoglycaemic patients, however, should be avoided as there is some evidence that this can aggravate neuronal damage.

If there is a history of alcoholism or other compromised nutritional state, 250 mg thiamine (for example, as the high-potency intravenous formulation Pabrinex®, 10 ml of which contains 250 mg) should also be given intravenously. This is particularly important if glucose has also been administered, as a glucose infusion increases the risk of Wernicke encephalopathy in susceptible patients. Intravenous high-dose thiamine should be given slowly (for example, 10 ml of high-potency Pabrinex over 10 minutes), with facilities for treating the anaphylaxis which is a potentially serious side-effect of Pabrinex infusions.

## Acidosis and other metabolic abnormalities

Lactic acidosis is common, and is largely caused by convulsive movements and hyperthermia. These can usually be controlled by halting the motor activity by antiepileptic, anaesthetic or paralysing agents. If acidosis is severe, the administration of bicarbonate has been advocated in the hope of preventing shock, and mitigating the effects of hypotension and low cerebral blood flow. In most cases, however, this is unnecessary, and the rapid control of respiration and abolition of motor seizure activity are more effective. Correction of hypoglycaemia and electrolyte and other metabolic abnormalities should be active and rigorous.

## Magnesium sulphate

Although magnesium is effective at preventing eclampsia, there is no evidence that increasing magnesium serum concentrations to supranormal levels has any benefit in status epilepticus. Indeed, such a policy can result in motor paralysis and hypotension. However, serum magnesium can be low in alcoholics and patients with acquired immune deficiency syndrome (AIDS), and in these patients intravenous loading with 2–4 g magnesium sulphate over 20 minutes may help with seizure control and the prevention of arrhythmias.

## Pressor therapy

Hypotension can result from the status itself and also from drug treatment, and is a universal problem in severe status. Hypotension increases the risk of cerebral damage, as loss of cerebral autoregulation means that cerebral perfusion becomes directly proportional to systemic blood pressure. Maintenance of blood pressure, therefore, is of paramount importance.

Pressor agents are usually required. Dopamine is the most commonly used, given by continuous intravenous infusion. The dose should be titrated up to achieve the desired haemodynamic and renal responses (usually initially between 2 and 5 µg/kg/min, but this can be increased to over 20 µg/kg/min in severe hypotension). Dopamine should be given into a large vein as extravasation causes tissue necrosis. ECG monitoring is required, as conduction defects may occur, and particular care is needed in dosing in the presence of cardiac failure.

## Cardiac arrhythmia

Cardiac arrhythmias pose a substantial risk in severe status, caused by autonomic hyperactivity, metabolic derangement, and the infusion of high-dose antiepileptic and anaesthetic drugs. Continuous EEG monitoring is mandatory, and arrhythmias are treated in the conventional manner.

## Acute renal or hepatic failure

A number of factors can result in acute renal failure, including myoglobinuria, disseminated intravascular coagulation, hypotension and hypoxia. In the early stages infusion of mannitol and dopamine may be of some benefit. Acute hepatic failure can also have various causes, including hypersensitivity reactions to administered drugs.

**Table 4.4** Medical complications in tonic–clonic status epilepticus.

---

*Cerebral*
Hypoxic/metabolic cerebral damage
Seizure-induced cerebral damage
Cerebral oedema and raised intercranial pressure
Cerebral venous thrombosis
Cerebral haemorrhage and infarction

*Cardio-respiratory and autonomic*
Hypotension
Hypertension
Cardiac failure, tachy- and bradydysrhythmia, cardiac arrest, cardiogenic
    shock
Respiratory failure
Disturbances of respiratory rate and rhythm, apnoea
Pulmonary oedema, hypertension, embolism, pneumonia, aspiration
Hyperpyrexia
Sweating, hypersecretion, tracheobronchial obstruction
Peripheral ischaemia

*Metabolic and systemic*
Dehydration
Electrolyte disturbance (especially hyponatraemia, hyperkalaemia,
    hypoglycaemia)
Acute renal failure (especially acute tubular necrosis)
Acute hepatic failure
Acute pancreatitis

*Other*
Disseminated intravascular coagulopathy/multi-organ failure
Rhabdomyolysis
Fractures
Infections (especially pulmonary, skin, urinary)
Thrombophlebitis, dermal injury

---

Care should be taken to avoid these drugs in cases with a prior history of hypersensitivity.

### Other physiological changes and medical complications

Some of the complications encountered in tonic–clonic status are listed in Table 4.4. These often need emergency treatment in their own right. Failure to do so can perpetuate the status and worsen outcome. Active treatment is most commonly required for hypoxia, pulmonary oedema and hypertension, cardiac arrhythmias, cardiac failure, hyperpyrexia, rhabdomyolysis and DIC. Rhabdomyolysis can be prevented by artificial ventilation and muscle paralysis.

### Establish aetiology

The outcome of status to a great extent depends on the aetiology, and the urgent treatment of causative factors is vital. CT or MRI scanning and CSF examination are often necessary, but the choice of investigations depends on the clinical circumstances.

If the status epilepticus has been precipitated by drug withdrawal, the immediate restitution of the withdrawn drug, even at lower doses, will usually rapidly terminate the status epilepticus. Pyridoxine should also be given intravenously to children under the age of 3 years who have a prior history of epilepsy, and to all neonates.

### Intensive care and seizure/EEG monitoring

If seizures are continuing in spite of the initial emergency measures, the patient must be transferred to an intensive care setting, where intensive monitoring is desirable, including, for instance, intra-arterial blood pressure, capnography, oximetry, central venous pressure, and Swan–Ganz monitoring.

Convulsive movements diminish over time in tonic–clonic status and may cease altogether in spite of ongoing epileptic electrographic activity. Such electrographic activity is potentially damaging to the cortical neurones, and anaesthetic therapy is targeted to suppress it by the attainment of the anaesthetic level of burst suppression. Both ongoing epileptic activity and also burst suppression require neurophysiological monitoring, which can be provided by either a full EEG or a cerebral function monitor (CFM). The CFM has to be calibrated for each individual patient, but then has the advantage over EEG of simplicity of use. Burst suppression provides an arbitrary physiological target for the titration of barbiturate or anaesthetic therapy, with drug dosing commonly set at a level that aims to produce burst suppression with inter-burst intervals of between 2 and 30 seconds.

### Raised intracranial pressure and intracranial pressure (ICP) monitoring

If there is evidence of persisting, severe or progressively elevated intracranial pressure (ICP) monitoring may be required. The need for this is usually determined by the underlying cause rather than the status, and its use is more common in children. If the ICP is critically raised, intermittent positive pressure ventilation, high-dose corticosteroid therapy (4 mg dexamethasone every 6 hours), or mannitol infusion—usually reserved as a temporary measure—can be used to lower the pressure. Neurosurgical decompression is occasionally required.

### The drug treatment of tonic–clonic status epilepticus

In tonic–clonic status epilepticus, as mentioned above, if seizure activity is allowed to persist for more than 1.5–2 hours there is a substantial risk of seizure-induced cerebral damage, and this risk rises the longer the seizures continue. For this reason, the drug treatment of tonic–clonic status epilepticus is best divided into stages, with the final stage (anaesthesia) reached within 1.5–2 hours of initiating therapy. The choice of drug regimen is somewhat arbitrary because of the lack of good comparative studies, the diversity of advice from the published reviews, and contradictory anecdotal reports on individual drugs. Nevertheless, a

**Stage of early status** *(0–30 min)*

Lorazepam 4 mg IV bolus (can be repeated once)

↓ (If seizures continue after 30 min)

**Stage of established status** *(30–60/90 min)*

Phenobarbital IV infusion of 10 mg/kg at a rate of 100 mg/min
or
Phenytoin IV infusion of 15 mg/kg at a rate of 50 mg/min
or
Fosphenytoin IV infusion of 15 mg PE/kg at a rate of 100 mg PE/min
or
Valproate IV infusion of 25 mg/kg at a rate of 3–6 mg/kg/min

↓ (If seizures continue after 30–90 min)

**Stage of refractory status** *(> 60/90 min; general anaesthesia)*

Propofol: IV bolus of 2 mg/kg, repeated if necessary, and then followed by a continuous infusion of 5–10 mg/kg/h initially reducing to a dose sufficient to maintain a burst-suppression pattern on the EEG (usually 1–3 mg/kg/h)
or
Thiopental: IV bolus of 100–250 mg given over 20 s with further 50 mg boluses every 2–3 min until seizures are controlled, followed by a continuous IV infusion at a dose sufficient to maintain a burst-suppression pattern on the EEG (usually 3–5 mg/kg/h)
or
Midazolam: IV bolus of 0.1–0.3 mg/kg at a rate not exceeding 4 mg/min initially, followed by a continuous IV infusion at a dose sufficient to maintain a burst-suppression pattern on the EEG (usually 0.05–0.4 mg/kg/h)

When seizures have been controlled for 12 h, the drug dosage should be slowly reduced over a further 12 h. *If seizures recur*, the general anaesthetic agent should be given again for a further 12 h, and then withdrawal attempted again. This cycle may need to be repeated until seizure control is achieved

**Figure 4.3** Protocol for the treatment of tonic–clonic status epilepticus in adults.
This is the author's personal protocol, and other published protocols exist with equal claims to effectiveness.

systematic organized approach is important in this emergency situation, and the simple fact of having a protocol has been shown to reduce morbidity and mortality, regardless of the protocol treatment options. The protocol favoured by the author is shown in Figure 4.3, and details of the drugs used are given in Tables 4.5 and 4.6 and on pp. 225–30.

### Premonitory stage, and stage of early status epilepticus

In many cases of status epilepticus, there is a premonitory stage. During this period there is a gradual increase in the frequency of tonic–clonic seizures or of myoclonic jerking. Parenteral drug treatment in this phase will often prevent the development of full-blown status, and the earlier treatment is given the more successful it is. If the patient is at home, antiepileptic drugs should be administered before transfer to hospital, or in the casualty department before transfer to the ward. Carers can be trained in the administration of emergency therapy. However, acute parenteral therapy will cause drowsiness or sleep, and occasionally cardio-respiratory collapse, and should therefore be carefully supervised. Out-of-hospital therapy can be with either rectal diazepam or paraldehyde, or buccal or intramuscular midazolam. All are highly effective, and the choice will depend on local circumstances. Rectal diazepam is available in a very convenient formulation with an already prepared syringe and catheter (Stesolid). Similarly, buccal midazolam is easy and quick to administer, and is especially useful for children. This is an off-label indication, but a convenient formulation exists packaged with a syringe and catheter (Epistat®). If intravenous therapy can be given in the premonitory stage, lorazepam is the drug of choice (see below).

The early stage of status epilepticus is defined as the first 30 minutes of status. It is usual to initiate intravenous treatment with a fast-acting benzodiazepine drug. Lorazepam is the drug of choice, given as a bolus injection at a dose of 4 mg in adults (0.1 mg/kg in children), and this can be repeated within 30 minutes if necessary. Alternatives include intravenous diazepam (Diazemuls) at a dose of 10 mg in adults or an intravenous bolus dose of phenytoin or of lidocaine; the latter drug may be preferable in patients with respiratory disease. The IV injection of subanaesthetic doses of propofol have also been tried. In most episodes of status, initial therapy treatment will be highly effective. Even if seizures cease, 24-hour inpatient observation should follow. In persons without a previous history of epilepsy, chronic antiepileptic drug treatment should be introduced,

**Table 4.5** Drugs used in the initial management of convulsive status epilepticus.

| Drug | Route | Adult dose | Paediatric dose |
|------|-------|-----------|-----------------|
| Diazepam at 2–5 mg/min[a] | IV bolus | 10–20 mg at 2–5 mg/min[a] | 0.25–0.5 mg/kg |
| | Rectal administration | 10–30 mg[a] | 0.5–0.75 mg/kg[a] |
| Midazolam | IM or rectally | 5–10 mg[a] | 0.15–0.3 mg/kg[a] |
| | IV bolus | 0.1–0.3 mg/kg at 4 mg/min[a] | |
| | IV infusion | 0.05–0.4 mg/kg/h | |
| Paraldehyde | Rectally or IM | 5–10 ml (approx 1 g/ml) in equal vol. of water[a] | 0.07–0.35 ml/kg[a] |
| | IV | 5–10 ml/h as a 5% solution in 5% dextrose | |
| Clomethiazole | IV infusion of 0.8% solution | 40–100 ml at 5–15 ml/min, then 0.5–20 ml/min | 0.1 ml/kg/min increasing every 2–4 h |
| Clonazepam | IV bolus | 1–2 mg at 2 mg/min[a] | 250–500 µg |
| Fosphenytoin | IV bolus | 15–20 mg PE/kg at 150 mg PE/min | |
| Lidocaine | IV bolus | 1.5–2.0 mg/kg at 50 mg/min[a] | |
| | IV infusion | 3–4 mg/kg/h | |
| Lorazepam | Rectally | | 0.05–0.1 mg/kg |
| | IV bolus | 0.07 mg/kg (usually 4 mg)[a] | 0.1 mg/kg |
| Phenytoin | IV bolus/infusion | 15–20 mg/kg at 50 mg/min | 20 mg/kg at 25 mg/min |
| Phenobarbital | IV bolus | 10–20 mg/kg at 100 mg/min | 15–20 mg/kg |
| Valproate | IV bolus | 15–30 mg/kg | 20–40 mg/kg |

[a] May be repeated. IM, intramuscular; IV, intravenous; PE, phenytoin equivalents.

**Table 4.6** Anaesthetics for refractory status epilepticus.

| Drug | Adult dose | Comments |
|------|-----------|----------|
| Midazolam | 0.1–0.3 mg/kg at 4 mg/min bolus followed by infusion at 0.05–0.4 mg/kg/h | Elimination half-life of 1.5 h, but accumulates with prolonged use. Tolerance and rebound seizures can be problematic |
| Thiopental | 100–250 mg bolus over 20 s then further 50 mg boluses every 2–3 min until seizures are controlled. Then infusion to maintain burst suppression (3–5 mg/kg/h) | Complicated by hypotension. It has saturable pharmacokinetics, and a strong tendency to accumulate. Metabolized to pentobarbital. Can also cause pancreatitis, hepatic disturbance and hypersensitivity reaction |
| Pentobarbital | 10–20 mg/kg at 25 mg/min then 0.5–1 mg/kg/h increasing to 1–3 mg/kg/h | As above |
| Propofol | 2 mg/kg then 5–10 mg/kg/h | Large volume of distribution and short half-life. Rapid recovery. Can be complicated by lipaemia, acidosis and rhabdomyolysis especially in children. Rebound seizures with abrupt withdrawal |

and in those already on maintenance antiepileptic therapy, this should be reviewed.

### Stage of established status epilepticus

Once the seizures have continued for 30 minutes, in spite of the therapy outlined above, the stage of established status epilepticus is entered.

In the protocol used by the author, there are four alternative first-line treatment options (Figure 4.2), but each has drawbacks. The author's own current preference is for phenobarbital, but there are many potential advantages to IV valproate.

Subanaesthetic infusions of benzodiazepine drugs were once fashionable in the stage of established status.

However, because of the risk of drug accumulation (see pp. 212–13), sudden respiratory depression, cardiovascular collapse and/or severe hypotension can occur. For these reasons, continuous benzodiazepine infusions (or repeated bolus injections) at this stage should not be given (the exception is with midazolam, see below). Clomethiazole infusion carries similar risks. Lidocaine infusion is essentially a short-term therapy and so should not be employed at this stage.

### The stage of refractory status epilepticus

In most patients, if seizures continue for 60–90 minutes in spite of the therapy outlined above, full anaesthesia is required. In some emergency situations (e.g. post-operative status, severe or complicated convulsive status, patient already in ITU), anaesthesia can and should be introduced earlier. The prognosis is now much poorer, and there is a moderate risk of mortality and morbidity.

The most commonly used anaesthetics are the intravenous barbiturates thiopental or pentobarbital, the intravenous non-barbiturate infusional anaesthetics propofol or midazolam. There have been no randomized controlled studies comparing these treatment options, but a meta-analysis suggests no difference in terms of mortality, but that pentobarbital was more effective than midazolam at the expense of greater hypotension. Propofol and midazolam have significant pharmacokinetic advantages over the barbiturates. Other anaesthetics that can be used include isoflurane, etomidate and ketamine. Experience with these agents in status is, however, meagre. Ketamine particularly is theoretically an attractive option as it has a strong blocking action at NMDA receptors, which might provide neuroprotection.

It is imperative at this stage to have EEG monitoring of the patient, as a patient in a drug-induced coma, with little outward sign of convulsions, can yet have ongoing electrographic epileptic activity. The point of therapy is to abolish electrographic activity and the attendant risk of excitotoxic cerebral damage, and EEG monitoring (or cerebral function monitoring) can be the only way to detect such activity. The depth of anaesthesia should be that which abolishes all EEG epileptic activity, and commonly 'burst suppression' is the targeted level of anaesthesia. Burst suppression with interburst intervals of 2–30 seconds is an acceptable end-point because it supposedly represents membrane inactivity, but it can be difficult to achieve, because this degree of anaesthesia commonly leads to hypotension.

All the anaesthetic drugs are given in doses sufficient to induce deep unconsciousness; therefore assisted respiration, intensive cardiovascular monitoring, and the full panoply of intensive care are essential.

Once the patient has been free of seizures for 12–24 hours, and provided that there are adequate plasma levels of concomitant antiepileptic medication, then the anaesthetic can be slowly tapered. If one anaesthetic agent is ineffective then it should be substituted by another. There are some data to suggest that those who are loaded with phenobarbital do better than those who are not. If seizures recur, anaesthesia should be re-established. In severe cases anaesthesia may be required for weeks or even months. In this situation, trials of steroids are often given, and in patients in whom immunologically-based aetiologies are present, repeated courses of intravenous IgG are sometimes effective.

### Additional maintenance antiepileptic therapy

In addition to emergency drug therapy, it is important that maintenance antiepileptic drug treatment should continued via a naso-gastric tube. If this is forgotten, seizures will almost inevitably recur when the anaesthesia is lightened.

### Failure to respond to treatment

In the great majority of cases, the above measures will control seizures and the status will resolve. If drug treatment fails, there are often complicating factors. Common reasons for the failure to control seizures in status epilepticus are:

- Inadequate drug treatment
  - Insufficient emergency antiepileptic drug therapy. A particular problem is the administration of intravenous drugs at too low a dose (for instance phenobarbital or phenytoin).
  - Failure to initiate or continue maintenance antiepileptic drug therapy in parallel with the acute emergency therapy. This will result in a recrudescence of seizures once the effects of the emergency drug treatment have worn off.
- Medical factors
  - Medical complications can exacerbate seizures.
  - A failure to treat (or identify) the underlying cause can result in intractable status. This is particularly the case in acute progressive cerebral disorders and cerebral infections.
- Misdiagnosis
  - A common problem is the failure to diagnose pseudo-status epilepticus. Indeed, in specialist practice, this condition is more common than true epileptic status. The diagnosis can usually easily be made by clinical observation, once considered, and confirmed by EEG in cases of uncertainty.

### Treatment of tonic–clonic status in special circumstances
*Drug withdrawal*

Status epilepticus can result from antiepileptic drug withdrawal (or too rapid reduction of dose). This can be the result of injudicious medical advice or poor compliance. In this situation, the rapid reintroduction of the drug often effectively terminates the status epilepticus and obviates the need for the above more elaborate measures. The drug should be given intravenously where possible.

*Alcohol withdrawal*

Alcohol withdrawal can also result in status epilepticus in the 24–48 hours after withdrawal. The withdrawal of opiates, cocaine and other recreational drugs can have the same effect. Traditionally, benzodiazepine, paraldehyde or clomethiazole are given either as treatment or prophylactically, but these cases are best managed in a unit specializing in addiction.

*Drug overdose*

Status epilepticus can occur during drug overdose. The status is usually treated with midazolam infusion. Other aspects of management are directed at reducing the levels of the offending drug, at controlling complications, and general supportive measures.

## Epilepsia partialis continua

Epilepsia partialis continua (EPC) can be defined as spontaneous regular or irregular clonic twitching of cerebral cortical origin, sometimes aggravated by action or sensory stimuli, confined to one part of the body, and continuing for hours, days or weeks. It is a remarkable condition, with highly characteristic features, and has a number of underlying causes (Table 4.7).

The clonic jerks in EPC can affect any group of muscles. In some individuals they are confined to a single muscle or muscle group, but in others the distribution is more widespread, and the distribution of the jerks can vary over time.

Table 4.7 Causes of epilepsia partialis continua.

| Cerebral tumour | Primary (benign/malignant) Metastasis |
| --- | --- |
| Cerebral infection | Bacterial abscess, tuberculoma Parasitic infection (e.g. cysticercosis) Viral encephalitis, meningitis, HIV Whipple disease |
| Cerebral inflammatory disease | Cerebral vasculitis (any type) Rasmussen encephalitis Granuloma (any type) Paraneoplastic disease, coeliac disease |
| Cerebrovascular disease | Cerebral infarction/haemorrhage Arterio-venous malformation Venous thrombosis |
| Other cerebral disorders | Cortical dysplasia (many types) Mitochondrial disease Anoxic brain damage |
| Metabolic disturbance | Acute metabolic disturbance Hereditary or congenital (many types) |
| Drugs, toxins, poisoning | Many types |

Agonists and antagonists are affected together, and distal muscles are more commonly involved than the proximal musculature. The jerks are spontaneous, and often exacerbated by action, startle or sensory stimuli. They can be single or cluster, and may have a rhythmic quality with a wide range of frequencies and amplitudes. Some jerks recur only every few minutes and others are more frequent. In chronic cases the jerks can continue relentlessly for months or years.

Treatment should be largely directed at the underlying cause. The seizures can remit spontaneously in acute cases. In a well-established case, however, epilepsia partialis continua can be particularly resistant to therapy, and IV antiepileptic therapy even to the point of anaesthesia can produce only temporary respite. It is usual to prescribe oral antiepileptic drugs, to prevent secondary generalization, even if the EPC itself is not controlled. Any of the antiepileptic drugs can be used and treatment follows conventional lines. In addition, the oral corticosteroids are sometimes helpful. Where there is an inflammatory or post-infective cause, courses of high-dose IV IgG have been used, sometimes with startling benefit. Plasma exchange has been tried with little effect, as have other immunosuppressive therapies and zidovudine. The long-term outcome depends on the underlying cause, but in many cases the clonic movements continue in spite of medical therapy. Very occasionally, there is resort to surgical therapy, either resective or by multiple subpial transection.

## Complex partial status epilepticus

This form of non-convulsive status can be defined as a prolonged epileptic episode in which fluctuating or frequently recurring focal electrographic epileptic discharges result in a confusional state. There are highly variable clinical symptoms, and the focal epileptic discharges may arise in temporal or extratemporal cortical regions. Any condition causing complex partial seizures can also cause status, although structural defects in the frontal lobe seem particularly likely to result in episodes of status epilepticus.

### Clinical features

Confusion, which can fluctuate or be fairly continuous, is the leading clinical feature. The severity of the confusion can vary from profound stupor with little response to external stimuli in some cases, to others in whom subtle abnormalities on cognitive testing are the only sign. Amnesia is usual but not invariable. Associated with the confusion are behavioural changes, speech and language disturbance, and motor and autonomic features. These can be very variable and cause considerable diagnostic difficulty. Periods of complex partial status can last for days or even weeks, although typically an episode will persist for several hours. It is most common in adults, usually with long histories of complex partial epilepsy. Precipitating factors include menstruation, and alcohol and drug withdrawal, but not usually photic stimulation or overbreathing as in typical absence status. The onset and offset are usually less well defined than in absence status, and the response to intravenous therapy more gradual. Complex partial status may typically follow a secondary generalized tonic–clonic seizure (or cluster of seizures), but is rarely terminated by a generalized convulsion, in contrast to the case in typical absence status. Episodes of complex partial status are usually recurrent, and in a few patients there is a remarkable periodicity. Complex partial status can arise in focal epilepsies of widely varying aetiologies.

The abnormalities on scalp EEG findings may be slight, although the EEG is seldom normal. A whole range of EEG patterns are seen including continuous or frequent spike or spikes/slow wave, or spike-wave paroxysms, which are sometimes widespread or focal, and also episodes of desynchronization. The longer the status proceeds, the less likely is discrete ictal activity to be noticeable.

The prognosis of complex partial status is good. It is not usually life threatening, and resolves with oral or intravenous therapy or is self-limiting. There is, however, a strong tendency for recurrence. Permanent neurological or psychological sequelae are rare, in contrast to the poor prognosis of tonic–clonic status.

### Drug treatment of complex partial status epilepticus

How aggressively complex partial status epilepticus needs to be treated is a matter of some controversy. It is the author's view that in most cases there is little risk of cerebral damage due to the seizures, and for this reason intravenous therapy is not needed unless the condition is particularly severe or resistant. Others disagree and treat complex partial status using similar protocols to that described above for tonic–clonic status. There is, however, no good evidence that aggressive treatment improves the prognosis in this condition, and intravenous medication can result in hypotension, respiratory depression, and occasionally cardio-respiratory arrest. In one series of non-convulsive status epilepticus in the elderly, aggressive treatment carried a worse prognosis than no treatment.

At present, treatment with oral benzodiazepines is usually first-line therapy. Lorazepam or clobazam are the most commonly prescribed drugs. In patients who have repetitive attacks of complex partial status epilepticus (a common occurrence), oral clobazam over a period of 2–3 days given early at home can abort the status epilepticus, and such strategies should be discussed with the patient and carers. The response to benzodiazepines can be disappointing. Often there is only a slow and partial improvement, in marked contrast to the complete and rapid improvement in absence status epilepticus. In other patients there may be resolution of the electrographic status epilepticus without concomitant clinical improvement. Although the response to benzodiazepines is often not complete, most episodes are self-limiting, and will recover spontaneously.

Treatment of the underlying cause where this is possible (e.g. encephalitis or metabolic derangement) is of course paramount. The routine maintenance antiepileptic drug regimen should also manipulated to provide maximum control of seizures.

## Absence status epilepticus

Absence status can be best subdivided into various separate syndromes, albeit with overlapping clinical and EEG features. These should all be distinguished from complex partial status, which can take a somewhat similar clinical form. While this is a tidy classification scheme, there are transitional cases which do not fit easily into any particular category.

### Typical absence status epilepticus ('petit mal' status)

This occurs only in patients with idiopathic generalized epilepsy, usually as part of the subcategory childhood absence epilepsy, in which a history of absence status occurs in about 3–9%. The attacks can recur, and can last for hours or occasionally days. The episodes are typically precipitated by factors such as menstruation, withdrawal of medication, hypoglycaemia, hyperventilation, flashing or bright lights, sleep deprivation, fatigue, stress, or grief. The principle clinical feature is clouding of consciousness. This can vary from slight clouding to profound stupor. At one extreme patients have nothing more than slowed ideation and expression, and deficits in activities requiring sustained attention, sequential organization or spatial structuring; amnesia may be slight or even absent. At the other extreme there may be immobility, mutism, simple voluntary actions performed only after repeated requests, long delays in verbal responses, and monosyllabic and hesitant speech. Typically, the patient is in an expressionless, trance-like state with slow responses and a stumbling gait. Motor features occur in about 50% of cases, including myoclonus, atonia, rhythmic eyelid blinking, and quivering of the lips and face. Facial, especially eyelid, myoclonus is common in absence status, but rare in complex partial status. Episodes of absence status are often terminated by a tonic–clonic seizure. The diagnostic electrographic pattern is continuous or almost continuous bilaterally synchronous and symmetrical spike-wave activity, with little or no reactivity to sensory stimuli.

Typical absence status can usually be rapidly and completely abolished by benzodiazepine therapy given as intravenous bolus doses. The usual drugs are diazepam 0.2–0.3 mg/kg, clonazepam 1 mg (0.25–0.5 mg in children) or lorazepam 0.07 mg/kg (0.1 mg/kg in children). The bolus doses can be repeated if required. If this is ineffective, intravenous clomethiazole, phenytoin or valproate may be needed. In childhood absence epilepsy, maintenance therapy with valproate, ethosuximide or other agents is required once the status is controlled.

### Absence status in other forms of childhood and adolescent forms of idiopathic generalized epilepsy

Other forms of absence and myoclonic status are common in other syndromes of idiopathic generalized epilepsy. These include the syndromes of myoclonic-astatic epilepsy, epilepsy with myoclonic absences, eyelid myoclonia with absences, and juvenile absence epilepsy. Treatment is generally as outlined above for typical absence epilepsy.

### Atypical absence status

This form of status is common in patients with diffuse cerebral damage and is typically seen as part of the Lennox–Gastaut syndrome. Although the clinical phenomenology of typical and atypical absence status overlap greatly, there are important differences. The clinical context is very different: typical absence status occurs in patients with childhood absence epilepsy and without intellectual deterioration; atypical absence epilepsy occurs in the epileptic encephalopathies (typically the Lennox–Gastaut syndrome), with other seizure types, and in the context of intellectual disability. The episodes of atypical absence status are usually longer and more frequent, with a gradual onset and offset. Atypical absence status is often preceded by changes in motor activity, mood or intellectual ability, for hours or days before the overt seizures develop. This prodromal stage might be due to subclinical status. Atypical absence status tends to fluctuate, and minor motor, myoclonic or more typically tonic seizures interrupt, but do not terminate an episode. Tonic seizures usually last a few minutes but occur in series. In some patients the mental state fluctuates gradually in and out of this ill-defined epileptic state over long periods of time—days or weeks—with little distinction possible between ictal and interictal phases. In contrast to typical absence status, tonic–clonic seizures seldom occur at the beginning or end of the status episode, and atypical absence status often responds poorly to injection of a benzodiazepine. Indeed, antiepileptic drug therapy may have little effect, and the condition fluctuates, apparently uninfluenced by external factors. Atypical absence status is more likely to occur if the patient is drowsy or under-stimulated, and it is thus important not to over-medicate patients with the Lennox–Gastaut syndrome. The EEG during atypical absence status may show continuous irregular slow (2 Hz) spike-wave, or hypsarrhythmia, or more discrete ictal patterns.

In contrast to typical absence status epilepticus, this condition is usually poorly responsive to intravenous benzodiazepines, which should, in any case, be given cautiously, as they can induce tonic status epilepticus in susceptible patients. Oral rather than intravenous treatment is usually more appropriate, and the drugs of choice are valproate, lamotrigine, clonazepam, clobazam and topiramate. Levetiracetam also shows promise. Barbiturates, carbamazepine, gabapentin, tiagabine and vigabatrin can worsen the episode.

### *De novo* absence status of late life

This curious syndrome presents in late adult life. The leading symptom is confusion, although the other features of absence status can occur. Many patients have a history of absence epilepsy in early life, but which has been in long remission. Many cases are misdiagnosed as dementia or cerebrovascular disease, but the abrupt onset should suggest the possibility of absence status, and the diagnosis is easily confirmed by EEG. In most cases, psychotropic drug (particularly benzodiazepine) toxicity or withdrawal seems to be the antecedent cause of the episode. The condition is rapidly alleviated by intravenous lorazepam (4 mg) and tends not to recur. Long-term antiepileptic drug treatment is not usually required.

## Treatment of other forms of status epilepticus

### Autonomic status epilepticus

This is a form of SE which occurs typically in Panyiotopoulos syndrome. The exact prevalence of this syndrome is unclear, and estimates have ranged from 0 to 6% of all children with epilepsy. The seizures consist of episodes of nausea, retching and vomiting, and deviation of the eyes. There may or may not be altered awareness. Other autonomic features occur including incontinence of urine, pallor, hyperventilation and headache. The EEG shows occipital spiking or runs of 3 Hz spike-wave and there is also often evidence of photosensitivity. About half of the seizure last longer than 30 minutes and so are categorized as 'status epilepticus'. The prognosis of the syndrome is excellent and at least 50% of patients have only a single attack, and most require no treatment. If treatment is required, any of the conventional first-line antiepileptic drugs can be used in monotherapy.

### Tonic status epilepticus

Tonic status epilepticus occurs in patients with syndromes such as Lennox–Gastaut syndrome. The tonic seizures are usually short lived but are rapidly repeated and a series can persist for days. Tonic status epilepticus is poorly responsive to conventional treatment, and can be dramatically worsened by benzodiazepines, which should be used with care. Sedating medication can worsen all seizure types in the Lennox–Gastaut syndrome, and thus should be avoided. There is anecdotal evidence that stimulants such as methylphenidate can be effective. Lamotrigine, adrenocorticotropic hormone (ACTH) and corticosteroids are also sometimes effective.

### Myoclonic status epilepticus in coma

Myoclonic status epilepticus in coma is a well-recognized complication of the cerebral anoxia resulting from cardio-respiratory arrest (typically after a myocardial infarction or cardiac surgery). It is characterized by spontaneous and stimulus-sensitive myoclonus usually occurring within 24 hours of the coma. To what extent this is really an 'epileptic' state, or is simply a sign of a severely damaged brain, is arguable. The patients generally have burst suppression on their EEGs, are deeply unconscious, and have signs referable to cerebral oedema. The mortality rates are very high. Survivors are usually left with Lance–Adams type action myoclonus. Whether antiepileptic treatment influences the course of this condition is quite unclear. Some authorities recommend aggressive antiepileptic therapy, and others none at all. It is this author's practice to recommend aggressive anti-status therapy, including anaesthesia, for a 24-hour period, but at this stage, in the absence of any improvement, the antiepileptic therapy should be withdrawn. Barbiturate or non-barbituate infusional anaesthetic drugs are given.

### Other forms of myoclonic status epilepticus

Myoclonic status in the progressive myoclonic epilepsies and in primary generalized epilepsy does not usually require intravenous therapy, although if needed an intravenous benzodiazepine can be given. The preferred therapy is with oral valproate, benzodiazepine, levetiracetam or piracetam.

### Simple partial status epilepticus

Prolonged simple partial seizures are rare. Any condition causing simple partial seizures can also result in status, although, as is the case with complex partial status, epilepsies due to extratemporal structural defects in the frontal lobe are particularly likely to do so. Prolonged simple partial seizures are also quite characteristic of some of the benign partial epilepsy syndromes of childhood, particular the occipital and rolandic epilepsy syndromes. Emergency administration of benzodiazepines is traditionally given, and the principles of treatment are similar to those of complex partial status epilepticus.

### Other forms of generalized non-convulsive status epilepticus

Episodes of non-convulsive status in various conditions are not easily classified as either absence status or complex partial status, although their clinical forms are very similar. This applies particularly to the rare childhood epilepsy syndromes. Episodes of non-convulsive status are a particularly characteristic feature of ring chromosome 20 epilepsy syndrome. Generally speaking, treatment follows the same lines as that of atypical absence status epilepticus.

## ANTIEPILEPTIC DRUGS USED IN STATUS EPILEPTICUS

Many of the main-line antiepileptic drugs have been used in status epilepticus. The potential for use of the newer agents has been only partly explored, and both topiramate and levetiracetam, for example, show promise in experimental models, and in preliminary reports in human status. Among the anaesthetic agents ketamine has the potential advantage of antiglutaminergic action. which might confer neuro-

protectant properties, but it has not been extensively used. Harkeroside is a novel agent whose use in status epilepticus has been specifically investigated. Salient properties of the antiepileptic drugs most commonly used parenterally are briefly listed here.

### Clomethiazole

Clomethiazole has been used in the stage of established status epilepticus, although its role in modern therapy is limited by the risks of accumulation. It is given by IV bolus followed by a continuous infusion. The drug is rapidly redistributed and has a very rapid and short-lived initial action. Dosage can be initially titrated against response, on a moment-by-moment basis, a unique property among the drugs used in status. The danger of clomethiazole is that it accumulates on prolonged use, with the risk of sudden cardio-respiratory collapse, hypotension and sedation. There is also a danger of respiratory arrest and hypotension if the maximum rate of injection is exceeded. Other side-effects include cardiac rhythm disturbances, vomiting and thrombophlebitis, and there is a tendency for seizure recurrence on discontinuing therapy. Prolonged therapy carries the risk of fluid overload and electrolyte disturbance. There is limited published experience in status, particularly in children, and insufficient published data for neonatal use. Hepatic disease reduces the metabolism and elimination of the drug, and prolonged contact with plastic tubing (for instance in drip sets) results in substantial resorption.

#### *Usual preparation*
0.8% (8 mg/ml) solution of clomethiazole edisylate in 500 ml of 4% dextrose.

#### *Usual dosage*
IV infusion of 40–100 ml (320–800 mg), at a rate of 5–15 ml/min, followed by a continuous infusion, with dosage titrated according to response (usually 1–4 ml/min, range 0.5–20 ml/min) (adults). Initially 0.1 ml/kg/min (0.8 mg/kg/min), increasing progressively every 2–4 hours as required (children).

### Clonazepam

Clonazepam is an alternative to diazepam in stage of early status epilepticus, and there is little to choose between the two drugs. It has a similar onset of action, and a longer duration of action (half-life, 22–33 hours), and may have a lower incidence of late relapse. There is wide experience with the drug in adults and children, although not in neonates, and the drug has proven efficacy in tonic–clonic, partial, and absence status. Clonazepam accumulates on prolonged infusion, with the resulting risk of respiratory arrest, hypotension and sedation—a side-effect profile very similar to that of diazepam (see below). The drug has a negative inotropic action, and as with diazepam thrombophlebitis may occur. There is also a danger of sudden collapse if the recommended rate of injection is exceeded. A continuous infusion of clonazepam is not now recommended because of the dangers of accumulation, and respiratory and cardiovascular collapse.

### Usual preparation

A 1 ml ampoule containing 1 mg of clonazepam.

### Usual dosage

A 1–2 mg bolus injection over 30 seconds (adults). 250–500 µg (children), which can be repeated up to four times. The 1 ml ampoule of clonazepam is mixed with 1 ml of water for injection (provided as diluent) *immediately* before administration. The rate of injection should not exceed 1 mg in 30 seconds. The drug can also be given more slowly in a 5% dextrose or 0.9% sodium chloride solution (1–2 mg in 250 ml).

## Diazepam

Diazepam is useful in the premonitory stage or the stage of epilepsy status epilepticus. There is extensive clinical experience in adults, children and the newborn, and the drug has well-proven efficacy in many types of status, a rapid onset of action, and well-studied pharmacology and pharmacokinetics. It can be given by rectal administration, and the rectal tubule is a convenient preparation. Diazepam has two important disadvantages, however, which limit its usefulness in status. First, although it has a rapid onset of action, it is highly lipid-soluble and thus has a short duration of action—usually less than 1 hour—after a single injection. This means that there is a strong tendency for seizure relapse after initial control. Secondly, diazepam accumulates on repeated injections or after continuous infusion, and this accumulation carries a high risk of sudden respiratory depression, sedation and hypotension. The respiratory effect of diazepam can be pronounced, and a mean 28% fall in ventilatory capacity was noted in healthy persons after a 10 mg IV injection; the fall is likely to be greater in patients with ongoing seizures in whom respiration is already compromised. Hypotension is common, and a mean fall in blood pressure of 10 mmHg was noted in healthy persons in one study after a 10 mg IV injection. Mild sedation is common, too, with parenteral diazepam. Tolerance to the effects develops rapidly (often after 24 hours). Other disadvantages are its dependency on hepatic metabolism and its metabolism to an active metabolite, which can complicate prolonged therapy. Diazepam has a tendency to precipitate from concentrated solutions and to interact with other drugs, and is absorbed onto plastic on prolonged contact. The Diazemuls preparation should be used, as this minimizes the risk of thrombophlebitis.

Because of the risks of accumulation, respiratory and cardiovascular depression and tolerance, the drug should be used in short-term therapy only (a bolus dose given once or twice) and long-term infusions are not now recommended.

### Usual preparation

IV formulation: diazepam emulsion (Diazemuls), 1 ml ampoule containing 5 mg/ml, or IV solution 2 ml ampoule containing 5 mg/ml. Rectal formulation: 2.5 ml rectal tube (Stesolid), containing 2 mg/ml, or using the IV solution, 2 ml ampoule containing 5 mg/ml.

### Usual dosage

IV bolus (undiluted) 10–20 mg (adults); 0.25–0.5 mg/kg (children), at a rate not exceeding 2–5 mg/min. The bolus dosing can be repeated. Rectal administration 10–30 mg (adults); 0.5–0.75 mg/kg (children), which can be repeated.

## Fosphenytoin

Fosphenytoin is a prodrug of phenytoin, and is a drug of choice in the stage of established status epilepticus. It is converted in the plasma into phenytoin by widely distributed phosphatase enzymes. The half-life of conversion is about 15 minutes, and conversion is not affected by age, hepatic status, or by the presence of other drugs. Fosphenytoin is soluble in water and prepared in a TRIS buffer; it thus causes less thrombophlebitis than phenytoin when given intravenously. It can also be administered intramuscularly as prophylaxis in acute epilepsy (but absorption is too slow for its use in status epilepticus). Fosphenytoin itself is inert, and its action in status is entirely due to the derived phenytoin. When fosphenytoin is infused at 100 mg phenytoin equivalents (PE)/min, the rate at which free phenytoin levels are reached in the serum is similar to that achieved by a phenytoin infusion of 50 mg/min (although there is considerable individual scatter in the levels reached). Fosphenytoin can therefore be administered twice as fast as phenytoin, with equivalent risks of hypotension, cardiac arrhythmias and respiratory depression. Its rate of anti-epileptic action is also similar. The faster action and the lower incidence of local side-effects are the main advantages of fosphenytoin over phenytoin. A disadvantage is the confusing units in which the dose is expressed, and fatal mistakes in dosing in A&E departments have been made. Fosphenytoin is more expensive than phenytoin, but cost-effectiveness studies have shown that the two drugs have equivalent value.

### Usual preparation

Fosphenytoin is formulated in a TRIS buffer at physiological pH. Phials of 50 mg phenytoin equivalents (PE) are available for mixture with dextrose or saline.

### Usual dosage

The dosage of the drug is expressed in PEs (thus, 15 mgPE of fosphenytoin is the same as 15 mg phenytoin). It is administered at a dose of 15 mgPE/kg at a rate of between 100 and 150 mgPE/min (100 mgPE/min is, in the author's experience, safer, so the average adult dose of 1000 mgPE is administered in 10 minutes). The drug is currently not recommended for children aged under 5 years. For older children the mgPE/min dose is the same as for adults.

## Isoflurane

Where inhalational anaesthesia is used to treat the stage of refractory status epilepticus status (a rare option), isoflurane is the drug of choice. It has advantages over other inhalational anaesthetics such as halothane or enflurane: lower solubility, less hepatotoxicity or nephrotoxicity, less effect on cardiac output, fewer cardiac arrhythmias, less hypotension, less effect on cerebral blood flow and autoregulation, less increase in intracranial pressure, less convulsant effect, and linear kinetics. It has a very rapid onset of action and recovery, and no tendency to accumulate. Although hypotension is common it is generally mild. There is no hepatic metabolism, and the drug is unaffected by hepatic or renal disease. There is, however, little published experience in status or of long-term use, and the major disadvantage is logistical, as isoflurane requires the use of an anaesthetic system with a scavenging apparatus which is inconvenient in most ITU situations. The other facilities required are the usual ones of assisted ventilation, intensive care, and cardio-respiratory monitoring.

### *Usual preparation*

Nearly pure (99.9%) liquid, for use in a correctly calibrated vaporizer via an anaesthetic system.

### *Usual dosage*

Inhalation of isoflurane at doses producing end-tidal concentrations of 0.8–2%, with the dose titrated to maintain a burst-suppression pattern on the EEG.

## Lidocaine

Lidocaine is a second-line drug for use in the stage of early status epilepticus only. It is given as a bolus injection or short IV infusion. The clinical effects and pharmacokinetics have been extensively studied in patients of all ages, and the drug is highly effective. The main disadvantage of lidocaine is that its antiepileptic effects are short-lived, and seizures are controlled for a matter of hours only. Lidocaine is thus useful only while more definitive antiepileptic drug treatment is administered. The risk of drug accumulation is low, and the incidence of respiratory or cerebral depression and hypotension is lower than with other antiepileptics. The drug may be particularly valuable in patients with respiratory disease. Other disadvantages include a possible proconvulsant effect at high levels, an active metabolite which may accumulate on prolonged therapy, the need for cardiac monitoring, as cardiac rhythm disturbances are common,

and the dependency of the clearance of lidocaine on hepatic blood flow.

### *Usual preparation*

A 5 ml ready-prepared syringe containing lidocaine 20 mg/ml (2%) or a 10 ml ready-prepared syringe containing lidocaine 10 mg/ml (1%) (i.e. both syringes contain 100 mg). Lidocaine is also available as a 5 ml vial containing 20 mg/ml (2%) (i.e. 100 mg) lidocaine or a 5 ml vial containing 200 mg/ml (20%) (i.e. 1000 mg) lidocaine, and as ready-made 0.1% (1 mg/ml) and 0.2% (2 mg/ml) infusions (in 500 ml containers in 5% dextrose).

### *Usual dosage*

Intravenous bolus injections of 1.5–2.0 mg/kg (usually 100 mg in adults), at a rate of injection not exceeding 50 mg/min. The bolus injection can be repeated once if necessary. A continuous infusion can be given at a rate of 3–4 mg/kg/h (usually of 0.2% solution in 5% dextrose, for no more than 12 hours); 3–6 mg/kg/h (neonates).

## Lorazepam

Lorazepam is the drug of choice in the stage of early status epilepticus, given by IV bolus injection. A single injection is highly effective, and the drug has a longer initial duration of action and a smaller risk of cardio-respiratory depression than does diazepam. There is little risk of drug accumulation, and also a lower risk of hypotension. The duration of action of lorazepam after a single initral infection is about 12 hours. However, the main disadvantage of lorazepam is a stronger tendency for tolerance to develop, and it is thus usable only as initial therapy, and longer-term maintenance antiepileptic drugs must be given in addition. There is a large clinical experience in adults, children and the newborn, with well-proven efficacy in tonic–clonic and partial status, and the pharmacology and pharmacokinetics of the drug are well characterized. Lorazepam is a stable compound which is not likely to precipitate in solution, and is relatively unaffected by hepatic or renal disease.

### *Usual preparation*

A 1 ml ampoule containing 4 mg/ml for IV injection.

### *Usual dosage*

IV bolus of 0.07 mg/kg (usually 4 mg), repeated after 10 minutes if necessary (adults); bolus of 0.1 mg/kg (children). The rate of injection is not crucial.

## Midazolam

Midazolam is another benzodiazepine, and it can be used in: (a) the premonitory stage or stage of early status epilepticus; or (b) as an anaesthetic in the stage of refractory status epilepticus. It is a water-soluble compound whose ring structure closes when in contact with serum to convert it into a highly lipophilic structure. Its solubility in water provides one major advantage over diazepam, that is, it can be rapidly absorbed by intramuscular (IM) injection or by intra-nasal or buccal administration. It is therefore useful in situations in which IV administration is difficult or ill-advised. In early status, blinded comparisons of buccal midazolam and rectal diazepam show no differences in efficacy or speed of action. Although there is a danger of accumulation on prolonged or repeated therapy, this tendency is less marked than with diazepam. There is, however, only limited published experience in adults or children with status. Occasionally severe cardio-respiratory depression occurs after IM administration, and other adverse effects include hypotension, apnoea, sedation and thrombophlebitis. Like diazepam, the drug is short acting, and there is a strong tendency for seizures to relapse after initial control, and as with diazepam its metabolism is altered by hepatic disease. Its half-life is prolonged in hepatic disease or in the elderly.

The use of midazolam as an intravenous anaesthetic in status epilepticus has become fashionable in recent years, in spite of an absence of controlled data. It is the only widely-used benzodiazepine that can be given by continuous intravenous infusion without a risk of drug accumulation. It carries a lower risk of hypotension than pentobarbital or thiopental, but the rate of rebound seizures on drug reduction is greater.

### Usual preparation
A 5 ml ampoule containing 2 mg/ml midazolam hydrochloride.

### Usual dosage
IM or rectally, 5–10 mg (adults); 0.15–0.3 mg/kg (children). This can be repeated once after 15 minutes. Buccal instillation of 10 mg can be given by a syringe and catheter in children or adults. For purposes of anaesthesia, an IV bolus of 0.1–0.3 mg/kg, at a rate not exceeding 4 mg/min, which can be repeated once after 15 minutes, and followed by an IV infusion, can be given at a rate of 0.05–0.4 mg/kg/h.

## Paraldehyde

Paraldehyde still has a minor role in premonitory stage given rectally, as an alternative to the benzodiazepines in situations where facilities for resuscitation are not available. Paraldehyde is rapidly and completely absorbed after IM injection or rectally. The risk of drug accumulation, hypotension or cardio-respiratory arrest is small, and seizures do not often recur after control has been obtained. Paraldehyde has been used for many years in status, and although there is wide experience in patients of all ages in status, no modern pharmacokinetic or clinical studies have been carried out. Toxicity is unusual provided the solution is freshly made, used immediately, and correctly diluted. The use of decomposed or inadequately diluted IV solutions is dangerous, causing precipitation, microembolism, thrombosis or cardio-respiratory collapse. The IM injection of paraldehyde is painful, and can cause sterile abscess and sciatic nerve damage if wrongly placed. Other side-effects include cardio-respiratory depression, sedation, and metabolic or lactic acidosis. The drug rapidly binds to plastic, and glass tubing and syringes are advisable unless injected immediately upon drawing the solution up. The drug should not be exposed to light. The half-life of paraldehyde is markedly increased by hepatic disease.

### Usual preparation
Ampoules containing 5 ml paraldehyde (equivalent to approximately 5 g) in darkened glass.

### Usual dosage
Paraldehdye can be given rectally (or IM), 5–10 ml diluted by the same volume of water for injection (adults) or 0.07–0.35 ml/kg (children). This dose can be repeated after 15–30 minutes.

## Pentobarbital

Pentobarbital is an alternative to thiopental, as barbiturate anaesthesia in the stage of refractory status epilepticus. It shares many of the characteristics of thiopental, but has the advantages of a shorter elimination half-life than thiopental, non-saturable kinetics, and no active metabolite. It is a stable compound and is unreactive with plastic. There is a surprising dearth of published information about its value, in spite of widespread use. Indeed, published trials have shown a uniformly poor outcome. Respiratory depression and sedation are invariable, and hypotension and cardio-respiratory dysfunction are common. Decerebrate posturing and flaccid paralysis occur during induction of anaesthesia, and a flaccid weakness can persist for weeks in survivors. There is a tend-ency for seizures to recur when the drug is withdrawn. It requires intensive care, artificial ventilatory support, and EEG and cardiovascular monitoring. Blood-level monitoring is usually advised, although there is in fact only an inconsistent relationship between serum levels and seizure control.

### Usual preparation
100 mg in a 2 ml injection vial, formulated in propylene glycol 40% and ethyl alcohol 10%.

### Usual dosage
IV loading dose of 10–20 mg/kg, at a rate not exceeding 25 mg/min, followed by a continuous infusion of 0.5–1.0 mg/kg/h, increasing if necessary to 1–3 mg/kg/h. Additional 5–20 mg/kg boluses can be given if breakthrough seizures occur. The dose should be tapered 12 hours after the last seizure by 0.5–1 mg/kg/h every 4–6 hours (depending on blood level).

## Phenobarbital

Phenobarbital is the drug of choice in the stage of established status epilepticus. It is a reliable antiepileptic drug, with well-proven effectiveness in tonic–clonic and partial status, and there is extensive clinical experience in adults, children and neonates. Phenobarbital has a stronger anticonvulsant action than other barbiturates and an additional potential cerebral protective action. It has a rapid-onset and long-lasting action, and can be administered much faster than can phenytoin. Its safety at high doses has been established, and the drug can be continued as chronic therapy. The disadvantages of the drug relate to prolonged use, where because of the long elimination half-life there is a risk of drug accumulation and inevitable sedation, respiratory depression, and hypotension. Marked auto-induction may also occur.

### Usual preparation

A 1 ml ampoule containing phenobarbital sodium 200 mg/ml in propylene glycol (90%) and water for injection (10%).

### Usual dosage

IV loading dose of 10 mg/kg at a rate of 100 mg/min (usual adult dose 600–800 mg), followed by maintenance dose of 1–4 mg/kg (adults). IV loading dose of 15–20 mg/kg, followed by maintenance dose of 3–4 mg/kg (children and neonates). Higher doses can be given, with monitoring of blood concentrations.

## Phenytoin

Phenytoin is a drug of choice and a highly effective medication for the stage of established status epilepticus. Extensive clinical experience has been gained in adults, children and neonates, and phenytoin has proven efficacy in tonic–clonic and partial status. The drug has a prolonged action, with a relatively small risk of respiratory or cerebral depression and no tendency for tachyphylaxis. Its main disadvantages are the time necessary to infuse the drug and its delayed onset of action. Fosphenytoin is a prodrug of phenytoin which can be administered more quickly. The pharmacokinetics of phenytoin are problematic, with zero-order kinetics at conventional doses and wide variation between individuals. Toxic side-effects include cardiac rhythm disturbances, thrombophlebitis and hypotension. The risk of cardiac side-effects is greatly increased if the recommended rate of injection is exceeded, and cardiac monitoring is advisable during phenytoin infusion. There is a risk of precipitation if phenytoin is diluted in solutions other than 0.9% saline or if mixed with other drugs.

### Usual preparation

A 5 ml ampoule containing 250 mg stabilized in propylene glycol, ethanol and water (alternatives exist, e.g. phenytoin in TRIS buffer or in infusion bottles of 750 mg in 500 ml of osmotic saline).

### Usual dosage

In adults, a 15–18 mg/kg IV infusion. This can be given via the side arm of a drip or, preferably, directly via an infusion pump. The rate of infusion should not exceed 50 mg/min (20 mg/min in the elderly). In children a 20 mg/kg IV infusion is usually given, at a rate not exceeding 25 mg/min. The drug should never be given by IM injection.

## Propofol

Propofol is the anaesthetic agent of choice for non-barbiturate infusional anaesthesia in the stage of refractory status epilepticus. It is an excellent anaesthetic with very good pharmacokinetic properties. In status, it has a very rapid onset of action and rapid recovery. There are few haemodynamic side-effects, and the drug has been used in all ages. There is, however, only limited published experience of its use in status, or indeed of prolonged infusions. Unlike isoflurane, it is metabolized in the liver and affected by severe hepatic disease. As with all anaesthetics, its use requires assisted ventilation, intensive care and intensive care monitoring. It causes lipaemia and acidosis, and there have been complications and deaths associated with its use as a prolonged infusion in children, and because of this it is relatively contra-indicated in children and infants. Involuntary movements (without EEG change) can occur, and should not be confused with seizure activity. Rebound seizures are a problem when it is discontinued too rapidly, and a decremental rate of 1 mg/kg every 2 hours is recommended when the drug is to be withdrawn.

### Usual preparation

A 20 ml ampoule containing 10 mg/ml (i.e. 200 mg) as an emulsion.

### Usual dosage

A 2 mg/kg bolus, repeated if necessary, and then followed by a continuous infusion of 5–10 mg/kg/h initially, reducing to 1–3 mg/kg/h. When seizures have been controlled for 12 hours, the drug dose should be slowly tapered over 12 hours.

## Thiopental

Thiopental is, in most countries, the usual choice for barbiturate anaesthesia in the stage of refractory status epilepticus. It is a highly effective antiepileptic drug, with additional potential cerebral protective action. It reduces intracranial pressure and cerebral blood flow, and has a very rapid onset of action. Its principal metabolite is pentobarbital. The drug has a number of pharmacokinetic disadvantages including saturable kinetics, a strong tendency to accumulate, and a prolonged recovery time after anaesthesia is withdrawn. Blood-level monitoring of the parent drug and its active metabolite (pentobarbital) is advisable on prolonged therapy. There is often some tachyphylaxis owing to its sedative and to a lesser extent its anticonvulsant properties. Respiratory depression and sedation are inevitable, and hypotension is common. Other less common side-effects include pancreatitis, hepatic dysfunction, and spasm at the injection site. Full intensive care facilities with artificial ventilatory support and intensive EEG and cardiovascular monitoring are needed. It can react with co-medication, and with plastic giving sets, and is unstable when exposed to air. Autoinduction occurs, and hepatic disease prolongs the elimination of thiopental. Although it is extensively used in the treatment of status epilepticus, this is only on the basis of anecdotal published case series.

### Usual preparation

Injection of thiopental sodium 2.5 g with 100 ml, and 5 g with 200 ml diluent (to make 100 and 200 ml of a 2.5% solution). It is also available as 500 mg and 1 g vials to make 2.5% solutions.

### Usual dosage

100–250 mg IV bolus given over 20 seconds, with further 50 mg boluses every 2–3 minutes until seizures are controlled, followed by a continuous IV infusion to maintain a burst-suppression pattern on the EEG (usually 3–5 mg/kg/h). The dose should be lowered if systolic blood pressure falls below 90 mmHg despite cardiovascular support. Thiopental should be slowly withdrawn 12 hours after the last seizure.

## Valproate

Intravenous valproate has been shown to be effective by bolus intravenous injection in the stage of established epilepsy, albeit in uncontrolled open studies. It is an effective antiepileptic which is safe to use in children and adults. In small series it was shown to be rapidly effective after fast administration with remarkably few side-effects. On anecdotal evidence, it seems to be associated with much lower rates of drug-induced hypotension and drug-induced respiratory or cerebral depression than other drugs (e.g. phenytoin, fosphenytoin or phenobarbital), and these are significant advantages. It can also be infused rapidly (within 5–10 minutes in adults). In adults, a dose of 25 mg/kg produces levels which are generally therapeutic (above 100 mg/l).

### Usual preparation

Injection of 400 mg valproate powder with vial of 4 ml ampoule of water for injection (100 mg/ml).

### Usual dosage

25 mg/kg in adults and 30–40 mg/kg in children. The rate of injection should be between 3 and 6 mg/kg/min.

# 5 The surgical treatment of epilepsy

## INTRODUCTION

The evolution of the surgical treatment of epilepsy in the past century has been dependent on, and largely dictated by, technical developments. The first resective surgery was performed in 1880, following improvements in anaesthetics and surgical instrumentation. Surgical treatment remained a therapeutic curiosity, however, until the late 1930s, when the introduction of EEG ushered in a period of intensive development. EEG provided the first objective method for localizing epileptic tissue. EEG and clinical localization were combined and this approach, which is still the basis of epilepsy surgery today, improved both diagnostic accuracy and surgical outcome. Temporal lobe epilepsy became a focus of attention, and the first temporal lobectomy was carried out in the 1940s. The standard operation with removal of hippocampus, devised by Penfield, was carried out in 1951. Intracranial depth EEG was first carried out in 1944 and video and EEG-video telemetry in the mid-1960s.

Imaging at this stage was confined to skull radiology and air encephalographyasigns such as asymmetrical dilatation of the horns of the lateral ventricles or changes in middle fossa curvature–were relied upon to suggest hippocampal sclerosis (both signs now thoroughly discredited!), and air encephalography and angiography were used to diagnose tumours and vascular malformations. Computerized tomography (CT) was introduced in 1971 and allowed the visualization of vascular and mass lesions. In 1982 the first magnetic resonance imaging (MRI) image in an epileptic patient was reported. Since then, the use of MRI has simplified pre-surgical investigation and improved patient selection. Hippocampal sclerosis and cortical dysplasia, which are largely invisible to CT or other forms of X-ray imaging, are readily identified by MRI. As a result, there has been a considerable increase in the proportion of patients for whom resective surgery has become a realistic option. Surgical technique has also improved through technological advance. The first stereotactic atlas was published in 1957, the use of the operative microscope became widespread in the late 1960s, and MRI has provided audit feedback in resective neurosurgery. Neuro-anaesthesia has also improved progressively, allowing more targeted surgery with less morbidity.

Figures have varied, but at a conservative estimate between 2 and 5% of individuals with medically refractory partial epilepsy might benefit from epilepsy surgery. Thus, about 100–250 cases per million persons in a population would benefit from epilepsy surgery, with the addition of about 10–25 new patients per million persons per year.

### Epilepsy surgery

Epilepsy surgery is defined as surgery carried out specifically to control epileptic seizures. This will include operations on tumours and vascular lesions where epilepsy is the primary indication for surgery. There is clearly an overlap with lesional surgery carried out for other primary reasons, if the lesion is causing epilepsy, and even if the operation influences the epilepsy, such operations are not generally included in epilepsy surgery statistics. The distinction though is not always clear-cut and the control of epilepsy can be an important additional consideration in the decision to undertake surgery. The term epilepsy surgery also implies a particular mindset and a specific approach to pre-surgical assessment which is discussed further below.

There are five main types of surgical approach:
1 Focal resection for hippocampal sclerosis and other lesions in the mesial temporal lobe;
2 Focal resections for other overt lesions (lesionectomies) in temporal neocortex or other cortical areas;
3 Non-lesional focal resections (where there is no lesion on imaging, but epileptic tissue is localized by functional methods and/or on clinical grounds);
4 Hemispherectomy, hemispherotomy and other multi-lobar resections;
5 Functional procedures—multiple subpial transection, corpus callosectomy, focal ablation, focal stimulation, vagal nerve stimulation.

The frequency of these operations in contemporary UK surgical practice is shown in Table 5.1.

**Table 5.1** The approximate frequency of different forms of epilepsy surgery in modern surgical practice in the UK.

| | |
|---|---|
| Focal resections for hippocampal sclerosis (e.g. temporal lobectomy, amygdalohippocampectomy) | 65% |
| Focal resections for other lesions | 20% |
| Non-lesional focal resections | 5% |
| Hemispherectomy, hemispherotomy and multi-lobar resections | 5% |
| Functional procedures (e.g. corpus callosectomy, multiple subpial transection, vagal nerve stimulation) | 5% |

**Table 5.2** Aims of pre-surgical assessment for epilepsy surgery.

To confirm that the patient has epilepsy, and that the seizures are medically intractable

To define the outcome goals of the chosen surgical procedure (e.g. seizure freedom [usually], 50% reduction in seizures) and estimate the chances of attaining this successful outcome

To define the likely gains in terms of quality of life if surgery is carried out

To determine the risks of carrying out the surgical procedure—for instance in terms of mortality, neurological morbidity, psychological and social effects; also the risks of not operating

To determine that the person is medically fit for surgery

To counsel the patient appropriately about the outcome and risks

## PRE-SURGICAL ASSESSMENT—GENERAL POINTS

### Selection of patients

As a general rule, surgical treatment should be at least considered in any patient with partial seizures that are intractable to medical therapy. When surgery is to be contemplated, the patient should be referred to an experienced epilepsy surgery team for pre-surgical evaluation. The evaluation will depend on the type of surgery being proposed, but in general terms assessment has the aims listed in Table 5.2.

Pre-surgical assessment requires specialist knowledge and a specific approach to investigation that are not usually available outside a tertiary centre. This process is usually emotionally demanding and time-consuming. The patient should be made aware of this at the outset. Not infrequently, surgery will prove not to be possible, and this rejection can be devastating for a person who has made a considerable emotional investment in the process. The decision to proceed with surgery is, in view of its risks and uncertainties, often difficult, and the balance of risks and benefits seldom clear-cut. The decision must always be an individual one, and one made by the patient; the doctor's role is to provide information and to advise. The decision

should be a considered choice on the basis of the information provided. The patient must feel confident that sufficient information has been given, and that this information is accurate and unbiased. Surgery should never be performed if the patient is reluctant or undecided. The specific investigations and operations are covered in subsequent sections. However, a few general points can be made here.

### Medically intractable epilepsy

The definition of 'medically intractable' is arbitrary, and strictly speaking, epilepsy can be defined as intractable only in retrospect. For pragmatic reasons, in the author's usual practice, epilepsy is regarded as sufficiently intractable to contemplate surgery if it has been continuously active for 5 years (or less in severe epilepsy) in spite of adequate trials of therapy with three or more main-line antiepileptic drugs, and if seizures are frequent (more than one per month). The chances of further medical therapy controlling seizures after 5 years of intractability, thus defined, depend on the skills of the treating physician, but are generally less than 10–20% with currently available drugs. Other authorities have used different criteria. A recent trend has been to define intractability earlier—after 2 or 3 years of failure to respond to medical therapy—based on studies that show that an early failure of treatment is generally predictive of later intractability. However, common clinical experience shows that in some patients seizures are initially uncontrolled by drugs but do respond later. For this reason, it seems to this author at least that, in most cases, a 2–3 year history of epilepsy is too short a period to recommend proceeding to surgical therapy.

These criteria are guidelines only, and there will be patients in whom epilepsy surgery is appropriate, and yet who do not fulfil these criteria. For instance, some patients with lesional epilepsy may be operated upon after a single seizure. The merits of each case should be considered individually, and this requires skill and experience.

### Estimating the seizure outcome after surgery and the risks of surgery

The purpose of the pre-surgical evaluation is to provide an estimate of outcome in terms of seizure control and surgical risk. The estimate should be based both on the literature and where possible the audited record of the surgical unit. The estimate of outcome and risk depends on the nature of the epilepsy, the nature of the surgery being offered, and other factors (see below). Estimates are usually given in percentage terms. A common example is the 50–70% chance of freedom from seizures following a modified anterior temporal lobectomy in an uncomplicated case of mesial temporal epilepsy. The estimates of risk and outcome should be given in writing to the patient, who must be given time for careful consideration and who should also be offered the opportunity for discussion and counselling. The patient's family or carers should usually be included in the discussion, and it must be clear that the patient fully comprehends the risks.

One risk, poorly studied, is the possibility that resective surgery lowers 'cerebral reserve', and that over time this reduction in reserve capacity will lead to late deterioration. Certainly, one encounters patients who years after surgery have deteriorated intellectually, but there are no formal studies of this important issue.

### Quality of life gain

The prediction of the extent of the expected quality of life gain due to surgery is a key part of the pre-surgical assessment. Surgery should be offered only to those whose quality of life is seriously compromised by the occurrence of seizures and in whom the expected outcome of surgery is likely to result in major overall improvement in the quality of life. This may seem obvious, but it is in fact often difficult to decide. The focus of this assessment should be broader than simple seizure control. There are patients who have had surgery which successfully controls seizures but who regret having had the operation, and whose life has shown little improvement. Frequent seizures—for example mild seizures, simple partial seizures or seizures occurring only at night—are not necessarily disabling. In some situations, even severe seizures are not the key determinant of quality of life, for instance in patients with multiple disabling features. Emotional factors are important, and surgery that is successful in controlling seizures will not automatically alleviate other negative lifestyle aspects, even if these have been moulded by the epilepsy. Social structures and interpersonal relationships may be predicated on a lifetime of seizures, and their sudden cure by surgery may result in changes in personal circumstances that can be hard to adjust to (this has been termed 'the burden of normality'). Skilful counselling is vital in this area.

### Non-epileptic seizures

It is not uncommon for a patient to be referred for surgery who on investigation turns out to have non-epileptic seizures, either alone or in combination with genuine epileptic attacks. Generally speaking, non-epileptic attacks —even in combination with genuine attacks—are a contraindication for surgery. Therapy should be directed at the physical or psychological causes that underpin these attacks. If surgery is carried out in patients with a combination of attacks, the psychogenic attacks frequently worsen even if the genuine attacks are relieved. Once non-epileptic attacks have been successfully alleviated by psychological therapies, the question of surgery can be revisited. Decisions about surgical treatment in this area should be made only in a specialist setting.

### Learning disability, behavioural disorder and psychosis

Learning disability (a full-scale IQ < 70) is a complicating factor when considering surgical therapy, for a number of reasons. First, it often indicates widespread cerebral dysfunction and resective surgery is less likely to control seizures even if a single lesion is demonstrable. Furthermore, in multiply handicapped persons, epilepsy may not be the most important aspect of disability, and control of seizures will not necessarily lead to major gains in quality of life. Finally, 'cerebral reserve' may be lower in persons with learning disability. On the other hand, many patients with learning disability are severely handicapped by severe epilepsy and have the potential for great benefit from surgery. Expert evaluation of these issues is necessary for all affected individuals, and the risk–benefit equation needs careful formulation and discussion with the patient and carers. The ethical issues surrounding informed consent are extremely important, and can be difficult.

Surgery is generally also contra-indicated in individuals who show severely dysfunctional behaviour. It should not be contemplated if it is likely that the patient will not be able to tolerate the intensive investigation or hospitalization required for epilepsy surgery, nor make informed and considered judgements about the potential risks and benefits of epilepsy surgery, nor be able to exploit the opportunities afforded by successful surgery.

The presence of a chronic interictal psychosis is also generally a contra-indication to surgery, as the psychosis can worsen dramatically after surgery. Decisions about surgical treatment should not be made by severely depressed patients. Psychosis and depression may also prevent informed consent. Again, individual decisions in this situation require a detailed assessment by an experienced practitioner.

### Medical fitness and age

Some patients have added risks due to general medical problems, for instance cervical, spinal or vascular disease. Surgery should only be contemplated in those who can withstand prolonged anaesthesia.

Surgery is usually restricted to those under the age of 50 years. Above this age, lifestyle is often adapted well to the epilepsy and may be difficult to change. The risks of surgery may be greater, and in the ageing brain the adverse consequences can be more severe. The reduction in cerebral reserve can be more critical in older ages groups. Age, however, is only one factor, and the key assessment is the potential for quality of life gain, whatever the patient's age.

### The timing of epilepsy surgery

In recent years there has been a vogue for recommending surgery at an early stage in epilepsy, especially in children. This is to minimize the impact of the seizure disorder on education and social development, to minimize the potential for morbidity or death due to epileptic seizures, to prevent the possibility of secondary epileptogenesis (either through injury or 'kindling') and the possibility of progressive intellectual or behavioural decline, and to minimize the psychological impact of epilepsy.

The recommendation for early surgery applies particularly in children and seizures pose additional risks to the developing brain of infants and young children. Uncontrolled seizures also jeopardize the chances for an independent lifestyle, and children with intractable epilepsy are likely to be excluded from normal educational, social and vocational opportunities.

## Approach to investigation

There are a number of investigatory modalities used in assessing suitability for epilepsy surgery: interictal scalp EEG, ictal scalp EEG, intracranial EEG, MRI, neuropsychological tests, and functional imaging with single photon emission computed tomography (SPECT), positron emission tomography (PET), and fMRI (Table 5.3). The use of these should be protocol-driven, and tests should be performed to answer specific questions. Their role and value depend on the type of surgery being performed (see below), but the following general points apply to all resective surgery and underpin investigation in all forms of epilepsy surgery.

## The concept of the epileptogenic zone

The approach to resective surgery for epilepsy can, since the time of Horsley, be summarized as follows. In many cases of epilepsy, the seizures originate in a small area of brain (the epileptic focus). Surgery aims to resect this epileptogenic tissue, sufficient in extent to lead to the resolution of the seizures. Unfortunately, this is a simplistic view—a phrenological approach to brain function—and often patently incorrect. A clear-cut and restricted 'focus' of epileptic brain tissue does exist in some cases, particularly in epilepsy due to extra-temporal neocortical lesions. However, in many, seizures are in fact sustained by quite widespread and complex neuronal networks and circuits. In such cases, the concept of a discrete focus is both naïve and untenable. It is as a response to this problem that the concept of the *epileptogenic zone* has gained currency, but this concept too

**Table 5.3** The approach to pre-surgical investigation taken at the National Hospital for Neurology and Neurosurgery, London.

| | |
|---|---|
| Medical history and examination | All patients |
| Psychiatric assessment | All patients |
| 24-channel scalp EEG (and review of previous EEG) | All patients |
| Seizure recordings using video-EEG telemetry | 95% of patients |
| MRI imaging at 1.5 T1-weighted thin slice volumetric, T2 and FLAIR acquisitions | All patients |
| Regional measurement of hippocampal volume and of T2 signal intensity | All patients undergoing investigation with a view to hippocampal surgery. >50% of patients with extra-hippocampal lesions to determine outcome and guide surgical planning |
| Other MRI techniques are used, selected from the following: MR angiography, diffusion imaging, perfusion imaging, MR spectroscopy, fMRI, 3D reconstruction and rendering of the cortical surface, surface area/volume measurements. Co-registration with EEG, angiographic, SPECT or PET | All patients with normal MRI ('MRI-negative cases') being investigated with a view to resective surgery. In selected patients, techniques are selected to answer specific questions. MRS used mainly in hippocampal epilepsy, and other tests in extra-hippocampal epilepsy. Use of diffusion scanning, perfusion scanning, surface area/volume measurements fMRI and fMRI-EEG is still confined largely to research |
| Other neuroimaging techniques (CT, plain skull radiography, angiography) | In a few selected patients |
| Neuropsychological assessment of general intellectual ability, language and memory | All patients |
| Other neuropsychological tests | Selected patients to address specific questions. Used mainly in extra-hippocampal epilepsy |
| Sodium amytal test | Selected patients undergoing hippocampal surgery (about 10% of the total) |
| Intracranial EEG | 5–10% of patients (see text for indications) |
| Functional imaging using HMPAO-SPECT or FDG PET | 5–10% of patients (see text for indications) |
| Other functional imaging investigations (ligand or receptor PET, MEG, SISCOM), TMS | Use still confined largely to research |
| Individual counselling | All patients |

is fraught with difficulty and inconsistency. This term is defined as the anatomical area necessary and sufficient for initiating seizures and whose removal or disconnection is necessary for the abolition of seizures. The pre-surgical evaluation of a patient, therefore (it is argued), aims to define the anatomical boundaries of the epileptogenic zone, and having done so, the feasibility and risks of resection. Unfortunately, there are no preoperative clinical or laboratory tests that can define the area in any individual patient. It is only possible to ascertain whether an 'epileptogenic zone' was successfully resected after years of postoperative freedom from seizures—and even then without knowing how much unnecessary resection of additional brain tissue was carried out. This is unsatisfactory, and the concept of the epileptogenic zone, in the author's opinion, adds little to that of the epileptic focus. The concept, however, has one virtue—it emphasizes what has been known for more than half a century, that the amount of brain resection necessary often extends beyond the lesion visualized on neuroimaging or the cortical area that generates interictal spikes.

This latter area is often known as the *irritative zone*. The irritative zone can extend beyond the epileptogenic zone, and it is common for residual tissue left after surgery to exhibit active spiking on electrocorticography (ECoG). Furthermore, the apparent extent of the irritative zone will vary with differing types of EEG investigation. On ictal recordings the electrographic onset of a seizure is sometimes known as the *ictal onset zone*. This area provides a rough indication of where to target surgery, but again its value depends on the extent to which the epileptic network is localized, and the method of investigation employed.

It has been shown pragmatically that the incomplete resection of structurally abnormal areas of brain tissue often fails to control seizures, but even complete excision does not always result in seizure control. The chance of success depends on the aetiology of the lesion—the resection of most types of cortical dysplasia, for instance, has a much lower success rate than that of mesial temporal sclerosis. The reasons are complex. Subtle anatomical changes may be present beyond the resolution of neuroimaging. Also, complex neuronal networks can spread well beyond the anatomical or even pathological defects.

The complexity of seizure generation is well demonstrated in mesial temporal lobe epilepsy. Here there is good experimental and clinical evidence that the seizures involve a network that extends well beyond the mesial temporal lobe, yet resection of the hippocampus, which will remove only part of this network, is often successful in controlling seizures (although auras often remain—further evidence that the 'focus' of the epilepsy cannot be simply the abnormal hippocampus). Furthermore, the presence of residual spiking in the brain tissue adjacent to the resection (detected on per-operative ECoG) is not predictive of surgical outcome;

and many patients with residual spiking will be rendered completely seizure free.

In contrast to the situation in mesial temporal lobe epilepsy where restricted resections are often adequate, in neocortical areas, the bigger the resection, the more likely is seizure control (a 'more is better' surgical approach proposed many times since the introduction of epilepsy surgery). Nevertheless, even in apparently well-localized non-lesional frontal epilepsy, resection of large areas of frontal cortex will stop seizures in only a relatively small proportion of patients.

## The principle of concordance of investigations

An observation fundamental to pre-surgical assessment is that resective surgery is more likely to be successful if the findings from the different modalities of pre-surgical investigations are concordant—i.e. if each points to a similar localization of seizure onset. Conversely, if results are discordant, resective surgery is likely to be less successful. It follows that all patients require multi-modal investigation aimed at defining the seizure localization. There are four main components of investigation—radiological, neurophysiological, psychological and clinical. Different centres use different methods of investigation in these four areas (see below) but all four modalities should be carried out in the majority of patients being worked up for surgery. It follows also that incomplete or unfocused investigation has a higher failure rate. It is for these reasons that pre-surgical evaluation is best carried out in a designated centre with multi-disciplinary experience.

## The importance of aetiology

A key determinant of surgical outcome, independent of electroclinical localization, is the underlying aetiology. This is why MRI has proved so important in the surgical work-up. Indeed, because of this, MRI should be the starting point of all investigations. Resective surgery is best for those with well-localized lesions shown on MRI, especially those with unilateral mesial temporal lobe sclerosis, small cavernomas, or benign or low-grade tumours. The demonstration of aetiology is also of prognostic importance in other types of surgery, for instance for hemispherectomy and for corpus callosectomy.

## MRI as a screening test, and MRI-negative cases

Prior to the introduction of MRI many cases of epilepsy (including virtually all cases of hippocampal sclerosis) were 'non-lesional', in the sense that no lesion could be detected pre-operatively. The nature and extent of the surgery in these cases depended on clinico-electrographic localization, and thus on scalp and invasive EEG. It was realized even then that if no pathology was found in the pathological examination of the excised specimen, the prognosis for seizure control was likely to be poor.

The advent of MRI has radically altered the clinical approach, as pre-operative MRI can identify most previously occult lesions. The dependency on EEG for localization has been lost, and the requirement for invasive EEG has been greatly reduced. It has been shown that if MRI shows no lesion pre-operatively, a so-called MRI-negative epilepsy, the chances of successful surgery are greatly diminished, even after intensive work-up using other modalities. In routine practice, therefore, MRI has become in effect a screening test for further surgical evaluation and has now displaced EEG in this role. The question of surgery in MRI-negative cases is discussed further below.

## SURGERY IN EPILEPSY ARISING IN THE MESIAL TEMPORAL LOBE

### Pathology of mesial temporal lobe epilepsy

The most common pathology causing temporal lobe epilepsy is hippocampal sclerosis (more accurately known as mesial temporal sclerosis). The principal abnormality is hippocampal neuronal cell loss, which has a characteristic distribution with maximum loss in the CA1 and CA3 regions and in the hilar region of dentate gyrus, and relative sparing of the CA2 region (Figure 5.1). There is also dense fibrous gliosis. The cell loss and gliosis result in atrophy, and the hippocampus is shrunken and hardened. Another common abnormality is an alteration in the laminar arrangement of the dentate gyrus, with dispersal of cells or sometimes duplication of the laminar structure. There is extensive synaptic rearrangement, including recurrent innervation of dentate granule cells by their own neurones, which reinnervate instead of projecting into the hippocampus proper. This aberrant 'mossy fibre' innervation results in alterations in excitatory and inhibitory balance. A large number of neurochemical changes have been documented in the sclerotic hippocampus, although the extent to which these are primary changes or simply consequential to the hippocampal injury is often unclear. There are also pathological changes outside the hippocampus, including widespread subpial fibrillary gliosis (Chaslin gliosis) and nerve cell loss in the neocortex, and gliosis and volume loss in the entorhinal cortex and other mesial structures. Cerebellar atrophy and widespread cerebral atrophy are also not uncommon. In some series, over 70% of patients with hippocampal sclerosis also show some evidence of micro-dysgenesis. MRI morphometry has also recently shown, in cases of unilateral hippocampal sclerosis, a mean 15% reduction of the volume of the rest of the temporal lobe, reductions of similar magnitude in the parahippocampal gyrus and middle and inferior temporal gyri, and a 25% reduction in mean size of the superior temporal gyrus.

Mesial temporal lobe epilepsy can also be caused by tumours (in about 10–15% of all cases of surgically treated mesial temporal lobe epilepsy). The most common are low-grade gliomas, oligodendroglioma and other astrocytic or glial tumours. Cortical dysplasia, of various types is also associated with hippocampal sclerosis, even if the dysplasia does not itself involve the hippocampus. This accounts for a further 15–25% of cases. Trauma, cavernous haemangioma (cavernoma) and other vascular disease, and cerebral infections (meningitis or encephalitis) can also result in temporal lobe epilepsy. The latter two categories carry a generally poorer surgical prognosis by virtue of the more widespread epileptogenic changes.

### Which patients should be evaluated

The general rules mentioned above (pp. 232–4) apply. Usually, a patient will be referred with a history of temporal lobe seizures and an MRI showing a hippocampal lesion (most commonly hippocampal sclerosis). The process of pre-operative evaluation should follow the following standard protocol.

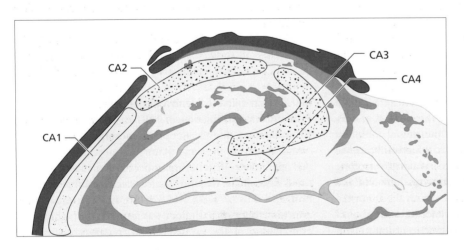

**Figure 5.1** The characteristic pattern of hippocampal cell loss in hippocampal sclerosis—note the severe pyramidal cell loss of the CA1, CA3 and CA4 regions, with relative sparing of CA2 region. Black lines are drawn to outline the boundaries of the regions.

## Clinical history and examination

A detailed history of the seizure disorder, its prior treatment and its causation must be obtained. Hippocampal sclerosis usually causes complex partial seizures of mesial temporal lobe type (see pp. 13–14). Additional secondary generalized tonic–clonic seizures are typically absent or infrequent, and indeed a history of secondarily generalized seizures is associated with poorer outcome following temporal lobe surgery. Other seizure types are not to be expected in hippocampal epilepsy, and their presence indicates an epileptogenic zone that extends beyond the mesial temporal lobe structures. A history of childhood febrile convulsions (especially if prolonged or focal) is very strongly associated with hippocampal sclerosis. The outcome of hippocampal surgery is better if such a history is present (and that of surgery for extra-hippocampal epilepsy is worse). The presence of a family history also worsens surgical outcome.

A detailed neurological history should include the following aspects: the observable features of the seizures, the aura and seizure manifestations as experienced by the patient, postictal features, lateralizing features, seizure precipitants, the onset and temporal evolution of the seizures, their pattern over time, seizure frequency and timing, family history, and response to therapy. The aetiology of the epilepsy can often be ascertained from the history and enquiry should be directed towards this. The clinical history may provide clues to the localization, and discordance between the clinical and investigatory localization should warn against surgery.

There are usually no signs on clinical examination, and indeed if motor or cognitive signs (other than memory defects —see below) are present, this implies extra-hippocampal damage. The examination should be meticulously recorded to document pre-operative deficit as a baseline for comparison with post-operative findings.

The patient's medical status and general suitability for a long anaesthetic and intracranial surgery should be assessed.

## Psychiatric assessment

A detailed neuropsychiatric evaluation is a vital part of the pre-surgical assessment and should be carried out routinely in the early stages of the assessment process. The structured clinical interview schedule can be backed up by the use of rating scales which might include: Neurobehavioural Inventory, State–Trait Anxiety Inventory, Beck Depression Inventory, Subjective Handicap of Epilepsy Scale, Quality of Life in Epilepsy Scale, and the Minnesota Multiphasic Personality Inventory. The evaluation has four purposes:

**1** To identify the presence of psychiatric contra-indications to surgery. Usually, surgery should not be performed in patients with ongoing interictal psychosis, severe personality disorder or psychopathy, co-morbid non-epileptic seizures, or ongoing alcohol or drug abuse. Peri-ictal psychosis is often considered to be a factor weighing on the side of epilepsy surgery, although this is not the author's experience. A history of severe depression or obsessive–compulsive disorder is also a relative contra-indication to surgery.

**2** To estimate the ability of the person to withstand the long process of surgical evaluation and any adverse consequences of surgery. Psychosocial support is often needed post-operatively, and surgery should not be offered to vulnerable individuals in the absence of such support.

**3** To confirm that the patient is able to provide informed consent for the procedure.

**4** To estimate the potential for psychological and psychiatric quality of life gains post-operatively, if seizure control is achieved. This requires judgement and experience, and the epilepsy rating scales can be helpful adjuncts. The patient should be encouraged to focus on this issue.

Psychiatry is, however, not an exact science, and the predictive value of premorbid psychiatric features is not fully established. This is a crucial deficiency, and high-quality research data in this area are largely lacking.

## Magnetic resonance imaging (MRI)

MRI is undertaken in all patients undergoing evaluation for epilepsy surgery. Indeed, it is now the primary screening test for entry into a programme of pre-surgical evaluation. The imaging must be of an appropriate quality and tailored to the visualization of mesial temporal pathologies. Substandard MRI, for instance with wide inter-slice intervals or sequences with poor grey/white differentiation, frequently fails to detect hippocampal sclerosis, which is then shown on better targeted imaging. For pre-surgical assessment in our own unit, the minimum MRI dataset applied, using high-quality 1.5-tesla scanning, is as follows:

• A volume acquisition T1-weighted coronal dataset that covers the whole brain in slices of 1 or 1.5 mm thickness (a sequence that provides approximately cubic voxels which can be used for reformatting in any orientation, quantitation of hippocampal volume and other morphological measures, three-dimensional reconstruction, and surface rendering).

• An oblique inversion recovery sequence, heavily T1 weighted, and oriented perpendicularly to the long axis of the hippocampus (a sequence that provides good hippocampal anatomical definition and contrast).

• An oblique T2-weighted sequence oriented perpendicularly to the long axis of the hippocampus (a sequence that provides the basis for regional hippocampal T2 intensity measurement).

• FLAIR or fast-FLAIR (sequences that increase the sensitivity of MRI to hippocampal sclerosis and other lesions).

This MRI approach can demonstrate hippocampal sclerosis with high specificity and sensitivity (Figure 5.2). The primary MRI signs of hippocampal sclerosis are loss

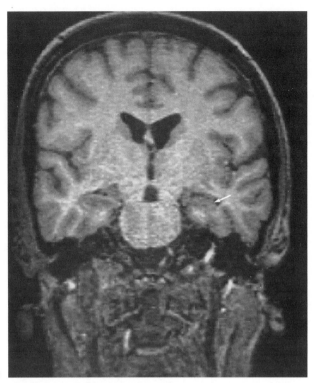

(a)

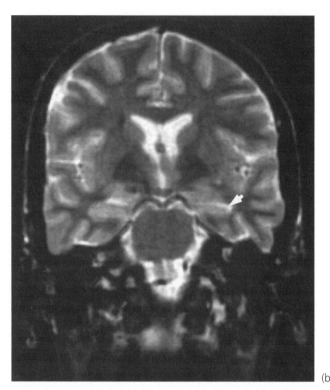

(b)

**Figure 5.2** (a) Left-sided hippocampal atrophy (arrowed), with low intensity within the hippocampus on $T_1$-weighted image. (b) $T_2$-weighted image at same location reveals minor signal-intensity increase of hippocampus on left (arrowed). It is interesting to note that there are only subtle T2 changes despite atrophy of over 50% on volumetry.

of volume on T1-weighted imaging and increased T2-weighted signal (the latter sign being less constant than the former). Other much less reliable signs are the loss of grey–white differentiation and loss of internal structure of the hippocampus. However, care must be taken not to misinterpret the MRI signs. On occasion, hippocampal atrophy is the result not the cause of epilepsy (e.g. after status epilepticus or in lesional cortical epilepsies). A swollen hippocampus on one side due to tumour can lead to the mistaken diagnosis of an atrophic contralateral hippocampus. Increased hippocampal T2 signal is a relatively non-specific sign which occurs also in patients with hippocampal tumour, vascular or developmental abnormalities, and in traumatic or post-infective lesions. Seizure activity, during or immediately before the scan, will occasionally also produce increased T2 signal. Also, in a sizeable number of patients, MRI will demonstrate more than one potentially causative lesion (so-called 'dual pathology'; see below).

Measuring the volume of the hippocampus (hippocampal volumetry) and hippocampal T2 values is also routinely undertaken in patients being assessed for hippocampal surgery (Figure 5.3). These measurements provide objective information about the severity of the hippocampal sclerosis and also the detection of bilateral damage. Volumetry is also used in many patients with extra-hippocampal lesions, as co-existing hippocampal atrophy worsens the prognosis

in extra-hippocampal lesional epilepsy and assists in deciding whether to include hippocampal resection during extra-hippocampal surgery.

Other techniques are used in selected cases, including MR angiography, diffusion imaging, perfusion imaging, MR spectroscopy, fMRI and three-dimensional reconstruction and rendering of the cortical surface, and surface area and volume measurements of other brain structures. Each technique assists in addressing specific issues and interpretation of the tests requires a good understanding of the clinical context. The importance of tailoring the MRI examination to address specific questions cannot be overemphasized, and in this sense MRI differs from CT. Co-registration of MRI and other investigatory modalities (such as EEG, angiography, fMRI, SPECT or PET) is used in complex cases to aid the localization of abnormal findings and to aid surgical planning.

### Other forms of neuroimaging

Computerized X-ray tomography (CT) still has a role in detecting small calcified lesions (e.g. small low-grade tumours in cysticercosis) which can be overlooked on MRI, and where MRI is contra-indicated (e.g. patients with pacemakers, aneurysm clips, metal plates, other metal implants). MRI is relatively contra-indicated in patients with vagal nerve stimulators, but CT can be safely used. Plain skull

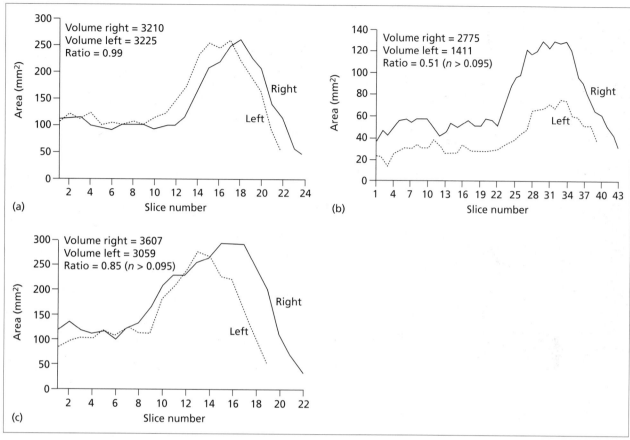

**Figure 5.3** Three graphs showing regional hippocampal volume. In the graphs, the cross-sectional areas of the hippocampus are measured from successive slices of volumetric T1-weighted coronal MRI images of the hippocampus covering the whole anterior to posterior extent of the hippocampus and amygdala. The MRI slices are spaced 1.5 mm apart. (a) Normal hippocampus. (b) Gross generalized hippocampal atrophy. (c) Focal anterior hippocampal atrophy.

radiography is now largely redundant. Conventional invasive angiography is still used, mainly to determine the anatomical features of blood supply to vascular malformations and also prior to depth electrode placement, where angiographic findings can be co-registered with other neuroimaging techniques to guide the positioning of electrodes. MRI angiography is likely to replace invasive angiography in these roles over the next few years.

### Interictal scalp EEG

Three aspect of the interictal scalp EEG should be emphasized:

**1** Clear-cut unilateral interictal abnormalities, when present, are a relatively good lateralizing sign in isolated mesial temporal lobe pathology (Figure 5.4). False localization occurs in less than 5% of such cases.

**2** In unilateral mesial temporal sclerosis, the interictal EEG often shows bilateral dependent or bilateral independent spikes even where pathology is well lateralized on MRI. Some authors consider that spike counting and the assessment of spike morphology or distribution may be inform- ative. If the ratio of the number of interictal spikes on the side of the hippocampal sclerosis compared with the normal side exceeds 8 : 1, seizures can be reliably assumed to be arising from the sclerotic side.

**3** Spikes arising outside the anterior temporal region carry a poorer surgical prognosis.

### Ictal scalp EEG and video-EEG telemetry

The ictal scalp EEG recording of a complex partial seizure remains a fundamental part of the pre-surgical evaluation (but see p. 242). Long recordings are usually performed with concurrent video (video-EEG telemetry). To catch seizures, recordings may need to be continued for days or even weeks. In unilateral hippocampal sclerosis, a clear-cut ictal unilateral temporal/sphenoidal rhythmic discharge of 5 Hz or faster within the first 30 seconds of the ictal record- ing occurs in about 50–60% of patients (Figure 5.5), and this is reliably localizing in about 90–95% of these cases (thus, in a small number of cases, the ictal EEG mislocalizes the epilepsy, owing to rapid undetected contralateral pro- pagation, which is important not to forget). About 30% of

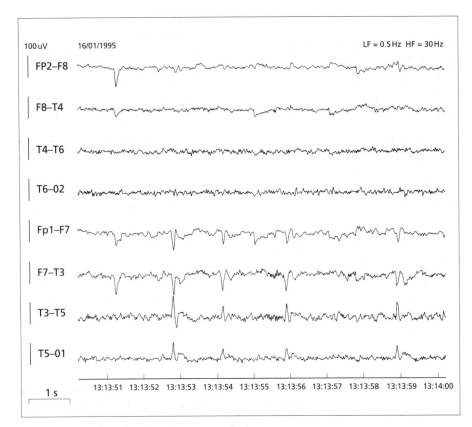

**Figure 5.4** Lateralized temporal sharp waves with phase reversal seen in the left mid-temporal region (T3). This is a common interictal finding in mesial temporal lobe epilepsy.

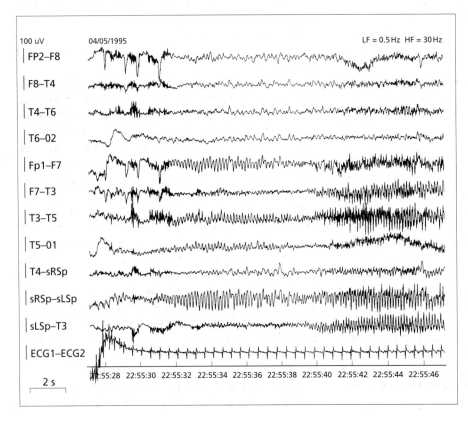

**Figure 5.5** Typical temporal lobe seizures with rhythmic lateralized epileptiform activity.

**Table 5.4** Clinical ictal features that predict side of seizure onset.

| Ictal feature | Side of onset |
|---|---|
| *Common signs that are reliable* | |
| Unilateral dystonic posturing | Contralateral to seizure onset |
| Unilateral automatisms | Ipsilateral to seizure onset |
| Ictal speech | Seizure onset in non-dominant hemisphere |
| Postictal dysphasia | Seizure onset in dominant hemisphere |
| *Less reliable (or rare) signs* | |
| Ictal blinking* | Ipsilateral to seizure onset |
| Ictal spitting* | Seizure onset in non-dominant hemisphere |
| Postictal nose wiping* | Ipsilateral to seizure onset |
| Head turning at onset of seizure (non-forced version) | Ipsilateral to seizure onset |
| Forced head version before secondary generalization | Contralateral to seizure onset |
| Ictal vomiting*,** | Seizure onset in non-dominant hemisphere |

*, Rare occurrences, where reliability is uncertain; **, applies to ictal vomiting, which is rare, but not to postictal vomiting, which is common.

patients show no lateralizing or localizing features in the scalp ictal recordings. Similar figures apply to other mesial temporal lesions (e.g. cavernoma, glioma, dysembryoplastic neuroepithelial tumour [DNET]).

Video telemetry allows detailed scrutiny of the clinical features of the seizure, and certain signs are reliable indicators of the side of onset of the seizure (Table 5.4).

In patients with concordant clinical, MRI and psychological features, interictal scalp EEG is often sufficient without the need to record seizures.

About 5% of patients with temporal lobe epilepsy show additional generalized spike-and-slow-wave discharges. These imply a genetically lowered seizure threshold, and their presence worsens post-surgical outcome.

### Intracranial ictal EEG

In some centres, intracranial (depth) EEG recordings used to be carried out in all patients with temporal lobe epilepsy being evaluated for epilepsy surgery (Figure 5.6). With the advent of MRI this practice seems now to be obsolete in most cases; indeed in our unit it is applied in less than 5% of cases. Depth EEG does record from otherwise functionally inaccessible cortex, but the EEG data come from only a small area around the electrode (< 1 cm core), and unless the electrodes are placed logically to address specific questions, results can be misleading.

In the work-up for surgery of hippocampal sclerosis, depth EEG is used in five main clinical situations:

1 To determine from which temporal lobe seizures are arising in patients with MRI evidence of bilateral hippocampal sclerosis.

2 To determine whether or not seizures are arising from the temporal lobe in patients in whom imaging shows 'dual pathology', and the scalp EEG is inconclusive.

3 To lateralize the seizure discharge in patients with discordant MRI and ictal or interictal EEG.

4 To lateralize seizure onset in patients with a unilateral hippocampal lesion on MRI but where ictal scalp EEG suggests bilateral seizure onsets.

5 In cases suggestive of mesial temporal lobe epilepsy, but with a normal MRI.

Electrodes are usually placed bitemporally, and in other sites as determined by the questions being addressed. There is a 1–2% risk of haemorrhage or infection from each electrode placement, and the overall risk of the procedure increases with the number of electrodes inserted. There is no place for the insertion of multiple electrodes without a prior idea about the most likely sites of seizure onset.

Foramen ovale electrode placement, in which the electrode tip is inserted through the foramen ovale to lie medial to the hippocampus, is a form of extracerebral intracranial electrode placement. It is a straightforward technique and does not require a craniotomy or stereotactic equipment, but has a significant complication rate, including facial pain, meningitis and vascular damage to the brainstem. There is probably little place for this in modern practice. Similarly, invasive sphenoidal recordings are generally no better than those from superficial sphenoidal electrodes, which carry lower morbidity.

In patients requiring depth EEG, a substantial number have findings that exclude surgery. Even where surgery can

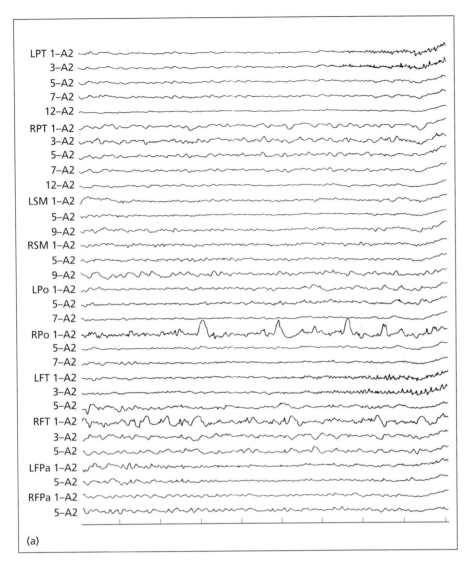

(a)

**Figure 5.6** (a,b) One typical mesial temporal seizure onset pattern is seen in these continuous electroencephalogram segments as low-voltage fast discharge in LPT 1,3 (left depth electrode contacts at tip). Simultaneous seizure onset of similar morphology is identified in distal contacts of left temporal subdural strip (LFT 1,3) overlying entorrhinal cortex. Electrode contacts are labelled from distal (1) to proximal. LPT, RPT, left and right hippocampal depth electrodes; LSM, RSM, supplementary motor subdural strips; LPo, RPo, LFT, RFT, LFPa, RFPa, left and right frontopolar, frontotemporal and frontoparietal subdural strips. Full scale, 1000 μV; each division, 1 s. (*continued on p. 243*)

be offered, the chances of seizure freedom are often lower than in cases in whom depth EEG is not needed. In other words, the yield of successful surgery is relatively small and it is important that this is fully appreciated before embarking on depth recordings.

### Other issues relating to MRI and EEG

The use of high-quality MRI is changing pre-surgical evaluation practice, and six specific issues are worth further consideration.

### *Are ictal recordings always required?*

In the past, it had been the rule that ictal recordings were required in all patients with temporal lobe epilepsy (TLE). Evidence now suggests that ictal recordings add little in one important category of patient with TLE—those with clear-cut MRI unilateral abnormalities, a concordant clinical history/psychometry, concordant lateralized interictal EEG,

and in whom there is no question of non-epileptic attacks. Thus, it is now current practice in some centres not to require ictal recordings in these patients. However, if there are any discordant or complicating features, seizures should be recorded.

### *Bilateral hippocampal sclerosis, demonstrated by MRI*

Significant bilateral pathological changes, albeit asymmetrical, in hippocampal structures are found in at least one-third of patients with hippocampal sclerosis. With the use of absolute volumetry and quantification of T2 measures, such bilateral sclerosis can now be detected radiographically. Bilateral changes occur most often in patients with a history of previous encephalitis or meningitis, and in such cases, seizures usually arise independently from both temporal lobes, and the chances of a good surgical outcome are poor. The presence of two clinical seizure types is even more suggestive of bilateral epileptogenesis.

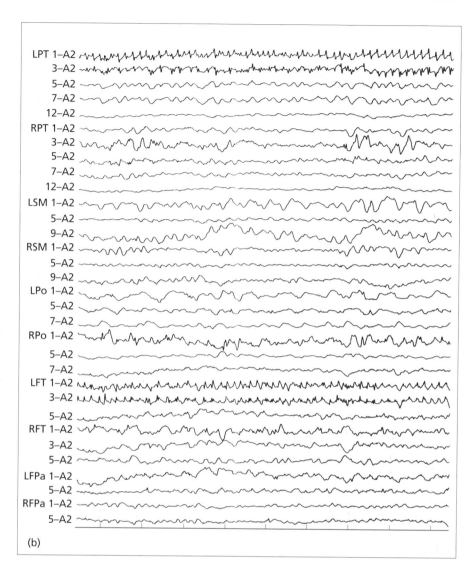

(b)

**Figure 5.6**  (*continued*)

The scalp ictal and interictal EEGs are much less reliable in bilateral than in unilateral hippocampal sclerosis. One study reported discordant ictal scalp EEG lateralization in nearly 20% of patients with asymmetric bilateral hippocampal sclerosis. If surgery is to be considered, most patients with bilateral hippocampal sclerosis require depth EEG. With clear-cut bilateral hippocampal atrophy, even after invasive EEG, surgery is usually not feasible because of bilateral epileptogenesis and also because of the risks of surgery to memory function.

### Bitemporal EEG changes

As emphasized above, in the absence of bilateral hippocampal abnormalities on MRI, bilateral interictal temporal spikes on scalp EEG do not necessarily indicate bilateral epileptogenesis or less good surgical outcome. Between 40% and 70% of patients with bilateral independent spikes on scalp EEG have unilateral seizures on depth EEG. In most centres, it is considered that patients with bitemporal inde-pendent interictal spikes on scalp EEG do not require depth EEG if the ratio of spikes over the affected side compared with the unaffected side is 8 : 1 or higher, and/or if surface recorded seizures arise over one temporal lobe and are concordant with MRI, neuropsychological, and other data.

Conversely, bilateral ictal onsets on scalp EEG should be taken as strong evidence of bilateral temporal epileptogenesis. Depth EEG is required in these patients if temporal lobectomy is to be considered. The usual policy in this situation is to record five or more seizures. If 80% or more arise in one temporal lobe, surgery can be offered with a good chance of improvement (but with a small chance only of seizure freedom). Surgical outcome is good particularly if other complementary tests strongly favour the resected side. It is also important to recognize that apparent bitemporal epileptogenesis may well be due to extratemporal seizure onset with bitemporal seizure spread. This is not infrequent in patients with parietal or occipital lobe epilepsies, in whom the onset of seizures may be difficult to identify on scalp EEG. Depth EEG with additional electrode placements may be helpful in this setting.

### *Hippocampal sclerosis with another pathology (dual pathology)*

The importance of so-called dual pathology has become apparent with the widespread application of MRI. Between 5% and 15% of patients with hippocampal sclerosis have evidence of additional pathology (mostly cortical dysplasia) and about 15% of extra-hippocampal lesions have co-incident hippocampal sclerosis (Figure 5.7). In one study hippocampal sclerosis was found in 30% of patients with porencephalic cysts, 20% of those with cortical dysgenesis, 9% of those with vascular abnormalities, and 2% of those with tumours. These are important to diagnose, for hippocampal resection alone in the presence of additional pathologies has a generally poor outcome. Patients with dual pathology will often require invasive monitoring.

### *'MRI-negative' patients*

A few patients are encountered with typical temporal lobe epilepsy in whom the MRI is normal. In such patients it is important to check that the MRI is of high enough quality, as poorly performed MRI will miss many cases of hippocampal sclerosis. If high-quality MRI is normal, the application of research techniques such as diffusion or perfusion imaging or MRS may demonstrate abnormalities, although currently the reliability of these techniques is unknown. Intensive EEG, including depth EEG, is almost always required in patients with normal MRI, but even then surgical outcome is generally poor with, in most circumstances, 30% or less of patients becoming free from seizures even if invasive recording demonstrates apparently localized seizure onset. There may also be a place for PET and SPECT (see below), although in MRI-negative adult cases, these techniques are seldom sensitive enough to localize the onset of seizures.

### *Discordant MRI and ictal EEG*

In occasional patients with hippocampal sclerosis demonstrable by MRI, the ictal EEG lateralizes to the contralateral side. In most of these cases, the EEG is falsely lateralizing (owing, usually, to rapid undetected contralateral propagation) and, with concordant clinical and other data, resection of the MRI abnormality results in seizure control in most patients. This is particularly the case in patients with very severe hippocampal sclerosis ('burned out' hippocampus). Currently, although resection of the MRI abnormality usually has a good outcome in terms of seizure control, invasive EEG is still advised.

### Neuropsychology

Neuropsychometric evaluation is a vital part of pre-surgical assessment, and it is shocking to encounter patients in whom this has been omitted. In mesial temporal lobe epilepsy, the minimum battery includes measures of intelligence, frontal executive skills, memory, attention, visuo-spatial skills and language. The dominant (usually left) temporal lobe mediates memory for verbal material such as names, word lists, stories or number sequences, and the non-dominant (usually right) temporal lobe mediates memory for material that cannot be verbalized readily, such as faces, places, music or abstract designs. Bilateral lesions can cause severe global memory deficits although profound memory impairment is rare, while a more restricted, material-specific deficit is frequent in patients with temporal lobe dysfunction. Core neuropsychology has two main functions:

1 To identify dysfunctioning cortex. If neuropsychological findings point to dysfunction that is discordant or more wide-ranging than the damage seen on MRI or from the EEG findings, the epileptogenic zone may extend beyond the damaged hippocampus and the outcome of surgery will generally be unfavourable. Broadly speaking, an overall IQ below 70 usually indicates widespread cerebral dysfunction and is a relative contra-indication to surgery. A discrepancy between verbal and non-verbal memory and learning tests

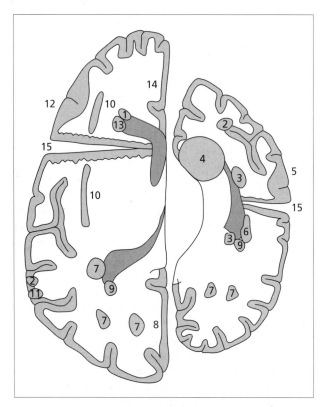

**Figure 5.7** Location of areas of cortical dysgenesis in 15 patients with dual pathology from a series of 100 patients with hippocampal sclerosis (cases 1, 3, 4, 6, 9, 13, subependymal heterotopia; cases 2 and 11, gyral abnormalities; case 8, focal cortical dysplasia; cases 5 and 12, macrogyria; cases 7 and 14, tuberous sclerosis; case 10, band heterotopia; case 15 schizencephaly).

also indicates lateralized dysfunction, which should be concordant with the side of the hippocampal sclerosis.

**2** To assess the risk of amnesia as a consequence of temporal lobe resection. The better the pre-operative verbal memory or learning abilities, the worse will be the memory outcome following dominant temporal lobectomy. Conversely, a poor verbal memory does not usually worsen after surgery, for poor verbal memory pre-operatively implies that hippocampal memory function is already damaged. A similar but less striking pattern is encountered in regard to non-verbal memory and the non-dominant temporal lobe. Bilateral hippocampal dysfunction should be suspected if both verbal and non-verbal memory tests are affected, and surgery in this situation carries the risk of severe amnesia, even if the pre-operative memory scores are low on the side to be operated upon.

### *Intracarotid amytal test (Wada test, sodium amytal test)*

The basic procedure consists of the intra-arterial injection of a fast acting barbiturate (usually sodium amobarbital) into the internal carotid artery (usually through a groin catheter). This barbiturate is absorbed into the injected hemisphere and 'anaesthetizes' it for a short period of time (5–8 minutes). During this time, neuropsychological tests are performed to test the ability of the contralateral (unanaesthetized) hemisphere in isolation. The injection is then performed on the other side and the tests repeated. The injection is made by a radiologist who has performed an arterial angiogram before the test to verify that there is no serious vascular anomaly and to predict the distribution of the drug. In most institutions an EEG is performed during the test, to confirm the lateralized effect of the drug. The test is invasive, and carries a risk of inducing focal cerebral spasm and infarction in about 1 in 200 cases.

The neuropsychological tests applied are basic language and memory tests. The memory testing consists of showing new material while only one hemisphere is functional, and testing memory for that material later, when the drug effects have worn off and both hemispheres are back to baseline functioning. Speech tests are simple and usually include naming, serial or automatic speech.

The test has two main purposes:

**1** To assess language dominance. This may be necessary in left-handed persons, or in other persons if the routine psychological testing suggests that speech is lateralized unexpectedly, or is bilaterally represented—a not infrequent situation in epilepsy.

**2** To confirm that resective surgery (imitated by the transient anaesthesia) will not result in severe memory disturbance. If a patient 'fails' the amytal, surgery is usually not carried out, on the basis that the risk of amnesia is too great.

Wada tests are also used in some centres for lateralizing seizure onset and for assessing the degree of post-operative memory loss. Their value in these situations is controversial.

In the past, the amytal test was performed in some centres on all patients being assessed for temporal lobe resection. However, in current practice, the test is increasingly being abandoned in favour of less invasive options. fMRI has already replaced the sodium amytal test to lateralize language dominance in uncomplicated cases, although where language is bilaterally represented, fMRI is at present too inconsistent to be relied upon. It is worth noting that even in cases where fMRI can lateralize language, it cannot localize it, and fMRI currently is not sensitive enough to map language or to replace invasive cortical mapping for this purpose. Attempts are also being made to develop fMRI tests of memory function, although currently these are too unreliable to be used for clinical purposes.

Finally, it is surprising to note that the predictive value of the amytal test for amnesia has never been formally validated, and there is an increasing feeling among psychologists that conventional neuropsychological testing provides reliable enough prediction without the need to resort to this test.

Currently, amytal testing is used in about 10% of all cases being assessed for temporal lobe surgery in our own unit, and its use is reserved to identify risks of amnesia in patients who already demonstrate significant memory deficits and in whom neuropsychological findings are complex or contradictory, and to lateralize language in patients in whom atypical or bilateral representation is suspected.

### Functional imaging using single photon emission computed tomography (SPECT) and positron emission tomography (PET)

The use of functional imaging techniques varies from centre to centre, and there is little agreement about the necessity of these investigations in mesial temporal surgery.

SPECT is the most commonly used functional imaging method. Interictal SPECT can show low-perfusion areas in the temporal lobe, although the value of the test has been shown to be limited by a low sensitivity of 44% and a false-positive rate of 7%. Ictal SPECT (obtained by injecting the ligand during a seizure) demonstrates hyperperfusion in the area of the epileptic focus. Certainly, perfusion changes do occur in mesial temporal complex partial seizures and the pattern has been well studied. During the initial phases of the seizure the whole temporal lobe is hyperperfused, and in the immediate postictal phase the mesial temporal structures remain hyperperfused, although the lateral temporal structures are hypoperfused. Within 2–15 minutes postictally, there is hypoperfusion of the whole temporal lobe, and a return to normal is seen in 10–30 minutes. SPECT can demonstrate these changes, and the sensitivity of the test is said by some authorities to be as high as 97%. However, its specificity is lower, and the predictive value of the test is uncertain. Also, depth EEG clearly shows that ictal activity not infrequently switches sides during a seizure, and in this situation ictal SPECT would be expected to falsely lateralize the seizure, with the hyperperfusion reflecting the propagated activity. The sensitivity of ictal SPECT localization during simple partial seizures is much lower. A recent development has been the comparison of ictal and interictal SPECT signals, and the resulting 'subtraction ictal SPECT' can be co-registered to MRI (this method is known as SISCOM). Abnormalities demonstrated using this method have been shown to be predictive of surgical outcome, but it is unclear how much this adds to more conventional investigatory methods in temporal lobe surgery.

The use of interictal 2-[$^{18}$F] fluoro-2-deoxyglucose-PET ($^{18}$FDG-PET) for detecting temporal lobe seizure foci (which appear as hypometabolic areas) has been well studied. The test has a sensitivity of 84% and a specificity of 86%, and it is interesting to note that the area of interictal hypoperfusion tends to be concordant with but smaller than the areas of hypometabolism. Interictal $^{18}$FDG-PET and ictal SPECT are both sensitive techniques for the detection of the epileptic focus, but ictal SPECT is probably more sensitive and specific than interictal $^{18}$FDG-PET and is easier to interpret and less expensive. For this reason, in most centres PET is not routinely used in temporal lobe epilepsy at least, although it can contribute to the investigation of patients with complex or discordant results on other modalities. Ictal PET is generally not feasible for practical reasons.

## The outcome of mesial temporal lobe surgery
### Seizure outcome
It is important not to take an over-optimistic view of temporal lobectomy, nor to assume that it guarantees long-term seizure control. The short-term outcome of temporal lobectomy has been carefully studied, but there is a serious lack of longer-term information, in spite of the fact that the operation has been performed now for over 50 years. At 1 year post-surgery, in published studies, 'seizure freedom' rates have generally ranged between 50 and 80% (median 70%), and at 5 years, rates have ranged between 50 and 70%. 'Seizure freedom' in these studies includes patients who continue to have auras (or other 'non-disabling' seizures) or seizures occurring only on drug withdrawal, and the rates for true 'complete seizure freedom' are lower. Furthermore, the quoted 5-year rates include patients who had been free from seizures for a year or more at the time of follow-up (only 50–55% of quoted patients had been seizure free for the whole of the 5-year period). Longer-term data are largely lacking, but one study showed a 7% drop—from 52 to 45%—in seizure freedom rates from 5 to 10 years after surgery. The proportion of 'seizure free' patients has increased by about 5–10% since the widespread use of MRI due to its impact on patient selection. If seizures are continuing at a point 12 months after surgery,

the chance of remission in the next 5 years is only about 10%.

A further 10–30% of patients, even if not completely free from seizures, achieve at least a 75% reduction in seizures in the year after surgery. The longer-term outcome of these patients has not been reported. Only 10–20% of patients do not experience any improvement after surgery, although in one series 18% of patients who had been operated on had at least monthly seizures at a point 5 years after the operation.

Generalized tonic–clonic seizures occurring in the first few weeks after surgery are generally considered to be of little prognostic significance to the long-term outcome, and may reflect the acute trauma of surgery. Similarly partial seizures may continue for a few months and then fade away (so-called run-down seizures). About 1% of patients develop recurrent convulsive seizures several years after surgery. These seizures are probably due to the surgical procedure and are usually readily controlled medically, but it is important that patients are warned about this prior to surgery.

### Immediate neurological complications and morbidity
Temporal lobectomy has a number of potential complications. The most common neurological deficit is a superior quadrantanopia, due to damage to the optic radiation, which loops through the posterior temporal lobe. Published rates for any field defect have varied between 2 and 50%, but in recent years, with modified operations, a functionally significant field defect has been found in less than 5% of cases. This is an important complication from the driving point of view and in Britain a quadrantanopic visual field cut that exceeds 15 degrees will prevent licensing. The risk of hemiplegia following temporal lobe surgery is about 1–2%, and is usually due to damage to the anterior choroidal artery and the pial vessels that lie on the surface of the midbrain mesial to the hippocampus. Selective hippocampectomy is a technically more difficult operation, and the risk of hemiplegia is slightly greater (up to 4%). A transient mild dysphasia is not uncommon with dominant temporal lobe resections, but a permanent dysphasia should occur in less than 1% of operated cases. Other risks of surgery include third-nerve palsy, meningitis, bone or scalp infection, vascular spasm, subdural haematoma or empyema, hydrocephalus and pneumocephalus. The overall risk of serious permanent neurological complications of temporal lobectomy (excluding quadrantanopia) in an experienced centre is in the order of 2–3%, and the mortality rate of surgery is less than 0.5%. These risks must be carefully explained to the patient prior to surgery, if possible in writing. It should not be forgotten, however, that uncontrolled epilepsy itself carries greater potential risks; for example, the annual mortality rate in persons with severe intractable epilepsy is between 5 and 10 per 1000 and is particularly high in patients experiencing convulsive attacks.

## Outcome in relation to memory

A temporal lobectomy involves the resection of much of the temporal lobe tissue thought to be involved in memory and learning. It is not surprising therefore that post-operative memory deficits, detectable on neuropsychological testing, are common. What is perhaps more remarkable is that these are generally mild, and a marked deterioration in memory should be a rare complication if patients are prudently selected. Indeed, memory and intellectual function can actually improve after surgery owing presumably to better seizure control and the need for fewer antiepileptic drugs. A profound amnesia occurs in less than 1% of cases in modern practice. The memory defects following temporal lobectomy involve verbal memory and learning in dominant lobe operations (usually left-sided operations), and non-verbal memory and learning deficits in non-dominant operations—the former are much more noticeable in daily life than the latter, and are the cause of more disability. The selective amygdalo-hippocampectomy was introduced to minimize memory disturbance, but in practice the rates of memory deficit seem to be broadly similar to those in more extensive operations.

The underlying pathology—particularly the pre-operative status of the hippocampus targeted for removal—is an important predictive factor. Hippocampal MRI volumetry is a vital test in this regard. In cases where there is unilateral hippocampal sclerosis with significant MRI volume loss, post-surgical memory deficit is usually minimal, perhaps because the target hippocampus is already so damaged that it performs little useful function in relation to memory. At the other extreme, if a normal sized hippocampus is to be removed as an adjunct to lesionectomy, some loss in memory function is inevitable. Lesional mesial temporal lobe surgery overall carries more risk to memory than surgery for hippocampal sclerosis. If the temporal lobe pathologies have been present since childhood, the risk of surgery to memory is also less, presumably owing to brain plasticity and the re-assignment of cerebral function away from the epileptic focus during the child's development.

## Psychiatric and cognitive outcome

Post-operative psychiatric disturbance is perhaps the biggest risk following temporal lobe surgery. Unfortunately, there are still considerable uncertainties about the extent of this problem. In early series, the incidence of schizophreniform illness following temporal lobectomy was about 15%, but in recent studies the incidence of *de novo* psychosis following temporal lobe surgery is much lower—less than 5%. This is probably because of better patient selection, and a pre-operative chronic psychosis is usually now considered a contra-indication, in most situations, to temporal lobe surgery. A depressive illness following surgery is more common, occurring in about 35% of patients in the first year after surgery. The rate may be higher after non-dominant

resections. The rates of psychiatric disease are significantly higher in those who are not seizure free following surgery; and these patients—with post-operative seizures and psychotic illness—pose a grave problem for post-operative rehabilitation. Less well studied are various behavioural changes after temporal lobe surgery. Changes in sexuality and obsessionality are not uncommon. Hyposexual changes are more frequent than hypersexuality, but both occur. Obsessional behaviour can reach disabling levels requiring psychotropic therapy. Case reports of striking personality change have been published, but this aspect of post-operative psychopathology has been poorly researched. Behaviour in children often improves following successful epilepsy surgery, perhaps due to a combination of the surgical resection, drug reduction, alleviation of seizures and social effects. In adult cases, behavioural improvements are less common. It is important to stress that epilepsy surgery must not be conducted with the primary aim of behavioural modification. On ethical grounds, such surgery should be considered to be a form of psycho-surgery, thus requiring complex oversight and a careful ethical regulatory framework; these do not exist in most epilepsy surgery programmes.

Another quantified risk is that of late deterioration owing to lack of 'cerebral reserve', and longer follow-up studies are urgently required to assess the extent of this risk, particularly in cases operated upon in mid- or late-adult life.

## Psychosocial outcome

After successful surgery, a major readjustment is needed to a life without epilepsy. This can be difficult and painful, as is the realization that the problems of life are not automatically resolved. There is often a sense of anticlimax, at least in the first 12 months following the operation. Furthermore, if the operation fails, disappointment and depression are almost inevitable. Seizure freedom will not immediately reverse years of social isolation, a lack of self-confidence or of a strong sense of identity, or missed educational or career opportunities. Becoming seizure free can alter interpersonal relationships, which might have been based on dependence or a 'sick-role'. Appropriate pre-operative counselling can help to prepare people, and in some cases a structured post-operative rehabilitation programme can be helpful.

However, when freedom from seizures is obtained, and where patients have been carefully selected, the temporal lobectomy can have an extraordinarily positive effect, allowing the patient, often for the first time, to engage in all aspects of life with confidence and unencumbered by the constant fear of seizures. This can be profoundly beneficial.

## Different surgical approaches to temporal lobe surgery

Because of the rate of complications, operative techniques have been modified to try to avoid some of the adverse

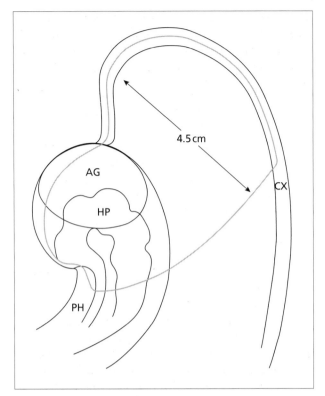

**Figure 5.8** A standard temporal lobectomy. Transverse plane showing the habitual extent of temporal resections (cortical and limbic) in the dominant hemisphere. AG, amygdala; CX, neocortex; HP, hippocampus; PH, parahippocampus; grey line, extent of resection.

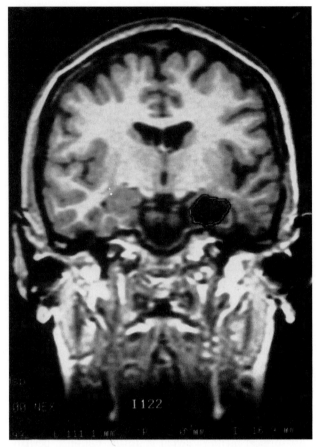

**Figure 5.9** Post-operative magnetic resonance imaging studies following stereotactic amygdalohippocampectomy via a lateral temporal neocortical approach. The coronal postoperative magnetic resonance image demonstrates the focal mesial resection that is possible with this technique, while sacrificing the minimum of temporal lobe neocortex, and shows complete resection of the mesial temporal structures.

effects. The standard temporal lobectomy extends for 4–5 cm behind the temporal pole in the dominant temporal lobe (Figure 5.8) and up to 6 cm in the non-dominant temporal lobe, sparing the posterior part of the superior temporal gyrus. Most of the hippocampus, the amygdala, and some surrounding mesial structures are removed. Modified temporal lobectomies have also been devised, and in the most common type 3 cm only of the temporal tip is removed, providing good access to the amygdala and hippocampal formation, which are then resected in their entirety. This is now the most common operation performed.

The selective amygdalo-hippocampectomy is carried out either stereotactically (Figure 5.9) through the middle temporal gyrus or occipital cortex or by an approach along the Sylvian fissure. This preserves much of the lateral cortex. However, there is little convincing evidence that the selective amygdalo-hippocampectomy actually has a better outcome in regard to memory function or cognition, and as the operation is technically more difficult to perform, the rates of vascular disturbance and hemiplegia are higher than in temporal lobectomy. The selective operations do have a lower risk of dysphasia or visual-field defect.

Furthermore, the rates of long-term seizure freedom, although not adequately studied, appear at an anecdotal level to be slightly less good than after standard or modified temporal lobectomy.

A recent development has been the use of radio-surgery with the gamma knife to ablate mesial temporal lobe structures. This can be performed on an outpatient basis. Preliminary experience is promising, but anxieties remain about the risk of deterioration owing to late progressive radiation-induced necrosis. Conflicting results are reported. In a European study of 21 patients given a dose of 24 Gy, 65% were seizure free at 2 years, and no serious long-term neurological deficits, apart from visual-field deficits, were recorded. A report from the Cleveland Clinic, however, of five patients treated with 20 Gy showed that none achieved seizure freedom, and all required subsequent operation. Gamma-knife surgery must at present be considered an experimental procedure, but shows promise and is likely

**Table 5.5**  Follow-up protocol for patients without complications after successful temporal lobe epilepsy surgery.

| | |
|---|---|
| Neurosurgical follow-up | 6 weeks, 1 year, and then annually |
| Neurological follow-up | 3, 6, 9, 12 months, then annually |
| Psychiatry | 1, 6, 12 months, and then annually |
| Psychology | 3, 12 months |
| Field testing | 6 months |
| MRI | 3 months |
| Counselling | 3, 12 months |

This is based on the protocol used by the author.

to be increasingly used. The use of the 'proton pencil beam' is another technique currently in development.

Follow-up following successful temporal lobe surgery should be protocol-driven, and that adopted in the author's own unit is shown in Table 5.5.

## SURGERY IN EPILEPSY ARISING IN EXTRA-TEMPORAL REGIONS AND IN THE TEMPORAL NEOCORTEX

Mesial temporal resection is the most common form of resective surgery for epilepsy. However, with the widespread use of MRI, lesions causing focal epilepsy are now also frequently demonstrated in the temporal neocortex and extra-temporal cortex. The lesions most commonly treated by epilepsy surgery are small slow-growing or benign tumours, small arteriovenous malformations (AVMs), and cavernomas. Although the investigatory approach has similarities to that in mesial temporal epilepsy, there are differences in emphasis. Two key determinants of surgical outcome are aetiology and the extent of the resection.

### Aetiology
#### Tumours
Epilepsy occurs in approximately 50% of patients with intracerebral neoplasms (see pp. 46–7). The surgical management of rapidly growing tumours depends on factors other than epilepsy. For small benign tumours, however, surgery is sometimes indicated with the primary aim of controlling epilepsy.

#### Gliomas in patients presenting with epilepsy: the role of surgery and radiotherapy
Not uncommonly, gliomas are identified on CT or MRI in patients who have presented with new-onset seizures with-

out other neurological signs. The management of these cases crucially depends on the histological grade of the glioma. In patients under the age of 50 years, MRI is now sufficiently reliable to predict this with a greater than 90% degree of accuracy (CT is less reliable) but the rate of diagnostic error on MRI and CT is greater in older patients. On MRI, low-grade gliomas (grades I and II) are generally non-enhancing whilst high-grade gliomas (grades III and IV) usually enhance markedly and have an irregular outline, necrotic centre and vasogenic oedema. However, low grade gliomas have as strong tendency to 'transform' to become more malignant over time, sometimes after many years of quiescence. This transformation is unpredictable, and because of this the surgical management of low-grade tumours can be difficult and contentious.

The author's usual practice in regard to the management of an MRI-defined low-grade glioma presenting with epilepsy is as follows:

**1** In patients over 50 years of age—biopsy is usually carried out (in view of the greater risk of diagnostic error).

**2** In patients under 50 years of age in whom MRI suggests a low-grade glioma-biopsy with a view to resection is advised only if the tumour is small and in a non–dominant polar location. In other cases, biopsy and/or resection are usually deferred and the lesion is assessed by serial scanning—initially at 3 months and then at 6 and 12 monthly intervals. Serial scanning is continued as long as the MRI appearances to not change.

**3** In patients in whom new clinical signs develop, or in whom serial MRI shows changing size or new enhancement even in the absence of new signs, biopsy is advised, with a view to resection.

**4** When resection is performed, it should be as complete as is possible without causing neurological deficit.

**5** Radiotherapy is usually reserved for those with evidence of malignant transformation, or occasionally in patients whose epilepsy is wholly intractable and in whom resection is not possible.

**6** The epilepsy is treated initially medically, along conventional lines. If the seizures persist or are severe enough to warrant surgical intervention, epilepsy surgery is considered (see below).

In patients with MRI findings suggestive of a high-grade gliomas, and in all patients with increasing neurological signs and/or signs of increased intracranial pressure, urgent surgical referral with a view to tumour resection is advised. The resection should be as extensive as possible, and the surgery is usually followed by immediate radiotherapy. Adjunctive chemotherapy with sometimes advised in glioblastomas, and currently oral temozolomide is the most commonly used agent. More experimental approaches using biodegradable polymers containing BCNU inserted into the resection cavity are also under investigation.

In patients with gliomas, a multidisciplinary approach to treatment should be taken, with neurological, oncological and neurosurgical input. The patient should be fully involved in what are often difficult decisions, and fully informed of the potential risks and benefits of the various treatment options.

### Benign tumours: the role of epilepsy surgery

The beneficial effect of epilepsy surgery in patients with medically refractory partial seizures associated with small benign tumours is well established. In well-selected cases, about 50–80% can expect to be seizure free after surgery, and seizures are reduced in most other cases. The outcome of the surgical treatment of tumoural epilepsy is influenced largely by the underlying pathology (often possible to determine only after surgery) and how complete the resection of the lesion is. Seizure-free rates of 70% or so are reported in patients with low-grade astrocytomas (completely resected) but rates are lower in more malignant tumours. Total excision of gangliogliomas and dysembryoplastic neuroepithelial tumours (DNETs) relieves seizures in 80% of cases. Seizure-free rates are generally less if the resection is incomplete, although this does not apply in the case of DNETs, in which epileptogenesis is often intrinsic to the tumour.

The necessity to investigate the extent of surrounding epileptogenicity in the resective surgery of tumours by EEG, where complete lesional resection is possible, has not been clearly established, but most patients undergo ancillary epilepsy-related investigations (see below). Exactly what these add to surgical outcome, however, is unclear, and in most cases extensive EEG or functional testing is not required. The main exception to this rule is the not uncommon situation in which extra-hippocampal lesions are associated with hippocampal sclerosis, which occurs especially when the tumour is situated in the temporal lobe. Resection of the lesion alone in these cases has a lower chance of seizure control, and hippocampectomy is often carried out in conjunction with the lesionectomy. Hippocampal resection should generally not be performed if the hippocampus shows no radiological signs of atrophy, especially in the dominant temporal lobe, as resection of healthy hippocampal tissue is associated with a significant loss of memory skills. The other complications and outcome are similar to that in hippocampal sclerosis.

### Arteriovenous malformations

Epilepsy is the presenting symptom in 20–40% of cases of cerebral arteriovenous malformation, and is present in over 60%. The effect on epilepsy of surgical resection of the AVM depends largely on its size and location. The complete resection of a small AVM, particularly if sited in the temporal lobe, will frequently control seizures completely. However, the resection of large AVMs, which anyway is often incomplete, has little chance of controlling epilepsy and should not usually be performed for this purpose.

Stereotactic radiosurgery is accepted alternative therapy for small lesions in which the nidus measures less than 2.5–3 cm in diameter, particularly if located deeply in the brain. This technique induces endothelial proliferation and ultimately causes obliteration of the lumen over a period of 1–2 years. Stereotactic radiosurgery is non-invasive and can be administered on an outpatient basis. The pathological changes induced by radiation, and thus also the clinical benefits, take months to develop. Studies have shown that stereotactic radiosurgery will obliterate all lesions with a diameter less than 2 cm within 3 years after treatment but only 50% of lesions with a diameter greater than 2.5 cm. In open studies epilepsy has been shown to improve in over two-thirds of cases after radiosurgery, and seizures are improved even before complete occlusion of the nidus. In one series of 160 AVMs, 48 patients had epilepsy. At 2-year follow-up, 38% of these cases were seizure free, 22% had improved seizure control and 6% were worse.

Endovascular embolization is also available for the treatment of cerebral AVMs. It can be used as a primary treatment or as a prelude to surgery. However, it often does not achieve permanent obliteration of the malformation owing to the high rate of recanalization. It can also induce acute haemodynamic changes in the treated region, and multiple procedures may be required to complete the treatment. The complication rate for this procedure has been estimated to be about a 1.5% risk of severe deficit, a 1–2% risk of death, a 10% risk of haemorrhage (including 3% first time haemorrhage) and a 3% risk of new-onset seizures. Embolization probably has little effect on the frequency or severity of existing seizures.

### Cavernous haemangiomas (cavernomas)

Cavernomas (see pp. 51–2) are vascular malformations consisting of closely clustered enlarged capillary channels ('caverns') with a single layer of endothelium without normal intervening brain parenchyma or mature vessel wall elements, ranging in size for a few millimetres to several centimetres. The characteristic lesion on MRI is of mixed signal intensity with a central reticulated core surrounded by a dark ring. The latter is presumed to be haemosiderin deposition from prior haemorrhage (Figure 5.10). There is a risk of haemorrhage from these lesions of between 0.5 and 2% per year, thus, although the per-annum risk of haemorrhage is lower than that of AVMs, the cumulative lifetime risk for younger patients is not insubstantial. It is generally acknowledged that such risk is higher for patients with documented previous haemorrhage. Several published series show that excisional surgery can be accomplished with low morbidity, with excellent or good results achieved. A meta-analysis of surgical outcome of 268 supra-tentorial cavernous haemangiomas, in retrospective series, revealed

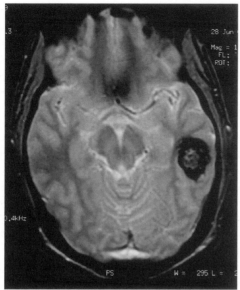

(a)

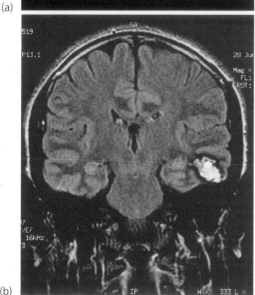

(b)

**Figure 5.10** (a) MRI of a left temporal cavernous angioma causing complex partial seizures in a 27-year-old man. The scan shows the typical appearances of a hypo-intense haemosiderin halo with a mixed-signal core on a T2-weighted image. (b) Same cavernoma on a T1-weighted coronal view.

that 84% of patients were seizure free after surgery and 21% were improved; there was no change in only 6%, and 2% were worse. A long duration of epilepsy negatively affected the outcome of surgery, suggesting that resection should be performed sooner rather than later. However, in a more recent prospective series, outcome was poorer, with only 42% becoming seizure free.

Focused radiosurgery (e.g. with the gamma knife) can also be used to treat cavernomas. However, if the lesion is surgically accessible and the risk of surgical morbidity is low, surgery is the preferred option, as it offers a better

chance of controlling seizures and less risk of rebleeding, which has been shown to be as high as 33% in one study following radiosurgery. However, one recent multicentre study suggested that, despite the failure to protect against the risk of further haemorrhage, there was a beneficial effect on epilepsy. Out of 49 patients treated with radiosurgery 26 (53%) were seizure free, two (4%) had occasional auras and 10 (19%) had a significant decrease in the number of seizures. Cavernomas in the mesiotemporal region were associated with a poor outcome, whereas location in the latero-temporal and central regions was associated with significantly better results.

Cavernomas are sometimes multiple and surgical resection of individual lesions in such cases is only advisable if epilepsy can be clearly localized. Surgical resection for epilepsy in familial cavernoma is possible where there is a single accessible lesion, but generally the lesions are multiple and develop over time, and surgery to individual lesions has limited value.

### Cerebral infections
#### Encephalitis or meningitis
In general, surgical therapy for chronic post-meningitic or post-encephalitic epilepsy carries a poor outcome for seizure control. Even if an apparently single lesion is uncovered on imaging (for example, apparently unilateral hippocampal atrophy following herpes simplex encepahlitis) there is usually more subtle widespread diffuse damage in other areas of the brain, and localized resection will fail to control seizures. This may be because the boundaries of the destructive process in post-infective lesions are seldom sharply defined, and it is these boundary areas that contribute most to epileptogenesis.

#### Acute brain abscess
The same applies to epilepsy following acute brain abscess (Figure 5.11). Although surgery is usually carried out in the acute phase, the optimal surgical management of brain abscess depends on the type of infecting organism and the immunological state of the patient. Various procedures are utilized, including continuous tube drainage, stereotacticor open aspiration, marsupialization of the abscess, and craniotomy with complete excision. Unfortunately, epilepsy follows brain abscess, whether surgically treated or not, in between 40 and 80% of cases, and is often severe and intractable. Surgical resection of the cavity in an attempt to control the seizures can be attempted, but the results are generally disappointing. Corpus callosotomy (see below) is sometimes used in severe intractable seizures following a frontal brain abscess.

#### Neurocysticercosis
Neurocysticercosis with a solitary or small number of cerebral lesions is a self-limiting infestation with a pattern of

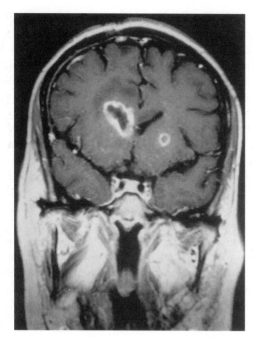

**Figure 5.11** *Aspergillus* abscesses in 38-year-old immunocompromised man.

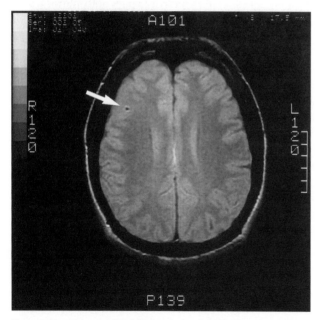

**Figure 5.12** A 36-year-old right-handed male with seizures since age 15 years, including sensations of heat or cold and forced head-turning to the left, with no loss of consciousness or postictal confusion. Axial proton-density magnetic resonance image demonstrates a small lesion with low signal intensity in the right frontal lobe (arrowed). Surgical resection demonstrated a calcified degenerated cysticercal cyst.

spontaneous resolution (Figure 5.12). Resection of persisting calcified lesions to control seizures is hardly ever required.

The main debate about surgical intervention for neuro-cysticercosis has revolved around the need for biopsy for

diagnostic purposes, especially in patients in endemic areas presenting with seizures and a solitary enhancing CT lesion. Assuming there are no other clinical features, over 90% of these lesions turn out to be due to neurocysticercosis, and biopsy is now largely abandoned. The epilepsy (pp. 49–50) is usually treated medically with antiepileptic drugs, and imaging is repeated at 12–16 weeks. If there is no resolution, or if the lesion has increased in size, diagnosis should be reconsidered and anticysticercal therapy instituted. Stereo-tactic or image-guided excision should be reserved for lesions that enlarge or persist.

Surgical excision is also indicated where cysts exert a local mass effect or cause raised intracranial pressure, for subarachnoid cysts refractory to albendazole, cysts in the parasellar region, and large racemose cysts. These forms do not present with epilepsy.

### *Tuberculosis*

Tuberculoma (see p. 50) is one of the most common lesions causing focal epilepsy in some parts of the developing world, and in immunocompromised patients (for instance with HIV infection). Medical treatment with antitubercu-lous drugs is the therapy of choice. A stereotactic biopsy is sometimes necessary to establish the diagnosis (usually to differentiate tuberculoma from neurocysticercosis). Occa-sionally excision of the residual cerebral lesion is necessary to control chronic intractable seizures.

### Rasmussen chronic encephalitis

This is a syndrome of uncertain pathogenesis, but which has the histological appearances of a chronic encephalitis. It presents as intractable focal epilepsy, often with periods of EPC, and progressive neurological deficit including hemiplegia, aphasia and hemionopia. Wide lobar excision or hemispherectomy will be curative if the lesion is com-pletely excised without causing unacceptable neurological deficit (see pp. 260–3).

### Trauma

As is the case in post-infectious epilepsy, the physiological changes causing refractory seizures after closed head trauma are often widespread and ill-defined. The MRI lesions do not necessarily correlate well with the extent of the histological changes, and limited surgical resection is often ineffective. In open trauma (including depressed fracture with dural breach), emergency débridement of the lesion will often pre-vent or reduce the intensity of subsequent epilepsy and should be carried out wherever possible. The wide débride-ment of established chronic lesions, including the resection of haemosiderin-lined cavities, will also sometimes improve chronic refractory epilepsy, although in general the results of surgery are disappointing, even where the damage appears to be relatively circumscribed. In penetrating head injury, surgery to remove bone fragments is also important to prevent abscess formation, which can cause severe epilepsy. Abscess development can be very delayed after penetrating head injury, and cases presenting 10–15 years after the injury have been reported.

## Pre-surgical assessment

Small indolent lesions, such as cavernomas, indolent gliomas and dysembryoplastic neuroepithelial tumours (DNETs), are readily recognized on neuroimaging and increasingly such patients are undergoing limited lesional resections (lesionectomy) to control seizures. Pre-surgical assessment is usually triggered by scanning with MRI or CT, which demonstrates the visible lesion.

The discovery of an intracerebral lesion in a patient with epilepsy does not inevitably mean that the lesion is causing the epilepsy, and the main purposes of the pre-surgical evaluation are to confirm that the lesion is responsible for the epilepsy and to define the extent of the epileptogenic zone.

The extent of resection is a key factor in lesional epilepsy. For most lesions, incomplete resection has a low chance of controlling seizures, whatever EEG or other investigations show. This should not be contemplated except as a last resort if the purpose of surgery is to control seizures, although it is often carried out for oncological reasons or to lower the risk of haemorrhage from AVMs. Only in the case of DNETs does incomplete resection seem routinely to control seizures.

As the most important determinants of outcome are the extent of resection and the nature of the underlying lesion, imaging is the primary investigation. Concordance with the clinical features of the epilepsy will provide reassurance that the lesion is responsible for the seizures, and EEG and other functional tests have only a subsidiary role. However, EEG remains important in difficult cases, cases where previous surgery has failed, or in cases where there is a strong clinical suggestion of epileptogenesis beyond the visible limits of the lesion (particularly in post-traumatic or post-infective epilepsy). Functional assessments are usually included in epilepsy lesional surgery, but their value is less than in mesial temporal lobe epilepsy.

## Clinical assessment

The clinical features of partial seizures are a reliable indicator of the anatomical localization of seizure onset. The most frequent type of seizure associated with lesional epilepsy is the complex partial seizure, occurring in almost all patients with epileptogenic lesions in the temporal lobe and three-quarters of patients with extra-temporal lesions. Simple partial seizures are often even more useful in localizing seizure onset. This 'clinical localization' is of fundamental importance, and discordant findings are associated with much poorer surgical outcome.

Generalized epilepsy worsens outcome. Lesionectomy rarely controls epilepsy in childhood epilepsy syndromes

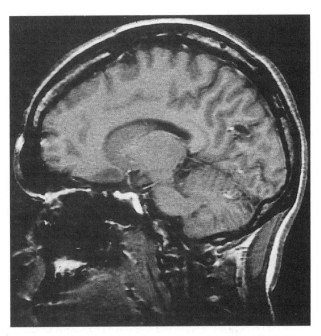

**Figure 5.13** Magnetic resonance image scan showing small parasagittal parieto-occipital lesion (biopsy-proven oligodendroglioma) in a patient with brief complex partial seizures characterized by visual disturbance, arrest of activity and loss of awareness.

(e.g. Lennox–Gastaut syndrome [pp. 23–5] or West syndrome [pp. 22–3]), even where these are associated with obvious lesions.

## Magnetic resonance imaging (MRI)

MRI should be carried out in all cases, whether or not a lesion has been demonstrated by CT. Particular MRI characteristics help to identify the underlying pathology, but the histological or pathological features of a lesion cannot be predicted with absolute accuracy. If MRI shows a cortically based tumour with sharply defined borders, little or no surrounding oedema, and little or no contrast enhancement, the tumour is likely to be benign (although exceptions occur) (Figure 5.13). Some lesions may have characteristic distinguishing features, for example DNETs, gangliogliomas, cavernomas, tuberculomas, neurocysticercosis, hypothalamic hamartomas, AVMs, and the lesions in tuberous sclerosis or Sturge–Weber syndrome.

Volumetric measurements of the hippocampi should now be routine in lesional epilepsy in order to characterize the possible extent of the epileptogenic zone(s), especially given the possibility of dual pathology.

## Interictal scalp EEG

In the presence of a neocortical lesion EEG often is unhelpful. The spatial distribution of an EEG focus coincides with lesion localization in less than one-third of patients, and can

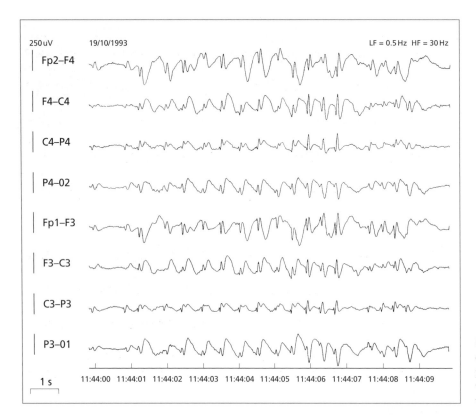

**Figure 5.14** Interictal electroencephalograph from the patient illustrated in Fig. 5.13 showing widespread bilateral slow spike and wave discharges.

indeed be widely discrepant (Figures 5.13 and 5.14). This is due to the rapid and wide propagation of seizure discharges in neocortical regions. Bilateral changes occur in many patients with unilateral hemispheric lesions, and indeed even large lesions may sometimes be associated with scalp EEG changes that predominate over the contralateral side. The nature of the lesion is important. In cortical dysplasia the interictal EEG is often widely distributed. In tumours and infective lesions it has more specificity but still often lacks reliability. In tumours or other lesional epilepsy there are few data to indicate which neurophysiological factors should influence the extent of resection. The site of the lesion also influences the interictal EEG. In lesional parietal or occipital lobe epilepsy, for example, only a minority of lesions show interictal spikes well correlated to the site of the lesion. Lesions in the temporal neocortex are more often associated with concordant EEG data. The EEG in lesional frontal lobe epilepsy often shows either no interictal spiking or apparently widespread or bilateral epileptiform discharges.

### Ictal scalp EEG

Ictal recordings (with video-EEG telemetry) are more informative than interictal EEG, but still lack critical reliability (Figures 5.15 and 5.16). However, in cases where clinico-EEG data correlate well with the visible lesion, the data are usually sufficient to proceed to surgery without invasive monitoring or other investigation. Some claim that

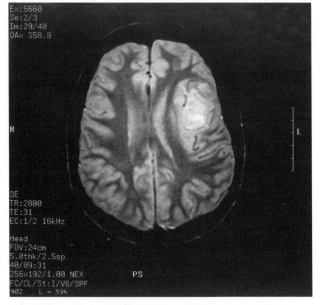

**Figure 5.15** Patient with a large left temporal lobe structural abnormality with apparently discordant ictal electroencephalograph.

concordant ictal fast activity particularly predicts a good surgical outcome. However, the potential for misleading or multifocal scalp EEG changes in patients with surgically resectable focal structural lesions should be recognized in planning investigative strategies, and surgery should

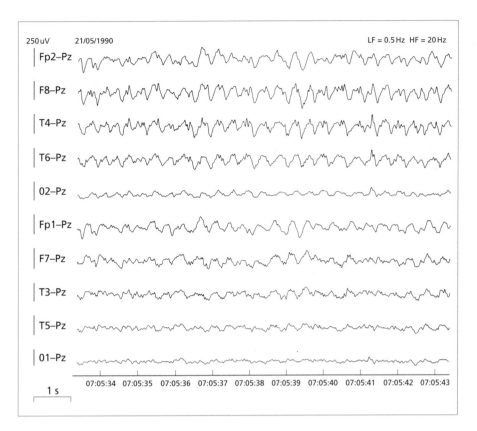

250 uV     21/05/1990                                                                LF = 0.5 Hz  HF = 20 Hz

Fp2–Pz

F8–Pz

T4–Pz

T6–Pz

02–Pz

Fp1–Pz

F7–Pz

T3–Pz

T5–Pz

01–Pz

07:05:34  07:05:35  07:05:36  07:05:37  07:05:38  07:05:39  07:05:40  07:05:41  07:05:42  07:05:43

1 s

**Figure 5.16** Ictal electroencephalograph findings from the patient illustrated in Fig. 5.15 with widespread rhythmic activity over the right hemisphere, and irregular slowing over the left temporal region (the site of the known large structural lesion).

certainly not be rejected merely because of discordant scalp electrographic findings.

### Intracranial EEG

The use of intracranial EEG in extra-hippocampal lesional epilepsy varies from centre to centre, as do the techniques employed. Intracranial EEG is needed in patients with lesional extra-hippocampal epilepsy for the following reasons:
• Non-localizing or discordant ictal scalp recordings suggest that the lesion might not be responsible for the seizures.
• It is necessary to decide whether or not to carry out hippocampal resection in patients with lesions adjacent to it, who are at risk of memory decline following surgery.
• It is necessary to define the margins of the epileptogenic zone to guide the extent of resection (although other strategies such as ECoG, radiological or pathological evaluation of margins may be used). The epileptogenicity of cortical dysplasia and post-traumatic lesions, particularly, tend to extend beyond the radiologically demonstrable lesion.
• For cortical stimulation for brain mapping with lesions overlying or adjacent to the eloquent cortex (see below).

Depth electrodes subdural strip electrodes, subdural grid electrodes and epidural electrodes are all used for invasive EEG (Figure 5.17, a–e), and indeed the techniques are often combined. The recording type is tailored to the individual patient, and the neurophysiological question being addressed. These tests carry significant morbidity, and their usefulness depends on the nature and site of the lesion. Formal studies have shown surprisingly little value from depth recordings.

EEG localization needs only to be regionally concordant and consistent, and precise localization around a lesion is not usually required. On depth recordings, interictal spikes do not show the same localizing significance as ictal spikes. Ictal discharges should be at the onset of or precede clinical seizures, whereas in scalp recordings seizure discharges are localizing if they occur within 30 seconds of the clinical discharge. In occipital or parietal lesions depth EEG is often non-localizing.

### Cortical mapping

Cortical mapping of functionally important cortex is a vital function where neurosurgical procedures are planned in sensory, motor or speech areas, and is required to identify eloquent areas and thus avoid post-surgical neurological deficit. Techniques vary but all include the placement of grids over the proposed resection site, and the observation of the clinical effects of electrical stimulation of each cortical contact. Ictal and interictal EEG can be recorded at the same time. Mapping is important because lesions commonly alter or distort the normal topography of the cerebral cortex and vascular landmarks. Acute intra-operative mapping can be carried out under local anaesthetic, but less elaborate

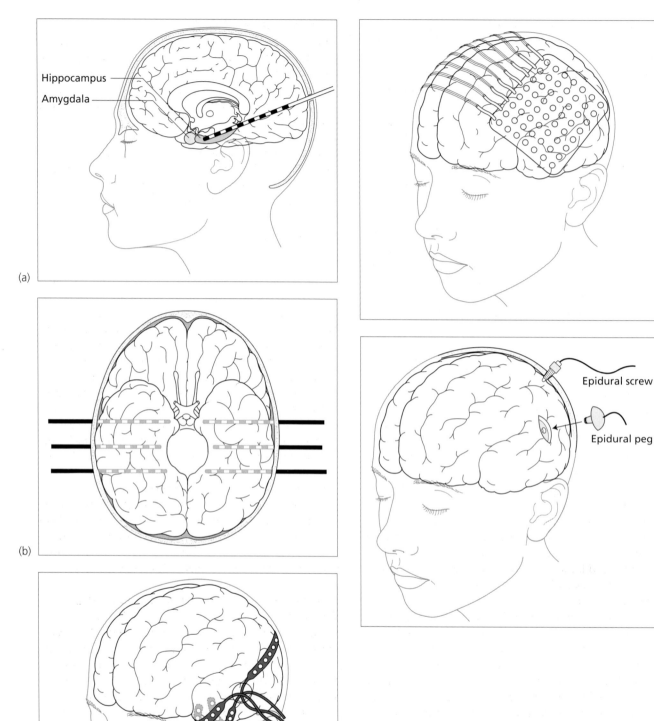

Hippocampus

Amygdala

(a)

(b)

(c)

(d)

Epidural screw

Epidural peg

(e)

**Figure 5.17** (a) Longitudinal depth electrode inserted in an anteroposterior fashion from the occipital lobe toward the ipsilateral hippocampus. (b) Orthogonal depth electrodes inserted transversely from lateral to medial temporal lobe at various locations. (c) Subdural strip electrodes inserted through a temporal burr hole to study lateral and medial temporal neocortex. (d) Subdural grid electrode implanted for localization of the epileptogenic zone and functional topographic mapping. (e) A percutaneous epidural screw tightened into a twist drill hole through the cranium and an epidural peg electrode placed in another twist drill hole.

functional tasks can be evaluated than in chronic longer-term pre-operative mapping. Subdural grids of electrodes have also been used for recording cortical somatosensory evoked potentials from peripheral nerve stimulation, to locate the somatosensory cortex. fMRI has the potential to replace cortical mapping in the identification of the primary motor areas, but currently cannot localize speech or language areas with sufficient accuracy to be practically useful.

### Neuropsychology

A battery of standard neuropsychological tests, aimed at lateralizing and localizing the area(s) of functional abnormality, are also routinely used in the pre-operative evaluation. However, the value of the tests for localizing lesions is limited. In a recent study, neuropsychological findings were congruent with the lateralization of the lesion in 56% but incongruent in 14%; furthermore, localization corresponded with the lobe of the lesion in 26% but was misleading in 30%. Neuropsychology also helps to predict post-operative deficit, but its value is generally less in extra-temporal than in temporal lobe surgery.

### SPECT and PET

The value of these functional imaging methods in lesional extra-hippocampal epilepsy has not been fully established. What is clear is that ictal SPECT is more useful than interictal SPECT, and indeed the sensitivity of ictal SPECT for demonstrating at least regional changes in extra-temporal seizures has been reported to be as high as 90%. In extra-temporal lesional epilepsy, if subtraction ictal SPECT coregistered on MRI (SISCOM) localizes a seizure accurately enough, and with concordance with other modalities, then about 40% of patients can expect to be seizure free following surgery and a further 40% to have a favourable surgical outcome. In one study SISCOM localization was concordant with the site of the surgical excision in 52.8%, non-concordant in 13.9% and non-localizing in 33.3% of cases.

Interictal or peri-ictal PET using 2-[$^{18}$F] fluoro-2-deoxyglucose (FDG-PET) is included routinely in the pre-surgical evaluation protocols of many epilepsy surgery programmes. However, PET findings, characterized by the increased or decreased uptake of FDG, reflect the neuronal activity not only at the site of the ictal onset but also in areas of ictal spread and postictal depression. Interictal PET has been shown to be more sensitive than MRI in detecting foci of gliotic tissue with decreased metabolic uptake of FDG, but gliotic tissue does not necessarily correlate with an epileptogenic region. Only one-third of patients with extra-temporal seizures have relevant hypometabolic abnormalities concordant with an abnormal EEG focus, and these regions of hypometabolic activity are frequently widely distributed and poorly localized. Overall, FDG-PET does not appear to provide additionally clinically useful information in the majority of patients with lesional extra-temporal epilepsy.

### Electrocorticography (ECoG)

Intraoperative EEG recording directly from the cortex (ECoG) can be used to identify and resect epileptogenic tissue surrounding a lesion, and has been used for at least 50 years. Its value, however, still remains controversial. In one study of patients with low-grade gliomas and intractable epilepsy who underwent ECoG during surgery and in whom resection was guided by ECoG, 41% of the adults and 85% of the children were rendered seizure free. Others have found that ECoG has no predictive value and does not assist surgery. Perhaps surprisingly, the complete resection of all spiking areas identified at corticography seems by no means always to succeed in stopping seizures, nor does incomplete resection always fail.

### Stereotactic surgical methods

Stereotactic neurosurgery has greatly improved the surgical approach to small lesions and has improved surgical accuracy. Stereotaxis usually relies on co-registration of MRI and other data, and is often computer directed. Stereotactic lesionectomy is now routinely performed in many centres.

Depth electrode implantation is now best carried out using computer-guided stereotaxis. This is currently frame-based although developments in frameless stereotaxy may well prove it to be a safer and more convenient option. The overall risk of serious complication from each electrode implantation is about 2%, the major dangers being haemorrhage and infection. There are recorded cases of transmission of prion disease, but this is now usually avoided by using disposable electrodes (albeit at great expense).

Finally, there is considerable interest in stereotactic radiosurgery, using the gamma knife or the X-knife. These techniques have, not surprisingly, caught the public imagination. The best evaluated techniques have used radiosurgery to obliterate small AVMs or cavernomas.

### Surgical treatment of epilepsy due to cortical dysplasia

Cortical dysplasia is an important cause of medically intractable seizures. MRI scanning detects brain malformations in 5–10% of patients with refractory epilepsy and up to 15% of children with refractory epilepsy and learning disability. These figures are, however, likely to underestimate the true incidence, as histologically proven dysplasia is sometimes found on examination of tissue removed at surgery in patients with refractory epilepsy and normal conventional MRI. 'MRI-negative' cases currently account for about one-quarter of all cases with refractory epilepsy, and it is likely that a proportion have occult 'dysplasia'. In most cases, epileptic discharges are generated within dysplastic cortex as well as in adjacent tissue. This is an important difference from the epilepsy caused by foreign tissue lesions, in which the seizures are generated entirely from adjacent tissue, and may account for the poorer surgical results in incomplete resections.

Epilepsy surgery in cortical dysplasia is generally disappointing. The best outcome is reported following complete resection of focal cortical dysplasia (Taylor dysplasia), with short-term seizure-free rates of about 50% of cases, and there are no data about longer-term outcome. Resection of small areas of subcortical heterotopia also alleviate epilepsy in a reasonable number of cases. Other types of dysplasia, however, fare worse, and the comparatively poor outcome of all types of dysplastic lesion must reflect widespread epileptogenesis which extends beyond the margins of the lesions visible on conventional MRI scanning. Furthermore, brain anatomy is often abnormal in patients with cortical dysplasia, and cortical mapping shows aberrant location of functional cortex, and surgical morbidity can be greater than is the case in surgery for other cortical lesions. In focal cortical dysplasia and subcortical heterotopia, a good outcome requires at least the complete resection of the visible lesion. In one series a seizure-free outcome was achieved in 58% with complete resection compared with 27% of those with incomplete resection. It is also likely that the larger the resection, the better the chances of seizure control, although studies on this point are few. Better methods for detecting subtle cortical dysplastic lesions currently invisible on conventional MRI are needed, and only with these is epilepsy surgery likely to be routinely available to patients with even apparently focal lesions. In tuberous sclerosis the resection of single lesions can

successfully control seizures in well-selected cases. Resective surgery for more widespread lesions such as polymicrogyria, schizencephaly, periventricular heterotopia or lissencephaly is currently not recommended.

The pre-surgical assessment of patients with cortical dysgenesis is generally conducted in a similar manner to that of 'MRI-negative' cases (even if a dysplastic lesion is visible), for it is likely that the extent of the dysplastic lesion exceeds that visualized. The clinical history and examination will certainly not reveal the extent of the epileptogenic zone, although severe intellectual impairment suggests diffuse damage. Thus investigation must be multimodal. A striking feature of studies of surgical outcome, however, is the lack of predictive utility of EEG. Interictal scalp EEG often shows widespread, generalized or multifocal interictal spiking, and ictal EEG is often poorly localized. Indeed, even in those with clear-cut MRI lesions, ictal EEG is localized in less than 50%, and often ictal onsets appear to be diffuse or multifocal, and discordant with MRI lesions. The lack of specificity of EEG, conversely, means that some patients have good outcomes after resective surgery even if the interictal and ictal scalp EEG show widespread changes (Figure 5.18). The role of intracranial recordings is uncertain, and surgical outcome in most series does not correlate well with intracranial EEG findings. ECoG is widely used to guide resections per-operatively but the results from

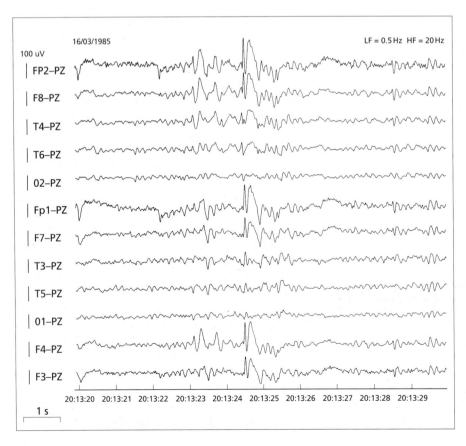

**Figure 5.18** Widespread bilateral anteriorly predominant interictal spikes recorded from a patient with an area of localized macrogyria in the left motor cortex.

different studies are contradictory. To a large extent, the effects of surgery are therefore unpredictable, and this uncertainty must be conveyed to the patient. Making prognostic predictions in terms of percentage chances (as is usually done, for instance, prior to surgery for hippocampal sclerosis) seems inappropriate given the small number of published cases, and the individual variation.

Interictal PET can identify brain malformations that are invisible to MRI but are histologically verified at operation. In paediatric practice PET may have a clinical role, revealing abnormalities that are otherwise difficult to detect, and leading to successful surgical intervention, particularly in young children undergoing large excisions for overwhelming epilepsy. MRI is normal in many of these cases. In adults, though, the utility of PET in pre-surgical evaluation is poorly studied. Ictal SPECT may not be as reliable in extra-temporal epilepsy due to cortical dysplasia as it is in hippocampal epilepsy. Hyperperfusion during seizures may be a useful sign, particularly if MRI is normal or inconclusive, and SPECT can also provide a guide to invasive monitoring. New imaging methods hold promise, and in the future better definition of the extent of epileptogenic tissue may be possible.

### Hypothalamic hamartoma

The surgery of hypothalamic hamartoma requires special mention. These lesions are a cause of severe epilepsy (including gelastic epilepsy, see p. 47). MRI must be very carefully performed. Large lesions are easily seen, but small lesions are often overlooked, particularly when confined to the tuber cinereum. High-quality T1-weighted images produce the best visualization, although the lesions are often isodense on T1 and T2 images. The EEG is usually non-localizing, and has limited value. Resection of this lesion results in complete seizure remission in about 50% of cases, and early operation will prevent learning disability, behavioural disturbance, and precocious puberty as well as evolution into intractable epilepsy. Various approaches have been attempted, including thermocoagulation, gamma-knife radiosurgery, and open or stereotactic resection via a transcallosal and other approaches. The choice of approach depends on the location and size of the hamartoma, and the experience of the surgeon.

## SURGERY WHERE NO LESION IS APPARENT ON NEUROIMAGING

Prior to MRI many cases of epilepsy (including virtually all cases of hippocampal sclerosis and cortical dysgenesis) were considered 'non-lesional'. The nature and extent of the surgery in these cases depended heavily on scalp and invasive EEG. It was realized, even then, that if no pathology was found in the operated specimen the prognosis for seizure control was poor. Often, however, small lesions were found and the prognosis was good.

Since the advent of MRI the situation has radically altered, as many of these previously occult lesions can be clearly demonstrated pre-operatively. Where the MRI is normal the chances of finding a 'lesion' in operated tissue are greatly reduced, and thus surgery must be considered a treatment of last resort. It should be offered only to patients with severe epilepsy, and usually only to patients experiencing secondarily generalized tonic–clonic seizures (on the basis that these carry greater risk if left untreated). It would be unusual to operate on individuals with partial seizures only, unless they were particularly handicapping. The pre-surgical assessment needs to be tailored to individual cases, but a number of general principles apply.

1 MRI studies should be of adequate quality. It is important to stress that a patient should not be considered MRI-negative unless a detailed MRI examination has been made, applying appropriate sequences and techniques. A critical approach is needed. Many patients with apparently normal MRI scans using inappropriate examinations show clear lesions when scanned using the epilepsy-orientated MRI protocols—this is especially true of patients harbouring such lesions as hippocampal atrophy, small vascular lesions or tumours, or cortical dysplasia. These 'pseudo-MRI-negative' cases emphasize the importance of a tailored MRI approach. Advanced scanning should include multi-sequence MRI, hippocampal volumetry, T2 quantitation, and a detailed scrutiny of high-resolution anatomical images, including multiplanar reformatting and three-dimensional rendering of cortical surface.

2 If MRI is normal, multimodal functional investigations are an absolute requirement. These should always include ictal scalp recordings and, in adults, neuropsychometric assessment. SPECT or PET is also usually carried out. The interictal EEG is seldom helpful in localization. Ictal scalp EEG will help to define where invasive EEG monitoring should be undertaken, and seldom will invasive EEG be contemplated if the scalp ictal EEG shows no localizing features. Although invasive EEG is often conceived as a gold standard, it should also be realized that only small areas of cortical tissue are sampled around implanted electrodes; the scalp EEG surveys a bigger territory. Invasive EEG should never be undertaken blindly (a 'fishing expedition'), and electrode placement should address specific questions and be guided by other clinical or investigatory findings. In one series ictal scalp EEG, ictal SPECT, and interictal PET allowed surgery to be carried out in 41 MRI-negative cases, of whom 39% were free from seizures at 1 year, and the ictal scalp EEG predicted good outcome more often than the other tests (70% vs 43% vs 33%, respectively). In another study only five out of 40 MRI-negative cases were found after intensive investigation to have localized lesions, and only three could be offered surgery.

**3** The bigger the resection, the better is the outcome. In young children particularly, large resections carry less functional penalty as brain plasticity allows reallocation of function during subsequent development. Thus, in young children with devastating epilepsy, large-scale resections, guided for example by interictal PET hypoperfusion, are considered appropriate even where no lesion or focal EEG disturbance is present. It has also become clear, however, that operating on adults without MRI changes, even in the presence of a clear-cut EEG focus, and even after a wide resection (e.g. a frontal lobectomy for epilepsy originating in anterior frontal regions), carries a generally poor prognosis, and fewer than 30% of patients can expect any great improvement in seizure frequency.

**Table 5.6** Approximate frequencies of underlying aetiologies treated by hemispherectomy.

| | |
|---|---|
| Rasmussen chronic encephalitis | 35% |
| Perinatal insult (usually vascular, leading to unilateral porencephaly) | 30% |
| Hemimegencephaly | 10% |
| Migrational disorder | 5% |
| Sturge–Weber disease | 5% |
| Viral or bacterial infection | 5% |
| Cerebral trauma | 5% |
| Postnatal cerebrovascular event | 5% |

## HEMISPHERECTOMY, HEMISPHEROTOMY AND OTHER LARGE RESECTIONS

The term 'hemispherectomy' is used here to cover a variety of operations in which one cerebral hemisphere is excised or disconnected from the other. These are operations carried out in children or adolescents (and occasionally adults) with medically refractory seizures due to severe unilateral hemisphere damage. The operations are nowadays carried out only to improve the control of epilepsy, although originally hemispherectomy was performed as a form of tumoural surgery.

### Pre-operative assessment

The suitability of any individual for hemispherectomy depends upon aetiology, clinical features, the neurological examination, the scalp EEG, and the results of neuroimaging. The assessment aims to examine the diseased hemisphere, and also the status of the 'good' hemisphere.

### Aetiology

The usual aetiologies in patients undergoing hemispherectomy are shown in Table 5.6. It is imperative to ascertain that the cerebral damage is wholly or very largely confined to one hemisphere. Even where the primary pathology is unilateral—for instance after a vascular or traumatic event—secondary bihemispheric damage can result from prolonged anoxia or coma. The results of surgery where there is bilateral damage are far less good.

### Seizures

Only patients with severe epilepsy, intractable to medical therapy, should be considered for this operation. Most patients going forward for hemispherectomy will have multi-ple seizure types and frequent (more than five) seizures each day. The seizures must have a focal onset in the damaged hemisphere. The condition in which focal motor seizures are most frequently seen is epilepsia partialis continua, usually secondary to Rasmussen encephalitis. Commonly, com-binations of secondarily generalized tonic–clonic seizures, drop attacks, and focal motor seizures co-exist. Complex partial seizures are not common in the types of pathology for which hemispherectomy is appropriate.

### Neurological status

The great majority of suitable candidates for hemispherectomy have a pre-operative fixed hemiplegia, reflecting the severity of the hemispheric damage. This can be associated with other signs, such as hemionopia or hemisensory loss, and most patients have some degree of mental and psychomotor retardation.

The operation is almost always carried out only where the hemiparesis is severe enough to impair the performance of individual finger movements. The pre-operative ability to perform gross movements of the fingers, or at other major joints (e.g. shoulder, elbow, hip, knee) is not a contraindication to surgery. These movements are not usually worse after a hemispherectomy, nor is a pre-existing spastic gait, although there may be a transient worsening for weeks after the operation. Lesser degrees of disability will deteriorate post-operatively. Occasionally patients with lesser defects are offered hemispherectomy, if they have a progressive disorder that, it is deemed, will inevitably lead to hemiplegia. In such children social and intellectual development will be accelerated with improved seizure control resulting from the operation, so that early hemispherectomy can be considered despite the inevitable worsening of motor function that will be caused by the operation. Hemionopia is usually but not always complete in the cases being considered. Its absence should not be considered an absolute contra-indication to hemispherectomy, although the operation will inevitably result in a

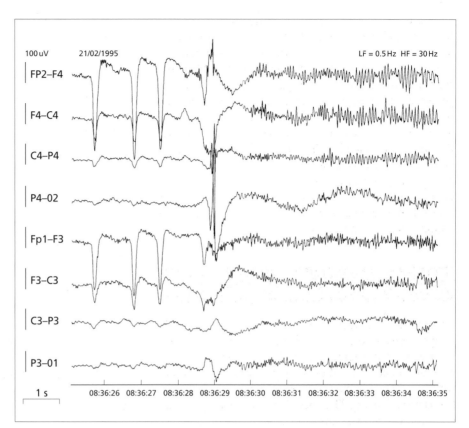

**Figure 5.19** Ictal scalp electroencephalograph from the patient illustrated in Fig. 5.20. Note the rhythmic activity evident over both hemispheres but of higher amplitude over the normal hemisphere.

complete hemionopia—but this deficit is not usually severely disabling. The presence or absence of sensory loss is not usually a consideration in deciding whether or not to proceed to surgery, as hemispherectomy rarely results in any marked change in sensory function.

The degree of intellectual impairment of patients suitable for hemispherectomy will vary, and is a good index of the functional status of the 'good' hemisphere. Severe psychomotor retardation should be interpreted as reflecting bilateral cerebral damage, and in this situation the outcome of hemispherectomy will be less good. Pathologies present early in life are generally associated with better preservation of function owing to brain plasticity.

Finally, if this operation is performed on the language-dominant hemisphere, permanent aphasia will result unless language functions can be transferred to the other side of the brain by processes of cortical plasticity and development. These processes are age dependent. It is possible to carry out dominant hemispherectomy before the age of 5 years without any impairment of language functions. Recovery of language after dominant hemispherectomy in children with later onset seizures (after the age of 5 years) is, however, rarely complete although some transfer of language functions is possible until the early teens. Language lateralization in older children can be confirmed preoperatively by the intracarotid amytal test (p. 245).

### EEG

Interictal scalp EEG is usually sufficient, and invasive EEG is not usually required, in the pre-operative assessment for hemispherectomy. Ideally, the EEG should show low-amplitude slow activity and epileptic discharges confined to the affected hemisphere, but this is not always the case (Figure 5.19). Sometimes the damaged hemisphere is incapable of generating sufficiently strong electrical signals to be detectable on scalp EEG, and discharges appear to be of higher amplitude on the side of the normal hemisphere. In about 50% of cases, secondary or independent epileptiform abnormalities occur in the 'good' hemisphere. Although these raise the possibility of bilateral damage, they are not an absolute contra-indication to the operation. Even apparently independent epileptic spikes originating from the 'good' hemisphere usually disappear after hemispherectomy.

### MRI and CT scanning

The appearances depend on the aetiology. Often unilateral hemispheric atrophy is present, with increased skull thickness, enlarged sulci and ventricles, and a small cerebral peduncle (Figure 5.20). Calcification, porencephaly, hemimegalencephaly, signal change, dysgenesis, or other lesions can be demonstrated on radiology. The contralateral hemisphere should show no major lesions.

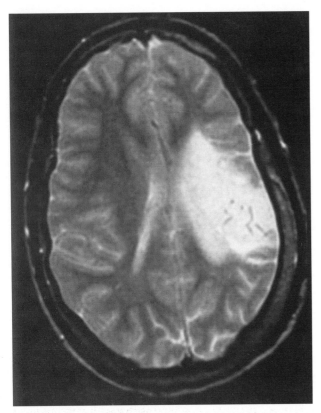

**Figure 5.20** Pre-operative magnetic resonance image scan in a patient subsequently undergoing a left hemispherectomy showing cerebral infarction, occurring in early childhood, leading to medically intractable seizures.

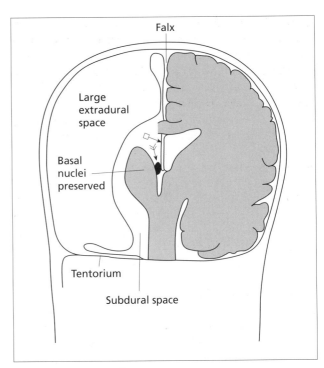

**Figure 5.21** Modified hemispherectomy: diagrammatic representation of the extent of excision. The arrows show the muscle plug and the foramen of Monro.

## Surgical techniques and surgical outcome
### Surgical techniques

The original surgical operation (the so-called 'anatomical hemispherectomy', Figure 5.21) has been shown in recent years to have serious late post-operative complications (see below). It has, therefore, been largely abandoned, and a variety of new surgical techniques have been developed. The anatomical hemispherectomy consisted of the complete removal of the affected cerebral hemisphere with or without the basal ganglia, either en bloc or in fragments. The modified hemispherectomy links this operation with procedures to eliminate communication of CSF with the hemispherectomy cavity by creating a largely extradural cavity and obstructing the foramen of Monro with a piece of muscle (Figure 5.21). The operations of hemidecortication and hemicorticectomy consist of excision of the cortex with the preservation of as much white matter as possible. The functional hemispherectomy consists of a subtotal anatomical hemispherectomy with complete physiological disconnection. The technique involves a large central removal including parasagittal tissue, and exposure of the whole length of the corpus callosum. All fibres entering the corpus callosum are then interrupted by undercutting from within the lateral ventricle in a parasagittal plane. The residual frontal and parieto-occipital lobes are disconnected by aspiration of white and grey matter in the posterior frontal region to the level of the sphenoid wing, and in the parieto-occipital region down to the tentorium. A large temporal lobectomy, including excision of medial structures, is finally carried out. The hemispherotomy and peri-insular hemispherotomy are variations on this principle, allowing cortical disconnection via alternative operative routes.

The choice of surgical method depends on the experience and preference of the surgeon, but functional hemispherectomy and hemispherotomy are now widely preferred to the anatomical hemispherectomy because of the smaller risks of morbidity.

### Early surgical morbidity

Fatal complications include brain swelling and tentorial herniation, and the overall mortality of hemispherectomy, which is often carried out in very young children, is in the region of 2–10%. Early morbidity includes haemorrhage and infection. Early hydrocephalus develops in 5–30% of cases and will require CSF shunting. Transient worsening of motor or speech function occurs but usually resolves.

### Late surgical morbidity

The traditional anatomical hemispherectomy is associated with two specific late complications—superficial cerebral haemosiderosis and late hydrocephalus. Superficial cerebral haemosiderosis results in a gradual neurological deterioration evident at a mean of 8 years after surgery. The pathological findings are obstructive hydrocephalus due to aqueduct stenosis, gliosis and ependymitis, while the hemispherectomy cavity is lined with a membrane similar to that found in a chronic subdural haematoma. The fluid in the ventricle is brownish and of 'machine oil' appearance. This complication is due to chronic bleeding into the subdural hemisherectomy cavity, and occurs in at least 30–50% of cases, leading eventually to disability and death. Late hydrocephalus is presumably produced by a similar mechanism. Patients who have had the operation require regular brain scans for early warning of these complications. The newer operations, and in particular the functional operations, are not followed by these disastrous complications.

### Outcome for seizure control and behaviour

Hemispherectomy is a very effective operation in carefully selected patients. Complete seizure control is expected in about 70–80%, and an improvement in seizures of at least 80% in 90–95% of suitably selected and competently operated cases. Even in carefully selected cases, however, 5% of operated patients will show no worthwhile benefit.

The primary indication of the operation is to control seizures. Secondary gains in terms of behaviour and psychosocial development usually also occur. Severely abnormal behaviour patterns are common in the sorts of children with severe epilepsy who undergo surgery. Typically taking the form of aggression and regressive behaviour, these are often a consequence of repeated seizures, subclinical EEG activity and drug treatment. A remarkable improvement can be expected post-operatively in children whose seizures have been controlled, and there are also gains in social development and intellectual function. Children whose seizures are controlled almost always integrate better into their family and school, and demonstrate greatly improved abilities to learn and concentrate. The intellectual deterioration which is inevitable without the operation is usually halted. Some children will develop to the stage where independent living and work are possible.

### Other large resections

A basic principle of the surgery of extra-temporal neocortical epilepsy is that the wider the excision around an epileptic focus, the more likely is complete seizure control to be achieved. This 'more is better' philosophy has characterized the surgical approach to epilepsy in non-eloquent cortical regions. A large frontal lobectomy, for example, can be carried out with no gross deficit and only an approximately 3% risk of hemiparesis. The inferior central region, over the face area, can be resected without sensory or motor deficit, presumably due to bilateral cortical representation, although resections in the hand or leg areas of the cortex do result in monoplegia. Similarly, a large resection of the non-dominant parietal lobe can be carried out with minor sensory deficit only. Dominant parietal resections carry a risk of profound sensory loss and apraxia. These large lobar resections are less common now because the MRI localization of structural disease has allowed more precise surgical planning.

### Sturge–Weber syndrome

In selected cases, resective surgery in this syndrome can have an excellent result. This should be carried out as early as is feasible in view of the danger of progressive neurological impairment caused by episodes of status epilepticus in this condition (see p. 38). Hemispherectomy can be carried out in patients with extensive lesions, and lesionectomy or lobectomy in smaller lesions. Corpus callosotomy has been used as a palliative procedure, but where possible resective surgery is preferable. MRI is the main pre-surgical investigation, and neither pre-operative EEG nor corticography has much influence on surgical procedure or outcome. The outcome after appropriate resective surgery is good, with at least 80% seizure control. The outcome for behaviour and intellectual development is also improved by early surgery.

## CORPUS CALLOSECTOMY (CORPUS CALLOSUM SECTION, CORPUS CALLOSOTOMY)

This operation, the transection of the corpus callosum, can be carried out in either a one- or two-staged procedure. Although first performed in 1940, even now neither the precise physiological rationale for the surgery not its indications are clearly defined.

It was originally proposed that section of the corpus callosum would prevent the rapid spread of epileptic activity from one hemisphere to the other, but in fact seizure activity can propagate widely via non-callosal pathways. It is simplistic to assume that the operation prevents secondary generalization, but it does have a desynchronizing effect on epileptic activity, and can inhibit seizures, although exactly how or why is unclear. In recent years the number of patients undergoing callosectomy has declined.

### Indications

The operation is now primarily reserved for patients with severe secondarily generalized epilepsy manifest by frequent drop attacks causing injury, in whom medical therapy is ineffective and in whom other surgical procedures are not possible. The procedure therefore is mostly considered in patients with tonic or atonic seizures, many of whom have additional seizure types and moderate or severe learning disability; many have the Lennox–Gastaut syndrome. However, it has also been shown to have an effect in complex partial seizures, some myoclonic seizures, and in tonic–clonic seizures. It can also be used in combination with resective surgery, and the operation can have a particular role, combined with frontal lobe resection, in patients with severe frontal lobe damage following trauma or abscess. In any of these indications, there seems little way of selecting out those patients who will do well from those who will not. This lack of predictability combined with its generally disappointing effects and its potential hazards render the corpus callosectomy a last ditch operation now only infrequently carried out. Vagal nerve stimulation carries far less risk, and many patients who would previously have been considered for corpus callosectomy are currently referred instead, initially at least, for vagal nerve stimulation.

### Pre-operative assessment

EEG, MRI and psychometric assessment are usually carried out. Patients with pre-operative EEG showing bilateral synchronous epileptic discharges or lateralized abnormalities tend to have a better outcome than those with multifocal EEG discharges.

### Operative procedure

In most centres corpus callosectomy is carried out as a two-stage procedure. In the first stage the anterior two-thirds of the corpus callosum are sectioned (Figure 5.22). If this is ineffective, the section can be completed at a second operation. The two-stage procedure has a lower morbidity. Actual surgical technique varies and improvements in recent times have lowered the rate of complications. EcoG is sometimes used to guide the extent of the first-stage resection. A recent development has been the use of focused radiosurgery with the gamma knife to carry out an anterior callosal section, and this may become the method of choice.

### Outcome

The operation must be considered a palliative procedure, intended to reduce seizure severity and in particular to reduce injuries due to falls. No patient should undergo the procedure on the assumption that epileptic seizures will stop completely. Short-term freedom from seizures does occur in about 5–10% of cases, but there is a strong tendency to relapse over months or years. Nevertheless, the number of generalized seizures or seizures with falls is usually reduced by the operation (albeit sometimes with an increase in the number of partial seizures).

Both the single- and the two-stage operation carry significant risks of neurological deficit. Hemiparesis can be due to traction per-operatively or to vascular infarction due to damage to the pericallosal arteries or venous thrombosis. A transient and highly distinctive disconnection syndrome with mutism, urinary incontinence and bilateral leg weakness is a not uncommon consequence of a single-stage complete callosal section. It is present in the immediate post-operative period and usually resolves after a matter of weeks, although in 5% of cases it can be permanent; the pathophysiology of this effect is not clear. A posterior disconnection syndrome in which complex motor tasks become impossible occurs in about 5% after a one-stage procedure. After the completed transection, most patients will exhibit elements of a 'split brain' profile on neuropsychological testing, although remarkably this causes little disability in everyday living. Other recorded complications include extradural haematoma, air embolism, infection, and an increase in the frequency or intensity of partial seizures or the appearance of new hemiclonic seizures. Callosectomy does not seem to affect overall behaviour or personality. Overall, the risks of permanent severe sequelae after corpus callosum section, either neurological or neuropsychological, are of the order of 5–10%, and there is a mortality rate of about 1–5%.

## MULTIPLE SUBPIAL TRANSECTION

This operation is also referred to as the Morrell procedure. Parallel rows of 4–5 mm deep cortical incisions are ploughed perpendicular to the cortical surface. This is done on the theoretical basis that the transections sever horizontal cortical connections and thus disrupt the lateral recruitment of neurones, which is essential for the production of synchronized epileptic discharges (Figure 5.23). At the same time normal function is preserved, as this is supported largely by vertically oriented afferent and efferent connections. There are many critics of this theory, and it is not clear whether or not this is a valid explanation of the post-operative consequences. The procedure has, theoretically, one major advantage—it can be used when the epileptogenic zone involves eloquent brain cortex, in which resection would result in significant neurological deficit. It has thus been principally applied to patients with epileptic foci in language, or primary sensory or motor cortex. In many cases it has been combined with a lesion resection in or adjacent to the eloquent cortex.

The procedure has been the subject of only a rather limited evaluation, and its true role is yet to be defined. A meta-analysis of data in 211 patients from six centres has been published. Fifty-three underwent the procedure without resection. In those in whom it was combined with resection, a short-term excellent result (≥ 95% reduction in seizures) was observed in 87% of those with generalized seizures and 68% of those with simple and complex partial seizures; in those who underwent the procedure without resection the figures were 71%, 62% and 63%, respectively. Neurological deficits occurred post-operatively in 23% of those operated with resection and 19% of those who had multiple subpial transection alone. These results are certainly encouraging, but only limited information regarding long-term seizure

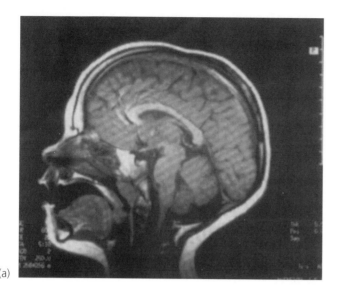

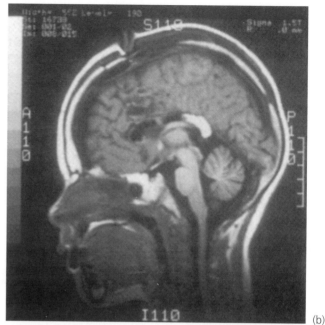

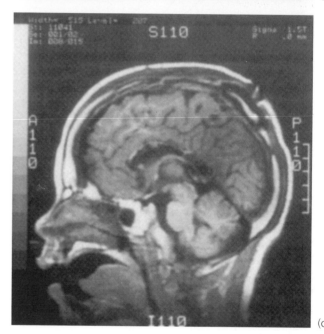

**Figure 5.22** MRI showing sagittal cuts through the corpus callosum in a 9-year-old patient. (a) Pre-operative, (b) after anterior two-thirds corpus callosotomy and (c) after callosotomy completion.

control is available, and at present the procedure should be reserved for patients with severe frequent seizures arising from the eloquent cortex in whom all alternative strategies have been exhausted. The operation, however, has a particular role in EPC and in the Landau–Kleffner syndrome.

Multiple subpial transection has been successfully carried out in Broca's area, the pre-central and post-central gyrus, and in Wernicke's area without noticeable loss of function. There is also a risk of haemorrhage, and a proportion of patients will experience severe motor, sensory, and language deficits. The overall morbidity of this opera-

tion in routine surgical practice has not been clearly established, and its use seems to be declining.

## VAGUS NERVE STIMULATION

In 1997 vagus nerve stimulation was approved by the US FDA for use as adjunctive therapy for adults and adolescents over 12 years of age whose partial-onset seizures are refractory to antiepileptic medications. Vagus nerve stimulation was then also approved in European Union countries

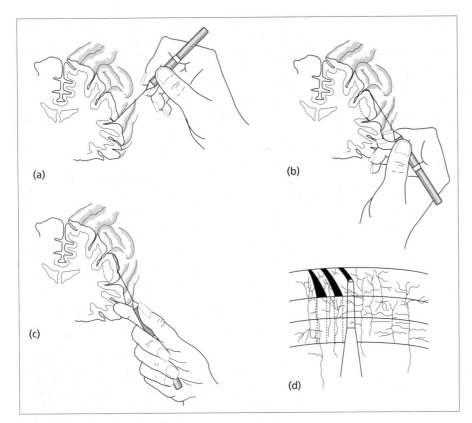

**Figure 5.23** Technique of multiple subpial transection. (a) After a tiny incision is created in the pia, a hook is inserted down one gyral edge. (b) It is then swept across the full width of the gyrus. (c) The hook is brought back to its starting point such that the tip is just visible under the pia as it crosses the gyrus. (d) The procedure is repeated at intervals of less than 5 mm along the gyrus leaving thin but visible scars. Thus, the transverse fibres only are sectioned, preserving the columnar organization.

for use in reducing the frequency of seizures in patients of any age whose epileptic disorder is dominated by partial seizures (with and without secondary generalization) or generalized seizures. Its use has grown rapidly in the past 5 years, and it is now the second most common epilepsy surgery procedure carried out in Great Britain (after temporal lobectomy). By August 2003 over 22,000 patients had been implanted with vagus nerve stimulation worldwide. There is no clear idea how vagus nerve stimulation influences epileptic seizures (which are, after all, a cortical phenomenon) but there is considerable experimental and clinical data now confirming that there is an observable, albeit modest, effect.

### The operative procedure

The operation comprises the implantation of a stimulator below the skin in the chest wall with bipolar electrodes wrapped around the left vagus nerve (Figure 5.24). The latest version of the stimulator box is an hermetically sealed titanium generator weighing 25 g, and measuring 52 mm in diameter and 6.9 mm deep. The operation takes only 1–2 hours to perform and is often carried out as a day case. It is a relatively minor procedure, lacking the inherent risks of intracranial surgery, hence its immediate attraction to physicians and patients alike.

The stimulation parameters can be set via a programming wand beaming radio-frequency signals to the

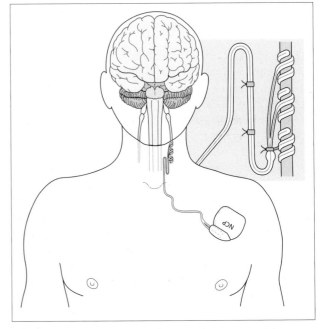

**Figure 5.24** Schematic drawing of the general placement of the NCP vagus nerve stimulation system and bipolar stimulating lead.

**Table 5.7** Available stimulation parameter settings in vagus nerve stimulation (Model 102 VNS Therapy).

| Stimulation parameter | Available settings |
|---|---|
| Output current | 0–3.5 mA ± 10%, in 0.25 mA steps |
| Signal frequency | 1, 2, 5, 10, 15, 20, 25, 30 Hz |
| Pulse width | 130, 250, 500, 750, 1000 µs ± 10% |
| Signal ON time | 7, 14, 21, 30, 60 s |
| Signal OFF time | 0.2, 0.3, 0.5, 0.8, 1.1, 1.8, 3 min, and 5–180 min (5–6 min in 5-min steps; 60–180 min in 30-min steps) |

generator. The wand is further used to perform diagnostic checks of wand–generator communications, lead impedance, programmed current, and an estimate of the remaining generator battery life. Once implanted, the stimulation parameters are slowly ramped up during the first 12 months after implantation. The ramp-up procedure and settings are tailored according to individual response and side-effects (Table 5.7). Patients can also trigger the stimulator at any time by applying a magnet to the skin over the generator. The generator in the current models should provide between 6 and 11 years of operation, after which it can be replaced, which involves only a minor procedure performed under local anaesthesia.

### Efficacy of vagus nerve stimulation

The effectiveness and safety of vagus nerve stimulation were investigated in clinical trials in a manner identical to that applied to new antiepileptic drugs. This was a copybook example of a regulatory trial programme, the only example in epilepsy surgery, and was highly successful.

Single-blind pilot studies in patients with refractory partial seizures were followed by two pivotal multicentre, double-blind, randomized, parallel, group-controlled trials, with vagus nerve stimulation added as adjunctive therapy. Two different vagus nerve stimulation protocols—high stimulation (30 Hz, 30 s on, 5 min off, 500 ms pulse width) and low stimulation (1 Hz, 30 s on, 90–180 min off, 130 ms pulse width)—were compared, the low stimulation protocol acting as an 'active control'. Individuals were monitored over a 12–16-week prospective baseline period, and then randomized to high- or low-stimulation groups. Over the next 2 weeks those in the high-stimulation group had their generator output current increased to as high a level as was tolerated, and those in the low-stimulation group had the current increased until stimulation could just be perceived. Efficacy was then assessed during the remaining 12 weeks of the treatment phase. The patient characteristics were similar to those in antiepileptic drug trials.

In both studies the primary efficacy analysis was percentage change in seizure frequency during treatment compared with baseline. In one trial the mean reduction in the high- and low-stimulation groups was 24.5 and 6.1%, respectively, and this difference was significant at a level of $P = 0.01$. In the second the mean per cent decreases in seizure frequency during treatment compared with baseline were 28 and 15% for the high- and low-stimulation groups, a statistically significant result at a level of $P = 0.039$. Secondary efficacy measures in both studies showed statistically significant effects in favour of high stimulation. In the first study 31% of patients in the high-stimulation group had a reduction in seizures of at least 50% compared with 13% of patients in the low-stimulation group ($P = 0.02$). In the second study 11% of patients in the high-stimulation group had a reduction in seizure frequency of at least 75% vs 2% for patients in the low-stimulation group ($P = 0.01$). On the basis of these results, the device was licensed for use. A study was then carried out in 60 children aged 3–18 years with pharmaco-resistant epilepsy. After 6 months of vagus nerve stimulation treatment ($n = 55$), the median reduction in seizure frequency was 31%. The corresponding figures at 12 and 18 months were 34% ($n = 51$) and 42% ($n = 46$), respectively. Other studies, some controlled, have shown progressive (but modest) falls in seizure rates over the longer term and a progressive decrease in the number of antiepileptic drugs needed as co-therapy. Studies have also been carried out in generalized epilepsy, in the Lennox–Gastaut syndrome, in the elderly, in children with epileptic encephalopathy, and in those with learning disability. In all these studies positive effects were noted.

### Safety and tolerability of vagus nerve stimulation

The implantation of a vagus nerve stimulator and its use with high-stimulation protocols can both cause adverse effects. Peri-operative complications include infection, left vocal cord paralysis, lower facial muscle paresis, pain, and fluid accumulation over the generator requiring aspiration. The rates of side-effects in the first double-blind study are shown in Table 5.8. Dyspnoea and hoarseness of the voice were the only adverse events that were reported significantly more often with high stimulation than with low stimulation. Longer-term effects were studied in a cohort of 444 patients who entered a long-term trial following participation in a short-term clinical study of vagus nerve stimulation. Ninety-seven per cent of patients continued for at least 1 year, and 85% and 72% continued for at least 2 and 3 years, respectively. The most commonly reported side-effects at the end of the first year of vagus nerve stimulation were, during 'on' periods, hoarseness (29%) and paresthesiae (12%); at the end of 2 years the most reported side-effects were hoarseness (19%) and cough (6%); and at 3 years, shortness of breath (3%) was the most frequent side-effect.

**Table 5.8** Adverse events among patients treated with low or high vagus nerve stimulation in randomized double-blind study.

| Adverse event | Low stimulation (n = 103) number (%) | High stimulation (n = 95) number (%) |
|---|---|---|
| Voice alteration | 31 (30.1) | 63 (66.3) |
| Cough | 44 (42.7) | 43 (45.3) |
| Pharyngitis | 26 (25.2) | 33 (34.7) |
| Pain | 31 (30.1) | 27 (28.4) |
| Dyspnoea | 11 (10.7) | 24 (25.3) |
| Headache | 24 (23.3) | 23 (24.2) |
| Dyspepsia | 13 (12.6) | 17 (17.9) |
| Vomiting | 14 (13.6) | 17 (17.9) |
| Paraesthesia | 26 (25.2) | 17 (17.9) |
| Nausea | 21 (20.4) | 14 (14.7) |
| Accidental injury | 13 (12.6) | 12 (12.6) |
| Fever | 19 (18.4) | 11 (11.6) |
| Infection | 12 (11.7) | 11 (11.6) |

Only adverse events that occurred in more than 10% of high-stimulation patients are listed.

Quality of life measures have also been assessed. These demonstrate an apparent improvement in energy, memory, daytime sleepiness, social aspects, mental effects and fear of seizures, and these effects occur whether or not seizures have been improved. The common sedative side-effects of new drugs do not occur, and this is of course a very important difference and a major attraction of the procedure to patients. There is some evidence that vagus nerve stimulation has an antidepressant action, but currently the procedure is not licensed for this indication. Positive effects on mood and behaviour in children with learning disability and epilepsy have also been recorded.

Vagus nerve stimulation carries the potential for serious adverse effects. One concern has been the possibility that vagus nerve stimulation might induce cardiac arrhythmia owing to the vagus innervation of the heart. Changes in heart rate and heart rate variability have been observed in treated patients, and episodes of asystole have also been recorded. However, mortality rates have been published and are no different from historical controls with epilepsy. The published rate of sudden unexpected death in epilepsy (SUDEP) in treated patients is 4.1 per 1000 person-years. Chronic stimulation can also mildly impair swallowing and increase the risk of aspiration in vulnerable persons. Other side-effects recorded include posture-dependent stimula-

tion of the phrenic nerve and worsening of pre-existing obstructive sleep apnoea.

### Clinical role for vagus nerve stimulation

There seems to be no doubt that vagus nerve stimulation can exert a modest antiepileptic action. It has the advantage of not being a drug, and so patients can escape the cognitive and CNS side-effects associated with all conventional antiepileptic medication. Furthermore, the stimulator can be simply implanted with low operative morbidity—and certainly none of the risk of intracranial surgery. However, the effectiveness of the procedure has not, in the opinion of many, lived up to the promise apparent from the clinical trials. Few patients have gained seizure freedom from the technique, and there appears often to be little or no effect at all. The problem of assessing the procedure is compounded both by the large number of possible variations in stimulation parameters that can be tried, and also the suggestion that effects on seizure frequency may be delayed and become observable weeks or months after the initiation of therapy.

The indications for the procedure are not fully explored, but currently it is used in patients who have failed to respond to conventional medical therapy, and in whom resective surgical therapy is not appropriate. There is no clear evidence that one seizure type does better than any other, although the use of vagus nerve stimulation in generalized epilepsy is currently evinced only by open, uncontrolled studies.

The usual initial target parameters are shown in Table 5.9. Programming is commenced a few weeks after implantation. The ramping up of stimulation parameters typically is performed at outpatient follow-up visits with a specially trained nurse, every 1–2 weeks over the next several months. At these visits the current is usually increased by 0.25 mA increments, or more, to the maximum tolerated settings or until reduction in seizure frequency exceeds 50% compared with the pre-implantation baseline. If side-effects become intolerable or do not resolve following a change of stimulation parameters, the current is reduced by 0.25 mA decrements as necessary. Reducing the pulse width may also improve tolerability.

**Table 5.9** Usual initial target stimulation parameters for VNS stimulation in patients with epilepsy.

| Stimulation parameter | Setting |
|---|---|
| Output current | 1.5 mA |
| Signal frequency | 20–30 Hz |
| Pulse width | 250–500 µs |
| Signal ON time | 30 s |
| Signal OFF time | 5 min |

The patient can override stimulation patterns with the magnet, which can be used to trigger stimulation or to suppress programmed activity. If seizures have not improved after 6–9 months of stimulation, the 'off time' is usually decreased from 5 to 3 minutes. Subsequent staged reductions of the 'off time' to 1.8 and 0.2 minutes, with an associated decrease of 'on time' to 7 seconds ('rapid cycle') can be tried. If within 12–18 months there is no improvement, the device is usually switched off and the box subsequently removed. This is an outpatient procedure carried out under local anaesthesia. The electrodes usually have to be left *in situ* as surgical removal often damages the nerve. No long-term deleterious effects on the vagus nerve have been reported. The initial cost of vagus nerve stimulation is high, and much higher than the initial costs of pharmacotherapy and attempts have been made to demonstrate long-term cost effectiveness.

## OTHER FUNCTIONAL SURGICAL PROCEDURES

Stereotactic neurosurgery is a fast-moving area with the potential for a major impact on epilepsy surgery, in a number of different ways.

Both stereotactic ablation and deep-brain stimulation have been used, in small numbers of patients, in an attempt to control or modify seizures since the 1930s. Targets have included the amygdala, various thalamic nuclei, the fields of Forel, the anterior commissure, the fornix, and the posterior limb of the internal capsule. The results of these operations in the past were generally poor, and this type of functional surgery had until recently been largely abandoned.

There has been a recent resurgence of interest in deep brain stimulation (DBS), encouraged by both the improved anatomical precision of stereotaxy made possible by MRI, better surgical instrumentation and stimulation technology, and also by the success of these procedures in other conditions such as Parkinson disease and in pain. Targets that are most favoured include the caudate nucleus, the centromedian nucleus of the thalamus, the anterior thalamic nucleus, the mamillary bodies and the subthalamic nucleus. Direct stimulation of the epileptic focus, in both the neocortex and the hippocampus, has also been attempted. All these approaches have had encouraging results in animal experimentation, and there are small human case reports and small series. Pioneering double-blind studies in small numbers of patients with severe epilepsy have been reported. In six of nine patients, stimulation of the subthalamic nuclear resulted in an > 80% reduction in seizures, and in a study of five patients, stimulation of the anterior thalamus produced an average 54% seizure reduction after a mean follow-up of 15 months. Centromedian nucleus stimulation has also

shown promising results with stimulation settings in the range 60–130 Hz, 2.5–5.0 V, 0,2–1.0 ms duration for 1 minute in every 5. A greater than 50% reduction in seizures occurred in an open investigation of amygdalo-hippocampal stimulation in three patients. However, well-controlled and blinded studies of cerebellar stimulation and hippocampal stimulation have shown no benefit. One research direction is the combination of brain stimulation with seizure-detection technology, so that the stimulator is turned on at the onset, or just before, the initiation of a seizure. DBS carries risks, notably of infection and haemorrhage (a rate of about 5%), and as yet none of these techniques is in routine clinical usage in any major centre.

A related technique is transcranial magnetic stimulation (TMS), which has been used to treat myoclonus and partial seizures. Anecdotal case reports are encouraging, and in one open study eight of nine patients with myoclonus showed a seizure reduction of 39%. A recent study of 24 patients with frequent partial and secondary generalized seizures has been published. Low-frequency, repetitive transcranial magnetic stimulation on five consecutive days resulted in a mean reduction of only 16% in seizures, which was not significant. The parameters of the stimulation can be varied considerably, and there is no agreement on the optimal settings and methods.

Gamma-knife or proton-pencil beam surgery are also under investigation for use in focal ablations and other forms of functional surgery. There is also research interest in the possibility of stem-cell and neural transplantation, and in the possibility of stereotactic drug implantation. None of these procedures is yet at a stage where surgery in routine clinical practice is possible.

A note of caution is needed, however, when considering functional surgical approaches to epilepsy. Over the past century various functional procedures have been practised, usually without proper evaluation, which are now considered worthless (Table 5.10). The current vogue

**Table 5.10** A lesson from history—'functional operations' still being performed for epilepsy, 1900–1930.

| |
|---|
| Trepanation |
| Trephination |
| Carotid artery occlusion |
| Bilateral vertebral artery occlusion |
| Cervical sympathectomy |
| Castration |
| Circumcision |
| Hysterectomy/oopherectomy |
| Adrenalectomy |
| Dural splitting |
| Colectomy and other bowel resections |
| Arterialization of internal jugular vein |

**Table 5.11** The characteristics of level 1 and level 2 epilepsy centres.

| | Level 1 centres | Level 2 centres |
|---|---|---|
| Patients | Adults | Adults and children (in some centres) |
| Type of surgery | Anterior temporal lobectomy | A full range of epilepsy surgical procedures |
| General facilities | Full range of neurological and neurosurgical facilities, and neurosurgical ITU | As for level 1 |
| MRI facilities | 1.5 Tesla with facilities for thin slice volumetric imaging | As for level 1, with additional facilities where possible for fMRI, MRS and post-processing |
| Other neuroimaging facilities | CT and angiography | As for level 1, with access to other procedures such as PET, SPECT, SISCOM |
| Neuropsychological facilities | Routine neuropsychology and facilities for WADA testing | As for level 1 |
| EEG facilities | Routine scalp EEG, video telemetry and corticography | As for level 1, with additional facilities for intracranial recording and stimulation |
| Staffing | Access to: neurology, neurosurgery, clinical neurophysiology, neuroradiology, neuropsychiatry, neurorehabilitation, neuropathology, counselling, full technical support | As for level 1, with additional paediatric specialities if paediatric surgery is being performed |
| Audit | An audit of surgical volume and results should be available where possible | As for level 1 |

for functional surgery requires careful evaluation to avoid similar mistakes.

## THE ORGANIZATION OF EPILEPSY SURGERY CARE: THE EPILEPSY SURGERY CENTRE

It should be clear that epilepsy surgery is a specialized area which requires, for almost every patient, an input from specialists in different non-surgical areas—for example neurology, neurophysiology, neuroradiology, neuropaediatrics, neurorehabilitation, neuropsychology and psychiatry. The input is needed to select suitable patients for surgery, to counsel patients adequately about the potential risks and benefits of surgery, and to follow-up patients after surgery. A full range of necessary facilities and expertise is likely to be available only in designated centres, and standards for such centres have been defined by the ILAE Commission on Neurosurgery.

It has been proposed that there should be two levels of epilepsy surgery centre: basic epilepsy surgery centres (level 1), and reference epilepsy surgery centres (level 2). Both should be sited within a comprehensive neuroscience centre, and the typical characteristics of each level are shown in Table 5.11. In the age of clinical governance and audit, it is inevitable as well as desirable that epilepsy surgery services are organized in such a formal and regulated fashion.

# Pharmacopoeia

Use of antiepileptic drugs in different seizure types and syndromes.

| | Partial and secondarily generalized tonic–clonic seizures* | Tonic–clonic seizures (primary generalized)** | Absence seizures† | Myoclonic seizures†† | West syndrome††† | Lennox–Gastaut syndrome†††† |
|---|---|---|---|---|---|---|
| Carbamazepine | + | + | | | | |
| Clobazam | + | + | + | + | | + |
| Clonazepam | + | + | + | + | + | + |
| Ethosuximide | | | + | | | |
| Gabapentin | + | | | | | |
| Lamotrigine | + | + | +[1] | +[1,2] | | + |
| Levetiracetam | + | +[1] | +[1] | +[1] | | |
| Oxcarbazepine | + | + | | | | |
| Phenobarbital | + | + | + | + | | |
| Phenytoin | + | + | | | | |
| Pregabalin | + | | | | | |
| Primidone | + | + | | | | |
| Tiagabine | + | | | | | |
| Topiramate | + | + | +[1] | +[1] | +[1] | + |
| Valproate | + | + | + | + | + | + |
| Vigabatrin | + | | | | + | |
| Zonisamide | + | +[1] | | +[3] | +[1] | +[1.] |

+ Reasonable clinical experience of effectiveness.

* At the time of writing, gabapentin, levetiracetam, pregabalin, tiagabine and vigabatrin are licensed only for use as add-on therapy in most countries. However, there is extensive published experience of off-label use in monotherapy (in all except pregabalin, which has been introduced into practice only recently).

** Primary generalized tonic–clonic seizures, usually in the syndrome of idiopathic generalized epilepsy (IGE).

† Typical absence seizures (petit mal) as part of the syndrome of idiopathic generalized epilepsy (IGE); Other effective drugs include acetazolamide and felbamate.

†† Other drugs effective in myoclonic seizures include acetazolamide, felbamate and piracetam.

††† Other drugs effective in West syndrome include ACTH, corticosteroids and felbamate.

†††† Drugs commonly used are listed. Other effective drugs include felbamate, rufinamide and corticosteroids.

+[1] Off-label indication currently, but with clinical trial evidence to support use.

+[2] Off-label indication currently; effect variable with myoclonus, in some cases worsened.

+[3] Off-label indication currently, but with clinical trial evidence to support its use in progressive myoclonic epilepsies. Less evidence for any on myoclonus in idiopathic generalized epilepsies.

Usual dosing regimens in adults.

| | Initial dose (mg/day) | Drug initiation: usual dose increment[1] (mg/day) | Usual maintenance dose on monotherapy (mg/day) | Usual maximum dose in monotherapy (mg/day) | Dosing intervals (per day) | Drug reduction: usual dose decrement[2] (mg/day) | Maintenance doses can differ in polytherapy |
|---|---|---|---|---|---|---|---|
| Carbamazepine† | 100 | 100–200 | 400–1600 | 2000 | 2 | 200 | Yes |
| Clobazam | 10 | 10 | 10–30 | 30 | 1–2 | 10 | |
| Clonazepam | 0.25 | 0.25–0.5 | 0.5–4 | 4 | 1–2 | 1 | |
| Ethosuximide | 250 | 250 | 750–1500 | 1500 | 2–3 | 250 | Yes |
| Gabapentin | 300–400 | 300–400 | 900–2400 | 3200 | 2–3 | 300 | |
| Lamotrigine | 12.5–25 | 25–100 | 100–400 | 600 | 2 | 100 | Yes |
| Levetiracetam | 125–250 | 250–500 | 500–1500 | 4000 | 2 | 500 | |
| Oxcarbazepine | 600 | 300 | 600–2400 | 3000 | 2 | 300 | Yes |
| Phenobarbital | 30 | 30–60 | 60–120 | 180 | 1–2 | 30 | Yes |
| Phenytoin | 200 | 25–100 | 200–300 | 450 | 1–2 | 50 | Yes |
| Pregabalin | 150 | 50–100 | 150–600 | 600 | 2–3 | 150 | |
| Primidone | 62.5–125 | 125–250 | 250–1000 | 1500 | 1–2 | 125 | Yes |
| Tiagabine | 4–5 | 4–15 | 15–30 | 56–60 | 2–3 | 5 | Yes |
| Topiramate | 25–50 | 50–100 | 100–300 | 600 | 2 | 50 | Yes |
| Valproate | 200–500 | 200–500 | 600–1500 | 3000 | 2–3 | 200 | Yes |
| Vigabatrin | 1000 | 500 | 1000–2000 | 4000 | 2 | 500 | |
| Zonisamide | 100 | 50 | 200–400 | 600 | 1–2 | 100 | Yes |

(Values in this table are based on the author's own practice, and may vary from those published elsewhere.)

[1] In routine situations, the dose is stepped up every 2 weeks;

[2] In routine situations, the dose is stepped down every 2–4 weeks;

† Values are for the slow-release formulation, which is the formulation of choice, particularly at high doses.

Usual dosing regimens and licensing of antiepileptic drugs for use in children.

| | Usual daily maintenance dose | Dosing interval | Licence for add-on therapy[1] | Licence for monotherapy (Europe) |
|---|---|---|---|---|
| Carbamazepine | < 1 year, 100–200 mg<br>1–5 years, 200–400 mg<br>5–10 years, 400–600 mg<br>10–15 years, 600–1000 mg | 2–4 | Yes (with no age restriction) | Yes (with no age restriction) |
| Clobazam | 3–12 years : 5–10 mg/day | 1–2 | ≥ 3 years (can be used in children over 6 months of age in exceptional circumstances) | No |
| Clonazepam | < 1 year: 1 mg/day<br>1–5 years: 1–2 mg/day<br>5–12 years: 1–3 g/day | 1–2 | Yes (with no age restriction) | Yes (with no age restriction) |
| Ethosuximide | 20–40 mg/kg/day | 2–3 | Yes (with no age restriction) | Yes (with no age restriction) |
| Gabapentin | 50–100 mg/kg | 2–3 | ≥ 6 years | No |
| Lamotrigine | See tables on page 141 | | ≥ 2 years | ≥ 12 years |
| Levetiracetam | – | | Not licensed for use in children | No |
| Oxcarbazepine | 30–60 mg/kg | 2 | ≥ 6 years | ≥ 6 years |
| Phenobarbital | 3–4 mg/kg | 1–2 | Yes (with no age restriction) | Yes (with no age restriction) |
| Phenytoin | 10 mg/kg | 1–2 | Yes (with no age restriction) | Yes (with no age restriction) |
| Pregabalin | – | | Not licensed for use in children | No |
| Primidone | 10–20 mg/kg | 1–3 | Yes (with no age restriction) | Yes (with no age restriction) |
| Tiagabine | | | ≥ 12 years | No |
| Topiramate | 5–9 mg/kg | 2 | ≥ 2 years | ≥ 6 years |
| Valproate | Under 20 kg: 20–40 mg/kg<br>Over 20 kg: 20–30 mg/kg/day | 2–3 | Yes (with no age restriction) | Yes (with no age restriction) |
| Vigabatrin | 10–15 kg: 40 mg/kg or 500–1000 mg<br>15–30 kg: 1000–1500 mg<br>> 30 kg: 1500–3000 mg | 2 | Yes (with no age restriction) | Yes (with no age restriction) |
| Zonisamide | 4–8 mg/kg | 1–2 | Not licensed for use in children[2] | No |

[1] Licensing in UK and in most of Europe (at time of writing). Similar rules apply elsewhere, although exact licensing regulations differ in different countries.

[2] Licensed in other countries for use in children.

Common and/or important side-effects of antiepileptic drugs.

| | Common and/or important adverse effects |
|---|---|
| Carbamazepine | Drowsiness, fatigue, dizziness, ataxia, diplopia, blurring of vision, sedation, headache, insomnia, gastrointestinal disturbance, tremor, weight gain, impotence, effects on behaviour and mood, hepatic disturbance, rash and other skin reactions, bone marrow dyscrasia, leucopenia, hyponatraemia, water retention, endocrine effects |
| Clobazam | Sedation, dizziness, weakness, blurring of vision, restlessness, ataxia, aggressiveness, behavioural disturbance, withdrawal symptoms |
| Clonazepam | Sedation (common and may be severe), cognitive effects, drowsiness, ataxia, personality and behavioural changes, hyperactivity, restlessness, aggressiveness, psychotic reaction, seizure exacerbations, hypersalivation, tone changes, leucopenia, withdrawal symptoms |
| Ethosuximide | Gastrointestinal symptoms, drowsiness, ataxia, diplopia, headache, dizziness, hiccups, sedation, behavioural disturbances, acute psychotic reactions, extrapyramidal symptoms, blood dyscrasia, rash, lupus-like syndrome, severe idiosyncratic reactions |
| Gabapentin | Drowsiness, dizziness, seizure exacerbation, ataxia, headache, tremor, diplopia, nausea, vomiting, rhinitis |
| Lamotrigine | Rash (sometimes severe), headache, blood dyscrasia, ataxia, asthenia, diplopia, nausea, vomiting, dizziness, somnolence, insomnia, depression, psychosis, tremor, hypersensitivity reactions |
| Levetiracetam | Somnolence, asthenia, infection, dizziness, headache, irritability, aggression, behavioural and mood changes |
| Oxcarbazepine | Somnolence, headache, dizziness, diplopia, ataxia, rash, hyponatraemia, weight gain, alopecia, nausea, gastrointestinal disturbance |
| Phenobarbital | Sedation, ataxia, dizziness, insomnia, hyperkinesis (children), mood changes (especially depression), aggressiveness, cognitive dysfunction, impotence, reduced libido, folate deficiency, vitamin K and vitamin D deficiency, osteomalacia, Dupuytren contracture, frozen shoulder, connective tissue abnormalities, rash. Risk of dependency. Potential for abuse |
| Phenytoin | Ataxia, dizziness, lethargy, sedation, headaches, dyskinesia, acute encephalopathy (phenytoin intoxication), hypersensitivity, rash, fever, blood dyscrasia, gingival hyperplasia, folate deficiency, megaloblastic anaemia, vitamin K deficiency, thyroid dysfunction, decreased immunoglobulins, mood changes, depression, coarsened facies, hirsutism, peripheral neuropathy, osteomalacia, hypocalcaemia, hormonal dysfunction, loss of libido, connective tissue alterations, pseudolymphoma, hepatitis, vasculitis, myopathy, coagulation defects, bone marrow hypoplasia |
| Pregabalin | Somnolence, dizziness, ataxia asthenia, weight gain, blurred vision, diplopia, tremor |
| Primidone | As for phenobarbital. Also dizziness and nausea on initiation of therapy |
| Tiagabine | Dizziness, tiredness, nervousness, tremor, diarrhoea, nausea, headache, confusion, psychosis, flu-like symptoms, ataxia, depression, word-finding difficulties, encephalopathy, non-convulsive status epilepticus |
| Topiramate | Dizziness, ataxia, headache, paraesthesia, tremor, somnolence, cognitive dysfunction, confusion, agitation, amnesia, depression, emotional lability, nausea, diarrhoea, diplopia, weight loss |
| Valproate | Nausea, vomiting, hyperammonaemia and other metabolic effects, endocrine effects, severe hepatic toxicity, pancreatitis, drowsiness, cognitive disturbance, aggressiveness, tremor, weakness, encephalopathy, thrombocytopenia, neutropenia, aplastic anaemia, hair thinning and hair loss, weight gain, polycystic ovarian syndrome |
| Vigabatrin | Mood change, depression, psychosis, aggression, confusion, weight gain, insomnia, changes in muscle tone in children, tremor, diplopia, severe visual field constriction |
| Zonisamide | Somnolence, ataxia, dizziness, fatigue, nausea, vomiting, irritability, anorexia, impaired concentration, mental slowing, itching, diplopia, insomnia, abdominal pain, depression, skin rashes, hypersensitivity. Significant risk of renal calculi. Weight loss, oligohidrosis and risk of heat stroke |

Pharmacokinetic parameters of antiepileptic drugs (average adult values).

| | Oral bioavailability | Volume of distribution | Time to peak level | Metabolism | Half-life† | Protein binding | Active metabolite |
|---|---|---|---|---|---|---|---|
| Carbamazepine | Moderate | High | 4–8 h | Hepatic | 5–26 h[5] | 75% | CBZ-epoxide |
| Clobazam | Moderate | High | 1–4 h | Hepatic | 10–77 h (50 h[1]) | 83% | *N*-desmethyl clobazam |
| Clonazepam | Moderate | High | 1–4 h | Hepatic | 20–80 h | 86% | None |
| Ethosuximide | High | Moderate | < 4 h | Hepatic | 30–60 h[5] | < 10% | None |
| Gabapentin | Variable | High | 2–3 h | None | 5–7 h | None | None |
| Lamotrigine | High | High | 1–3 h | Hepatic | 12–60 h[5] | 55% | None |
| Levetiracetam | High | Moderate | 1–2 h | Non-hepatic | 6–8 h | None | None |
| Oxcarbazepine | High | Moderate | 4–6 h | Hepatic | 8–10 h[1,5] | 38%[1] | MHD |
| Phenobarbital | Variable | Moderate | 1–3 h | Hepatic | 75–120 h[5] | 45–60% | None |
| Phenytoin | Variable | Moderate | 4–12 h | Hepatic | 7–42 h[2,5] | 85–95% | None |
| Pregabalin | High | Moderate | 1 h | None | 6 h | None | None |
| Primidone | High | High | 3 h | Hepatic | 5–18 h[5] (75–120 h[1]) | 25% | Phenobarbital |
| Tiagabine | High | High | 1–2 h[3] | Hepatic | 5–9 h[5] | 96% | None |
| Topiramate | High | High | 2–4 h | Hepatic | 19–25 h[5] | 15% | None |
| Valproate | High | Low | 0.5–8 h[4] | Hepatic | 12–17 h[5] | 85–95% | None |
| Vigabatrin | High | High | 0.5–2 h | None | 4–7 h | None | None |
| Zonisamide | High | High | 2–4 h | Hepatic | 49–69 h[5] | 30–60% | None |

The values in this table are approximate and relate to typical adult patients (individuals vary and values in children are often different).

| Bioavailablity: | | Volume of distribution: | |
|---|---|---|---|
| High | = > 90% | High | = > 0.8 l/kg |
| Moderate | = 70–90% | Moderate | = 0.5–0.8 l/kg |
| | | Low | = < 0.5 l/kg |

† Half-life in healthy adult.

[1] Value for active metabolite.

[2] Phenytoin has non linear kinetics, and so half-life can increase at higher doses.

[3] Absorption of tiagabine is markedly slowed by food, and it is recommended that the drug is taken at the end of meals.

[4] The time to peak concentration varies according to formulation (0.5–2 h for normal formulation, 3–8 h for enteric coated).

[5] Half-life varies with co-medication.

Mechanisms of antiepileptic drug action and principal pathways of metabolism.

| | Major mechanism of antiepileptic drug action | Phase 1 reactions | Phase 2 reactions | P450 enzymes identified in the phase 1 reactions[3] |
|---|---|---|---|---|
| Carbamazepine | Inhibition of voltage-dependent sodium conductance. Also action on monoamine, acetylcholine, and NMDA receptors | Epoxidation, hydroxylation | Conjugation | CYP3A4 CYP2C8 CYP1A2 |
| Clobazam | GABA-A receptor agonist | Demethylation, hydroxylation | Conjugation | |
| Clonazepam | GABA-A receptor agonist | Reduction, hydroxylation | Acetylation | CYP3A4 |
| Ethosuximide | Effects on calcium T-channel conductance | Oxidation | Conjugation | CYP3A4 |
| Gabapentin | Not known | Renal excretion without metabolism | | – |
| Lamotrigine | Inhibition of voltage-dependent sodium conductance | No phase one reaction | Conjugation | – |
| Levetiracetam | Action via binding to SV2A synaptic vesicle protein | Hydrolysis by non-hepatic enzymes | | CYP3A4 |
| Oxcarbazepine | Inhibition of voltage-dependent sodium conductance. Also effects on potassium conductance, N-type calcium channels, NMDA receptors | Reduction | Conjunction | CYP2C8 |
| Phenobarbital | Enhances activity of GABA-A receptor; also depresses glutamate excitability, and affects sodium, potassium, and calcium conductance | Oxidation, glucosidation, hydroxylation | Conjunction | CYP2C9 CYP2C19 CYP2E1 |
| Phenytoin | Inhibition of voltage-dependent sodium channels | Oxidation, glucosidation, hydroxylation | Conjunction | CYP2C9 CYP2C19 CYP3A4 |
| Pregabalin | Binds to alpha 2 delta subunit voltage-gated calcium channel. Also reduces release of glutamate and other excitatory neurotransmitters | Renal excretion without metabolism | | – |
| Primidone | – | Transformation to phenobarbital and a phenylethyl derivative, then metabolized as per phenobarbital | | |
| Tiagabine | Inhibits GABA reuptake | Oxidation | Conjunction | CYP3A4 |
| Topiramate[1] | Inhibition of voltage-gated sodium channels; potentiation of GABA-mediated inhibition at the GABA-A receptor; reduction of AMPA receptor activity; inhibition of high-voltage calcium channels; carbonic anhydrase activity | Hydroxylation, hydrolysis | Conjunction | |
| Valproate | Effects on GABA and glutaminergic activity, calcium (T) conductance and potassium conductance | Oxidation, hydroxylation, epoxidation, reduction[2] | Conjugation | CYP4B1 CYP2C9 CYP2A6 CYP2B6 CYP2C19 |
| Vigabatrin | Inhibition of GABA transaminase activity | Renal excretion without metabolism | | – |
| Zonisamide | Inhibition of voltage-gated sodium channel, T-type calcium currents, benzodiazepine GABA-A receptor excitatory glutaminergic transmission, carbonic anhydrase | Acetylation, reduction | Conjugation | CYP3A4 |

Conjugation (phase 1) is always by glucuronidation involving the UDPGT family enzymes.

[1] In non-induced patients, most topiramate is excreted renally without metabolism.

[2] Some of the biotransformation of valproate is via non-P450 enzyme systems.

[3] This lists known enzymes. Other enzymes, not yet fully characterized, play a part in the metabolism of many of these drugs.

Blood level monitoring.

| | 'Target level' (µ mol/l) | Value of blood level measurements in routine practice | Potential for drug interactions | Drug levels commonly affected by co-medication | Levels of oral contraceptive can be affected by co-medication | Levels of other commonly drugs affected by co-medication |
|---|---|---|---|---|---|---|
| Carbamazepine | 20–50 | *** | †† | Yes | Yes | Yes |
| Clobazam | | 0 | † | | | |
| Clonazepam | | 0 | † | | | |
| Ethosuximide | 300–700 | *** | †† | Yes | | |
| Gabapentin | | 0 | None | | | |
| Lamotrigine | 10–60 | ** | †† | Yes | Yes | Yes |
| Levetiracetam | | 0 | None | | | |
| Oxcarbazepine | 50–140[2] | * | †† | Yes | Yes | |
| Phenobarbital | 50–130 | ** | †† | Yes | Yes | Yes |
| Phenytoin | 40–80 | *** | †† | Yes | Yes | Yes |
| Pregabalin | | 0 | None | | | |
| Primidone | 25–50[1] | ** | †† | Yes | Yes | Yes |
| Tiagabine | | 0 | †† | Yes | | |
| Topiramate | 10–60 | * | †† | Yes | Yes | |
| Valproate | 300–700 | ** | †† | Yes | | Yes |
| Vigabatrin | | 0 | None | | | |
| Zonisamide | 30–140 | * | †† | Yes | | |

*** Very useful—measurements should be frequently made.

** Useful—measurements often required.

* Limited usefulness—measurements occasionally required.

0 Not useful.

[1] Primidone levels—measurement of derived phenobarbital levels is more useful.

[2] MHD derivative.

†† Many interactions, frequently of clinical relevance and many require dose modification.

† Minor interactions common, but not usually of much clinical relevance.

# Further reading

The purpose of this section is to provide guidance for further reading on the topics in this book. This is not intended to be a comprehensive list of citations (in the age of PubMed, this seems not really necessary), but simply a selection of recent reviews, key articles and important summary papers. Where data are cited in the text, the source is also included here. The list should be sufficient for the interested reader to follow up any aspect of particular interest. The key text from which this book borrows is the sister book, *The Treatment of Epilepsy*, 2nd edn (Shorvon SD, Perucca E, Fish D, Dodson E, eds. Blackwell Publishing, 2004)—most of the chapters in the book have comprehensive citation lists and these are an invaluable source for further study. Other textbooks that provide comprehensive citations are also listed below. The citations to articles in the scientific journals are biased towards recently published papers.

## SECTION 1—THE CLINICAL FORMS AND CAUSES OF EPILEPSY

### Books

Arzimanoglou A, Guerrini R, and Aicardi J. 2003. *Aicardi's Epilepsy in Children* (3rd edn). Lippencott, Williams and Wilkins, Philadelphia.

Engel J and Pedley TA (eds). 1997. *Epilepsy: A Comprehensive Textbook*. Raven Press, New York.

Panayiotopoulos CP. 2005. *The Epilepsies: Seizures, Syndromes and Management*. Bladon Medical Publishing, Chipping Norton.

Shorvon SD, Perucca E, Fish D, and Dodson E (eds). 2004. *The Treatment of Epilepsy* (2nd edn). Blackwell Publishing, Oxford.

Wallace SJ and Farrell K (eds). 2004. *Epilepsy in Children*. Arnold, London.

### Articles in scientific journals

American Academy of Pediatrics. 1999. Committee on Quality Improvement, Subcommittee on febrile seizures. Practice parameter: Long-term treatment of the child with simple febrile seizures. *Pediatrics*, **103**: 1307–9.

Antunes NL. 2003. Seizures in children with systemic cancer. *Pediatr Neurol*, **28**: 190–3.

Avanzini G. 2003. Musicogenic seizures. *Ann N Y Acad Sci*, **999**: 95–102.

Barkovich AJ and Raybaud CA. 2004. Neuroimaging in disorders of cortical development. *Neuroimaging Clin N Am*, **14**: 231–54.

Baulac S, Gourfinkel-An I, Nabbout R, *et al.* 2004. Fever, genes, and epilepsy. *Lancet Neurol*, **3**: 421–30.

Bautista JF, Foldvary-Schaefer N, Bingaman WE, *et al.* 2003. Focal cortical dysplasia and intractable epilepsy in adults: clinical, EEG, imaging, and surgical features. *Epilepsy Res*, **55**: 131–6.

Beghi E. 2003. Overview of studies to prevent post-traumatic epilepsy. *Epilepsia*, **44** (Suppl. 10): 21–6.

Binnie CD. 2003. Cognitive impairment during epileptiform discharges: is it ever justifiable to treat the EEG? *Lancet Neurol*, **2**: 725–30.

Camilo O and Goldstein LB. 2004. Seizures and epilepsy after ischemic stroke. *Stroke*, **35**: 1769–75.

Caviness JN and Brown P. 2004. Myoclonus: current concepts and recent advances. *Lancet Neurol*, **3**: 598–607.

Cendes F. 2004. Febrile seizures and mesial temporal sclerosis. *Curr Opin Neurol*, **17**: 161–4.

Chan EM, Andrade DM, Franceschetti S, *et al.* 2005. Progressive myoclonus epilepsies: EPM1, EPM2A, EPM2B. *Adv Neurol*, **95**: 47–57.

Chang BS, Lowenstein DH, and the Quality Standards Subcommittee of the American Academy of Neurology. 2003. Practice parameter: antiepileptic drug prophylaxis in severe traumatic brain injury: report of the Quality Standards Subcommittee of the American Academy of Neurology. *Neurology*, **60**: 10–6.

Chong JY, Rowland LP, and Utiger RD. 2003. Hashimoto encephalopathy: syndrome or myth? *Arch Neurol*, **60**: 164–71.

Cleary P, Shorvon S, and Tallis R. 2004. Late-onset seizures as a predictor of subsequent stroke. *Lancet*, **363**: 1184–6.

Cockerell OC, Johnson AL, Sander JWAS, *et al.* 1997. Prognosis of epilepsy: further analysis of the first nine years of the British National General Practice Study of Epilepsy, a prospective population-based study. *Epilepsia*, **38**: 31–46.

Combi R, Dalpra L, Tenchini ML, *et al.* 2004. Autosomal dominant nocturnal frontal lobe epilepsy: a critical overview. *J Neurol*, **251**: 923–34.

Comi AM. 2003. Pathophysiology of Sturge–Weber syndrome. *J Child Neurol*, **18**: 509–16.

Commission on Classification and Terminology of the International League Against Epilepsy. 1981. Proposal for revised clinical and electroencephalographic classification of epileptic seizures. *Epilepsia*, **22**: 489–501.

Commission on Classification and Terminology of the International League Against Epilepsy. 1989. A revised proposal for the classification of epilepsies and epileptic syndromes. *Epilepsia*, **30**: 389–99.

Conry JA. 2004. Pharmacologic treatment of the catastrophic epilepsies. *Epilepsia*, **45** (Suppl. 5): 12–6.

Covanis A. 2005. Eyelid myoclonia and absence. *Adv Neurol*, **95**: 185–96.

Crino PB. 2004. Malformations of cortical development: molecular pathogenesis and experimental strategies. *Adv Exp Med Biol*, **548**: 175–91.

d'Orsi G, Tinuper P, Bisulli F, *et al.* 2004. Clinical features and long-term outcome of epilepsy in periventricular nodular heterotopia: simple compared with plus forms. *J Neurol Neurosurg Psychiatry*, **75**: 873–8.

Dravet C, Bureau M, Oguni H, *et al.* 2005. Severe myoclonic epilepsy in infancy: Dravet syndrome. *Adv Neurol*, **95**: 71–102.

Dulac O, Chiron C, Luna D, *et al.* 1991. Vigabatrin in childhood epilepsy. *J Child Neurol*, **6** (Suppl. 2): S30–S37.

Eisermann MM, DeLaRaillere A, *et al.* 2003. Infantile spasms in Down syndrome: effects of delayed anticonvulsive treatment. *Epilepsy Res*, **55**: 21–7.

Freeman JL, Coleman LT, Wellard RM, *et al.* 2004. MR imaging and spectroscopic study of epileptogenic hypothalamic hamartomas: analysis of 72 cases. *Am J Neuroradiol*, **25**: 450–62.

Frey LC. 2003. Epidemiology of post-traumatic epilepsy: a critical review. *Epilepsia*, **44** (Suppl. 10): 11–7.

Gaitanis JN and Walsh CA. 2004. Genetics of disorders of cortical development. *Neuroimaging Clin N Am*, **14**: 219–29.

Garcias Da Silva LF, Nunes ML, *et al.* 2004. Risk factors for developing epilepsy after neonatal seizures. *Pediatr Neurol*, **30**: 271–7.

Genton P, Roger J, Guerrini R, *et al.* 2005. History and classification of 'myoclonic' epilepsies: from seizures to syndromes to diseases. *Adv Neurol*, **95**: 1–14.

Gourfinkel-An I, Baulac S, Nabbout R, *et al.* 2004. Monogenic idiopathic epilepsies. *Lancet Neurol*, **3**: 209–18.

Guerrini R and Aicardi J. 2003. Epileptic encephalopathies with myoclonic seizures in infants and children (severe myoclonic epilepsy and myoclonic-astatic epilepsy). *J Clin Neurophysiol*, **20**: 449–61.

Guerrini R, Carrozzo R, Rinaldi R, *et al.* 2003. Angelman syndrome: etiology, clinical features, diagnosis, and management of symptoms. *Paediatr Drugs*, **5**: 647–61.

Guerrini R, Moro F, Andermann E, *et al.* 2003. Non-syndromic mental retardation and cryptogenic epilepsy in women with double cortin gene mutations. *Ann Neurol*, **54**: 30–7.

Hancock E and Cross H. 2003. Treatment of Lennox–Gastaut syndrome. *Cochrane Database Syst Rev*, (3): CD003277.

Hedges D, Jeppson K, and Whitehead P. 2003. Antipsychotic medication and seizures: a review. *Drugs Today (Barc)*, **39**: 551–7.

Hillbom M, Pieninkeroinen I, and Leone M. 2003. Seizures in alcohol-dependent patients: epidemiology, pathophysiology and management. *CNS Drugs*, **17**: 1013–30.

Hindmarsh JT. 2003. The porphyrias, appropriate test selection. *Clin Chim Acta*, **333**: 203–7.

Hrachovy RA and Frost JD Jr. 2003. Infantile epileptic encephalopathy with hypsarrhythmia (infantile spasms/West syndrome). *J Clin Neurophysiol*, **20**: 408–25.

Jallon P. 2004. Mortality in patients with epilepsy. *Curr Opin Neurol*, **17**: 141–6.

Jallon P, Loiseau P, and Loiseau J. 2001. Newly diagnosed unprovoked epileptic seizures: presentation at diagnosis in CAROLE study. Coordination Active du Réseau Observatoire Longitudinal de l'Epilepsie. *Epilepsia*, **42**: 464–75.

Johnston MV. 2004. Clinical disorders of brain plasticity. *Brain Dev*, **26**: 73–80.

Johnston MV, Mullaney B, and Blue ME. 2003. Neurobiology of Rett syndrome. *J Child Neurol*, **18**: 688–92.

Kasper BS, Stefan H, and Paulus W. 2003. Microdysgenesis in mesial temporal lobe epilepsy: a clinicopathological study. *Ann Neurol*, **54**: 501–6.

Kauppinen R. 2004. Molecular diagnostics of acute intermittent porphyria. *Expert Rev Mol Diagn*, **4**: 243–9.

Kohelet D, Shochat R, Lusky A, *et al.* and the Israel Neonatal Network. 2004. Risk factors for neonatal seizures in very low birthweight infants: population-based survey. *J Child Neurol*, **19**: 123–8.

Lhatoo SD, Sander JW, and Shorvon SD. 2001. The dynamics of drug treatment in epilepsy: an observational study in an unselected population based cohort with newly diagnosed epilepsy followed up prospectively over 11–14 years. *J Neurol Neurosurg Psychiatry*, **71**: 632–7.

MacDonald BK, Cockerell OC, Sander JWAS *et al.* 2000. The incidence and lifetime prevalence of neurological disorders in a prospective community-based study in the UK. *Brain*, **123**: 665–76.

Manford M, Hart YM, Sander JW, *et al.* 1992. The National General Practice Study of Epilepsy. The syndromic classification of the International League Against Epilepsy applied to epilepsy in a general population. *Arch Neurol*, **49**: 801–8.

Manning JP, Richards DA, and Bowery NG. 2003. Pharmacology of absence epilepsy. *Trends Pharmacol Sci*, **24**: 542–9.

Markand ON. 2003. Lennox–Gastaut syndrome (childhood epileptic encephalopathy). *J Clin Neurophysiol*, **20**: 426–41.

Mason WP. 2003. Anticonvulsant prophylaxis for patients with brain tumours: insights from clinical trials. *Can J Neurol Sci*, **30**: 89–90.

Mturi N, Musumba CO, Wamola BM, *et al.* 2003. Cerebral malaria: optimising management. *CNS Drugs*, **17**: 153–65.

Muhle R, Trentacoste SV, and Rapin I. 2004. The genetics of autism. *Pediatrics*, **113**: 472–86.

Najm I, Ying Z, Babb T, Crino PB, *et al.* 2004. Mechanisms of epileptogenicity in cortical dysplasias. *Neurology*, **62** (6 Suppl. 3): S9–S13.

Nelson KB and Lynch JK. 2004. Stroke in newborn infants. *Lancet Neurol*, **3**: 150–8.

Neubauer BA, Hahn A, Doose H, *et al.* 2005. Myoclonic-astatic epilepsy of early childhood: definition, course, nosography, and genetics. *Adv Neurol*, **95**: 147–55.

Neul JL and Zoghbi HY. 2004. Rett syndrome: a prototypical neurodevelopmental disorder. *Neuroscientist*, **10**: 118–28.

Ohtahara S and Yamatogi Y. 2003. Epileptic encephalopathies in early infancy with suppression-burst. *J Clin Neurophysiol*, **20**: 398–407.

Palmini A, Najm I, Avanzini G, *et al.* 2004. Terminology and classification of the cortical dysplasias. *Neurology*, **62** (Suppl. 3): S2–S8.

Panayiotopoulos CP. 2004. Autonomic seizures and autonomic status epilepticus peculiar to childhood: diagnosis and management. *Epilepsy Behav*, **5**: 286–95.

Panayiotopoulos CP, Obeid T, and Tahan AR. 1994. Juvenile myoclonic epilepsy: a 5-year prospective study. *Epilepsia*, **35**: 285–96.

Poser CM and Brinar VV. 2003. Epilepsy and multiple sclerosis. *Epilepsy Behav*, **4**: 6–12.

Riikonen R. 2004. Infantile spasms: therapy and outcome. *J Child Neurol*, **19**: 401–4.

Riley T and White AC Jr. 2003. Management of neurocysticercosis. *CNS Drugs*, **17**: 577–91.

Rodriguez D and Young Poussaint T. 2004 Neuroimaging findings in neurofibromatosis type 1 and 2. *Neuroimaging Clin N Am*, **14**: 149–70.

Ryvlin P and Kahane P. 2003. Does epilepsy surgery lower the mortality of drug-resistant epilepsy? *Epilepsy Res*, **56**: 105–20.

Satishchandra P. 2003. Hot-water epilepsy. *Epilepsia*, **44** (Suppl. 1): 29–32.

Shevell M, Ashwal S, Donley D, *et al.*, and the Quality Standards Subcommittee of the American Academy of Neurology; Practice Committee of the Child Neurology Society. 2003. Practice parameter: evaluation of the child with global developmental delay: report of the Quality Standards Subcommittee of the American Academy of Neurology and The Practice Committee of the Child Neurology Society. *Neurology*, **60**: 367–80.

Shorvon SD. 1984. The temporal aspects of prognosis in epilepsy. *J Neurol Neurosurg Psychiatry*, **47**: 1157–65.

Sloviter RS. 2005. The neurobiology of temporal lobe epilepsy: too much information, not enough knowledge. *C R Biol*, **328**: 143–53.

Siegel AM. 2003. Parietal lobe epilepsy. *Adv Neurol*, **93**: 335–45.

Smirniotopoulos JG. 2004. Neuroimaging of phakomatoses: Sturge–Weber syndrome, tuberous sclerosis, von Hippel–Lindau syndrome. *Neuroimaging Clin N Am*, **14**: 171–83.

Smith MC and Hoeppner TJ. 2003. Epileptic encephalopathy of late childhood: Landau–Kleffner syndrome and the syndrome of continuous spikes and waves during slow-wave sleep. *J Clin Neurophysiol*, **20**: 462–72.

Steinlein OK. 2004. Genes and mutations in human idiopathic epilepsy. *Brain Dev*, **26**: 213–18.

Striano P, Orefice G, Brescia Morra V, *et al.* 2003. Epileptic seizures in multiple sclerosis: clinical and EEG correlations. *Neurol Sci*, **24**: 322–8.

Taylor I, Scheffer IE, and Berkovic SF. 2003. Occipital epilepsies: identification of specific and newly recognized syndromes. *Brain*, **126**: 753–69.

Torres FR, Montenegro MA, Marques-De-Faria AP, *et al.* 2004. Mutation screening in a cohort of patients with lissencephaly and subcortical band heterotopia. *Neurology*, **62**: 799–802.

Vivarelli R, Grosso S, Calabrese F, *et al.* 2003. Epilepsy in neurofibromatosis 1. *J Child Neurol*, **18**: 338–42.

Walker DG and Kaye AH. 2003. Low grade glial neoplasms. *J Clin Neurosci*, **10**: 1–13.

Zupanc ML. 2004. Neonatal seizures. *Pediatr Clin North Am*, **51**: 961–78.

## SECTION 2—THE PRINCIPLES OF DRUG TREATMENT

### Books

Engel J, Pedley TA (eds). 1997. *Epilepsy: A Comprehensive Textbook*. Raven Press, New York.

Morrell MJ (ed). 2003. *Women with Epilepsy*. Cambridge University Press, Cambridge.

Murphy PA. 2001. *Treating Epilepsy Naturally*. Keats Publishing, Chicago.

Shorvon SD, Perucca E, Fish D, Dodson E (eds). 2004. *The Treatment of Epilepsy* (2nd edn). Blackwell Publishing, Oxford.

Wallace SJ, Farrell K (eds). 2004. *Epilepsy in Children*. Arnold, London.

### Articles in scientific journals

Adab N, Kini U, Vinten J, Ayres J, *et al.* 2004. The longer term outcome of children born to mothers with epilepsy. *J Neurol Neurosurg Psychiatry*, **75**: 1575–83.

Adab N, Tudur SC, Vinten J, Williamson P, and Winterbottom J. 2004. Common antiepileptic drugs in pregnancy in women with epilepsy. *Cochrane Database Syst Rev*, (3): CD004848.

American Academy of Pediatrics. Committee on Quality Improvement, Subcommittee on Febrile Seizures. 1999. Practice parameter: long-term treatment of the child with simple febrile seizures. *Pediatrics*, **103**: 1307–9.

Arts WF, Brouwer OF, Peters AC, *et al.* 2004. Course and prognosis of childhood epilepsy: 5-year follow-up of the Dutch study of epilepsy in childhood. *Brain*, **127**: 1774–84.

Baram TZ, Mitchell WG, Tournay A, *et al.* 1996. High-dose corticotropin (ACTH) versus prednisone for infantile spasms: a prospective, randomized, blinded study. *Pediatrics*, **97**: 375–9.

Bauer J, Jarre A, Klingmuller D, *et al.* 2000. Polycystic ovary syndrome in patients with focal epilepsy: a study in 93 women. *Epilepsy Res*, **41**: 163–7.

Brodie MJ, Overstall PW, and Giorgi L. The UK Lamotrigine Elderly Study Group. 1999. Multicentre, double-blind randomised comparison between lamotrigine and carbamazepine in elderly patients with newly diagnosed epilepsy. *Epilepsy Res*, **37**: 81–7.

Buck D, Baker GA, Jacoby A, Smith DF, *et al.* 1997. Patients' experiences of injury as a result of epilepsy. *Epilepsia*, **38**: 439–44.

Cendes F. 2004. Febrile seizures and mesial temporal sclerosis. *Curr Opin Neurol*, **17**: 161–4.

Chadwick D, Taylor J, and Johnson T. 1996. Outcomes after seizure recurrence in people with well-controlled epilepsy and the factors that influence it. The MRC Antiepileptic Drug Withdrawal Group. *Epilepsia*, **37**: 1043–50.

Chiron C, Dumas C, Jambaque I, *et al.* 1997. Randomized trial comparing vigabatrin and hydrocortisone in infantile spasms due to tuberous sclerosis. *Epilepsy Res*, **26**: 389–95.

Cockerell OC, Johnson AL, Sander JWAS, *et al.* 1994. Mortality from epilepsy: results from a prospective population-based study. *Lancet*, **344**: 918–21.

Coppola G. 2004. Treatment of partial seizures in childhood: an overview. *CNS Drugs*, **18**: 133–56.

Coulter DL. 1997. Comprehensive management of epilepsy in persons with mental retardation. *Epilepsia*, **38** (Suppl. 4): 24–31.

Craig I and Tallis R. 1994. The impact of sodium valproate and phenytoin on cognitive function in elderly patients: results of a single-blind randomised comparative study. *Epilepsia*, **35**: 381–90.

Czeizel AE. 2004. Folic acid and the prevention of neural-tube defects. *N Engl J Med*, **350**: 2209–11.

De Silva M, MacArdle B, McGowan M, *et al.* 1996. Randomized comparative monotherapy trial of phenobarbitone, phenytoin, carbamazepine, or sodium valproate for newly diagnosed childhood epilepsy. *Lancet*, **347**: 709–13.

Duncan S, Blacklaw J, Beastall GH, *et al.* 1999. Antiepileptic drug therapy and sexual function in men with epilepsy. *Epilepsia*, **40**: 197–204.

Fejerman N, Caraballo R, and Cersosimo R. 2005. Ketogenic diet in patients with Dravet syndrome and myoclonic epilepsies in infancy and early childhood. *Adv Neurol*, **95**: 299–305.

First Seizure Trial Group. 1993. Randomized clinical trial of the efficacy of antiepileptic drugs in reducing the risk of relapse after a first unprovoked tonic–clonic seizure. *Neurology*, **43**: 478–83.

Forsgren L, Edvinsson S-O, Blomquist HK, *et al.* 1990. Epilepsy in a population of mentally retarded children and adults. *Epilepsy Res*, **6**: 234–48.

Freeman JM, Vining EPG, Pillas DJ, *et al.* 1998. The efficacy of the ketogenic diet—1998: a prospective evaluation of intervention in 150 children. *Pediatrics*, **102**: 1358–63.

Goldstein LH. 1990. Behavioural and cognitive–behavioural treatments for epilepsy: a progress review. *Br J Clin Psychol*, **29** (Pt 3): 257–69.

Haller CA, Meier KH, Olson KR. 2005. Seizures reported in association with use of dietary supplements. *Clin Toxicol*, **43**: 23–30.

Hart YM, Sander JWAS, Johnson Al, *et al.*, for the NGPSE (National General Practice Study of Epilepsy). 1990. Recurrence after a first seizure. *Lancet*, **336**: 1271–4.

Heller AJ, Chesterman P, Elwes RDC, *et al.* 1995. Phenobarbitone, phenytoin, carbamazepine or sodium valproate for newly diagnosed adult epilepsy: a randomized comparative monotherapy trial. *J Neurol Neurosurg Psychiatry*, **58**: 44–50.

Hermanns G, Noachtar S, Taxhorn I, *et al.* 1996. Systematic testing of medical intractability for carbamazepine, phenytoin and phenobarbital or primidone in monotherapy for patients considered for epilepsy surgery. *Epilepsia*, **37**: 675–9.

Hertz D, Berg A, Bettis D, *et al.* 2003. Practice parameter: treatment of the child with a first unprovoked seizure. Report of the Quality Standards Subcommittee of the American Academy of Neurology and the Practice Committee of the Child Neurology Society. *Neurology*, **60**: 166–75.

Kang HC, Chung da E, Kim DW, *et al.* 2004. Early- and late-onset complications of the ketogenic diet for intractable epilepsy. *Epilepsia*, **45**: 1116–23.

Kanner AM. 2000. Psychosis of epilepsy: a neurologist's perspective. *Epilepsy Behav*, **1**: 219–27.

Kaplan PW. 2004. Reproductive health effects and teratogenicity of antiepileptic drugs. *Neurology*, **63** (Suppl. 4): S13–S23.

Knudsen FU, 1996. Febrile seizures: treatment and outcome. *Brain Dev*, **18**: 438–99.

Kossoff EH. 2004. More fat and fewer seizures: dietary therapies for epilepsy. *Lancet Neurol*, **3**: 415–20.

Kossoff EH, Pyzik PL, McGrogan JR, *et al.* 2002. Efficacy of the ketogenic diet for infantile spasms. *Pediatrics*, **109**: 780–3.

Krishnamoorthy ES. 2001. Psychiatric issues in epilepsy. *Curr Opin Neurol*, **14**: 217–24.

Kwan P and Brodie MJ. 2000. Early identification of refractory epilepsy. *N Engl J Med*, **342**: 314–19.

Kwan P and Brodie MJ. 2005. Potential role of drug transporters in the pathogenesis of medically intractable epilepsy. *Epilepsia*, **46**: 224–35.

Langan Y, Nashef L, and Sander JWAS. 2000. Sudden unexpected death in epilepsy: a series of witnessed deaths. *J Neurol Neurosurg Psychiatry*, **68**: 211–13.

Loiseau J, Loiseau P, Duche B, *et al.* 1996. A survey of epileptic disorders in southwest France: seizures in elderly patients. *Ann Neurol*, **27**: 232–7.

Loiseau P, Duche B, and Pedespan J-M. 1995. Absence epilepsies. *Epilepsia*, **36**: 1182–7.

Lux AL, Edwards SW, Hancock E, *et al.* 2004. The United Kingdom Infantile Spasms Study comparing vigabatrin with prednisolone or tetracosactide at 14 days: a multicentre, randomised controlled trial. *Lancet*, **364**: 1773–8.

Manford M, Hart YM, Sander JWAS, *et al.* 1992. The National General Practice Study of Epilepsy. The syndromic classification of the International League Against Epilepsy applied to epilepsy in a general population. *Arch Neurol*, **49**: 801–8.

Mattson RH, Cramer JA, Collins JF, *et al.* 1985. Comparison of carbamazepine, phenobarbital, phenytoin, and primidone in partial and secondarily generalized tonic–clonic seizures. *N Engl J Med*, **13**: 145–51.

Mattson RH, Cramer JA, Collins JF, and the Department of the Veteran Affairs Epilepsy Cooperative Study Group. 1992. A comparison of valproate with carbamazepine for the treatment of complex partial seizures and secondarily generalized tonic–cloic seizures in adults. *N Engl J Med*, **327**: 765–71.

McCorry D, Chadwick D, Marson A. 2004. Current drug treatment of epilepsy in adults. *Lancet Neurol*, **3**: 729–35.

Meador KM, Loring DW, Huh K, *et al.* 1990. Comparative cognitive effects of anticonvulsants. *Neurology*, **40**: 391–4.

Medical Research Council Antiepileptic Drug Withdrawal Study Group. 1991. Randomized study of antiepileptic drug withdrawal in patients in remission. *Lancet*, **337**: 1175–80.

Medical Research Council Antiepileptic Drug Withdrawal Study Group. 1993. Prognostic index for recurrence of seizures after remission of epilepsy. *Br Med J*, **306**: 1374–8.

Moran NF, Poole K, Bell G, Solomon J, 2004. Epilepsy in the United Kingdom: seizure frequency and severity, antiepileptic drug utilization and impact on life in 1652 people with epilepsy. *Seizure*, **13**: 425–33.

Morrell MJ. 1998. Guidelines for the care of women with epilepsy. *Neurology*, **51** (Suppl. 4): S21–S27.

Murphy K and Delanty N. 2000. Primary generalized epilepsies. *Curr Treat Options Neurol*, **2**: 527–42.

Musico M, Beghi E, Solair A, *et al.*, for the First Seizure Trial Group (FIRST Group). 1997. Treatment of first tonic–clonic seizure does not improve the prognosis of epilepsy. *Neurology*, **49**: 991–8.

Nashef L, Fish DR, Garner S, *et al.* 1995. Sudden death in epilepsy: a study of incidence in a young cohort with epilepsy and learning difficulty. *Epilepsia*, **36**: 1187–94.

Nashef L, Garner S, Sander JWAS, *et al.* 1998. Circumstances of death in sudden death in epilepsy: interviews of bereaved relatives. *J Neurol Neurosurg Psychiatry*, **64**: 349–52.

Nashef L, Sander JWAS, and Shorvon SD. Mortality in epilepsy. In: Pedley T and Meldrum BS (eds). 1995. *Recent Advances in Epilepsy 6*. Churchill Livingstone, Edinburgh: pp. 271–87.

Nashef L, Walker F, Allen P, Sander JWAS, Shorvon SD, and Fish DR. 1996. Apnoea and bradycardia during epileptic seizures: relation to sudden death in epilepsy. *J Neurol Neurosurg Psychiatry*, **60**: 297–300.

Neufeld MY, Vishne T, Chistik V, *et al.* 1999. Life-long history of injuries related to seizures. *Epilepsy Res*, **34**: 123–7.

Nilsson L, Farahmand BY, Persson PG, *et al.* 1999. Risk factors for sudden unexpected death in epilepsy: a case–control study. *Lancet*, **353**: 888–93.

Panayiotopoulos CP. 1999. Early-onset benign childhood occipital seizure susceptibility syndrome: a syndrome to recognize. *Epilepsia*, **40**: 621–30.

Patsalos PV and Perucca E. 2003. Clinically important drug interactions in epilepsy: general features and interactions between antiepileptic drugs. *Lancet Neurol*, **2**: 347–56.

Pennell PB. 2004. Pregnancy in women who have epilepsy. *Neurol Clin*, **22**: 799–820.

Penovich PE. 2000. The effects of epilepsy and its treatment on sexual and reproductive function. *Epilepsia*, **41** (Suppl. 2): S53–S61.

Perucca E, Beghi E, Dulac O, Shorvon SD, and Tomson T. 2000. Assessing risk to benefit ratio in antiepileptic drug therapy. *Epilepsy Res*, **41**: 107–39.

Perucca E, Gram L, Avanzini G, *et al.* 1998. Antiepileptic drugs as a cause of worsening seizures. *Epilepsia*, **39**: 5–17.

Posner EB, Mohamed K, and Marson AG. 2003. Ethosuximide, sodium valproate or lamotrigine for absence seizures in children and adolescents. *Cochrane Database Syst Rev*, (3): CD003032.

Ramaratnam S, Baker GA, and Goldstein L. 2001. Psychological treatments for epilepsy (Cochrane Review). *Cochrane Database Cyst Rev*, (4): CD002029.

Riikonen R. 2001. Long-term outcome of patients with West syndrome. *Brain Dev*, **23**: 683–7.

Riikonen R. 2004. Infantile spasms: therapy and outcome. *J Child Neurol*, **19**: 401–4.

Sabers A, Buchholt JM, Uldall P, *et al.* 2001. Lamotrigine plasma levels reduced by oral contraceptives. *Epilepsy Res*, **47**: 151–4.

Sander JWAS, Hart YM, Johnson AL, *et al.*, for the NGPSE. 1990. National General Practice Study of Epilepsy: newly diagnosed epileptic seizures in a general population. *Lancet*, **336**: 1267–71.

Sato S, White BG, Penry JK, *et al.* 1982. Valproic acid versus ethosuximide in the treatment of absence seizures. *Neurology*, **32**: 157–63.

Scottish Intercollegiate Guidelines Network. 1997. *Diagnosis and Management of Epilepsy in Adults. A national clinical guideline recommended for use in Scotland*. Royal College of Physicians of Edinburgh, Edinburgh: p. 14.

Shorvon SD. 2004. Longer term outcome of children born to mothers with epilepsy. *J Neurol Neurosurg Psychiatry*, **75**: 1517–8.

Sillanpää M, Jalava M, Kaleva O, *et al.* 1998. Long-term prognosis of seizures with onset in childhood. *N Engl J Med*, **338**: 1715–22.

Spitz MC, Towbin JA, Shantz D, *et al.* 1994. Risk factors for burns as a consequence of seizures in persons with epilepsy. *Epilepsia*, **35**: 764–7.

Tallis RC, Craig I, Hall G, *et al.* 1991. How common are epileptic seizures in old age? *Age Ageing*, **20**: 442–8.

Tomson T, Beghi E, Sundqvist A, *et al.* 2004. Medical risks in epilepsy: a review with focus on physical injuries, mortality, traffic accidents and their prevention. *Epilepsy Res*, **60**: 1–16.

Tomson T, Gram L, Sillanpaa M, *et al.*, and Johannassen SI. 1997. *Epilepsy and Pregnancy*. Wrightson Biomedical Publishing, Petersfield.

Vainionpää L, Rättyä J, Knip M, *et al.* 1999. Valproate induced hyperandrogenism during pubertal maturation in girls with epilepsy. *Ann Neurol*, **45**: 444–50.

Vecht CJ, Wagner GL, and Wilms EB. 2003. Interactions between antiepileptic and chemotherapeutic drugs. *Lancet Neurol*, **2**: 404–9.

Verity CM, Hosking G, and Easter DJ, on behalf of the Pediatric EPITEG Collaborative Group. 1995. A multicentre comparative trial of sodium valproate and cabamazepine in paediatric epilepsy. *Dev Med Child Neurol*, **37**: 97–108.

Vestergaard P, Rejnmark L, and Mosekilde L. 2004. Fracture risk associated with use of antiepileptic drugs. *Epilepsia*, **45**: 1330–7.

Villeneuve N, Soufflet C, Plouin P, *et al.* 1998. Treatment of infantile spasms with vigabatrin as first-line therapy and in monotherapy: apropos of 70 infants. *Arch Pediatr*, **5**: 731–8.

Vining EPG. 1999. Clinical efficacy of the ketogenic diet. *Epilepsy Res*, **37**: 181–90.

Vining EPG, Freeman JM, Ballaban-Gil K, *et al.* 1998. A multicentre study of the efficacy of the ketogenic diet. *Arch Neurol*, **55**: 1433–7.

Wallace H, Shorvon S, and Tallis RC. 1998. Age-specific incidence and prevalence rates of treated epilepsy in an unselected population of 2,052,922 and age-specific fertility rates of women with epilepsy. *Lancet*, **352**: 1970–3.

Wheless JW. 2001. The ketogenic diet: an effective medical therapy with side effects. *J Child Neurol*, **16**: 633–5.

Zahn CA, Morrell MJ, Collins SD, *et al.* 1998. Management issues for women with epilepsy: a review of the literature. *Neurology*, **51**: 949–56.

## SECTION 3—THE ANTIEPILEPTIC DRUGS

### Books

Levy R, Mattson RH, Meldrum BS, and Perucca E (eds). 2002. *Antiepileptic Drugs* (5th edn). Lippencott, Williams and Wilkins, Philadelphia.

Shorvon SD, Perucca E, Fish D, and Dodson E (eds). 2004. *The Treatment of Epilepsy* (2nd edn). Blackwell Publishing, Oxford.

### Articles in scientific journals

Anhut H, Ashman P, Feuerstein TJ, *et al.* 1994. Gabapentin (Neurontin) as add-on therapy in patients with partial seizures: a double-blind, placebo-controlled study: the International Gabapentin Study Group. *Epilepsia*, **35**: 795–801.

Arroyo S, Anhut H, Kugler AR, *et al.* 2004. Pregabalin add-on treatment: a randomized, double-blind, placebo-controlled, dose–response study in adults with partial seizures. *Epilepsia*, **45**: 20–7.

Bang L and Goa K. 2003. Oxcarbazepine: a review of its use in children with epilepsy. *Paediatr Drugs*, **5**: 557–73.

Barcs G, Walker EB, D'Souza J, *et al.* 2000. Oxcarbazepine placebo-controlled, dose ranging trial in refractory epilepsy. *Epilepsia*, **41**: 1597–607.

Battino D, Estienne M, and Avanzini G. 1995. Clinical pharmacokinetics of antiepileptic drugs in pediatric patients. II. Phenytoin, carbamazepine, sulthiame, lamotrigine, vigabatrin, oxcarbazepine, felbamate. *Clin Pharmacokinet*, **29**: 341–69.

Ben-Menachem E. 2004. Pregabalin pharmacology and its relevance to clinical practice. *Epilepsia*, **45** (Suppl. 6): 13–18.

Ben-Menachem E and Falter U, for the European Levetiracetam Study Group. 2000. Efficacy and tolerability of levetiracetam 3000 mg/day in patients with refractory partial seizures: a multicenter, double-blind, responder-selected study evaluating monotherapy. *Epilepsia*, **41**: 1276–83.

Ben-Menachem E, Henriksen O, Dam M, *et al.* 1996. Double blind, placebo-controlled trial of topiramate as add-on therapy in patients with refractory partial seizures. *Epilepsia*, **37**: 539–43.

Beran RC, Berkovic SF, Vajda F, *et al.* 1996. A double blind placebo-controlled cross over study of vigabatrin 2 g/day and 3 g/day in uncontrolled partial seizures. *Seizure*, **5**: 259–65.

Betts T, Waegemans T, and Crawford P. 2000. A multicentre, double-blind, randomized, parallel group study to evaluate the tolerability and efficacy of two oral doses of levetiracetam, 2000 mg daily and 4000 mg daily, without titration in patients with refractory epilepsy. *Seizure*, **9**: 80–7.

Beydoun A, Sachdeo RC, Rosenfeld WE, *et al.* 2000. Oxcarbazepine monotherapy for partial onset seizures: a multicenter, double-blind, clinical trial. *Neurology*, **54**: 2245–51.

Bialer M, Johannessen SI, Kupferberg HJ, *et al.* 2004. Progress report on new antiepileptic drugs: a summary of the Seventh Eilat Conference (EILAT VII). *Epilepsy Res*, **61**: 1–48.

Binnie CD, Debets RM, Engelsman M, *et al.* 1989. Double blind cross-over trial of lamotrigine (Lamictal) as add on therapy in intractable epilepsy. *Epilepsy Res*, **4**: 222–9.

Biton V, Edwards KR, Montouris GD, *et al.* 2001. Topiramate titration and tolerability. *Ann Pharmacother*, **35**: 173–9.

Boas J, Dam M, Friis M, *et al.* Controlled trial of lamotrigine (Lamictal) for treatment of resistant partial seizures. 1996. *Acta Neurol Scand*, **94**: 247–52.

Britzi M, Perucca E, Soback S, *et al.* 2005. Pharmacokinetic and metabolic investigation of topiramate disposition in healthy subjects in the absence and in the presence of enzyme induction by carbamazepine. *Epilepsia*, **46**: 378–84.

Brodie MJ. 2004. Pregabalin as adjunctive therapy for partial seizures. *Epilepsia*, **45** (Suppl. 6): 19–27.

Brodie MJ, Chadwick D, Anhut H, *et al.* 2002. Gabapentin vs lamotrigine monotherapy: a double blind comparison in newly diagnosed epilepsy. *Epilepsia*, **45**: 993–1000.

Brodie MJ, Duncan R, Vespignani H, 2005. Dose-dependent safety and efficacy of Zonisamide: a randomized, double-blind, placebo-controlled study in patients with refractory partial seizures. *Epilepsia* **46**: 31–41.

Brodie MJ, Richens A, and Yuen AWC, for the UK Lamotrigine/ Carbamazepine Monotherapy Trial Group. 1995. Double-blind comparison of lamotrigine and carbamazepine in newly diagnosed epilepsy. *Lancet*, **345**: 476–9.

Canadian Clobazam Cooperative Group. 1991. Clobazam in the treatment of refractory epilepsy: the Canadian experience—a retrospective survey. *Epilepsia*, **32**: 407–16.

Canadian Study Group for Childhood Epilepsy. 1998. Clobazam has equivalent efficacy to carbamazepine and phenytoin as monotherapy for childhood epilepsy. *Epilepsia*, **39**: 952–9.

Cereghino JJ, Biton V, Abou-Khalil B, *et al.* 2000. Levetiracetam for partial seizures: results of a double-blind, randomised clinical trial. *Neurology*, **55**: 236–42.

Chadwick D, Anhut H, Murray GH, *et al.* 1998. A double-blind trial of gabapentin monotherapy for newly diagnosed partial seizures. *Neurology*, **51**: 1282–8.

Chadwick D, for the Vigabatrin European Monotherapy Study Group. 1999. Safety and efficacy of vigabatrin and carbamazepine in newly diagnosed epilepsy: a multicentre randomised double-blind study. *Lancet*, **354**: 13–19.

Chadwick D. 1994. Gabapentin. *Lancet*, **343**: 89–91.

Chadwick D and Marson T. 2002. Zonisamide add-on for drug resistant partial epilepsy (Cochrane Review). In: *The Cochrane Library*, Issue 4. Oxford Update Software, Oxford.

Chadwick D, Leiderman DB, Sauerman W, *et al.* 1996. Gabapentin in generalized seizures. *Epilepsy Res*, **25**: 191–7.

Chung WH, Hung SI, Hong HS, *et al.* 2004. Medical genetics: a marker for Stevens–Johnson syndrome. *Nature*, **428**: 486.

Cook RJ and Sackett DL. 1995. The number needed to treat: a clinically useful measure of treatment effect. *Br Med J*, **310**: 452–4 (published erratum *Br Med J*, 310: 1056).

Cramer JA, Fisher R, Ben-Menachem E, *et al.* 1999. New antiepileptic drugs: comparison of key clinical trials. *Epilepsia*, **40**: 590–600.

Dalby NO and Nielsen EB. 1997. Comparison of the preclinical anticonvulsant profiles of tiagabine, lamotrigine, gabapentin and vigabatrin. *Epilepsy Res*, **28**: 63–72.

Dean C, Mosier M, and Penry K. 1999. Dose response study of vigabatrin as add-on therapy in patients with uncontrolled complex partial seizures. *Epilepsia*, **40**: 74–82.

De Silva M, MacArdle B, McGowas M, *et al.* 1996. Randomised comparative monotherapy trial of phenobarbitone, phenytoin, carbamazepine and sodium valproate for newly diagnosed childhood epilepsy. *Lancet*, **347**: 709–13.

DeVane CL. 2003. Pharmacokinetics, drug interactions, and tolerability of valproate. *Psychopharmacol Bull*, **37** (Suppl. 2): 25–42.

Duncan JS, Shorvon SD, and Trimple MR. 1988. Withdrawal symptoms from phenytoin, carbamazepine and sodium valproate. *J Neurol Neurosurg Psychiatry*, **51**: 924–8.

Faught E, Ayala R, Montouris GG, *et al.*, and the Zonisamide 922 Trial Group. 2001. Randomized controlled trial of zonisamide for the treatment of refractory partial-onset seizures. *Neurology*, **57**: 1774–9.

Faught E, Wilder BJ, Ramsey RE, *et al.* 1996. Topiramate placebo controlled dose-ranging trial in refractory partial epilepsy using 200-, 400-, and 600-mg daily dosages. *Neurology*, **46**: 1684–90.

Fitton A and Goa KL. 1995. Lamotrigine. *Drugs*, **50**: 691–713.

Flicker L and Grimley Evans J. 1999. Piracetam for dementia or cognitive impairment. *The Cochrane Library*, **1**: 1–43.

French JA, Kanner AM, Bautista J, *et al.* 2004. Efficacy and tolerability of the new antiepileptic drugs. I. Treatment of new onset epilepsy: report of the Therapeutics and Technology Assessment Subcommittee and Quality Standards Subcommittee of the American Academy of Neurology and the American Epilepsy Society. *Neurology*, **62**: 1252–60.

French JA, Kanner AM, Bautista J, *et al.* 2004. Efficacy and tolerability of the new antiepileptic drugs. II. Treatment of refractory epilepsy: report of the Therapeutics and Technology Assessment Subcommittee and Quality Standards Subcommittee of the American Academy of Neurology and the American Epilepsy Society. *Neurology*, **62**: 1261–73.

French JA, Kugler AR, Robbins JL, *et al.* 2003. Dose–response trial of pregabalin adjunctive therapy in patients with partial seizures. *Neurology*, **27**: 1631–7.

French JA, Mosier M, Walker S, *et al.*, and the Vigabatrin Protocol 024 Investigative Cohort. 1996. A double-blind, placebo controlled study of vigabatrin 3 g/day in patients with uncontrolled complex partial seizures. *Neurology*, **46**: 54–61.

Gil-Nagel A. 2003. Review of new antiepileptic drugs as initial therapy. *Epilepsia*, **44** (Suppl. 4): 3–10.

Glauser TA, Migro M, D'Souza J, *et al.* 2000. Adjunctive therapy with oxcarbazepine in children with partial seizures. *Neurology*, **54**: 2237–44.

Gouliaev AH and Senning A. 1994. Piracetam and other structurally related nootropics. *Brain Res Rev*, **19**: 180–2.

Grant SM and Heel RC. 1991. Vigabatrin: a review of its pharmacodynamic and pharmacokinetic properties, and therapeutic potential in epilepsy. *Drugs*, **41**: 889–926.

Grunwald RA, Thompson PJ, Corcoran RS, *et al.* 1994. Effect of vigabatrin on partial seizures and cognitive function. *J Neurol Neurosurg Psychiatry*, **57**: 1057–63.

Guerreiro MM, Vigonius U, Pohlmann H, *et al.* 1997. A double-blind controlled clinical trial of oxcarbazepine versus phenytoin in children and adolescents with epilepsy. *Epilepsy Res*, **27**: 205–13.

Hancock E and Cross H. 2003. Treatment of Lennox–Gastaut syndrome. *Cochrane Database Syst Rev*, (3): CD003277.

Heller AJ, Chesterman P, Elwes RD, *et al.* 1995. Phenobarbitone, phenytoin, carbamazepine, or sodium valproate for newly diagnosed adult epilepsy: a randomized comparative monotherapy study. *J Neurol Neurosurg Psychiatry*, **58**: 44–50.

Jawad S, Richens A, Goodwin G, *et al.* 1989. Controlled trial of lamotrigine (Lamictal) for refractory partial seizures. *Epilepsia*, **30**: 356–63.

Johannessen CU and Johannessen SI. 2003. Valproate: past, present, and future. *CNS Drug Rev*, **9**: 199–216.

Kälviäinen R and Nousiainen I. 2001. Visual field defects with vigabatrin: epidemiology and therapeutic implications. *CNS Drugs*, **15**: 217–30.

Kälviäinen R, Brodie MJ, Chadwick D, *et al.* 1998. A double-blind, placebo-controlled trial of tiagabine given three times daily as add-on therapy for refractory partial seizures. *Epilepsy Res*, **30**: 31–40.

Kälviäinen R, Nousiainen I, Mäntyjärvi M, *et al.* 1999. Vigabatrin, a gabaergic antiepileptic drug, causes concentric visual field defects. *Neurology*, **53**: 922–6.

Kasteleijn-Nolst Trenite DG *et al.* 1996. Photosensitive epilepsy: a model to study the effects of antiepileptic drugs—evaluation of the piracetam analogue, levetiracetam. *Epilepsy Res*, **25**: 225–30.

Koskiniemi M, Van Vleymen B, Hakamies L, Lamusuo S, and Taalas J. 1998. Piracetam relieves symptoms in progressive myoclonus epilepsy: a multicentre, randomised, double blind, crossover study comparing the efficacy and safety of three dosages of oral piracetam with placebo. *J Neurol Neurosurg Psychiatry*, **64**: 344–8.

Kwan P and Brodie MJ. 2004. Phenobarbital for the treatment of epilepsy in the 21st century: a critical review. *Epilepsia*, **45**: 1141–9.

Leach JP and Brodie MJ. 1998. Tiagabine. *Lancet*, **351**: 203–7.

Leppik IE. 1999. Zonisamide. *Epilepsia*, **40** (Suppl. 5): S23–9

Leppik IE, Gram L, and Deaton R. 1999. Safety of tiagabine: summary of 53 trials. *Epilepsy Res*, **33**: 235–46.

Liu M, Hurn PD, and Alkayed NJ. 2004. Cytochrome P450 in neurological disease. *Curr Drug Metab*, **5**: 225–34.

Loiseau P, Yuen AW, Duche B, *et al.* 1990. A randomised double blind placebo controlled cross-over add on trial of lamotrigine in patients with treatment resistant partial seizures. *Epilepsy Res*, **7**: 136–45.

Lotze TE and Wilfong AA. 2004. Zonisamide treatment for symptomatic infantile spasms. *Neurology*, **62**: 296–8.

Marson A, Beghi E, Berg A, *et al.*, on behalf of the Cochrane Epilepsy Network. 1996. The Cochrane Collaboration: systematic reviews and their relevance to epilepsy. The Cochrane Epilepsy Network. *Epilepsia*, **37**: 917–21.

Marson AG, Hutton JL, Leach JP, *et al.* 2001. Levetiracetam, oxcarbazepine, remacemide and zonisamide for drug resistant localization-related epilepsy: a systematic review. *Epilepsy Res*, **46**: 259–70.

Marson AG, Kadir ZA, Hutton JL, *et al.* 1997. The new antiepileptic drugs: a systematic review of their efficacy and tolerability. *Epilepsia*, **38**: 859–80.

Matsuo F, Bergen D, Faught E, *et al.* 1993. Placebo-controlled study of the efficacy and safety of lamotrigine in patients with partial seizures: U.S. Lamotrigine Protocol 0.5 Clinical Trial Group. *Neurology*, **43**: 2284–91.

Mattson RH, Cramer JA, Collins JF, *et al.* 1985. Comparison of carbamazepine, phenobarbital, phenytoin, and primidone in partial and secondarily generalized tonic–clonic seizures. *N Engl J Med*, **313**: 145–51.

Mattson RH, Cramer JA, and Collins JF, the VA Epilepsy Cooperative Study Group. 1986. Connective tissue changes, hypersensitivity rash, and blood laboratory test changes associated with antiepileptic drug therapy. *Ann Neurol*, **20**: 119–20.

Mattson RH, Cramer JA, and Collins JF. 1992. A comparison of valproate with carbamazepine for the treatment of complex partial seizures and secondarily generalized tonic–clonic seizures in adults. The Department of Veterans Affairs Epilepsy Cooperative Study. *N Engl J Med*, **327**: 765–71.

McCorry D, Chadwick D, and Marson A. 2004. Current drug treatment of epilepsy in adults. *Lancet Neurol*, **3**: 729–35.

Meador KJ, Loring DW, Ray PG, *et al.* 1999. Differential cogn-itive effects of carbamazepine and gabapentin. *Epilepsia*, **40**: 1279–85.

Messenheimer J, Ramsay RE, Willmore LJ, *et al.* 1994. Lamotrigine therapy for partial seizures: a multicenter, placebo-controlled, double-blind, cross-over trial. *Epilepsia*, **35**: 113–21.

Messina S, Battino D, Croci D *et al.* 2005. Phenobarbital pharmacokinetics in old age: a case-matched evaluation based on therapeutic drug monitoring data. *Epilepsia*, **46**: 372–7.

Montenegro MA, Cendes F, Noronha AL, *et al.* 2001. Efficacy of clobazam as add-on therapy in patients with refractory partial epilepsy. *Epilepsia*, **42**: 539–42.

Motamedi GK and Meador KJ. 2004. Antiepileptic drugs and memory. *Epilepsy Behav*, **5**: 435–9.

Mula M, Trimble MR, and Sander JW. 2004. Psychiatric adverse events in patients with epilepsy and learning disabilities taking levetiracetam. *Seizure*, **13**: 55–7.

Onat F and Ozkara C. 2004. Adverse effects of new antiepileptic drugs. *Drugs Today (Barc)*, **40**: 325–42.

Ortinski P and Meador KJ. 2004. Cognitive side-effects of antiepileptic drugs. *Epilepsy Behav*, **5** (Suppl. 1): S60–S65.

Patsalos PN. 2004. Clinical pharmacokinetics of levetiracetam. *Clin Pharmacokinet*, **43**: 707–24.

Patsalos PN and Perucca E. 2003. Clinically important drug interactions in epilepsy: general features and interactions between antiepileptic drugs. *Lancet Neurol*, **2**: 347–56.

Patsalos PN and Perucca E. 2003. Clinically important drug interactions in epilepsy: interactions between antiepileptic drugs and other drugs. *Lancet Neurol*, **2**: 473–81.

Pellock JM, Smith MC, Cloyd JC, Uthman B, and Wilder BJ. 2004. Extended-release formulations: simplifying strategies in the management of antiepileptic drug therapy. *Epilepsy Behav*, **5**: 301–7.

Perucca E and Tomson T. 1999. Monotherapy trials with the new antiepileptic drugs: study designs, practical relevance and ethical implications. *Epilepsy Res*, **33**: 247–62.

Privitera M. 1997. Topiramate: a new antiepileptic drug. *Ann Pharmacother*, **31**: 1164–73.

Privitera M, Fincham R, Penry J, *et al*. 1996. Topiramate placebo-controlled dose-ranging trial in refractory partial epilepsy using 600-, 800-, and 1000-mg daily dosages. *Neurology*, **46**: 1678–83.

Reunanen M, Dam M, and Yuen AW. 1996. A randomized open multicentre comparative trial of lamotrigine and carbamazepine as monotherapy in patients with newly diagnosed or recurrent epilepsy. *Epilepsy Res*, **23**: 149–55.

Richens A, Chadwick DW, Duncan JS, *et al*. 1995. Adjunctive treatment of partial seizures with tiagabine: a placebo-controlled trial. *Epilepsy Res*, **21**: 37–42.

Richens A, Davidson DL, Cartlidge NE, *et al*. 1994. A multicentre comparative trial of sodium valproate and carbamazepine in adult-onset epilepsy. Adult EPITEG Collaborative Group. *J Neurol Neurosurg Psychiatry*, **57**: 682–7.

Rogawski MA and Loscher W. 2004. The neurobiology of antiepileptic drugs. *Nat Rev Neurosci*, **5**: 553–64.

Sachdeo R, Reife R, Lim P, and Pledger G. 1997. Topiramate monotherapy for partial onset seizures. *Epilepsia*, **38**: 294–300.

Sachdeo RC, Leroy R, Krauss G, *et al*. 1997. Tiagabine therapy for complex partial seizures: a dose–frequency study. *Arch Neurol*, **54**: 595–601.

Sackellares JC, Ramsay RE, Wilder BJ, *et al*. 2004. Randomized, controlled clinical trial of zonisamide as adjunctive treatment for refractory partial seizures. *Epilepsia*, **45**: 610–17.

Sankar R and Holmes GL. 2004. Mechanisms of action for the commonly used antiepileptic drugs: relevance to antiepileptic drug-associated neurobehavioral adverse effects. *J Child Neurol*, **19** (Suppl. 1): S6–S14.

Sato S, White BG, Penry K, *et al*. 1982. Valproate versus ethosuximide in the treatment of absence seizures. *Neurology*, **32**: 157–63.

Schachter SC. 1995. Tiagabine monotherapy in the treatment of partial epilepsy. *Epilepsia*, **36** (Suppl. 6): S2–S6.

Schachter SC, Vazquez B, Fisher RS, *et al*. 1999. Oxcarbazepine: double-blind, randomized, placebo-controlled, monotherapy trial for partial seizures. *Neurology*, **52**: 732–7.

Schapel GJ, Beran RG, Vajda FJ, *et al*. 1993. Double blind, placebo controlled, cross-over study of lamotrigine in treatment resistant partial seizures. *J Neurol Neurosurg Psychiatry*, **56**: 448–53.

Schmidt D, Jacob R, Loiseau P, *et al*. 1993. Zonisamide for add on treatment of refractory partial epilepsy: a European double blind trial. *Epilepsy Res*, **15**: 67–73.

Semah F, Picot MC, Derambure P, *et al*. 2004. The choice of antiepileptic drugs in newly diagnosed epilepsy: a national French survey. *Epileptic Disord*, **6**: 255–65.

Sharief M, Viteri C, Ben-Menachem E, *et al*. 1996. Double blind placebo-controlled study of topiramate in patients with refractory epilepsy. *Epilepsy Res*, **25**: 217–24.

Shorvon SD. 1995. Clobazam. In: Levy R, Mattson R, and Meldrum B (eds). *Antiepileptic Drugs* (4th edn). Raven Press, New York: pp. 763–78.

Shorvon SD. 1996. Safety of topiramate: adverse events and relationships to dosing. *Epilepsia*, **37**: S18–S22.

Shorvon SD. 2001. New drug classes: pyrrolidone derivatives. *Lancet*, **200**: 1885–92.

Shorvon SD, Löwenthal A, Janz D, *et al*. for the European Levetiracetam Study Group. 2000. Multicenter double-blind, randomized, placebo-controlled trial of levetiracetam as add-on therapy in patients with refractory partial seizures. *Epilepsia*, **41**: 1179–86.

Sillanpää M. 1981. Carbamazepine: pharmacology and clinical uses. *Acta Neurol Scand*, **88** (Suppl. 64): 1–202.

Silvenius J, Kälviäinen R, Ylinen A, *et al*. 1991. Double blind study of gabapentin in the treatment of partial seizures. *Epilepsia*, **32**: 539–42.

Smith D, Baker G, Davies G, Dewey M, *et al*. 1993. Outcomes of add on treatment with lamotrigine in partial epilepsy. *Epilepsia*, **34**: 312–22.

Smith DB, Mattson RH, Cramer JA, *et al*. 1987. Results of a nationwide Veterans Administration Cooperative Study comparing the efficacy and toxicity of carbamazepine, phenobarbital, phenytoin, and primidone. *Epilepsia*, **28** (Suppl. 3): 50–8.

Tassinari CA, Michelucci R, Chauvel P, *et al*. 1996. Double blind, placebo-controlled trial of topiramate (600 mg daily) for the treatment of refractory partial epilepsy. *Epilepsia*, **37**: 763–8.

Tomson T. 2004. Drug selection for the newly diagnosed patient: when is a new generation antiepileptic drug indicated? *J Neurol*, **251**: 1043–9.

Tomson T, Perucca E, and Battino D. 2004. Navigating toward fetal and maternal health: the challenge of treating epilepsy in pregnancy. *Epilepsia*, **45**: 1171–5.

Trojnar MK, Wierzchowska-Cioch E, Krzyzanowski M, *et al*. 2004. New generation of valproic acid. *Pol J Pharmacol*, **56**: 283–8.

Tyagi A and Delanty N. 2003. Herbal remedies, dietary supplements, and seizures. *Epilepsia*, **44**: 228–35.

UK Gabapentin Study Group. 1990. Gabapentin in partial epilepsy. *Lancet*, **335**: 1114–17.

US Gabapentin Study Group No. 5. 1993. Gabapentin as add-on therapy in refractory partial epilepsy: a double-blind, placebo-controlled, parallel-group study. *Neurology*, **43**: 2292–8.

Uthman B, Rowan J, Ahman PA, *et al.* 1998. Tiagabine for complex partial seizures: a randomised, add-on, dose–response trial. *Arch Neurol*, **55**: 56–62.

Vecht CJ, Wagner GL, and Wilms EB. 2003. Interactions between antiepileptic and chemotherapeutic drugs. *Lancet Neurol*, **2**: 404–9.

Vigevano F and Cilio MR. 1997. Vigabatrin versus ACTH as first-line treatment for infantile spasms: a randomized, prospective study. *Epilepsia*, **38**: 1270–4.

Vittorio CC and Muglia JJ. 1995. Anticonvulsant hypersensitivity syndrome. *Arch Intern Med*, **155**: 2285–90.

Waugh J and Goa KL. 2003. Topiramate as monotherapy in newly diagnosed epilepsy. *CNS Drugs*, **17**: 985–92.

## SECTION 4—THE EMERGENCY TREATMENT OF EPILEPSY

### Books

Shorvon SD. 1994. *Status Epilepticus: its Clinical Features and Treatment in Children and Adults.* Cambridge University Press, Cambridge.

### Articles in scientific journals

Agathonikou A, Panayiotopoulos CP, Giannakodimos S, *et al.* 1998. Typical absence status in adults: diagnostic and syndromic considerations. *Epilepsia*, **39**: 1265–76.

Alldredge BK, Gelb AM, Isaacs SM, *et al.* 2001 A comparison of lorazepam, diazepam, and placebo for the treatment of out-of-hospital status epilepticus. *N Engl J Med*, **345**: 631–7. [Erratum in: *N Engl J Med* 2001, **345**: 1860.]

Aminoff MJ and Simon RP. 1980. Status epilepticus: causes, clinical features and consequences in 98 patients. *Am J Med*, **69**: 657–66.

Brenner RP. 2004. EEG in convulsive and non-convulsive status epilepticus. *J Clin Neurophysiol*, **21**: 319–31.

Cereghino JJ, Mitchell WG, Murphy J, *et al.* 1998. Treating repetitive seizures with a rectal diazepam formulation: a randomized study. The North American Diastat Study Group. *Neurology*, **51**: 1274–82.

Chamberlain JM, Altieri MA, Futterman C, *et al.* 1997. A prospective, randomized study comparing intramuscular midazolam with intravenous diazepam for the treatment of seizures in children [see comments]. *Pediatr Emerg Care*, **13**: 92–4.

Claassen J, Hirsch LJ, Emerson RG, *et al.* 2002. Treatment of refractory status epilepticus with pentobarbital, propofol, or midazolam: a systematic review. *Epilepsia*, **43**: 146–53.

Cockerell OC, Rothwell J, Thompson PD, *et al.* 1996. Clinical and physiological features of epilepsia partialis continua: cases ascertained in the UK. *Brain*, **119** (Pt 2): 393–407.

Cockerell OC, Walker MC, Sander JW, *et al.* 1994. Complex partial status epilepticus: a recurrent problem. *J Neurol Neurosurg Psychiatry*, **57**: 835–7.

Coeytaux A, Jallon P, Galobardes B, *et al.* 2000. Incidence of status epilepticus in French-speaking Switzerland: (EPISTAR). *Neurology*, **55**: 693–7.

Corsellis JA and Bruton CJ. 1983. Neuropathology of status epilepticus in humans. *Adv Neurol*, **34**: 129–39.

DeLorenzo RJ, Hauser WA, Towne AR, *et al.* 1996. A prospective, population-based epidemiologic study of status epilepticus in Richmond, Virginia. *Neurology*, **46**: 1029–35.

DeLorenzo RJ, Waterhouse EJ, Towne AR, *et al.* 1998. Persistent non-convulsive status epilepticus after the control of convulsive status epilepticus. *Epilepsia*, **39**: 833–40.

Dreifuss FE, Rosman NP, Lloyd JC, *et al.* 1998. A comparison of rectal diazepam gel and placebo for acute repetitive seizures. *N Engl J Med*, **338**: 1869–75.

Fischer JH, Patel TV, and Fischer PA. 2003. Fosphenytoin: clinical pharmacokinetics and comparative advantages in the acute treatment of seizures. *Clin Pharmacokinet*, **42**: 33–58.

Hesdorffer DC, Logroscino G, Cascino G, *et al.* 1998. Incidence of status epilepticus in Rochester, Minnesota, 1965–1984. *Neurology*, **50**: 735–41.

Hesdorffer DC, Logroscino G, Cascino G, *et al.* 1998. Risk of unprovoked seizure after acute symptomatic seizure: effect of status epilepticus. *Ann Neurol*, **44**: 908–12.

Kapur J and Macdonald RL. 1997. Rapid seizure-induced reduction of benzodiazepine and $Zn^{2+}$ sensitivity of hippocampal dentate granule cell GABA-A receptors. *J Neurosci*, **17**: 7532–40.

Knake S, Rosenow F, Vescovi M, *et al.* 2001. Incidence of status epilepticus in adults in Germany: a prospective, population-based study. *Epilepsia*, **42**: 714–18.

Knoester PD, Jonker DM, Van Der Hoeven RT, *et al.* 2002. Pharmacokinetics and pharmacodynamics of midazolam administered as a concentrated intranasal spray: a study in healthy volunteers. *Br J Clin Pharmacol*, **53**: 501–7.

Leppik IE, Derivan AT, and Homan RW. 1983. Double-blind study of lorazepam and diazepam in status epilepticus. *JAMA*, **249**: 1452–4.

Lothman E. 1990. The biochemical basis and pathophysiology of status epilepticus. *Neurology*, **40** (Suppl. 2): 13–23.

Mahmoudian T and Zadeh MM. 2004. Comparison of intranasal midazolam with intravenous diazepam for treating acute seizures in children. *Epilepsy Behav*, **5**: 253–5.

Mayer SA, Claassen J, Lokin J, *et al.* 2002. Refractory status epilepticus: frequency, risk factors, impact on outcome. *Arch Neurol*, **59**: 205–10.

Meldrum BS. 1983. Endocrine consequences of status epilepticus. *Adv Neurol*, **34**: 399–403.

Meldrum BS and Brierley JB. 1973. Prolonged epileptic seizures in primates: ischemic cell change and its relation to ictal physiological events. *Arch Neurol*, **28**: 10–17.

Meldrum BS and Horton RW. 1973. Physiology of status epilepticus in primates. *Arch Neurol*, **28**: 1–9.

Meldrum BS, Vigouroux RA, and Brierley JB. 1973. Systemic factors and epileptic brain damage: prolonged seizures in paralysed, artificially ventilated baboons. *Arch Neurol*, **29**: 82–7.

Prensky AL, Raff MC, Moore MJ, *et al.* 1967. Intravenous diazepam in the treatment of prolonged seizure activity. *N Engl J Med*, **276**: 779–84.

Schwagmeier R, Alincic S, and Striebel HW. 1998. Midazolam pharmacokinetics following intravenous and buccal administration. *Br J Clin Pharmacol*, **46**: 203–6.

Scott RC, Besag FM, and Neville BG. 1999. Buccal midazolam and rectal diazepam for treatment of prolonged seizures in childhood and adolescence: a randomised trial [see comments]. *Lancet*, **353**: 623–6.

Shaner DM, McCurdy SA, Herring MO, *et al.* 1988. Treatment of status epilepticus: a prospective comparison of diazepam and phenytoin versus phenobarbital and optional phenytoin. *Neurology*, **38**: 202–7.

Shorvon S. 2005. The classification of status epilepticus. *Epileptic disorders*, **7**: 1–3.

Shorvon SD. 2005. The definition and classification of non-convulsive status epilepticus. *Epileptic disorders*, **7** (in press).

Simon RP. 1985. Physiologic consequences of status epilepticus. *Epilepsia*, **26** (Suppl. 1): S58–S66.

Singhi S, Murthy A, Singhi P, *et al.* 2002. Continuous midazolam versus diazepam infusion for refractory convulsive status epilepticus. *J Child Neurol*, **17**: 106–10.

Thomas P, Lebrun C, and Chatel M. 1993. De novo absence status epilepticus as a benzodiazepine withdrawal syndrome. *Epilepsia*, **34**: 355–8.

Tinuper P, Aguglia U, and Gastaut H. 1986. Use of clobazam in certain forms of status epilepticus and in startle-induced epileptic seizures. *Epilepsia*, **27** (Suppl. 1): S18–S26.

Tomson T, Svanborg E, and Wedlund JE. 1986. Nonconvulsive status epilepticus: high incidence of complex partial status. *Epilepsia*, **27**: 276–85.

Treiman DM, Meyers PD, Walton NY, *et al.* 1998. A comparison of four treatments for generalized convulsive status epilepticus. Veterans Affairs Status Epilepticus Cooperative Study Group. *N Engl J Med*, **339**: 792–8.

Treiman DM, Walton NY, and Kendrick C. 1990. A progressive sequence of electroencephalographic changes during generalized convulsive status epilepticus. *Epilepsy Res*, **5**: 49–60.

Van-Ness PC. 1990. Pentobarbital and EEG burst suppression in treatment of status epilepticus refractory to benzodiazepines and phenytoin. *Epilepsia*, **31**: 61–7.

Walker MC, Howard RS, Smith SJ, *et al.* 1996. Diagnosis and treatment of status epilepticus on a neurological intensive care unit. *QJM*, **89**: 913–20.

Walker MC, Tong X, Brown S, *et al.* 1998. Comparison of single- and repeated-dose pharmacokinetics of diazepam. *Epilepsia*, **39**: 283–9.

Williamson PD, Spencer DD, Spencer SS, *et al.* 1985. Complex partial status epilepticus: a depth-electrode study. *Ann Neurol*, **18**: 647–54.

# SECTION 5—THE SURGICAL TREATMENT OF EPILEPSY

## Books

Engel J (ed). 1993. *Surgical Treatment of the Epilepsies* (2nd edn). Raven Press, New York.

Luders H and Comair Y (eds). 2001. *Epilepsy Surgery* (2nd edn). Lippencott, Williams and Wilkins, Philadelphia.

Shorvon SD, Perucca E, Fish D, and Dodson (eds). 2004. *The Treatment of Epilepsy* (2nd edn). Blackwell Publishing, Oxford.

## Articles in scientific journals

Alarcon G, Garcia Seoanne J, Binnie C, *et al.* 1997. Origin and propagation of interictal discharges in the acute electrocorticogram: implications for pathophysiology and surgical treatment of temporal lobe epilepsy. *Brain*, **120**: 2259–82.

Antel SB, Li LM, Cendes F, *et al.* 2002. Predicting surgical outcome in temporal lobe epilepsy patients using MR1 and MRSI. *Neurology*, **28**: 1505–12.

Arzimanoglou AA, Andermann F, Aicardi J, *et al.* 2000. Sturge–Weber syndrome: indications and results of surgery in 20 patients. *Neurology*, **55**: 1472–9.

Avoli M, Bernasconi A, Mattia D, *et al.* 1999. Epileptiform discharges in the human dysplastic neocortex: in vitro physiology and pharmacology. *Ann Neurol*, **46**: 816–26.

Awad IA, Katz A, Hahn JF, *et al.* 1989. Extent of resection in temporal lobectomy for epilepsy. I. Interobserver analysis and correlation with seizure outcome. *Epilepsia*, **30**: 756–62.

Awad IA, Nayel MH, and Luders H. 1991. Second operation after the failure of previous resection for epilepsy. *Neurosurgery*, **28**: 510–18.

Barkovich AJ, Kuzniecky RI, *et al.* 1996. A classification scheme for malformations of cortical development. *Neuropediatrics*, **27**: 59–63.

Baulac M, De Grissac N, Hasboun D, *et al.* 1998. Hippocampal developmental changes in patients with partial epilepsy: magnetic resonance imaging and clinical aspects. *Ann Neurol*, **44**: 223–33.

Bautista RE, Cobbs MA, Spencer DD, *et al.* 1999. Prediction of surgical outcome by interictal epileptiform abnormalities during intracranial EEG monitoring in patients with extrahippocampal seizures. *Epilepsia*, **40**: 880–90.

Ben-Menachem E, Hellstrom K, *et al.* 1999. Evaluation of refractory epilepsy treated with vagus nerve stimulation for up to 5 years. *Neurology*, **52**: 1265–7.

Ben-Menachem E, Manon-Espaillat R, Ristanovic R, *et al.* 1994. Vagus nerve stimulation for treatment of partial seizures. I. A controlled study of effect on seizures. *Epilepsia*, **35**: 616–26.

Berger MS, Ghatan S, Haglund MM, *et al.* 1993. Low grade gliomas associated with intractable epilepsy: seizure outcome utilizing electrocorticography during tumor resection. *J Neurosurg*, **79**: 62–9.

Bertram EH. 2003. Why does surgery fail to cure limbic epilepsy? Seizure functional anatomy may hold the answer. *Epilepsy Res*, **56**: 93–9.

Bien CG, Kurthen M, Baron K, *et al.* 2001. Long-term seizure outcome and antiepileptic drug treatment in surgically treated temporal lobe epilepsy patients: a controlled study. *Epilepsia*, **42**: 1416–21. PMID: 11879344 [PubMed—indexed for MEDLINE.]

Bingaman WE. 2004. Surgery for focal cortical dysplasia. *Neurology*, **62** (Suppl. 3): S30–S34.

Blume WT, Girvin JP, and Kaufman JCE. 1982. Childhood brain tumors presenting as chronic uncontrolled focal seizure disorders. *Ann Neurol*, **12**: 538–41.

Cascino GD, Hulihan JF, Sharbrough FW, *et al.* 1993. Parietal lobe lesional epilepsy: electroclinical correlation and operative outcome. *Epilepsia*, **34**: 522–7.

Cendes F, Li LM, Watson C, *et al.* 2000. Is ictal recording mandatory in temporal lobe epilepsy? Not when the interictal electroencephalogram and hippocampal atrophy coincide. *Arch Neurol*, **57**: 497–500.

Chassoux F, Devaux B, Landre E, *et al.* 2000. Stereoelectroencephalography in focal cortical dysplasia: a 3D approach to delineating the dysplastic cortex. *Brain*, **123**: 1733–51.

Cohen-Gadol AA, Britton JW, Wetjen NM, *et al.* 2003. Neuro-stimulation therapy for epilepsy: current modalities and future directions. *Mayo Clin Proc*, **78**: 238–48.

Cohen-Gadol AA, Leavitt JA, Lynch JJ, *et al.* 2003. Prospective analysis of diplopia after anterior temporal lobectomy for mesial temporal lobe sclerosis. *J Neurosurg*, **99**: 496–9.

Cook MJ, Fish DR, Shorvon SD, *et al.* 1992. Hippocampal volumetric and morphometric studies in frontal and temporal lobe epilepsy. *Brain*, **115**: 1001–15.

Cook SW, Nguyen ST, Hu B, *et al.* 2004. Cerebral hemispherectomy in pediatric patients with epilepsy: comparison of three techniques by pathological substrate in 115 patients. *J Neurosurg Spine*, **100**: 125–41.

Daniel RT and Villemure JG. 2003. Hemispherotomy techniques. *J Neurosurg*, **98**: 438–9.

Daniel RT and Villemure JG. 2003. Peri-insular hemispherotomy: potential pitfalls and avoidance of complications. *Stereotact Funct Neurosurg*, **80**: 22–7.

Daumas-Duport C, Scheithauer BW, Chodkiewicz JP, *et al.* 1988. Dysembryoplastic neuroepithelial tumor: a surgically curable tumor of young patients with intractable partial seizures: report of thirty-nine cases. *Neurosurgery*, **23**: 545–56.

Daumas-Duport C, Varlet P, Bacha S, *et al.* 1999. Dysembryoplastic neuroepithelial tumors: non-specific histological forms—a study of 40 cases. *J Neurooncol*, **41**: 267–80.

Del Brutto OH, Santibanez R, Noboa CA, *et al.* 1992. Epilepsy due to neurocysticercosis: analysis of 203 patients. *Neurology*, **42**: 389–92.

Devlin AM, Cross JH, Harkness W, *et al.* BG. 2003. Clinical outcomes of hemispherectomy for epilepsy in childhood and adolescence. *Brain*, **126** (Pt 3): 556–66.

Drake CG. 1979. Cerebral AVMs: considerations for and experience with surgical treatment in 166 cases. *Clin Neurosurg*, **26**: 145–208.

Dubeau F, Tampieri D, Lee N, *et al.* 1995. Periventricular and subcortical nodular heterotopia: a study of 33 patients. *Brain*, **118** (Pt 5): 1273–87.

Duchowny M, Jayakar P, Resnick T, *et al.* 1998. Epilepsy surgery in the first three years of life. *Epilepsia*, **39**: 737–43.

Duncan JS. 1997. Imaging and epilepsy. *Brain*, **120**: 339–77.

Edwards JC, Wyllie E, Ruggieri PM, *et al.* 2000. Seizure outcome after surgery for epilepsy due to malformation of cortical development. *Neurology*, **55**: 1110–14.

Elger CE, Helmstaedter C, and Kurthen M. 2004. Chronic epilepsy and cognition. *Lancet Neurol*, **3**: 663–72.

Engel J Jr, Wiebe S, French J, *et al.* 2003. Practice parameter: temporal lobe and localized neocortical resections for epilepsy: report of the Quality Standards Subcommittee of the American Academy of Neurology, in association with the American Epilepsy Society and the American Association of Neurological Surgeons. *Neurology*, **60**: 538–47.

Ferrier CH, Alarcon G, Engelsman J, *et al.* 2001. Relevance of residual histologic and electrocorticographic abnormalities for surgical outcome in frontal lobe epilepsy. *Epilepsia*, **42**: 363–71.

Fish DR, Smith SJ, Quesney LF, *et al.* 1993. Surgical treatment of children with medically intractable frontal or temporal lobe epilepsy: results and highlights of 40 years' experience. *Epilepsia*, **34**: 244–7.

Foldvary N, Nashold B, Mascha E, *et al.* 2000. Seizure outcome after temporal lobectomy for temporal lobe epilepsy. *Neurology*, **54**: 630–4.

Francione S, Vigliano P, Tassi L, *et al.* 2003. Surgery for drug resistant partial epilepsy in children with focal cortical dysplasia: anatomical–clinical correlations and neurophysiological data in 10 patients. *J Neurol Neurosurg Psychiatry*, **74**: 1493–501.

Frater JL, Prayson RA, Morris HH III, *et al.* 2000. Surgical pathologic findings of extratemporal-based intractable epilepsy: a study of 133 consecutive resections. *Arch Pathol Lab Med*, **124**: 545–9.

George R, Salinsky M, Kuzniecky R, *et al.* 1994. Vagus nerve stimulation for treatment of partial seizures. III. Long-term follow-up on first 67 patients exiting a controlled study. *Epilepsia*, **35**: 637–43.

Germano IM, Poulin N, and Olivier A. 1994. Reoperation for recurrent temporal lobe epilepsy. *J Neurosurg*, **81**: 31–6.

Gleißner U, Helmstaedter C, and Elger CE. 1998. Right hippocampal contribution to visual memory: a presurgical and postsurgical study in patients with temporal lobe epilepsy. *J Neurol Neurosurg Psychiatry*, **65**: 665–9.

Gleißner U, Helmstaedter C, Schramm C, *et al.* 2001. Memory outcome after selective amygdalohippocampectomy: a study in 140 patients with temporal lobe epilepsy. *Epilepsia*, **43**: 87–95.

Goldring S and Gregorie EM. 1984. Surgical management using epidural recordings to localize the seizure focus: review of 100 cases. *Neurosurgery*, **60**: 457–66.

Grote C, Van Slyke P, and Hoeppner J. 1999. Language dominance following multiple subpial transection for Landau–Kleffner syndrome. *Brain*, **122**: 561–6.

Guerrini R, Andermann E, Avoli M, *et al.* 1999. Cortical dysplasias, genetics, and epileptogenesis. *Adv Neurol*, **79**: 95–121.

Gupta A, Carreno M, Wyllie E, *et al.* 2004. Hemispheric malformations of cortical development. *Neurology*, **62** (6 Suppl. 3): S20–S26.

Hamandi K, Salek-Haddadi A, Fish DR, *et al.* 2004. EEG/functional MRI in epilepsy: The Queen Square Experience. *J Clin Neurophysiol*, **21**: 241–8.

Handforth A, DeGiorgio CM, Schachter SC, *et al.* 1998. Vagus nerve stimulation therapy for partial-onset seizures: a randomized active-control trial. *Neurology*, **51**: 48–55.

Helmstaedter C, Van Roost D, Clusmann H, *et al.* 2004. Collateral brain damage, a potential source of cognitive impairment after selective surgery for control of mesial temporal lobe epilepsy. *J Neurol Neurosurg Psychiatry*, **75**: 323–6.

Hennessy MJ, Elwes RD, Honavar M, *et al.* 2001. Predictors of outcome and pathological considerations in the surgical treatment of intractable epilepsy associated with temporal lobe lesions. *Neurol Neurosurg Psychiatry*, **70**: 450–8.

Hennessy MJ, Langan Y, Elwes RD, *et al.* 1999. A study of mortality after temporal lobe epilepsy surgery. *Neurology*, **53**: 1276–83.

Ho SS, Berkovic SF, Berlangieri SU, *et al.* 1995. Comparison of ictal SPECT and interictal PET in the presurgical evaluation of temporal lobe epilepsy. *Ann Neurol*, **37**: 738–45.

Hodaie M, Wennberg RA, Dostrovsky JO, *et al.* 2002. Chronic anterior thalamus stimulation for intractable epilepsy. *Epilepsia*, **43**: 603–8.

Holmes MD, Kutsy RL, Ojemann GA, *et al.* 2000. Interictal, unifocal spikes in refractory extratemporal epilepsy predict ictal origin and postsurgical outcome. *Clin Neurophysiol*, **111**: 1802–8.

Hosain S, Nikalov B, Harden C, *et al.* 2000. Vagus nerve stimulation treatment for Lennox–Gastaut syndrome. *J Child Neurol*, **15**: 509–12.

Irwin K, Birch V, Lees J, *et al.* 2001. Multiple subpial transection in Landau–Kleffner syndrome. *Dev Med Child Neurol*, **43**: 248–52.

Janszky J, Janszky I, Schulz R, *et al.* 2005. Temporal lobe epilepsy with hippocampal sclerosis: predictors for long-term surgical outcome. *Brain*, **128**: 395–404.

Janszky J, Jokeit H, Schulz R, *et al.* 2000. EEG predicts surgical outcome in lesional frontal lobe epilepsy. *Neurology*, **54**: 1470–6.

Jarrar RG, Buchhalter JR, Meyer FB, *et al.* 2002. Long-term follow-up of temporal lobectomy in children. *Neurology*, **26**: 1635–7.

Kanner AM, Kaydanova Y, Toledo-Morrell L, *et al.* 1995. Tailored anterior temporal lobectomy: relation between extent of resection of mesial structures and postsurgical seizure outcome. *Arch Neurol*, **52**: 173–8.

Khajavi K, Comair YG, Wyllie E, *et al.* 1999. Surgical management of pediatric tumor-associated epilepsy. *J Child Neurol*, **14**: 15–25.

Kim YD, Heo K, Park SC, *et al.* 2005. Antiepileptic drug withdrawal after successful surgery for intractable temporal lobe epilepsy. *Epilepsia*, **46**: 251–7.

Kirkpatrick PJ, Honavar M, Janota I, *et al.* 1993. Control of temporal lobe epilepsy following en bloc resection of low grade tumors. *J Neurosurg*, **78**: 19–25.

Koh S, Jayakar P, Dunoyer C, *et al.* 2000. Epilepsy surgery in children with tuberous sclerosis complex: presurgical evaluation and outcome. *Epilepsia*, **41**: 1206–13.

Kondziolka D, McLaughlin MR, and Kestle JRW. 1995. Simple risk predictions for arteriovenous malformation hemorrhage. *Neurosurgery*, **37**: 851–5.

Kossoff EH, Vining EP, Pillas DJ, *et al.* 2003. Hemispherectomy for intractable unihemispheric epilepsy etiology vs outcome. *Neurology*, **61**: 887–90.

Kothare SV, VanLandingham K, Armon C, *et al.* 1998. Seizure onset from periventricular nodular heterotopias: depth-electrode study. *Neurology*, **51**: 1723–7.

Kurita H, Kawamoto S, Suzuki I, *et al.* 1998. Control of epilepsy associated with cerebral arteriovenous malformations after radiosurgery. *J Neurol Neurosurg Psychiatry*, **65**: 648–55.

Kuzniecky R, Gilliam F, Morawetz R, *et al.* 1997. Occipital lobe developmental malformations and epilepsy: clinical spectrum, treatment and outcome. *Epilepsia*, **38**: 175–81.

Kuzniecky R, Ho SS, Martin R, *et al.* 1999. Temporal lobe developmental malformations and hippocampal sclerosis: epilepsy surgical outcome. *Neurology*, **52**: 479–84.

Labar D, Murphy J, and Tecoma E. 1999. Vagus nerve stimulation for medication-resistant generalized epilepsy. E04 VNS Study Group. *Neurology*, **52**: 1510–12.

Laich E, Kuzniecky R, Mountz J, *et al.* 1997. Supplementary sensorimotor area epilepsy: seizure localization, cortical propagation and subcortical activation pathways using ictal SPECT. *Brain*, **120**: 855–64.

Leblanc R, Tampieri D, Robitaille Y, *et al.* 1991. Surgical treatment of intractable epilepsy associated with schizencephaly. *Neurosurgery*, **29**: 421–9.

Lee HW, Hong SB, and Tae WS. 2000. Opposite ictal perfusion patterns of subtracted SPECT. Hyperperfusion and hypoperfusion. *Brain*, **123**: 2150–9.

Lee JY and Adelson PD. 2004. Neurosurgical management of pediatric epilepsy. *Pediatr Clin North Am*, **51**: 441–56.

Lehericy S, Cohen L, Bazin B, *et al.* 2000. Functional MR evaluation of temporal and frontal language dominance compared with the Wada test. *Neurology*, **54**: 1625–33.

Lesser RP, Arroyo S, Crone N, *et al.* 1998. Motor and sensory mapping of the frontal and occipital lobes. *Epilepsia*, **39** (Suppl. 4): 69–80.

Li LM, Cendes F, Antel SB, *et al.* 2000. Prognostic value of proton magnetic resonance spectroscopic imaging for surgical outcome in patients with intractable temporal lobe epilepsy and bilateral hippocampal atrophy. *Ann Neurol*, **47**: 195–200.

Li LM, Dubeau F, Andermann F, *et al.* 1997. Periventricular nodular heterotopia and intractable temporal lobe epilepsy: poor outcome after temporal lobe resection. *Ann Neurol*, **41**: 662–8.

Liporace J, Hucko D, Morrow R, *et al.* 2001. Vagal nerve stimulation: adjustments to reduce painful side effects. *Neurology*, **57**: 885–6.

Litt B, Esteller R, Echauz J, *et al.* 2001. Epileptic seizures may begin hours in advance of clinical onset: a report of five patients. *Neuron*, **30**: 51–64.

Liu KD, Chung WY, Wu HM, *et al.* 2005. Gamma knife surgery for cavernous hemangiomas: an analysis of 125 patients. *J Neurosurg*, **102** (Suppl.): 81–6.

Loring DW, Meador K, Lee G, *et al.* 1994. Wada memory performance predicts seizure outcome following anterior temporal lobectomy. *Neurology*, **44**: 2322–4.

Luders H, Hanh JF, Lesser RP, *et al.* 1989. Basal temporal subdural electrodes in the evaluation of patients with intractable epilepsy. *Epilepsia*, **30**: 131–42.

Luessenhop AJ and Rosa L. 1985. Cerebral arteriovenous malformations: Indications for and results of surgery, and the role of intravascular techniques. *J Neurosurg*, **60**: 14–22.

Lutz MT, Clusmann H, Elger CE, *et al.* 2004. Neuropsychological outcome after selective amygdalohippocampectomy with transsylvian versus transcortical approach: a randomized prospective clinical trial of surgery for temporal lobe epilepsy. *Epilepsia*, **45**: 809–16.

Maehara T and Shimizu H. 2001. Surgical outcome of corpus callosotomy in patients with drop attacks. *Epilepsia*, **42**: 67–71.

Manchanda R, Schaefer B, McLachlan RS, *et al.* 1996. Psychiatric disorders in candidates for surgery for epilepsy. *J Neurol Neurosurg Psychiatry*, **61**: 82–9.

Mauguiere F and Ryvlin P. 2004. The role of PET in presurgical assessment of partial epilepsies. *Epileptic Disord*, **6**: 193–215.

McBride MC, Binnie CD, Janota I, *et al.* 1991. Predictive value of intraoperative electrocorticograms in resective epilepsy surgery. *Ann Neurol*, **30**: 526–32.

McIntosh AM, Kalnins RM, Mitchell LA, *et al.* 2004. Temporal lobectomy: long-term seizure outcome, late recurrence and risks for seizure recurrence. *Brain*, **127**: 2018–30.

McIntosh AM, Wilson SJ, and Berkovic SF. 2001. Seizure outcome after temporal lobectomy: current research practice and findings. *Epilepsia*, **42**: 1288–307.

McKhann GM. 2004. Novel surgical treatments for epilepsy. *Curr Neurol Neurosci Rep*, **4**: 335–9.

Moran NF, Fish DR, Kitchen M, *et al.* 1999. Supratentorial cavernous haemangiomas and epilepsy: a review of the literature and case series. *J Neurol Neurosurg Psychiatry*, **66**: 561–8.

Moran NF, Lemieux L, Kitchen ND, *et al*. 2001. Extrahippocampal temporal lobe atrophy in temporal lobe epilepsy and mesial temporal sclerosis. *Brain*, **124**: 167–75.

Morrell F, Whisler W, and Bleck T. 1989. Multiple subpial transection: a new approach to the surgical treatment of focal epilepsy. *J Neurosurg*, **70**: 231–9.

Morrell F, Whisler W, Smith M, *et al*. 1995. Landau–Kleffner syndrome: treatment with subpial intracortical transection. *Brain*, **118**: 1529–46.

Morris HH III, Luders H, Hahn JF, *et al*. 1986. Surgical treatment of primary brain tumors. *Ann Neurol*, **19**: 559–67.

Murphy JV. 1999. Left vagal nerve stimulation in children with medically refractory epilepsy. The Pediatric VNS Study Group. *J Pediatr*, **134**: 563–6.

Nash TE, Del Brutto OH, Butman JA, *et al*. 2004. Calcific neurocysticercosis and epileptogenesis. *Neurology*, **62**: 1934–8.

Nayel MH, Awad IA, and Luders H. 1991. Extent of mesiobasal resection determines outcome after temporal lobectomy for intractable complex partial seizures. *Neurosurgery*, **29**: 55–60.

Naylor AS, Rogvi-Hansen BA, *et al*. 1994. Psychiatric morbidity after surgery for epilepsy: short-term follow-up of patients undergoing amygdalohippocampectomy. *J Neurol Neurosurg Psychiatry*, **57**: 1375–81.

O'Brien TJ, So EL, Mullan BP, *et al*. 1998. Subtraction ictal SPECT co-registered to MRI improves clinical usefulness of SPECT in localizing the surgical seizure focus. *Neurology*, **50**: 445–54.

O'Brien TJ, So EL, Mullan BP, *et al*. 2000. Subtraction peri-ictal SPECT is predictive of extratemporal epilepsy surgery outcome. *Neurology*, **55**: 1668–77.

Oguni H, Olivier A, Andermann F, *et al*. 1991. Anterior callosotomy in the treatment of medically intractable epilepsies: a study of 43 patients with a mean follow-up of 39 months. *Ann Neurol*, **30**: 357–64.

Ojemann G, Ojemann J, Lettich E, *et al*. 1989. Cortical language localization in left, dominant hemisphere: an electrical stimulation mapping investigation in 117 patients. *J Neurosurg*, **71**: 316–26.

Ojemann GA. 1992. Different approaches to resective epilepsy surgery: standard and tailored. *Epilepsy Res Suppl*, **5**: 169–74.

Ondra SL, Troupp H, George ED, *et al*. 1990. The natural history of symptomatic arteriovenous malformations of the brain: a 24-year follow-up assessment. *J Neurosurg*, **73**: 387–91.

Orbach D, Romanelli P, Devinsky O, *et al*. 2001. Late seizure recurrence after multiple subpial transections. *Epilepsia*, **42**: 1130–3.

Osorio I, Frei MG, Sunderam S, *et al*. 2005. Automated seizure abatement in humans using electrical stimulation. *Ann Neurol*, **57**: 258–68.

Pacia SV and Ebersole JS. 1997. Intracranial EEG substrates of scalp ictal patterns from temporal lobe foci. *Epilepsia*, **38**: 642–54.

Pacia SV and Ebersole JS. 1999. Intracranial EEG in temporal lobe epilepsy. *J Clin Neurophysiol*, **16**: 399–407.

Packard AM, Miller VS, and Delgado MR. 1997. Schizencephaly: correlations of clinical and radiologic features. *Neurology*, **48**: 1427–34.

Palmini A, Andermann F, Olivier A, *et al*. 1991. Focal neuronal migration disorders and intractable partial epilepsy: results of surgical treatment. *Ann Neurol*, **30**: 750–7.

Palmini A, Gambardella A, Andermann F, *et al*. 1995. Intrinsic epileptogenicity of human dysplastic cortex as suggested by corticography and surgical results. *Ann Neurol*, **37**: 476–87.

Parker AP, Polkey CE, Binnie CD, *et al*. 1999. Vagal nerve stimulation in epileptic encephalopathies. *Pediatrics*, **103**: 778–82.

Pataraia E, Lurger S, Serles W, *et al*. 1998. Ictal scalp EEG in unilateral mesial temporal lobe epilepsy. *Epilepsia*, **39**: 608–14.

Patwardhan RV, Stong B, Bebin EM, *et al*. 2000. Efficacy of vagal nerve stimulation in children with medically refractory epilepsy. *Neurosurgery*, **47**: 1353–8.

Polkey CE. 2003. Alternative surgical procedures to help drug-resistant epilepsy: a review. *Epileptic Disord*, **5**: 63–75.

Polkey CE. 2003. Resective surgery for hypothalamic hamartoma. *Epileptic Disord*, **5**: 281–6.

Polkey CE. 2004. Clinical outcome of epilepsy surgery. *Curr Opin Neurol*, **17**: 173–8.

Ramsay RE, Uthman BM, Augustinsson LE, *et al*. 1994. Vagus nerve stimulation for treatment of partial seizures: 2. Safety, side effects, and tolerability. *Epilepsia*, **35**: 627–36.

Raymond AA, Fish DR, Boyd SG, *et al*. 1995. Cortical dysgenesis: serial EEG findings in children and adults. *Electroencephalogr Clin Neurophysiol*, **94**: 389–97.

Raymond AA, Fish DR, Sisodiya S, *et al*. 1994. Association of hippocampal sclerosis with cortical dysgenesis in patients with epilepsy. *Neurology*, **44**: 1841–4.

Raymond AA, Fish DR, Sisodiya S, *et al*. 1995. Abnormalities of gyration, heterotopias, tuberous sclerosis, focal cortical dysplasia, microdysgenesis, dysembryoplastic neuroepithelial tumour and dysgenesis of the archicortex in epilepsy: clinical, EEG and neuroimaging features in 100 adult patients. *Brain*, **118**: 629–60.

Regis J, Bartolomei F, de Toffol B, *et al*. 2000. Gamma knife surgery for epilepsy related to hypothalamic hamartomas. *Neurosurgery*, **47**: 1343–51.

Regis J, Bartolomei F, Rey M, *et al*. 1999. Gamma knife surgery for mesial temporal lobe epilepsy. *Epilepsia*, **40**: 1551–6.

Regis J, Rey M, Bartolomei F, *et al*. 2004. Gamma knife surgery in mesial temporal lobe epilepsy: a prospective multicentre study. *Epilepsia*, **45**: 504–15.

Rees J and Zrinzo L. 2005. What to do with the patient who had had a fit and the scan shows a glioma? *Practical Neurology*, **5**: 84–91.

Reutens DC, Bye AM, Hopkins IJ, *et al*. 1993. Corpus callosotomy for intractable epilepsy: seizure outcome and prognostic factors. *Epilepsia*, **34**: 904–9.

Riley T and White AC Jr. 2003. Management of neurocysticercosis. *CNS Drugs*, **17**: 577–91.

Ring HA, Moriarty J, and Trimble MR. 1998. A prospective study of the early post-surgical psychiatric associations of epilepsy surgery. *J Neurol Neurosurg Psychiatry*, **64**: 601–4.

Rydenhag B and Silander HC. 2001. Complications of epilepsy surgery after 654 procedures in Sweden, September 1990–1995: a multicenter study based on the Swedish National Epilepsy Surgery Register. *Neurosurgery*, **49**: 51–6.

Ryvlin P, Bouvard S, Le Bars D, *et al*. 1999. Transient and falsely lateralizing flumazenil-PET asymmetries in temporal lobe epilepsy. *Neurology*, **53**: 1882–5.

Salanova V, Andermann F, Olivier A, *et al*. 1992. Occipital lobe epilepsy: electroclinical manifestations, electrocorticography, cortical stimulation and outcome in 42 patients treated between 1930 and 1991. Surgery of occipital lobe epilepsy. *Brain*, **115**: 1655–80.

Salanova V, Morris HH III, Van-Ness PC, *et al.* 1993. Comparison of scalp electroencephalogram with subdural electrocorticogram recordings and functional mapping in frontal lobe epilepsy. *Arch Neurol*, **50**: 294–9.

Salek-Haddadi A, Friston KJ, Lemieux L, *et al.* 2003. Studying spontaneous EEG activity with fMRI. *Brain Res Brain Res Rev*, **43**: 110–33.

Savard G and Manchanda R. 2000. Psychiatric assessment of candidates for epilepsy surgery. *Can J Neurol Sci*, **27** (Suppl. 1): S44–S49.

Sawhney I, Robertson I, Polkey C, *et al.* 1995. Multiple subpial transection: a review of 21 cases. *J Neurol Neurosurg Psychiatry*, **58**: 344–9.

Schaller C, Jung A, Clusmann H, *et al.* 2004. Rate of vasospasm following the transsylvian versus transcortical approach for selective amygdalohippocampectomy. *Neurol Res*, **26**: 666–70.

Schallert G, Foster J, Lindquist N, *et al.* 1998. Chronic stimulation of the left vagal nerve in children: effect on swallowing. *Epilepsia*, **39**: 1113–14.

Schmidt D, Baumgartner C, and Loscher W. 2004. Seizure recurrence after planned discontinuation of antiepileptic drugs in seizure-free patients after epilepsy surgery: a review of current clinical experience. *Epilepsia*, **45**: 179–86.

Schulz R, Luders HO, Hoppe M, *et al.* 2000. Interictal EEG and ictal EEG propagation are highly predictive of surgical outcome in mesial temporal lobe epilepsy. *Epilepsia*, **41**: 564–70.

Schwartz TH, Bazil CW, Walczak TS, *et al.* 1997. The predictive value of intraoperative electrocorticography in resections for limbic epilepsy associated with mesial temporal sclerosis. *Neurosurgery*, **40**: 302–9.

Scott CA. 2002. Current role of scalp ictal EEG in evaluation for epilepsy surgery. M Phil degree, London University.

Seeck M. 2003. Surgical treatment of tumoral temporal-lobe epilepsy. *Lancet Neurol*, **2**: 722–3.

Selway R and Polkey C. 2000. Multiple subpial transections, clinical outcome in 34 patients. *Epilepsia*, **41** (Suppl. 7): 145–6.

Sirven JI, Malamut BL, O'Connor MJ, *et al.* 2000. Temporal lobectomy outcome in older versus younger adults. *Neurology*, **54**: 2166–70.

Sirven JI, Sperling M, Naritoku D, *et al.* 2000. Vagus nerve stimulation therapy for epilepsy in older adults. *Neurology*, **54**: 1179–82.

Sisodiya SM. 2004. Surgery for focal cortical dysplasia. *Brain*, **127**: 2383–4.

Smith DF, Hutton JL, Sandemann D, *et al.* 1991. The prognosis of primary intracerebral tumors presenting with epilepsy: the outcome of medical and surgical management. *J Neurol Neurosurg Psychiatry*, **54**: 915–20.

Smith JR, Sillay K, Winkler P, *et al.* 2004. Orbitofrontal epilepsy: electroclinical analysis of surgical cases and literature review. *Stereotact Funct Neurosurg*, **82**: 20–5.

So N, Gloor P, Quesney LF, *et al.* 1989. Depth electrode investigations in patients with bitemporal epileptiform abnormalities. *Ann Neurol*, **25**: 423–31.

Spencer SS. 1998. Substrates of localization-related epilepsies: biologic implications of localizing findings in humans. *Epilepsia*, **39**: 114–23.

Spencer SS and Spencer DD. 1994. Entorhinal–hippocampal interactions in medial temporal lobe epilepsy. *Epilepsia*, **35**: 721–7.

Spencer SS and Spencer DD. 1996. Implications of seizure termination location in temporal lobe epilepsy. *Epilepsia*, **37**: 455–8.

Spencer SS, Guimaraes P, Katz A, *et al.* 1992. Morphological patterns of seizures recorded intracranially. *Epilepsia*, **33**: 537–45.

Spencer SS, Schramm J, Wyler A, *et al.* 2002. Multiple subpial transection for intractable partial epilepsy: an international meta-analysis. *Epilepsia*, **43**: 141–5.

Spencer SS, Spencer DD, Sass K, *et al.* 1993. Anterior, total, and two-staged corpus callosum section: differential and incremental seizure responses. *Epilepsia*, **34**: 561–7.

Spencer SS, Spencer DD, Williamson PD, *et al.* 1988. Corpus callosotomy for epilepsy. I. Seizure effects. *Neurology*, **38**: 19–24.

Spencer SS, Spencer DD, Williamson PD, *et al.* 1990. Combined depth and subdural electrode investigation in uncontrolled epilepsy. *Neurology*, **30**: 74–9.

Spencer SS, Williamson PD, Bridges SL, *et al.* 1985. Reliability and accuracy of localization by scalp ictal EEG. *Neurology*, **35**: 1567–75.

Spencer SS, Williamson PD, Spencer DD, *et al.* 1987. Human hippocampal seizure spread studied by depth and subdural recording: the hippocampal commissure. *Epilepsia*, **28**: 479–89.

Sperling M and O'Connor M. 1989. Comparison of depth and subdural electrodes in recording temporal lobe seizures. *Neurology*, **39**: 1497–504.

Sperling M, Saykin A, Glosser G, *et al.* 1994. Predictors of outcome after anterior temporal lobectomy: the intracarotid amobarbital test. *Neurology*, **44**: 2325–30.

Srikijvilaikul T, Najm I, Foldvary-Schaefer N, *et al.* 2004. Failure of gamma knife radiosurgery for mesial temporal lobe epilepsy: report of five cases. *Neurosurgery*, **54**: 1395–402.

Swartz BE, Rich JR, Dwan PS, *et al.* 1996. The safety and efficacy of chronically implanted subdural electrodes: a prospective study. *Surg Neurol*, **46**: 87–93.

Swartz BE, Walsh GO, Delgado-Escueta AV, *et al.* 1991. Surface ictal electroencephalographic patterns in frontal vs. temporal lobe epilepsy. *Can J Neurol Sci*, **18**: 549–53.

Tassi L, Colombo N, Cossu M, *et al.* 2005. Electroclinical, MRI and neuropathological study of 10 patients with nodular heterotopia, with surgical outcomes. *Brain*, **128**: 321–37.

Tatum WO, Moore DB, Stecker MM, *et al.* 1999. Ventricular asystole during vagus nerve stimulation for epilepsy in humans. *Neurology*, **52**: 1267–9.

The Vagus Nerve Stimulation Study Group. 1995. A randomized controlled trial of chronic vagus nerve stimulation for treatment of medically intractable seizures. *Neurology*, **45**: 224–30.

Theodore WH, Gaillard WD, DeCarli C, *et al.* 2001. Hippocampal volume and glucose metabolism in temporal lobe epileptic foci. *Epilepsia*, **42**: 130–2.

Theodore WH, Sato S, Kufta C, *et al.* 1992. Temporal lobectomy for uncontrolled seizures: the role of positron emission tomography. *Ann Neurol*, **32**: 789–94.

Theodore WH, Sato S, Kufta C, *et al.* 1997. FDG-positron emission tomography and invasive EEG: seizure focus detection and surgical outcome. *Epilepsia*, **38**: 81–6.

Topper R, Jurgens E, Reul J, *et al.* 1999. Clinical significance of intracranial developmental venous anomalies. *J Neurol Neurosurg Psychiatry*, **67**: 234–8.

Tran TA, Spencer SS, Marks D, *et al.* 1995. Significance of spikes recorded on electrocorticography in non-lesional medial temporal lobe epilepsy. *Ann Neurol*, **38**: 763–70.

Van Paesschen W, Dupont P, Van Heerden B, *et al.* 2000. Self-injection ictal SPECT during partial seizures. *Neurology*, **54**: 1994–7.

Villemure JG. 1992. Anatomical to functional hemispherectomy from Krynauw to Rasmussen. *Epilepsy Res Suppl*, **5**: 209–15.

Villemure JG and Mascott C. 1995. Peri-insular hemispherectomy: surgical principles and anatomy. *Neurosurgery*, **37**: 975–81.

Vining EP, Freeman JM, Pillas DJ, *et al.* 1997. Why would you remove half a brain? The outcome of 58 children after hemispherectomy—the Johns Hopkins experience: 1968–1996. *Pediatrics*, 100: 163–71.

Walczak TS, Lewis DV, and Radtke R. 1991. Scalp EEG differs in temporal and extratemporal complex partial seizures. *J Epilepsy*, **4**: 25–8.

Wasay M, Kheleani BA, Moolani MK, *et al.* 2003. Brain CT and MRI findings in 100 consecutive patients with intracranial tuberculoma. *J Neuroimaging*, **13**: 240–7.

Weiner HL, Ferraris N, LaJoie J, *et al.* 2004. Epilepsy surgery for children with tuberous sclerosis complex. *J Child Neurol*, **19**: 687–9.

Wheless JW and Baumgartner J. 2004. Vagus nerve stimulation therapy. *Drugs Today (Barc)*, **40**: 501–15.

Wichert-Ana L, Velasco TR, Terra-Bustamante VC, *et al.* 2001. Typical and atypical perfusion patterns in peri-ictal SPECT of patients with unilateral temporal lobe epilepsy. *Epilepsia*, **42**: 660–6.

Wiebe S, Blume WT, Girvin JP, *et al.* 2001. A randomized, controlled trial of surgery for temporal-lobe epilepsy. *N Engl J Med*, **345**: 311–18.

Wieser HG. 1991. Selective amygdalohippocampectomy: indications and follow-up. *Can J Neurol Sci*, **4**: 617–27.

Wieshmann UC, Free SL, Everitt AD, *et al.* 1996. Magnetic resonance imaging in epilepsy with a fast FLAIR sequence. *J Neurol Neurosurg Psychiatry*, **61**: 357–61.

Wiggins GC, Elisevich K, and Smith BJ. 1999. Morbidity and infection in combined subdural grid and strip electrode investigation for intractable epilepsy. *Epilepsy Res*, **37**: 73–80.

Williamson PD, Boon PA, Thadani VM, *et al.* 1992. Parietal lobe epilepsy: diagnostic considerations and results of surgery. *Ann Neurol*, **31**: 193–201.

Williamson PD, French JA, Thadani VM, *et al.* 1993. Characteristics of medial temporal lobe epilepsy. II. Interictal and ictal scalp electroencephalography, neuropsychological testing, neuroimaging, surgical results and pathology. *Ann Neurol*, **34**: 781–7.

Williamson PD, Thadani VM, Darcey TM, *et al.* 1992. Occipital lobe epilepsy: clinical characteristics, seizure spread patterns and results of surgery. *Ann Neurol*, **31**: 3–13.

Wyllie E, Comair YG, Kotagal P, *et al.* 1998. Seizure outcome after epilepsy surgery in children and adolescents. *Ann Neurol*, **44**: 740–8.

Yang S. 1981. Brain abscess: a review of 400 cases. *J Neurosurg*, **55**: 794–9.

Zaatreh MM, Spencer DD, Thopson JL, *et al.* 2002. Frontal lobe tumoral epilepsy: clinical, neurophysiologic features and predictors of surgical outcome. *Epilepsia*, **43**: 727–33.

Zentner J, Wolf HK, Osterun B, *et al.* 1994. Gangliogliomas: clinical, radiological, and histopathological findings in 51 patients. *J Neurol Neurosurg Psychiatry*, **57**: 1497–502.

# Index